Endovascular and Hybrid Therapies for Structural Heart and Aortic Disease

Endovascular and Hybrid Therapies for Structural Heart and Aortic Disease

EDITED BY

Jacques Kpodonu, MD

Raney Zusman Medical Group
University of California Irvine
Cardiovascular Hybrid Interventions
Hoag Heart and Vascular Institute
Hoag Memorial Presbyterian Hospital
Newport Beach, CA, USA

Raoul Bonan, MD

Institut de Cardiologie de Montréal
University of Montréal
Montréal, Canada

WILEY-BLACKWELL
A John Wiley & Sons, Ltd., Publication

This edition first published 2013 © 2013 by John Wiley & Sons, Ltd

Wiley-Blackwell is an imprint of John Wiley & Sons, formed by the merger of Wiley's global Scientific, Technical and Medical business with Blackwell Publishing.

Registered Office
John Wiley & Sons, Ltd, The Atrium, Southern Gate, Chichester, West Sussex, PO19 8SQ, UK

Editorial Offices
9600 Garsington Road, Oxford, OX4 2DQ, UK
The Atrium, Southern Gate, Chichester, West Sussex, PO19 8SQ, UK
111 River Street, Hoboken, NJ 07030-5774, USA

For details of our global editorial offices, for customer services and for information about how to apply for permission to reuse the copyright material in this book please see our website at www.wiley.com/wiley-blackwell

Library of Congress Cataloging-in-Publication Data

Endovascular and hybrid therapies for structural heart and aortic disease / edited by Jacques Kpodonu, Raoul Bonan.
p. ; cm.
Includes bibliographical references and index.
ISBN 978-0-470-65639-6 (hardback : alk. paper)
I. Kpodonu, Jacques. II. Bonan, R.
[DNLM: 1. Aorta, Thoracic–surgery. 2. Aortic Diseases–surgery. 3. Endovascular Procedures. 4. Heart Defects, Congenital–surgery. 5. Heart Valve Diseases–surgery. WG 410]
617.4′12–dc23

2012044838

A catalogue record for this book is available from the British Library.

Wiley also publishes its books in a variety of electronic formats. Some content that appears in print may not be available in electronic books.

Cover image: Mike Austin
Cover design by OptaDesign.co.uk

Set in 9.5/12 pt Minion by SPi Publisher Services, Pondicherry, India
Printed and bound in Malaysia by Vivar Printing Sdn Bhd

1 2013

Contents

About the companion website

This book is accompanied by a companion website:

http://www.wiley.com/go/valverepair

The website includes:

- Additional video materials from the book

Contributor list

Ottavio Alfieri
Department of Cardiac Surgery
San Raffaele Hospital
Milan, Italy

Dabit Arzamendi, MD, MSc
Interventional Cardiology and Structural Heart Intervention
Department of Cardiology
Hospital de la Santa Creu i Sant Pau
Barcelona, Spain

Ricardo Aun, MD, PhD
Associate Professor in Vascular and Endovascular Surgery
Universidade de São Paulo
Hospital Albert Einstein
São Paulo, Brazil

Colin D. Bicknell, MD, FRCS
Regional Vascular Unit
St. Mary's Hospital
Imperial College London, UK

James H. Black, III, MD, FACS
Division of Vascular Surgery
and Endovascular Therapy
Johns Hopkins University School of Medicine
Baltimore, MA, USA

Nicholas J. W. Cheshire, MD, FRCS
Regional Vascular Unit
St. Mary's Hospital
Imperial College
London, UK

Howie Choset, PhD
Robotics Institute
Carnegie Mellon University
Pittsburgh, PA, USA

Timothy A. M. Chuter
Division of Vascular Surgery
University of California San Francisco
San Francisco, CA, USA

Paolo Denti
Department of Cardiac Surgery
San Raffaele Hospital
Milan, Italy

Volkmar Falk, MD
Clinic for Cardiovascular Surgery
University Hospital Zurich
Zurich, Switzerland

Anne Figel
Siemens AG Healthcare Sector
Angiography, Fluoroscopic and Radiographic Systems
Forchheim, Germany

Thierry Folliguet
Pôle Territorial Lorrain Chirurgie Cardiaque Vasculaire et Transplantation Institut
Lorrain du Coeur et des Vaisseaux Louis Mathieu Centre Hospitalier U
Vandoeuvre
Les Nancy Cedex 54511
France

Jurg Grunenfelder, MD
Clinic for Cardiovascular Surgery
University Hospital Zurich
Zurich, Switzerland

Mohamad S. Hamady
Regional Vascular Unit
St. Mary's Hospital
Imperial College
London, UK

Thomas Hartkens
Siemens AG Healthcare Sector
Angiography, Fluoroscopic and Radiographic Systems
Forchheim, Germany

Stéphan Haulon, MD, PhD
Hôpital Cardiologique
CHRU de Lille, France

Keith A. Horvath
NIH Heart Center at Suburban Hospital
Cardiothoracic Surgery Research Program
National Heart, Lung and Blood Institute
National Institutes of Health
Bethesda, MD, USA

Hasan Jilaihawi
Cedars-Sinai Heart Institute
Los Angeles, CA, USA

Saibal Kar
Cardiovascular Intervention Center Research
Cedars-Sinai Heart Institute
Los Angeles, CA, USA

Theodoros Kofidis, MD
Senior Consultant, Department of Cardiac,
Thoracic and Vascular Surgery
National University Heart Center
Singapore

Jacques Kpodonu, MD
Raney Zusman Medical Group
University of California Irvine
Cardiovascular Hybrid Interventions
Hoag Heart and Vascular Institute
Hoag Memorial Presbyterian Hospital
Newport Beach, CA, USA

François Laborde
Department of Cardiovascular Surgery
Institut Mutualiste Montsouris
Paris, France

Ruediger Lange, MD, PhD
Department of Cardiac Surgery
German Heart Center Munich
Munich, Germany

Gilles Lemesle, MD
Service de Cardiologie B et Centre Hémodynamique
Pôle de Cardiologie
Hôpital Cardiologique
CHRU de Lille, France

Ming Li
Cardiothoracic Surgery Research Program
National Heart, Lung and Blood Institute
National Institutes of Health
Bethesda, MD, USA

Mohsen Mahvash, PhD
Division of Cardiothoracic Surgery, BHS
Medical Robotics and Computer Assisted Surgery
(MRCAS) Laboratory
Harvard Medical School
Boston, MA, USA

Francesco Maisano, MD, FESC
Transcatheter Valve Interventions Program
Cardiothoracic and Vascular Institute
San Raffaele Hospital
Milan, Italy

Giuseppe Martucci, MD, FRCPC
Department of Interventional Cardiology at McGill
University Health Center (MUHC)
Royal Victoria Hospital
Montreal, Canada

Dumitru Mazilu
Cardiothoracic Surgery Research Program
National Heart, Lung and Blood Institute
National Institutes of Health
Bethesda, MD, USA

Thomas Modine, MD, PhD, MBA
Service de Chirurgie Cardio-vasculaire
Pôle de Chirurgie Cardio-vasculaire
Hôpital Cardiologique
CHRU de Lille, France

Friedrich W. Mohr, MD, PhD
Heart Center
Leipzig University
Leipzig, Germany

Darren Mylotte, MD, MRCPI
Department of Interventional Cardiology at McGill
University Health Center (MUHC)
Royal Victoria Hospital
Montreal, Canada

Georg Nollert
Siemens AG Healthcare Sector
Angiography, Fluoroscopic and Radiographic Systems
Forchheim
Clinic of Cardiac Surgery
University of Munich
Munich, Germany

Babak Orandi, MD, MSc
Department of Surgery
Johns Hopkins Hospital
Baltimore, MD, USA

Paolo Perini, MD
Vascular Surgery
Hôpital Cardiologique
CHRU de Lille, France

Mark D. Peterson, MD, PhD, FRCSC
Division of Cardiac Surgery
St. Michael's Hospital
University of Toronto
Toronto, Ontario, Canada

Nicolo Piazza, MD, PhD, FRCPC, FESC
Department of Interventional Cardiology at McGill University Health Center (MUHC)
Royal Victoria Hospital
Montreal, Canada
Department of Cardiac Surgery
German Heart Center Munich
Munich, Germany

Andre Plass, MD
Clinic for Cardiovascular Surgery
University Hospital Zurich
Zurich, Switzerland

Mark Reisman, MD
Swedish Heart and Vascular Institute
Swedish Medical Center
Seattle, WA, USA

Pascal Rheaume, MD
Vascular Surgery
Hopital St-Francois D'Assise
Quebec City, Canada

Celia V. Riga, MBBS, BSc
Regional Vascular Unit
St. Mary's Hospital
Imperial College
London, UK

Eduardo Keller Saadi, MD, PhD
Federal University of Rio Grande do Sul
Hospital de Clinicas de Porto Alegre
Chief, Center for Aortic Diseases
Hospital Mae de Deus
Porto Alegre, Brazil

Joerg Seeburger, MD
Heart Center
Leipzig University
Leipzig, Germany

Arnaud Sudre, MD
Service de Cardiologie B et Centre Hémodynamique
Pôle de Cardiologie
Hôpital Cardiologique
CHRU de Lille, France

Sabine Wich
Siemens AG Healthcare Sector
Angiography, Fluoroscopic and Radiographic Systems
Forchheim, Germany

Bobby Yanagawa, MD, PhD
Division of Cardiac Surgery
St. Michael's Hospital
University of Toronto
Toronto, Canada

Marco A. Zenati, MD, MSc
Harvard Medical School
Boston, MA, USA

Preface

Since the first reports of endovascular repair of abdominal aortic aneurysm (AAA) and transcatheter aortic valve replacement in the early 1990s and 2000s, there has been an explosion in the volume and complexity of endovascular and hybrid procedures for the treatment of aortic diseases and structural heart diseases. Endovascular and hybrid techniques and technologies have evolved from the initial devices and continue to evolve allowing for the treatment of most aortic pathologies and most structural heart pathologies. These new endoaortic surgical procedures and transcatheter valve therapies have proven to shorten hospitalization, reduce morbidity and mortality, speed recovery, and hasten return to normal life. The evolution and conceptual design of the endoaortic grafts and transcatheter valves used to treat these complex pathologies would obviously not be possible without the simultaneous explosion in medical imaging technologies and the development of advanced hybrid surgical rooms and hybrid surgical techniques, which has taken place over a similar time period.

With chapters written in a comprehensive yet concise manner and numerous illustrations, this book aims to engage readers further with additional video materials. We hope that this textbook will be a useful tool for practitioners planning to execute treatment on patients with these various aortic and structural heart pathologies as well as serve as a useful reference as the field of segment continues to evolve.

Jacques Kpodonu, MD
Raoul Bonan, MD

List of videos

PART I
Aorta

1

CHAPTER 1

Access techniques

Jacques Kpodonu
University of California Irvine,
Cardiovascular Hybrid Interventions, Hoag Heart and Vascular Institute, Newport Beach, CA, USA

Brachial access techniques used for aortic endografting

Brachial and radial access techniques allow the utilization of angiographic catheters to assist with proximal deployment of thoracic stent-grafts [1]. They allow for easy identification of the left subclavian artery, and angiography can be performed to avoid coverage with the proximal end of a thoracic stent. When coverage of the left subclavian artery is required for an adequate proximal landing zone, subclavian to carotid bypassing may be required. The radial or brachial access can therefore accommodate subclavian artery coil embolization to minimize the risk of type II endoleaks.

The brachial artery has an enveloping fascial sheath, therefore, when a hematoma does occur, brachial plexopathies are more common. In addition, upper extremity vessels tend to spasm more frequently during manipulation, making access more challenging. Brachial access does carry the added risk of distal ischemia and embolization over radial access. Although sheaths up to 6 or 7 Fr (3 Fr ≈ 1 mm) may be percutaneously placed in either vessel, radial access should be preferred over brachial because of a lower complication profile, and open access used for larger sheaths or on smaller patients.

The left brachial artery is preferred over the right so as to avoid the origin of the right common carotid artery. The technique requires that the arm be abducted on an arm board with the arm circumferentially prepped. The artery is palpated just proximal to the antecubital fossa where the biceps muscle thins out to its tendinous insertion. Percutaneous retrograde puncture of the brachial artery with a 21 gauge micropuncture kit is preferred to the 18 gauge due to the smaller size of the vessel (Fig. 1.1a). Catheter-over-wire exchange can then be performed to the desired sheath. Sheaths up to 6 Fr can be placed with relative safety (Fig. 1.1b). Long sheaths can help deal with the inherent vasospasm.

In tortuous aorta, the use of the brachio-femoral wire may be required to aid advancement and deployment of an endograft. Deployment of an endoluminal graft in a tortuous aorta may be difficult, requiring the use of a brachio-femoral wire (Fig. 1.2). Use of brachio-femoral access wires can help straighten the most angulated of vessels. The presence of a tortuous aorta requires brachio-femoral access to deploy an endoluminal graft (Fig. 1.3). Brachial access is obtained by a percutaneous retrograde puncture of the right brachial artery with an 18 gauge needle or a micropuncture needle. An extra long 450 cm, 0.035 inch angled glide wire is advanced through the brachial sheath into the tortuous thoracic aorta, snared and pulled out through the groin sheath. The technique requires that a protective guiding catheter be placed over the brachial artery to protect the subclavian artery from injury. It is important to have at least a 260 cm

Endovascular and Hybrid Therapies for Structural Heart and Aortic Disease, First Edition.
Edited by Jacques Kpodonu and Raoul Bonan.

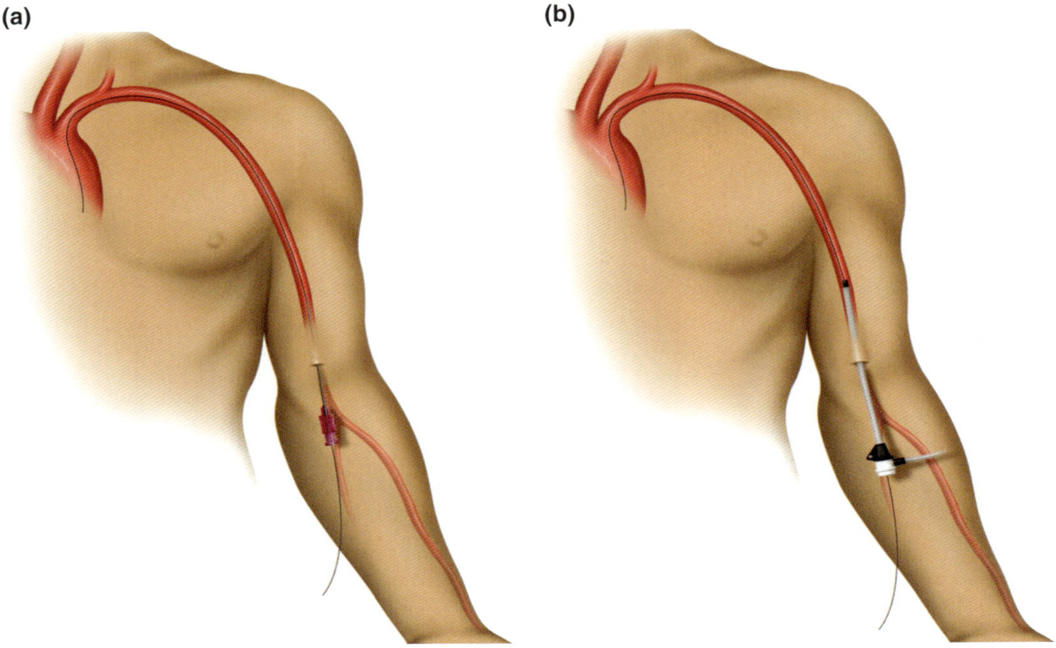

Fig. 1.1 (a) A retrograde percutaneous puncture of the brachial artery with (b) the placement of an introducer sheath.

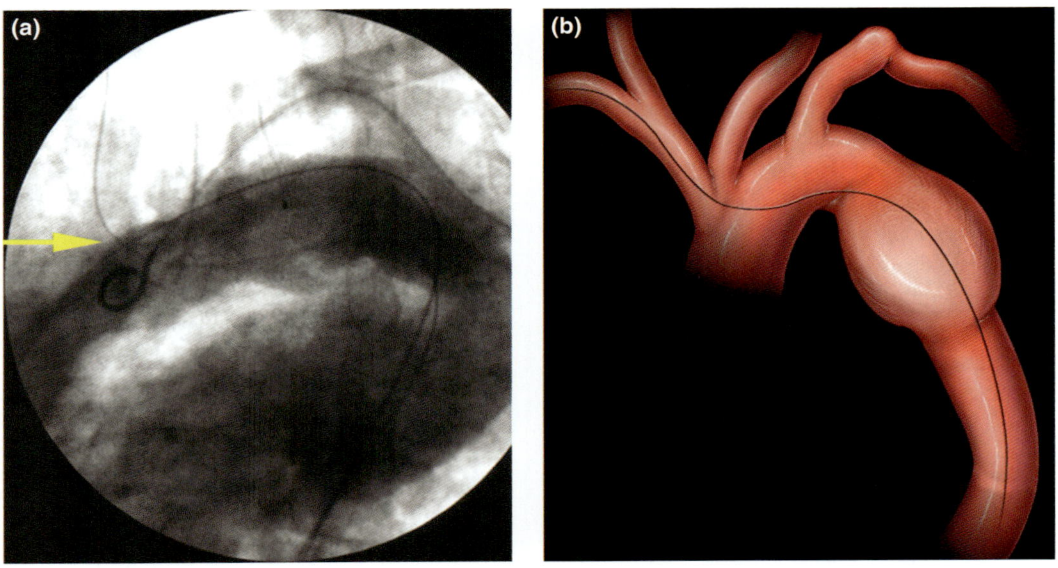

Fig. 1.2 (a) Angiogram and (b) illustration demonstrating advancement of a brachio-femoral wire in a tortuous thoracic aorta.

long wire and constant tension must be placed on both ends of the wire as the delivery sheath is passed into the aorta [2,3]. By pulling on both ends of the wire an endoluminal graft can be advanced up into the tortuous arch aorta with precise deployment of the endoluminal graft.

Techniques for constructing an endoconduit for aortic endografting

An endoconduit is an alternative percutaneous technique that can be used to deliver a thoracic endograft in a patient with a small, calcified, or tortuous

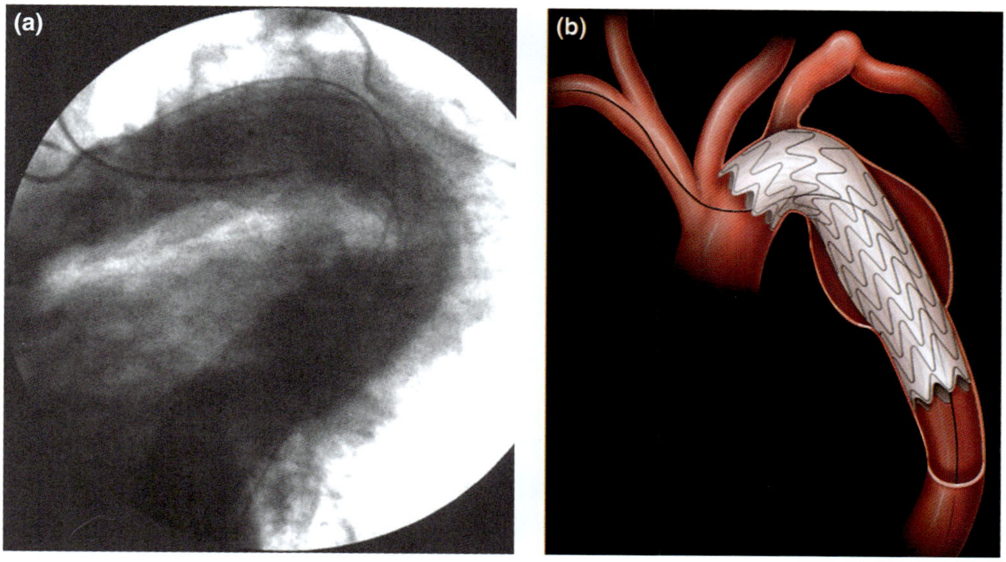

Fig. 1.3 (a) Angiogram and (b) illustration demonstration of deployment of a thoracic endograft using a brachio-femoral wire approach.

vessel instead of the conventional ilio-femoral conduit (Fig. 1.4). This technique can be applied in high-risk patients who have a relative contraindication to conventional open surgical techniques under general anesthesia. The endoluminal conduit technique allows aggressive balloon dilation of long segments of ilio-femoral stenosis without the risk of vessel rupture. The endoluminal graft conduit can be custom-assembled using graft diameters of at least 8 mm and preferably 10 mm, and can be backloaded into a delivery sheath and deployed via a femoral arteriotomy into the common iliac artery covering the origin of the internal iliac artery [2,4].

Retrograde percutaneous access of the common femoral artery is performed with an 18 gauge needle in the usual fashion and a 0.035 inch glide wire is advanced under fluoroscopic guidance into the distal thoracic aorta after heparin is administered. A 9 Fr sheath is then exchanged for the needle. A retrograde angiographic picture of the iliac vessels is performed noting the size, tortuosity, and calcification. The presence of a small, or severely calcific or tortuous, iliac vessel may preclude the introduction of a delivery sheath (Fig. 1.5). An attempt may be made to pass the delivery sheath, and if any resistance is noted the patient would require a retroperitoneal conduit or an endoconduit. Using the existing 9 Fr sheath, balloon angioplasty can be performed to

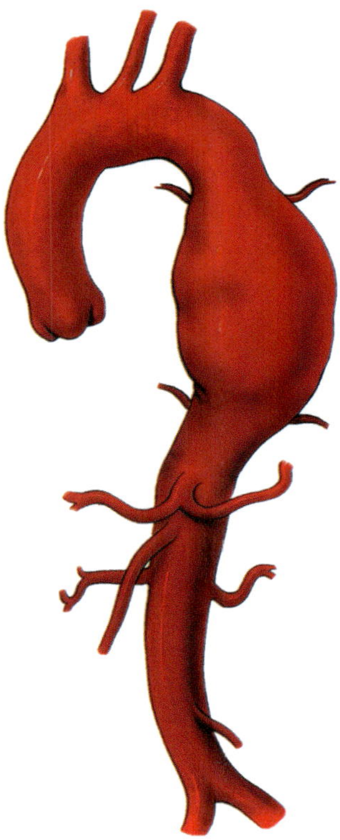

Fig. 1.4 Illustration of thoracic aorta.

gently dilate the vessel; subsequently, an endoluminal graft, most commonly (Viahbahn; W.L. Gore & Associates, Flagstaff, AZ), or an I-Cast stent-graft

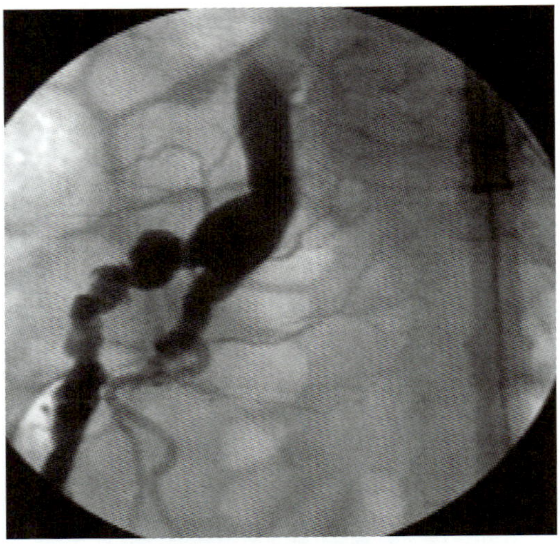

Fig. 1.5 Angiogram demonstrating a small, tortuous left iliac artery.

Table 1.1 Commercially available covered stents used for peripheral indications.

Stent	*Manufacturer*	*Indications*	*Type*
Fluency Plus	Bard	Tracheobronchial	Self-expanding
Jostent	Abbott	Coronary perforation	Balloon-expanded
Viabahn	Gore	Superficial femoral artery	Self-expanding
I-Cast	Atrium	Tracheobronchial	Balloon-expanded

(Atrium Medical, Hudson, NH) (Table 1.1) is deployed across the common iliac and external iliac artery covering the hypogastric vessels (Fig. 1.6). Post-deployment balloon angioplasty is subsequently performed with a balloon to expand the endoluminal graft; this technique has been referred to as cracking and paving. The 9 Fr sheath is subsequently exchanged to a 20–24 Fr delivery sheath that is required to deliver the thoracic endoluminal graft.

Transfemoral access techniques in aortic endografting

Percutaneous retrograde femoral artery access

Most right-handed physicians will prefer the patient's right groin for femoral access, although both groins should be prepped in case of inaccessibility.

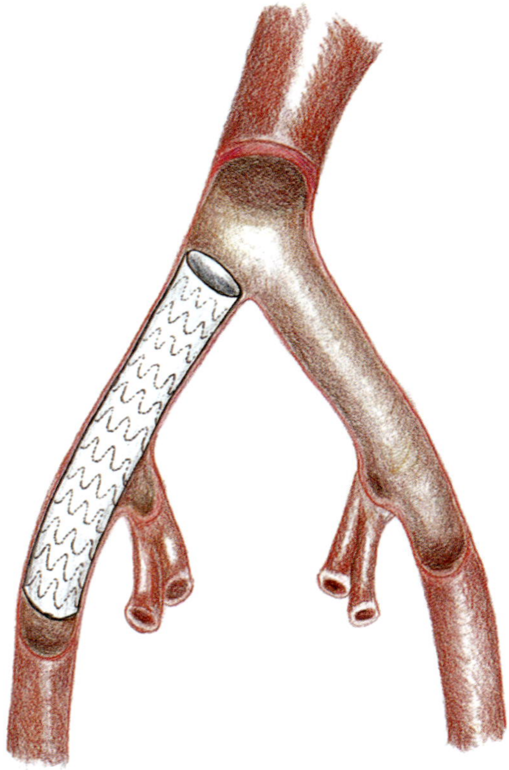

Fig. 1.6 Deployment of an endoconduit.

After the pulse is identified, the inguinal ligament is found by tracing a line between the anterior iliac spine and the pubic tubercle. Often, especially in obese individuals, the inguinal crease is inferior to this landmark. Access should be made below the inguinal ligament corresponding to the common femoral artery. One will find that if access is made too high, corresponding with the external iliac artery, hemostasis is difficult to achieve with manual pressure. In this case hemorrhage can occur after removal of devices and a retroperitoneal hematoma can develop. This is often insidious in onset. In addition, the risk of pseudoaneurysm formation is higher in an external iliac stick, again because direct manual pressure cannot be applied this superiorly.

A properly equipped endovascular suite will allow fluoroscopic imaging of the groin to identify all anatomic landmarks. In addition to surface landmarks, most physicians use the medial half of the femoral head to guide femoral artery access; this ensures common femoral artery entry

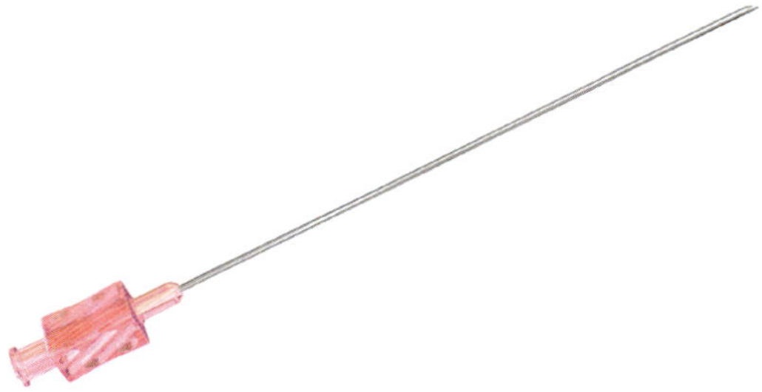

Fig. 1.7 An 18 gauge 7 cm Cook percutaneous needle.

and avoids the complications of a higher stick. It is also useful in the pulseless femoral artery. Most vascular access kits include an 18 gauge straight angiographic entry needle (Fig. 1.7). This is inserted using the dominant hand at a 45° angle while using the non-dominant hand for guidance using a Seldinger technique. Percutaneous arterial femoral access is usually obtained by the Seldinger technique. A careful palpation of the femoral pulse is performed and a beveled needle (usually 18 gauge) is introduced through the arterial wall. The needle is slowly withdrawn until return of arterial blood is achieved, signifying the intraluminal position of the needle. The presence of poor blood flow signifies that the tip is misplaced or the needle is too close to the arterial wall. A soft-tip angled 0.035 inch guide wire is then introduced through the central lumen of the needle under fluoroscopic guidance (Fig. 1.8). Progress of the guide wire intraluminally should be monitored with fluoroscopy to avoid diversion into branched vessels and dissection of the vessel. The presence of resistance in passing a guide wire signifies possible misdirection or dissection of the vessel wall. In instances where the vessel may be small, calcified, or tortuous, a smaller access needle may be desirable. A micropuncture kit (Cook Medical, Bloomington, IN) exists which includes a 21 gauge needle for initial access.

Once access is achieved a small nick is made in the skin with a no. 11 blade and a dilator, and an introducer sheath is then advanced over the glide wire with the dilator preceding the introducer sheath by a few inches, again under fluoroscopic visualization (Fig. 1.9). Once the introducer sheath is positioned the dilator is removed. A hemostatic valve at the end of the introducer

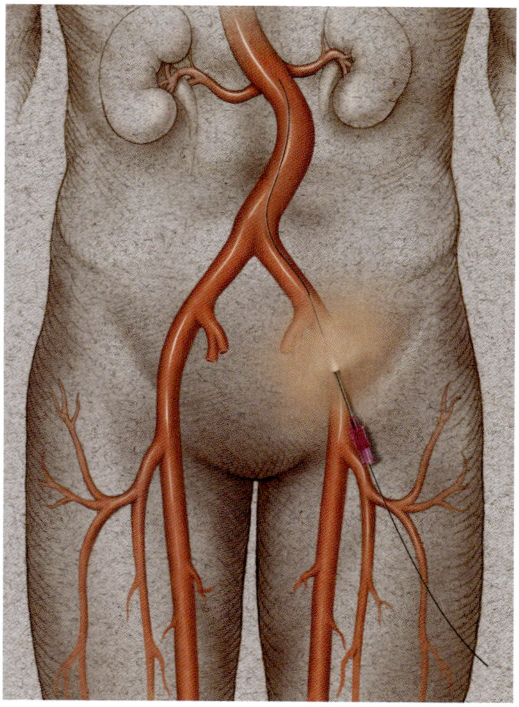

Fig. 1.8 Introduction of an angled glide wire through the 18 gauge needle.

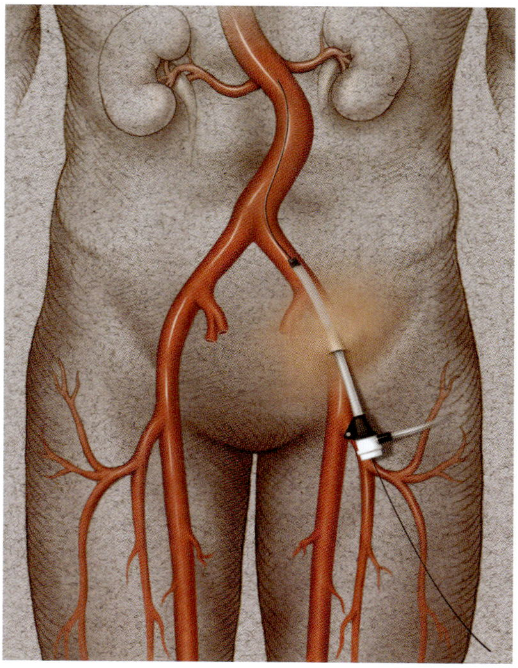

Fig. 1.9 Introduction of a 9 Fr 11 cm sheath in a retrograde percutaneous fashion through the common femoral artery.

sheath prevents leakage of blood. The introducer sheath permits various guide wires, balloons, and stents to be introduced safely within the arterial lumen. The introducer sheath can subsequently be upgraded to a larger delivery sheath for the deployment of an endograft. In patients with a femoral-to-femoral graft, percutaneous access can be performed either through the inflow limb of the femoral–femoral graft or above the inflow limb.

Contraindication to percutaneous femoral access

In patients with significant peripheral vascular disease, imaging studies using an angiogram or a CT scan are necessary for sizing and determination of calcification, as well as tortuosity of vessels which would make the femoral delivery of an endograft hazardous. The introduction of large sheaths in femoral vessels that are calcified, tortuous, small caliber, or a combination are predisposed to rupture.

Open retrograde access

The common femoral artery is usually exposed for retrograde cannulation and the introduction of various large-sized introducer sheaths, balloons, self-expandable and balloon-expandable stents, and endoluminal grafts.

A curvilinear incision is made two finger-breaths above the groin crease and over the palpable femoral pulse. The incision is carried down to the femoral sheath. Retraction is performed with a Gelpe retractor or a Wietlander retractor. The femoral sheath is incised to expose the common femoral artery. Heavy silk sutures are passed circumferentially round the various side branches. Adequate mobilization of the common femoral artery is desired to be able to achieve adequate proximal and distal control of the vessel. A Rummel tourniquet is applied to the common femoral artery to serve as a proximal control.

The fluoroscopic C-arm is then positioned over the exposed femoral artery. Retrograde cannulation of the common femoral artery is performed with a beveled needle (18 gauge) until pulsatile blood flow is visualized. A soft-tip angled guide wire is advanced in the vessels under fluoroscopy. The needle is then exchanged for a selected sized dilator and introducer sheath. The dilator is removed and the sheath flushed with heperanized saline. Open cannulation or retrograde percutaneous access can be similarly performed in the contralateral common femoral artery (Fig. 1.10a).

Once the procedure is completed all wires and sheaths are removed under fluoroscopic guidance to ensure no injury is caused to the vessel wall. The arteriotomy is then closed with a 5-0 prolene suture after proximal and distal control is achieved (Fig. 1.10b).

Complications of femoral access

Rupture

Attempts to introduce a delivery sheath in a small, tortuous, or calcified artery, or a combination, will lead to rupture of the access vessel typically at the junction of the external and internal iliac artery or at the aorto-iliac bifurcation. Rupture of an access vessel should be suspected if there is a drop in the blood pressure during advancement of the delivery sheath or during removal of the delivery sheath. The guide wire should be maintained at all times prior to removal of a delivery sheath and an iliac angiogram performed prior to removal of the introducer sheaths to confirm extravasation of contrast (Fig. 1.11a). Once rupture is confirmed, an appropriate length and diameter of a covered stent-graft should be chosen (Fig. 1.11b) and deployed across the area of rupture (Fig. 1.11c). In most instances coverage of the hypogastric artery is required.

Dissections

The introduction of guide wires, introduction and delivery sheaths may result in dissection of the access vessels. Similarly, balloon angioplasty of calcified access vessels may also result in a dissection flap of the resulting access vessels. Once a dissection is identified on angiogram, gentle balloon angioplasty may be performed to seal the dissecting septum or a covered or uncovered balloon-deployable stent may be used to seal off the dissection. Failure to recognize a dissection may result in thrombosis of the access vessels with resulting ischemia of the involved lower extremity [2].

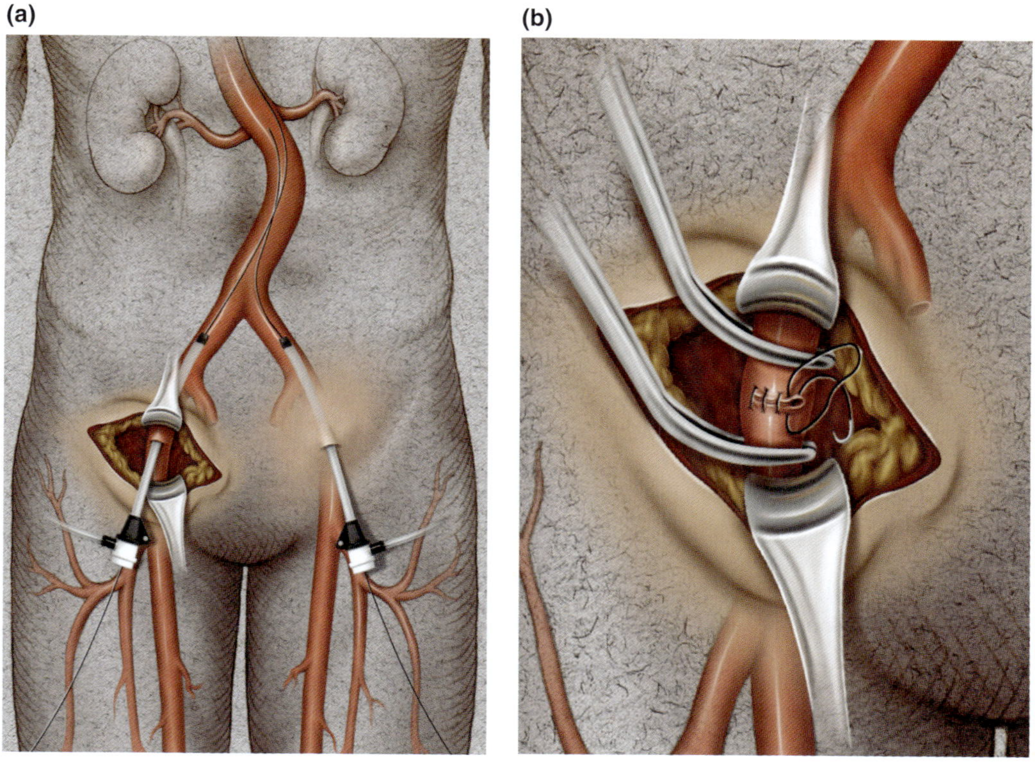

Fig. 1.10 (a) Open retrograde cannulation of the right common femoral artery and percutaneous retrograde cannulation of the left common femoral artery. (b) Closure of the arteriotomy after removal of the guide wire and introduction sheath.

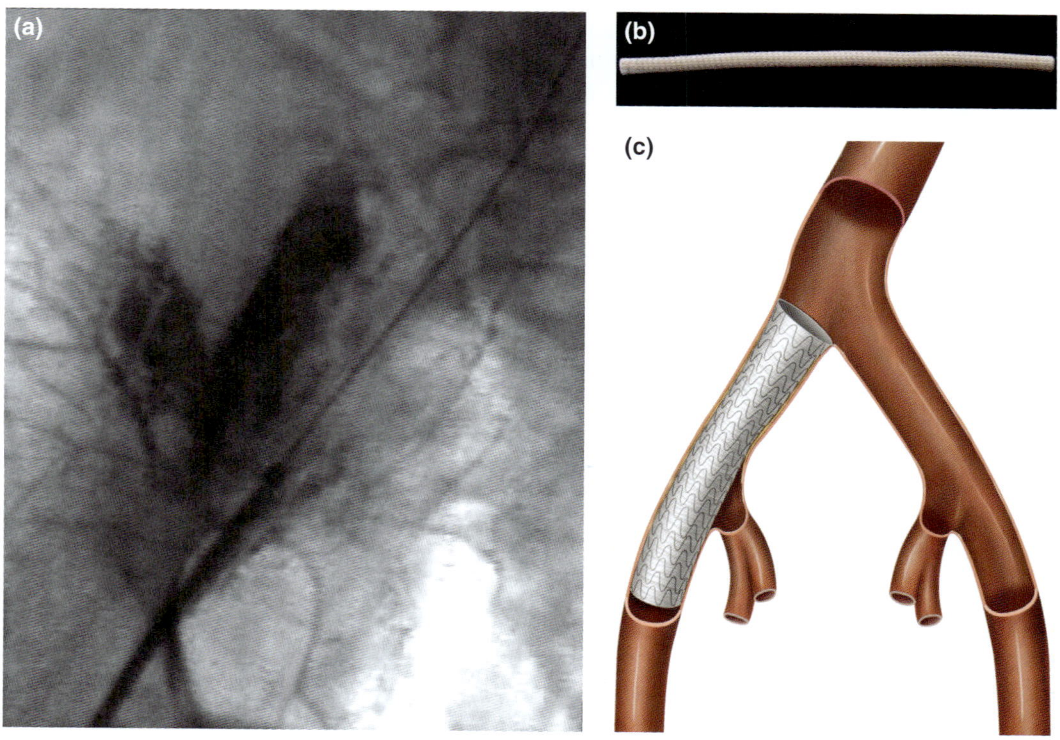

Fig. 1.11 (a) Angiogram demonstrating rupture of the right external iliac artery. (b) A covered stent-graft used to exclude the site of rupture. (c) A covered stent-graft deployed across a ruptured iliac artery.

Retroperitoneal access for aortic endografting

Introduction

Safe performance of thoracic endovascular procedures including thoracic stent-grafting of aneurysms, dissections, retrograde delivery of transcatheter aortic valves, and other complex endovascular procedures for structural heart disease requires zero tolerance for major access-related complications. Thorough preoperative planning, understanding the pathology of aorto-iliac occlusive disease, advanced endovascular skills, and ability to perform an iliac conduit via a retroperitoneal approach are necessary to achieve excellent results. Furthermore, deliverability of complex thoracic endovascular devices through tortuous anatomy or old graft material may be improved by the more proximal access provided by an iliac conduit [5].

Indications and preoperative planning

Patients undergoing thoracic aortic endografting require access with devices ranging between 18 and 25 Fr caliber. The external iliac artery is the size-limiting segment and, depending on the size of sheath required, a minimum diameter of 9 mm may be necessary for safe access via the common femoral arteries. Patients with calcified, tortuous, or small vessel size or a combination (Fig. 1.12) may not be candidates for delivery of these large sheaths through femoral arterial access and any attempts to deliver an introducer sheath or an endoluminal graft may result in an increased risk of iliac artery rupture or the "artery on a stick" phenomenon (Fig. 1.13). Iliac artery diameters of 7.6–9.2 mm are required to deliver most devices through the femoral approach safely without the requirement of a conduit (Tables 1.2 and 1.3). Retroperitoneal exposure with construction of a 10 mm ilio-femoral conduit permits delivery of large sheaths in patients with tortuous, calcified and small iliac vessels or vessels with severe ilio-femoral vascular occlusive disease.

Construction of a 10 mm retroperitoneal conduit

A 15 cm semi-lunar right flank incision is made four finger-breaths above the groin crease. Division of the external oblique, internal oblique and transversus abdominus muscles is performed in the direction of their fibers. The extraperitoneal fascia and peritoneum are then retracted medially and dissection is carried out in the avascular plane of the retroperitoneum down to the level of the psoas muscle. All of the abdominal contents are then retracted medially with the help of a handheld retractor or an Omni retractor, providing excellent exposure of the lower infrarenal aorta, common iliac artery, and iliac bifurcation. The right common iliac artery along with the hypogastric and the external iliac artery are identified and mobilized (Fig. 1.14a). Care is taken to spare the right urether which crosses the common iliac artery before diving deep into the pelvis. A Rummel tourniquet is applied to control the proximal common iliac artery, the external iliac artery, and origin of the hypogastric artery; alternatively, vascular clamps could be applied for control. Heparin is usually given to the patient prior to clamping the vessels. An arteriotomy is made on the common iliac artery with a no. 11 blade and extended with Pott's scissors close to the bifurcation of the hypogastric artery and the external iliac artery. A 10 mm conduit is then sewn in an end-to-side fashion using 5-0 prolene sutures (Fig. 1.14b). The 10 mm graft is subsequently tunneled through the retroperitoneal space beneath the inguinal ligament and brought out through the groin incision used to expose the common femoral artery. The graft is subsequently flashed and clamped at the groin incision with the Rummel tourniquets released from the common iliac artery, external iliac artery, and hypogastric artery. The 10 mm conduit is subsequently looped with a Rummel tourniquet and ready to be punctured with an 18 gauge needle for access and introduction of a guide wire and an introducer sheath (Fig. 1.14c). The introducer sheath is subsequently exchanged for a device sheath, which is advanced into the distal aorta (Fig. 1.14d). The endoluminal graft is then introduced into the delivery sheath and deployed to the target area. Wires and sheaths are removed from the 10 mm conduit and the conduit is clamped.

The conduit can either be trimmed to the appropriate length and the conduit tied off as a stump (Fig. 1.14e) or the distal end of the conduit can be sewn to the more distal iliac system in an

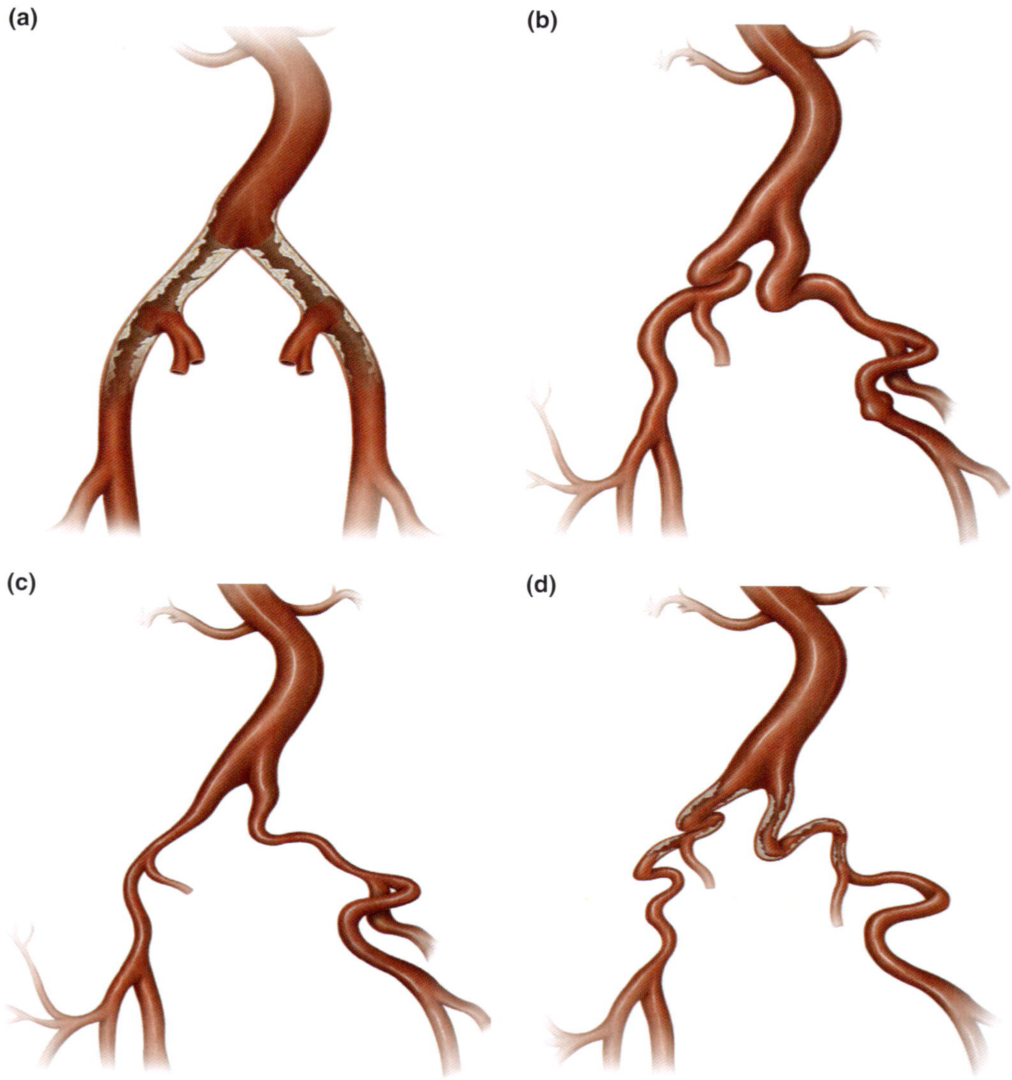

Fig. 1.12 Illustrations demonstrating calcified, tortuous, small tortuous, and small calcified tortuous iliac arteries which are contraindication for femoral access, requiring a retroperitoneal exposure with sewing of an iliac conduit for delivery of the endograft. (a) Calcified iliac artery. (b) Tortuous iliac artery. (c) Small tortuous iliac artery. (d) Small calcified tortuous iliac artery.

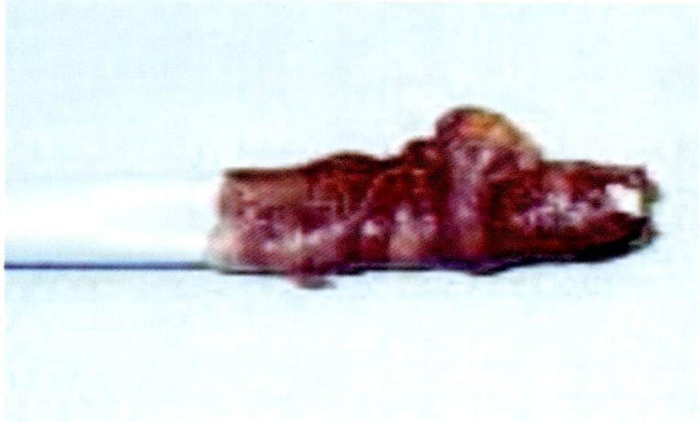

Fig. 1.13 Artery on a stick.

Table 1.2 Graft and delivery sheath sizes for descending thoracic aortic stent-grafts currently available in the United States.

Endograft	*Graft size available (diameter)*	*Sheath size required (diameter)*
Gore TAG	26–40 mm	20–24 Fr (7.6–9.2 mm)
Zenith TX1/TX2	28–42 mm	20–22 Fr (7.6–8.3 mm)
Talent	22–46 mm	22–25 Fr

end-to-end fashion as an interposition graft. Or, more commonly, the conduit can be brought to the groin by tunneling the conduit under the inguinal ligament and performing either an end-to-end anastomosis or an ilio-femoral conduit. The ilio-femoral conduit is performed by making an arteriotomy on the adequately exposed common femoral artery after adequate proximal and distal control is achieved. An end-to-side anastomosis is constructed with a 5-0 prolene suture with adequate flushing maneuvers performed prior to completion of the anastomosis (Fig. 1.14f). The ilio-femoral conduit is best for patients who may require further intervention for diffuse thoracic aneurysmal disease as the conduit may be reused through a simple infrainguinal incision in the future. The groin incision is approximated in layers. The right flank incision is irrigated, a 10 Fr Jackson–Pratt drain is placed in the retroperitoneal space and the incision closed in layers. The same technique can be applied to the infrarenal aorta and thoracic aorta. Similarly, end-to-side grafting of a conduit to the axillary artery, as described elsewhere, to facilitate deep hypothermic circulatory arrest also provides excellent access to the thoracic aorta via the innominate [2].

Table 1.3 Recommended iliac diameters for the introduction of Gore sheaths.

Size (Fr)	*ID (mm)*	*OD (mm)*
20	6.7	7.6
22	7.3	8.3
24	8.1	9.1

ID, inner diameter; OD, outer diameter.

Direct iliac artery access via a retroperitoneal approach

A 15 cm semi-lunar right flank incision is made four finger-breaths above the groin crease. Division of the external oblique, internal oblique,

(a) **(b)**

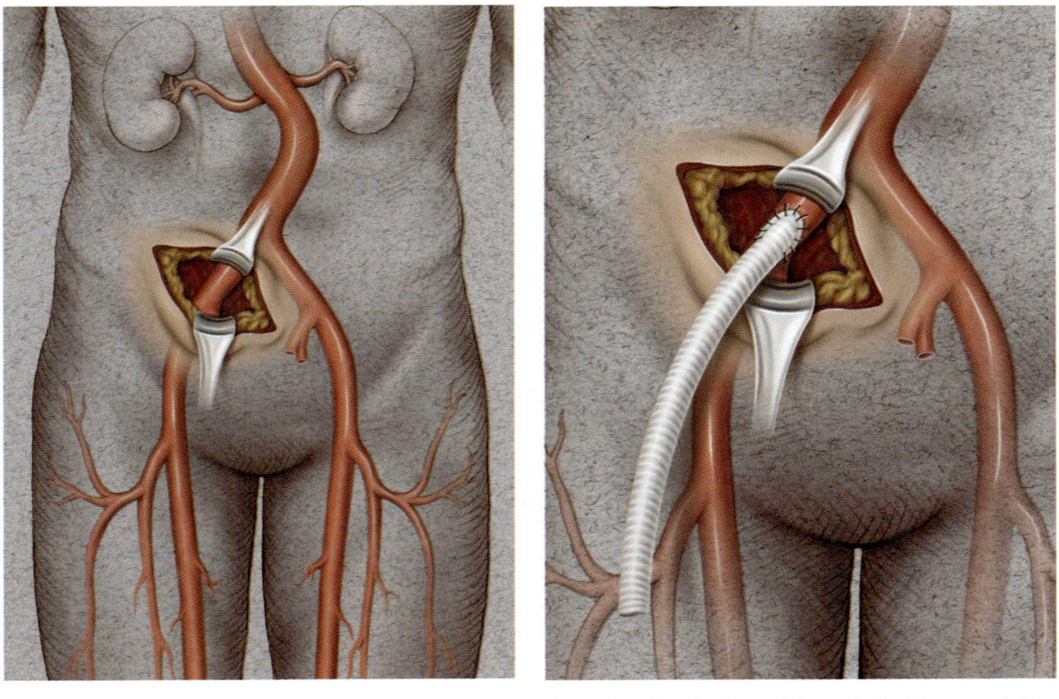

Fig. 1.14 (a) Retroperitoneal exposure. (b) A 10 mm conduit sewn to the iliac artery. (c) Conduit brought out of the incision with cannulation of the conduit with an introducer sheath. (d) Introducer sheath exchanged for a device sheath and advanced through the 10 mm conduit to the distal abdominal aorta. (e) Ligation of a 10 mm conduit. (f) Conduit tunneled and sewn to the femoral artery as an ilio-femoral conduit.

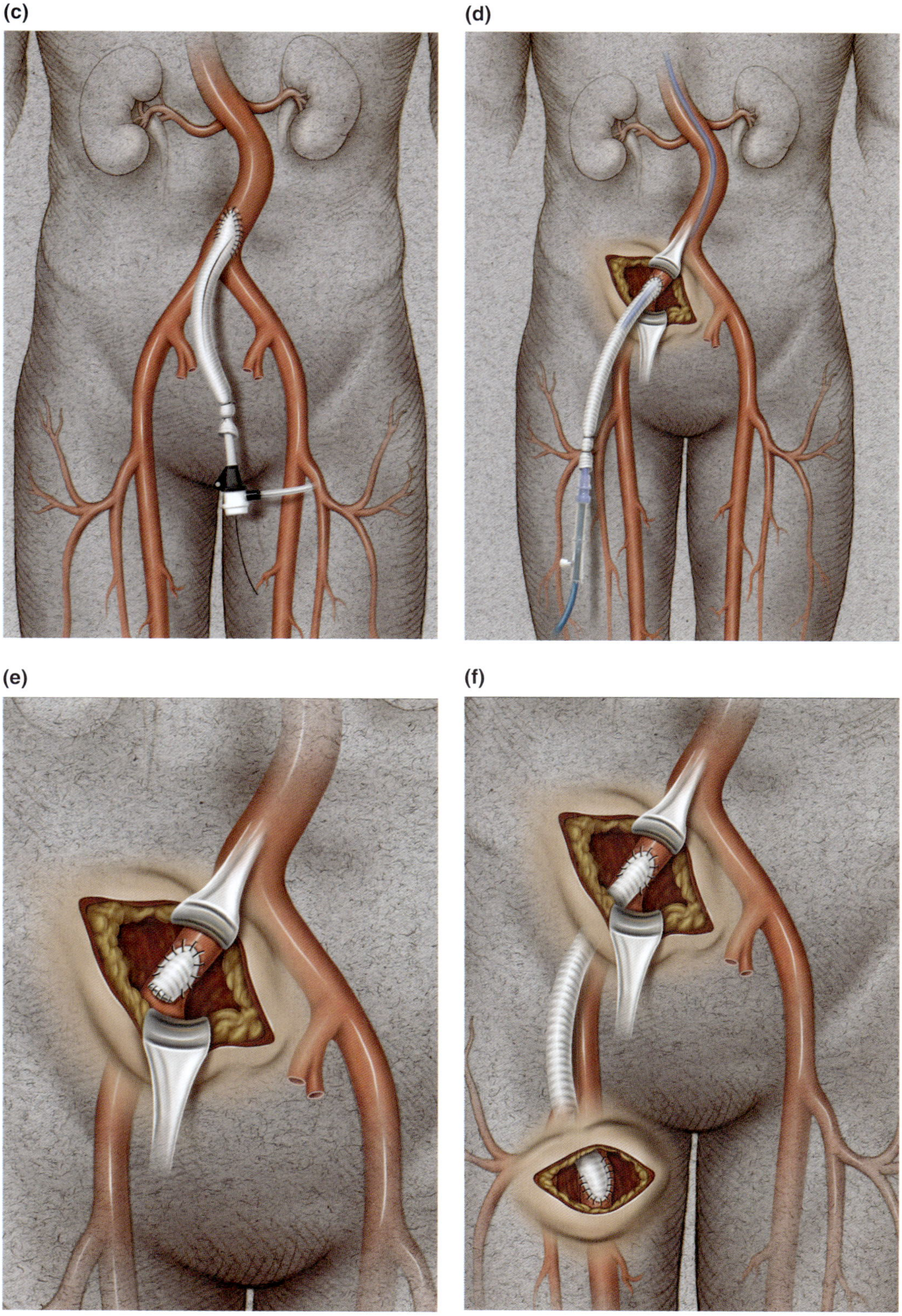

Fig. 1.14 *(Continued).*

and transversus abdominus muscle is performed. The peritoneum is identified and gently retracted medially with the help of a handheld retractor. The common iliac artery along with the hypogastric and external iliac artery are identified and mobilized. Care is taken to spare the right urether which crosses the common iliac artery before diving deep into the pelvis. A Rummel tourniquet is applied to control the proximal common iliac artery, the external iliac artery, and origin of the hypogastric artery; alternatively, vascular clamps could be applied for control. Heparin is usually given to the patient prior to clamping the vessels. An 18 gauge needle is used to access the common iliac artery close to the hypogastric artery bifurcation and a guide wire and an introducer sheath are advanced. The introducer sheath is subsequently exchanged for a device sheath, which is advanced into the distal aorta (Fig. 1.15). The endoluminal graft is then introduced into the delivery sheath and deployed to the target area. Wires and sheaths are removed and the arteriotomy repaired in a standard fashion (Fig. 1.16). The flank incision is

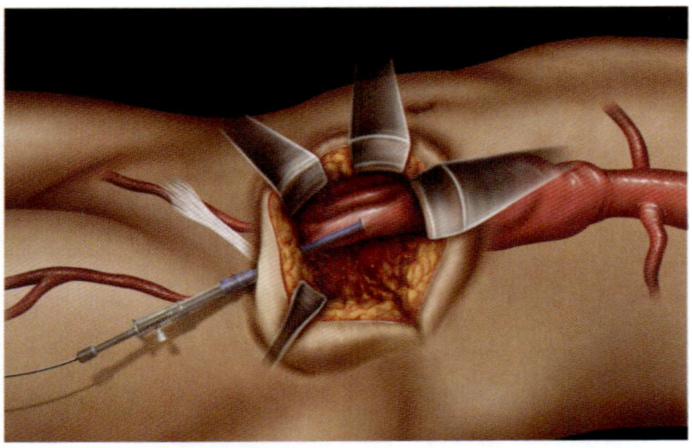

Fig. 1.15 Direct introduction of the device sheath through the common iliac artery through a retroperitoneal exposure.

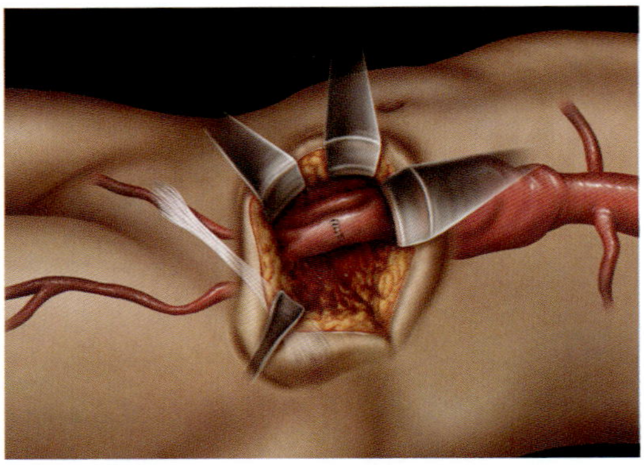

Fig. 1.16 Direct repair of the iliac artery.

irrigated, a 10 Fr Jackson–Pratt drain is placed in the retroperitoneal space, and the incision closed in layers.

References

1 Schneider PA. Endovascular Skills: Guidewire and Catheter Skills for Endovascular Surgery, 3rd edn. New York: Informa Healthcare, 2008.

2 Diethrich EB, Ramaiah VG, Kpodonu J, et al. Endovascular and Hybrid Management of the Thoracic Aorta. A case-based approach, 1st edn. Oxford: Wiley-Blackwell, 2008.

3 Kpodonu J, Rodriguez JA, Ramaiah VG, et al. Use of the right brachio-femoral wire approach to manage a thoracic aortic aneurysm in an extremely angulated and tortuous aorta with an endoluminal stent graft. Interact CardioVasc Thorac Surg 2008; 7:269–71.

4 Kpodonu J, Rodriguez JA, Ramaiah VG, et al. Cracking and paving: a novel technique to deliver a thoracic endograft despite ilio-femoral occlusive disease. J Card Surg 2009; 24(2):188–90.

5 Abu-Ghaida AM, Clair DG, Greenberg RK, et al. Broadening the applicability of endovascular aneurysm repair: the use of iliac conduits. J Vasc Surg 2002; 36:111–17.

CHAPTER 2

Equipment required for aortic endografting

Jacques Kpodonu
University of California Irvine,
Cardiovascular Hybrid Interventions, Hoag Heart and Vascular Institute, Newport Beach, CA, USA

Equipment lists

Main equipment

- Fluoroscope with digital angiography capabilities (C-arm or fixed unit):
  - non-obstructive table for imaging of chest and abdomen
  - power injector for fluoroscopic contrast studies
  - connecting tubing for power injector
  - digital subtraction angiography
  - road mapping
  - multiplane image system.
- High-resolution fluoroscopic imaging and the ability to record and recall at imaging.
- Surgical suite standby in the event that emergency surgery is necessary.
- Cell saver and/or autotransfuser (optional).
- Inflation device with pressure gauge.
- Needles.
- Radiopaque ruler with centimeter increments.
- Heparinized solution.
- Puncture needles 18 or 19 gauge.
- Assorted guide wires of at least 260 cm in length, including a stiff 0.035 inch wire to support the Xcelerant delivery system (Medtronic, Minneapolis, MN).
- Assorted angiographic, angioplasty, and graduated pigtail catheters.
- 12 Fr introducer system to be used with the Reliant stent-graft balloon catheter (Medtronic).
- Sterile introducer sheaths of 5 or 10 Fr for vascular access to femoral arteries and to perform diagnostic imaging.
- Radiopaque contrast media.
- Sterile silicone lubricant or mineral oil.

Supplementary equipment

- Nitinol goose neck snare (10–15 mm).
- Angioplasty catheters 8–40 mm (depending on case).
- Intravascular ultrasound unit with catheters.
- Sterile marker.
- 25–30 mm valvuloplasty balloons.
- Dilators.

Further equipment information

Percutaneous entry needle/devices

Endovascular procedures require the use of a percutaneous needle. Needles come in a variety of lengths and gauges. Each needle contains two parts: the hub used when attaching the needle to the syringe and the cannula, which is the hollow shaft of the needle. The most common gauge used is the 18 gauge needle (Fig. 2.1). The 18 gauge needle will accommodate a .035 inch guide wire. The length of

Endovascular and Hybrid Therapies for Structural Heart and Aortic Disease, First Edition.
Edited by Jacques Kpodonu and Raoul Bonan.

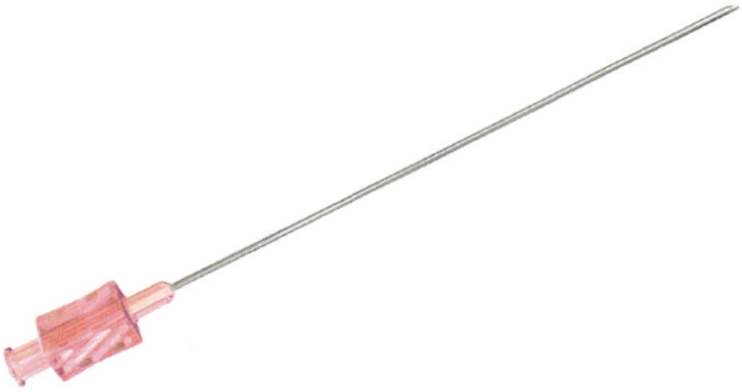

Fig. 2.1 18 gauge 7 cm Cook percutaneous needle.

needles varies between 2 and 3.5 inches. Other accessories include micropuncture sets and smart needles.

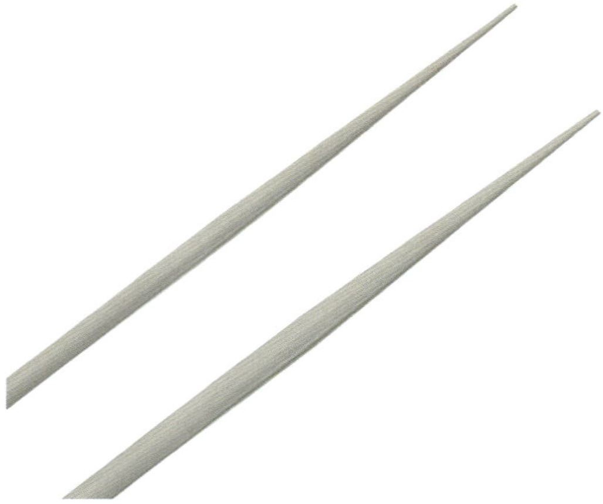

Fig. 2.2 Dilator sets.

Vessel dilators

These devices dilate the tract the needle has created, allowing large devices such as catheters and sheaths to be introduced into the vessel. They are placed over the guide wire that was introduced through the original puncture needle. Vessel dilators are measured in French sizes (1 Fr ≈ 0.33 mm) and are most commonly 15–20 cm in length. "Serial dilation" can be necessary when attempting to introduce large diameter sheaths, particularly with patients that have scar tissue build up in the common femoral artery (CFA) area. It is important not to overdilate the tract. Overdilating can allow blood to leak around your catheter or sheath, not allowing you to gain hemostatic control of the vessel. Dilator sets may vary from 4 to 22 Fr × 20 cm (Fig. 2.2).

Guide wires

Guide wires are used to access the vessel through the percutaneous needle [1]. In addition, they are used to help steer catheters and devices through the vascular anatomy. Guide wires are manufactured in several different ways: they are either solid steel core wires, or the steel core can be wrapped in a thin steel coil. The core can also be encased in a polymer-type jacket. Recently they have started using nitinol metal for the inner core material. Guide wires usually have a floppy tip with a stiff body. The tip configuration usually includes angled tips, straight tips, J-tips, and shapeable tips. The diameters of the wires are measured in thousandths of an inch, ranging from 0.014 to 0.038 inches. Lengths are measured in centimeters and can range from 80 to 300 cm. However, some specialty wires can come in lengths up to 450 cm.

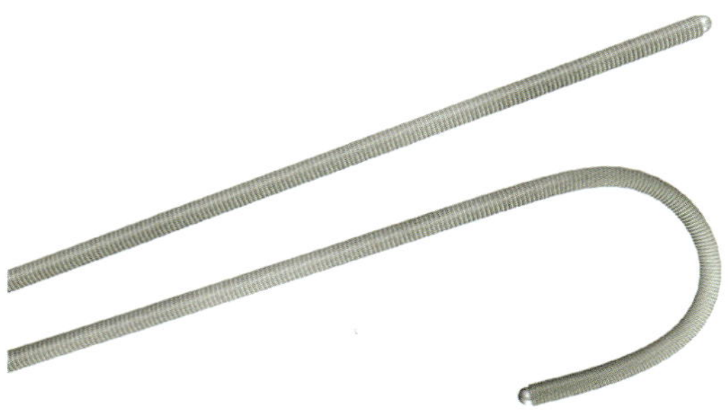

Fig. 2.3 Ultrastiff guide wires used in thoracic endografting.

Some guide wires may have a hydrophilic coating, making them slippery when wet. Hoag Hospital's primary workhorse guide wire is the 0.035 inch Terumo angled glide wire. This wire has a hydrophilic coating. It is constructed with a center core of superelastic metal alloy that tapers to a soft flexible tip. The kink-resistant core is coated with a polyurethane jacket. This jacket is bonded with a hydrophilic polymer that becomes slick when saline has been applied. There are many guide wire manufacturers, with hundreds, possibly thousands, of wires to choose from (Fig. 2.3). The wire selection is dependent on the location of the lesion, the tortuousity of the vessel, and the physician's preference.

Introducer sheaths

Sheaths are hemostatic conduits inserted into the vessel (Fig. 2.4). They allow the passage of guide wires, catheters, and interventional devices. The

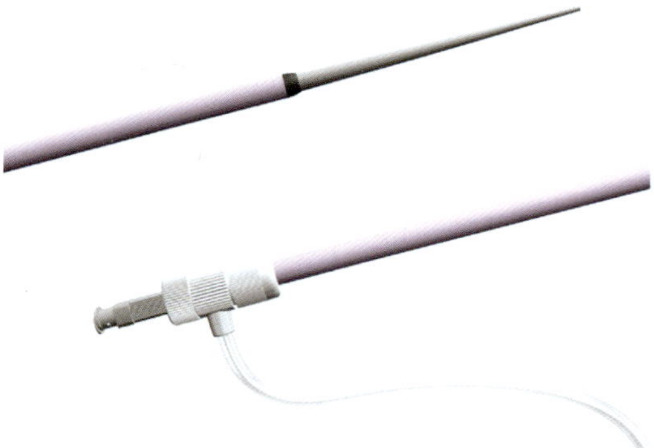

Fig. 2.4 Introducer sheaths commonly used in introducing balloons, catheters, and wires for thoracic endografting.

Box 2.1 Universal color coating

- 4 Fr = red
- 5 Fr = grey
- 6 Fr = green
- 7 Fr = orange
- 8 Fr = blue
- 9 Fr = black
- 10 Fr = violet
- 11 Fr = yellow

sheath allows these to be passed in and out of the body without damaging the vessel and reduces the blood loss. Some sheaths may have a braided wire construction to reduce kinking in acute angles. They may have a radiopaque tip for visualization under fluoroscopy. Sheaths are measured by the inner diameter in French sizes. They are universally color coated (Box 2.1). They range in sizes from 4 to 24 Fr. Larger sized sheaths may require the surgeon to "cut down" and expose the CFA in order to repair the large arteriotomy post procedure.

Flush/diagnostic/guiding catheters

Catheters have three primary purposes: to delivery contrast for arteriography images, to assist in directing wires through target lesions needing intervention, and to give shaped support when trying to deliver devices to these target lesions (Box 2.2). Catheters are measured by the outer diameter in French sizes. The diagnostic catheters

Box 2.2 Types of catheters

- Cerebral catheters
- Visceral catheters
- Coronary catheters
- Exchange catheters
- Flush catheters
- Guiding catheters

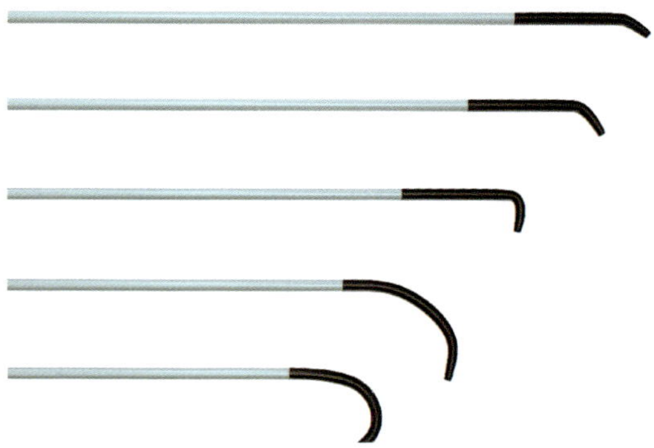

Fig. 2.5 Guiding catheters used in thoracic endografting.

are of 4–5 Fr diameters and are used to help maneuver guide wires through the vascular anatomy and to deliver contrast for angiograms (Fig. 2.5). The guide catheters are 6–12 Fr in diameter and are used to assist in the delivery of the interventional devices, such as stents and balloons. These catheters come in hundreds of shapes and lengths; they come in braided and non-braided construction. They have special features like hydrophilic coatings, radiopaque tips, and radiopaque markers used to help determine lesion lengths.

Angioplasty balloons

Angioplasty balloons are used for several different reasons. They are used to assist self-expanding stent-grafts with arterial wall apposition, which is called profile ballooning. They are also used to dilate lesions and for mounting stainless steel or cobalt chromium stents. These are expanded in the target lesion; this is called therapeutic ballooning. Balloons are measured by diameter (mm) and then length (mm or cm) (e.g. 5 × 10 balloon = 5 mm × 10 cm). The balloons

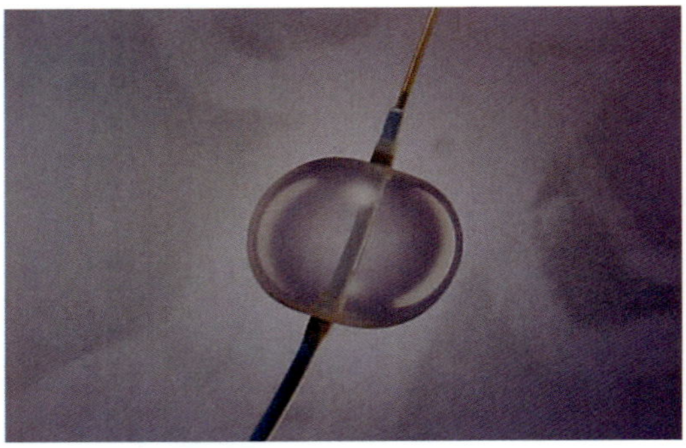

Fig. 2.6 Compliant Equalizer (Boston Scientific) balloon used for profiling of an endoluminal graft.

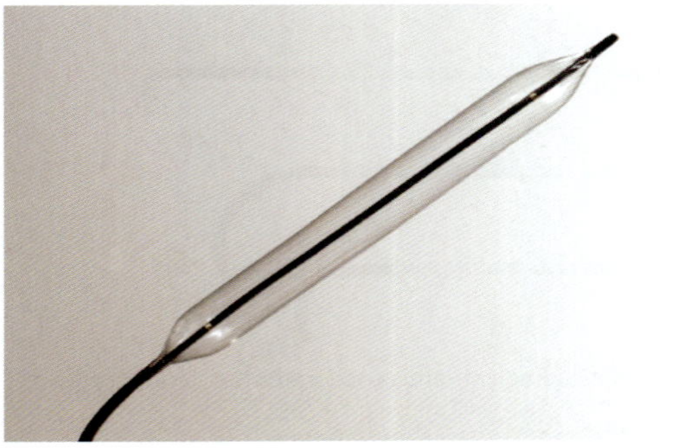

Fig. 2.7 Non-compliant balloon used for dilating calcified arteries.

come in many different shaft lengths and various crossing profiles. The balloons have pressure ratings called nominal and rated burst pressures. Nominal pressure is the amount of atmospheres it takes to expand the balloon to its listed diameter and length. Rated burst pressure is a conservative measurement, in which one out of 100 balloons tested ruptured at this atmospheric pressure. These rates, and the amount of growth the balloon has when the pressure exceeds the nominal pressure, determine how the balloons are classified. The classifications of the balloons are compliant (greater than 10% growth), semi-compliant (between 5% and 10% growth) and non-compliant (less than 5% growth). The more non-compliant the balloon, the stronger the balloon is for dilating hard calcified lesions (Fig. 2.6). The more compliant the balloon is, the more suitable it is for profile ballooning, or pulling a thrombus or an embolus out of a vessel (Fig. 2.7).

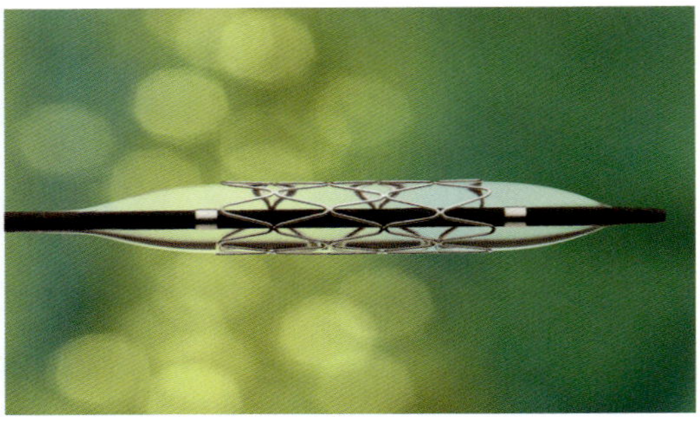

Fig. 2.8 Balloon-expandable stent.

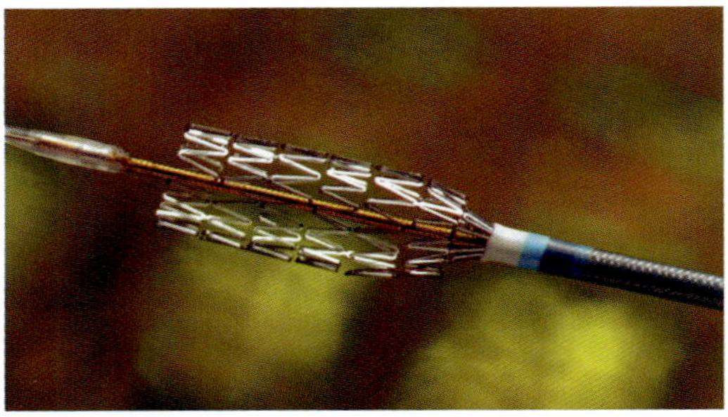

Fig. 2.9 Self-expandable stent.

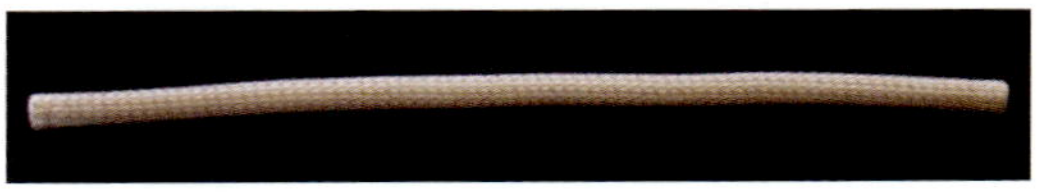

Fig. 2.10 Covered stent-graft.

Stents

Stents are metallic scaffolding used to permanently dilate a lesion. There are two different types of stents: balloon-expandable and self-expanding stents. The balloon-expandable stents (Fig. 2.8) are constructed of 316 L stainless steel. They have a high radial strength and are placed in ostial lesions where the vessel has low mobility, e.g. renal arteries and common iliac arteries. The stent is mounted on a balloon. When the stent has been placed so it is straddling the lesion, the balloon is inflated pressing the stent open. Self-expanding stents are constructed of nitinol (Fig. 2.9). Nitinol is a manmade metal created by the US Navy. When the nitinol is chilled, the metal can be compressed so the stent can be loaded into a delivery catheter system. This is done by the stent manufacturing company. When the stent is placed in the human body and the delivery system is deployed the stent expands due

Table 2.1 Technical features of some commercially available thoracic aortic devices (author's personal assessments).

Device	*Introducing sheath*	*Introducing system size (Fr)*	*Available diameter size (mm)*	*Available lengths (mm)*	*Bare proximal portion*	*Delayed deployment of more proximal stent*	*Radial force (*)*	*Flexibility (*)*	*MRI compatibility (images artifacting)*	*Delivery system*
TAG (Gore)	Y	20–24	26–40	20	N	N	+	++	Y	Pull-knob
Talent (Medtronic)	N	22–27	22–46	100	Y	N	++	+	Y	Pull-back
Valiant (Medtronic)	N	20–24	22–46	100–220 150–	Y	N	+++	++	Y	Pull-back Xcelerant System
Zenith TX2 (Cook Medical)	Y	20–22	22–42	100–216 150–	Y	Y	++	+	N	Pull-back
Relay (Bolton Medical)	N	22–26	22–46		Y	Y	++	+	Y	Pull-back

to the body temperature. The interesting property of nitinol is that it has memory, so it can be crushed and it will recover its manufactured specifications. Self-expanding stents are placed in lesions where the vessels are more mobile, e.g. near joints or in limbs. Most self-expanding stents have radiopaque markers that increase their visibility. Covered stent-grafts (Fig. 2.10) are alternatively used for arthero-occlusive disease, dissection, and rupture of vessels.

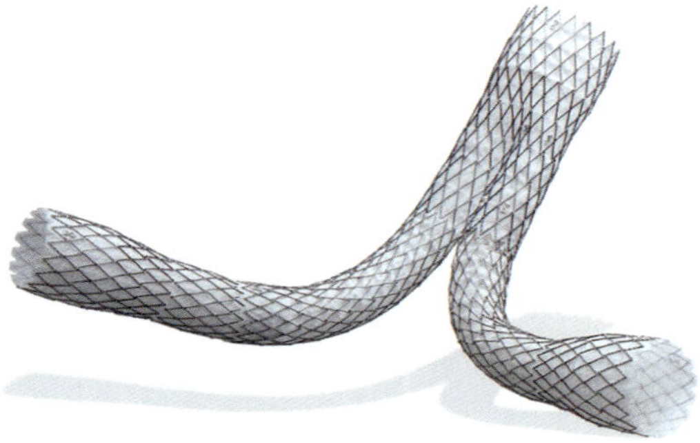

Fig. 2.11 Medtronic Aneurex abdominal endoluminal graft.

Endoluminal grafts

Endoluminal grafts (ELGs) are stents, primarily self-expanding, that are covered with polytetrafluoroethylene (PTFE) material or woven Dacron. They are most commonly used in the aorta to exclude aneurysms. They are used in both the abdominal and the thoracic aortas. The majority of grafts used in the abdominal aorta bifurcate and the limbs continue into the iliac system. Currently, there are three US Food and Drug Administration (FDA) approved thoracic endoluminal grafts. Most of these grafts require large sheaths to place into the body. Flexibility, conformability, ease of deployment, accuracy of deployment, durability, availability in a wide range of diameters and lengths, and low profile delivery systems are desirable attributes for the ideal endograft. Several types of thoracic aortic endograft are currently commercially available; these include the Gore TAG (W.L. Gore & Associates, Flagstaff, AZ), Zenith TX2 (Cook Medical, Bloomington, IN), Talent and Valiant (Medtronic, Minneapolis, MN), Relay (Bolton Medical, Sunrise, FL), Evita (Jotec, Hechingen, Germany) and Endofit (Endomed Phoenix, AZ).

The technical features of the most commonly used devices are presented in Table 2.1.

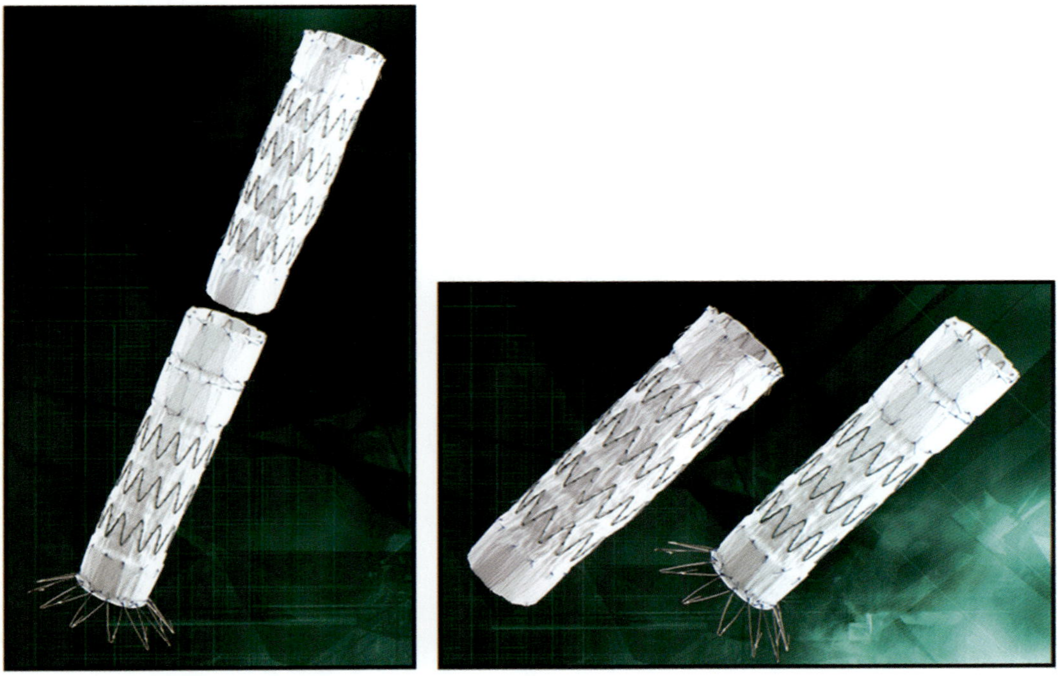

Fig. 2.12 Cook TX2 thoracic endoluminal graft.

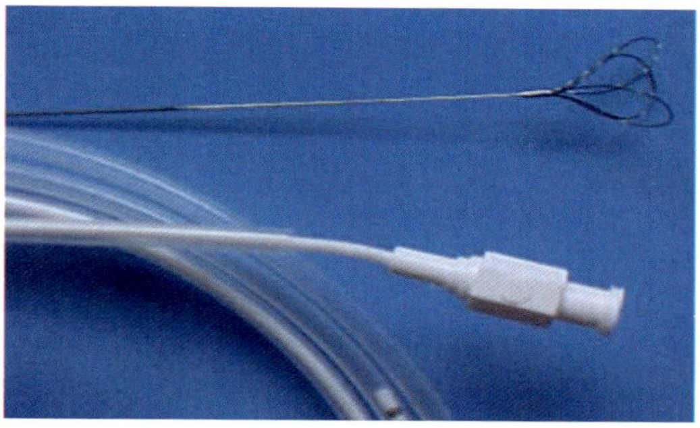

Fig. 2.13 Inter V Ensnare device.

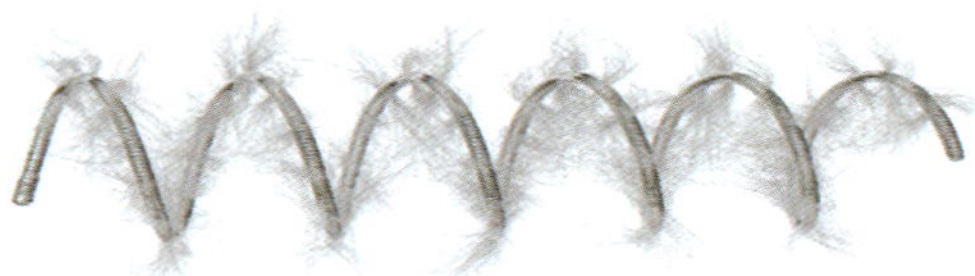

Fig. 2.14 Nestor (Cook) embolization coils used for arterial and venous embolization.

Endograft selection

The following statements can be made about the current devices: No device is perfect. There is no good quality scientific evidence that any one device is better than the others. The majority of devices are chosen on the basis of personal preference and experience. The nitinol stent-grafts are magnetic resonance compatible so that the risk of irradiation can be reduced for the follow-up examinations.

In general, devices are oversized by 10–20% for aneurysms and slightly less for acute dissection (e.g. 5–10%). When selecting a device diameter for use in dissections, the caliber of the aorta just proximal to the dissection should be used. This will generally be the diameter of the mid-aortic arch. In acute dissections, a device length should be chosen to cover the main entry tear. In chronic dissection, devices should extend from just proximal to the entry tear to the diaphragm (Figs 2.11 and 2.12).

Accessory tools

A variety of other tools may also be useful in thoracic aortic endografting procedures. Snares, such as the EV3 Gooseneck (EV3, Plymouth, MN) and Inter V Ensnare device (INTER-V, Gainesville, FL) (Fig. 2.13) are intended for use in thoracic endografting procedures to retrieve and manipulate foreign objects and are useful when establishing brachio-femoral guide wire access to assist with delivery of the thoracic stent in cases of severely tortuous aortas. Embolization coils (Fig. 2.14) may also be needed to treat a type II endoleak by coiling the origin of the left subclavian artery or to deposit the coils in the sac. Peripheral vascular stents and covered stents may be important tools when addressing iliac artery stenoses to help with delivery of the sheath and thoracic endoprosthesis.

Reference

1 Endovascular supplies 2010.

3

CHAPTER 3

Advanced computed tomography imaging, workstations, and planning tools

Paolo Perini[1], *Pascal Rheaume*[2] *& Stéphan Haulon*[1]

[1] Vascular Surgery, Hôpital Cardiologique, CHRU de Lille, France

[2] Vascular Surgery, Hopital St-Francois D'Assise, Quebec City, Canada

Multidetector row computed tomography (MDCT) has now replaced the old "gold standard" intra-arterial digital subtraction angiography (DSA) for assessing abdominal, thoracic, and cranial vasculature. MDCT raw data is captured in two-dimensional transverse sections; therefore to generate an angiographic display, a 3D workstation is required. To depict vascular anatomy on the workstation, specific anatomic projections must be created using one or more of the visualization techniques. The image projections must display the vascular region of interest in the correct viewing planes without being obscured by other vascular territories or non-cardiovascular structures. Furthermore, the resultant images must be rendered with the correct window, level, and lighting settings to accurately depict normal anatomy and pathology. The volumetric data acquired enable the acquisition of views from any angle and perspective. MDCT has a superior diagnostic accuracy in comparison with intra-arterial DSA in characterizing the neck of the abdominal aortic aneurysm (AAA), identifying accessory renal arteries, and characterizing renal arterial stenoses.

The implantation of an infrarenal endoprosthesis is a relatively simple procedure, requiring preoperative length and diameter measurements and accurate longitudinal device placement. However, designing and implanting a device which will accommodate the aortic branches is more complex: inappropriate orientation of the visceral branches will preclude successful endovascular repair. Essential information needed for preoperative assessment of aortic aneurysms includes the relationship of the aneurysm to the aortic branches, the degree of iliac arterial involvement with the aneurysm, the presence of other coexisting iliac arterial or aortic aneurysms, the presence of supernumerary or aberrant aortic branches, and the presence of coexistent iliac arterial occlusive disease.

On currently available 3D workstations, there are four principal visualization techniques: multiplanar (axial, sagittal, coronal, oblique) reconstruction (MPR), curved planar reformation (CPR), maximum intensity projection (MIP), and 3D volume rendering (VR) (Fig. 3.1). Automated and semi-automated vessel analysis tools are integrated to run these techniques. The generation of a center line of flow image allows the visualization of a tortuous aorta as if it were straightened or stretched out and aids greatly in the design of the endoprosthesis, particularly in accurately measuring the correct length of the graft between key anatomic targets such as branch locations and vessel bifurcations (Fig. 3.2).

Endovascular and Hybrid Therapies for Structural Heart and Aortic Disease, First Edition.
Edited by Jacques Kpodonu and Raoul Bonan.

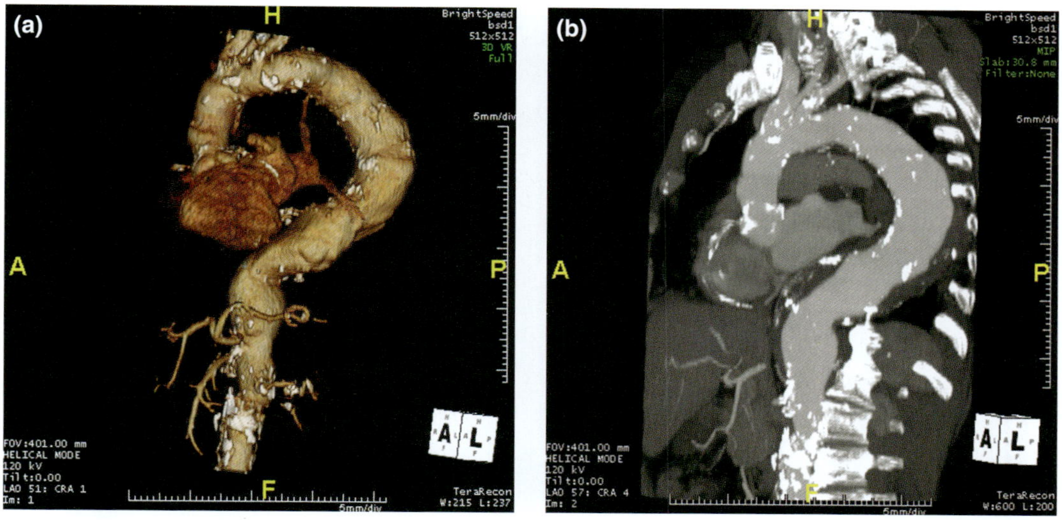

Fig. 3.1 (a) MIP and (b) 3D-VR reconstructions of a descending thoracic aortic aneurysm. From Atlas of Advanced Endoaortic Surgery. Copyright Springer.

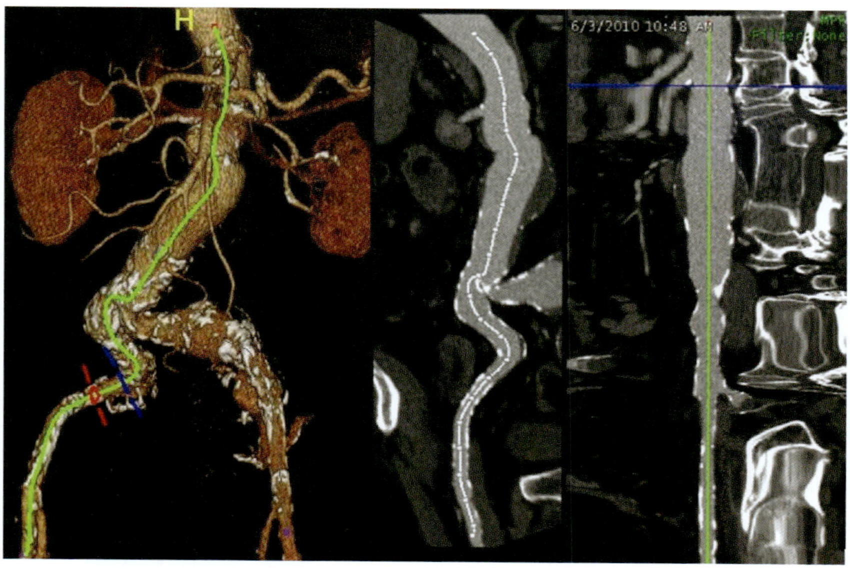

Fig. 3.2 Practical steps for the generation of a "stretched" aorta using a center line technique: a center line of flow (green line on the left image) is generated by the workstation. Before a stretched reconstruction is obtained (right image), the center line can be modified by adding, retrieving, or moving the numerous dots of the line (middle image). From Atlas of Advanced Endoaortic Surgery. Copyright Springer.

Three-dimensional workstations are now intuitive and "user-friendly" in order to be accessible to cardiovascular surgeons and not only to experienced radiologists. Reliable default VR and MIP templates and quick access to advanced segmentation algorithms that automatically edit and grow vessel territories are essential (Fig. 3.3).

Vessel caliber, patency, tortuosity, and burden of calcium and thrombus are important vascular features to assess preoperatively (Fig. 3.4). Diameters, lengths, and angles are often necessary dimensions to measure (Fig. 3.5). Although much of this imaging information can be visualized on conventional axial images, 3D-VR, multiplanar, and

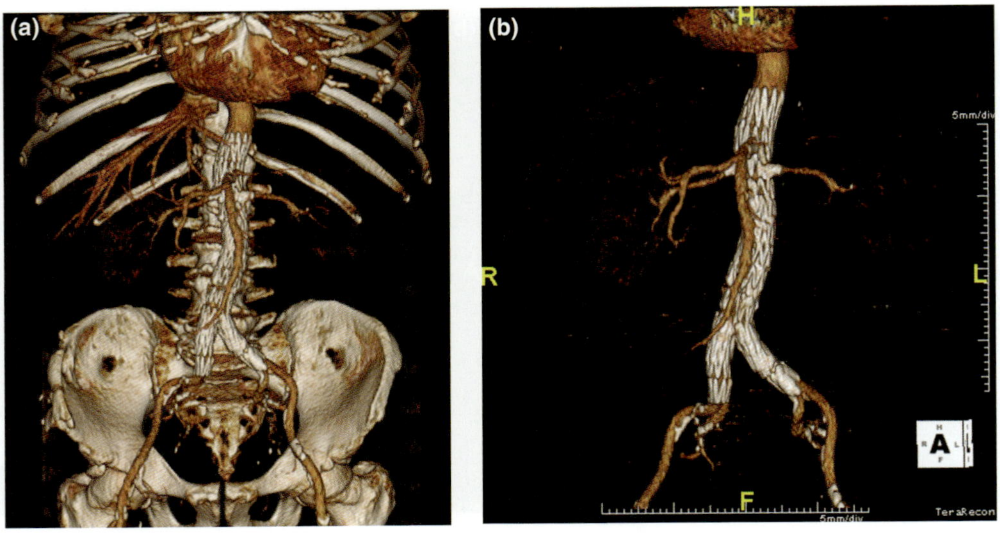

Fig. 3.3 3D-VR of a juxtarenal abdominal aortic aneurysm treated with a fenestrated endograft before (a) and after (b) running the "bone removal" algorithm. From Atlas of Advanced Endoaortic Surgery. Copyright Springer.

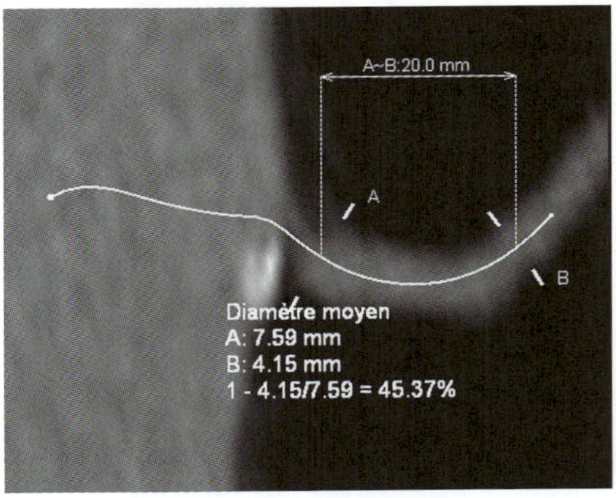

Fig. 3.4 CPR of a renal artery used for planning a fenestrated endograft depicting a severe stenosis at the origin of the vessel. From Atlas of Advanced Endoaortic Surgery. Copyright Springer.

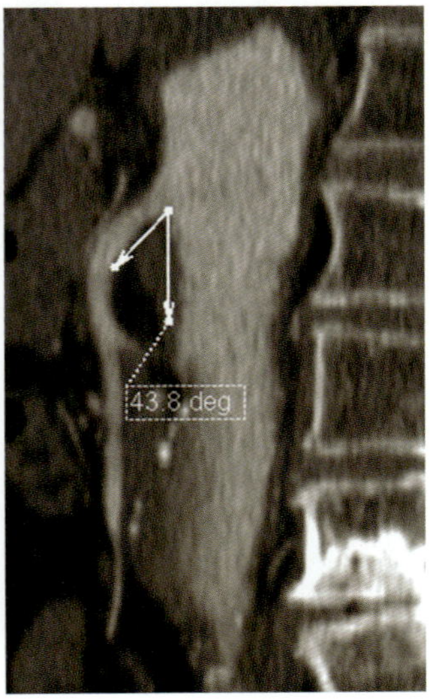

Fig. 3.5 Sagittal MPR showing the superior mesenteric artery and its angle with the aorta. The catheterization of this vessel via a femoral approach during fenestrated endovascular aortic repair (EVAR) is anticipated to be challenging (angle of the target vessel to the aortic wall <60°). From Atlas of Advanced Endoaortic Surgery. Copyright Springer.

curved planar reconstructions provide quick and clear visualization of the complex relationships of anatomy and pathology (Fig. 3.6). The combined use of the various visualization techniques is critical in surgical planning.

The advantage of VR is the accurate spatial perception through a complete 3D angiographic overview. Care however must be taken in interpreting these reformatted images; for example, a critical stenosis may appear like a complete occlusion. It is important to correlate 3D findings with the corresponding two-dimensional images in order to

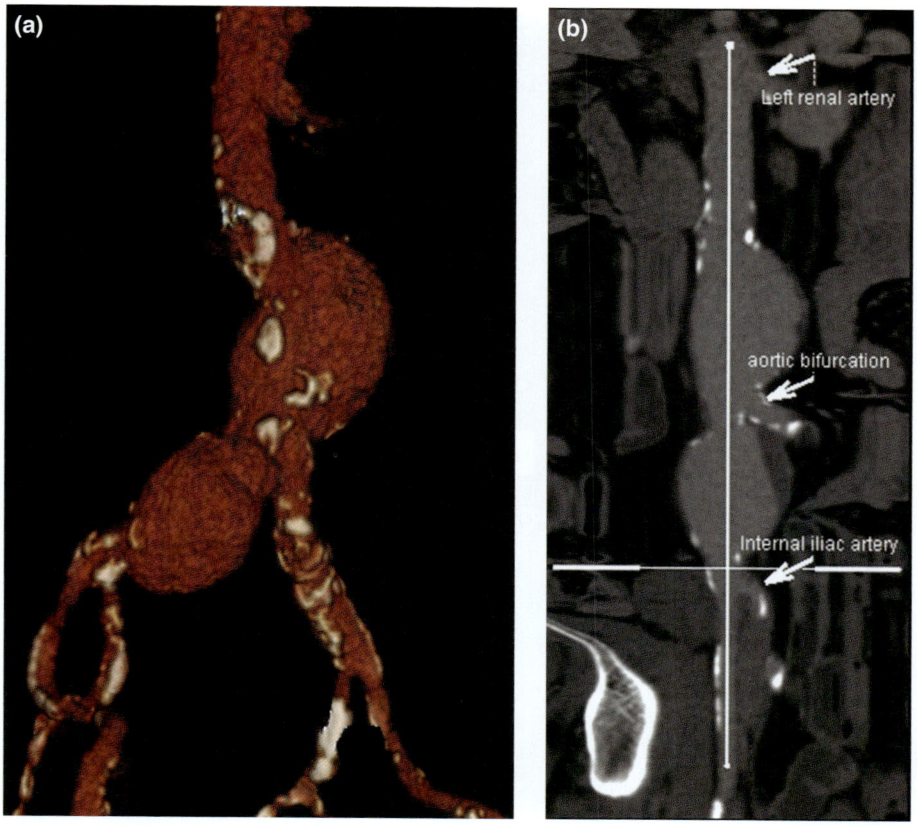

Fig. 3.6 (a) 3D-VR and (b) stretched CPR of an infrarenal aortic aneurysm associated with a right common iliac aneurysm. The combination of the various visualization techniques is vital to properly size and plan the endograft. From Atlas of Advanced Endoaortic Surgery. Copyright Springer.

avoid such pitfalls. With MPR, a two-dimensional analysis through the original dataset is performed in axial, coronal, sagittal, or oblique orientations. Analysis of the vessel wall and the flow lumen with accurate display of stenosis, occlusions, and calcification can be performed. The only disadvantage is the limited spatial display. MIP is also a two-dimensional analysis option for an angiographic overview, but semi-automated or complete manual editing is required to remove structural overlay. It can be useful to depict small caliber vessels and poorly enhanced vessels. Its accuracy is, however, limited in calcified vessels. Confirmation of stenosis and vessel caliber measurements should always be done with orthogonal MPR. As vessels curve in and out of the planes, standard MPRs cannot display an entire vascular territory and flow lumen in one image. To obtain a complete longitudinal vessel display, the solution is to generate a longitudinal cross-section using either two-dimensional or rotating CPR techniques.

The measurements required for accurate planning of branched and fenestrated endografts are complex and beyond the scope of what can be achieved accurately with standard two-dimensional axial images and table positions to measure aortic lengths and the relative positions of visceral arteries. Indeed, there is significant potential for error when trying to measure aortic lengths using a combination of coronal and sagittal images of the angulated aorta. The evolution of modern workstations has consigned these difficulties to history with rapid generation of accurate 3D images now feasible in real time (Figs 3.7 and 3.8). It is likely that some of the ongoing improvements in clinical outcomes that are continuously being reported in the endovascular literature are in part attributable to more accurate graft design with consequent

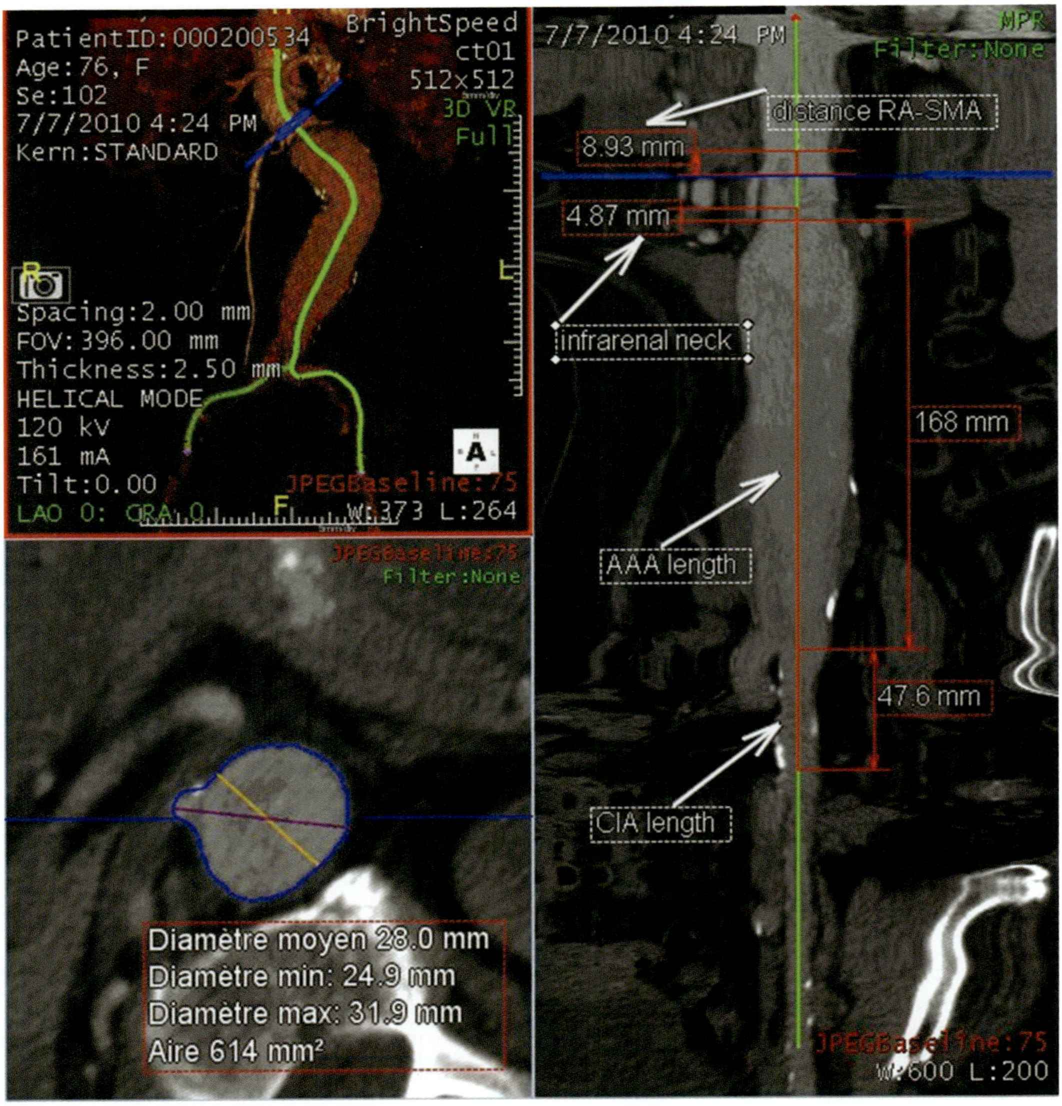

Fig. 3.7 Various phases of the planning of a fenestrated endograft using a workstation. On the upper left the 3D-VR is generated. The center line is drawn in green, and is used to generate the stretched CPR on the right of the screen. The two-dimensional image on the lower left is the reconstruction perpendicular to the center lumen line. It is used to precisely assess the diameter of the aorta. From Atlas of Advanced Endoaortic Surgery. Copyright Springer.

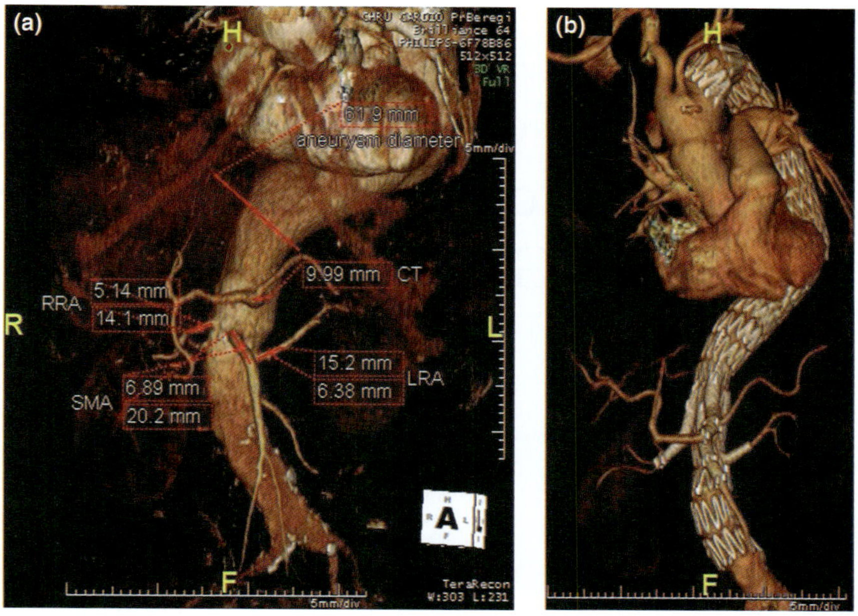

Fig.3.8 (a) A meticulous analysis of the preoperative CT scan on the workstation was mandatory to design an endograft that perfectly matched the aortic anatomy. (b) Postoperative 3D-VR of a type II thoraco-abdominal aneurysm treated with a four-branch endograft. The length and diameter of the sealing zone in each target vessel has also been evaluated. From Atlas of Advanced Endoaortic Surgery. Copyright Springer.

benefits in terms of improved target vessel perfusion rates, less graft migration/endoleak, and shorter procedure times. Clearly in striving to improve clinical outcomes it is incumbent on all endovascular surgeons to become comfortable with this remarkable technology.

4

CHAPTER 4

Technique of thoracic endografting for thoracic aneurysm using the approved Gore TAG device

Jacques Kpodonu
University of California Irvine,
Cardiovascular Hybrid Interventions, Hoag Heart and Vascular Institute, Newport Beach, CA, USA

The technique of thoracic endografting for the treatment of thoracic aortic aneurysm [1] using a Gore TAG device (W.L. Gore & Associates, Flagstaff, AZ) (Fig. 4.1) is preferably performed in a hybrid operating room (Fig. 4.2) or an endovascular suite provided the patient is an adequate candidate for endovascular repair. The procedure is performed under general anesthesia with spinal drainage selected for patients who have had a previous open surgical repair of an abdominal aortic aneurysm or patients considered high risk for paraplegia.

Percutaneous retrograde access of the common femoral artery is obtained in one groin and open retrograde cannulation of the contralateral common femoral artery performed with an 18 gauge needle (Fig. 4.3). An 0.035 inch soft-tip angled glide wire (Medi-tech/Boston Scientific, Natick, MA) is passed into the distal thoracic aorta (Fig. 4.4). A 9 Fr sheath is usually placed in the open common femoral artery and, similarly, 5 Fr sheath placed in the percutaneously accessed common femoral artery under fluoroscopic visualization. A dose of 5000 units of heparin is given to keep the activated clotted time at greater than 200 seconds. A 5 Fr pigtail catheter is advanced through the percutaneous sheath into the ascending thoracic aorta for an ascending and arch angiogram which is saved as a road map picture (Fig. 4.5). The fluoroscopic C-arm is positioned in a left anterior oblique angle and an oblique thoracic arch aortogram is performed to visualize the arch vessels and the descending thoracic aortic aneurysm (Fig. 4.6).

Intravascular ultrasound (IVUS) (Fig. 4.7) can be performed to provide more information on the proximal and distal neck diameter, length of thoracic aorta involved with the aneurysm, presence or absence of thrombus in the neck, and any other pathology that may have been missed on the angiogram or preoperative computed tomography (CT) angiogram of the thoracic aorta (see Fig. 4.1). The 5 Fr pigtail catether is exchanged for an extra stiff 260 cm double curve Lunderquist wire (Cook Medical, Bloomington, IN). The 9 Fr groin sheath in the open cannulated femoral artery is exchanged for an appropriate-sized device sheath which is advanced to the distal thoracic aorta (Fig. 4.8). The endograft is subsequently advanced through the device sheath and positioned into the thoracic aorta to exclude the thoracic aneurysm (Fig. 4.9). Prior to deployment, the proximal and distal landing zones identified are marked on

Endovascular and Hybrid Therapies for Structural Heart and Aortic Disease, First Edition.
Edited by Jacques Kpodonu and Raoul Bonan.

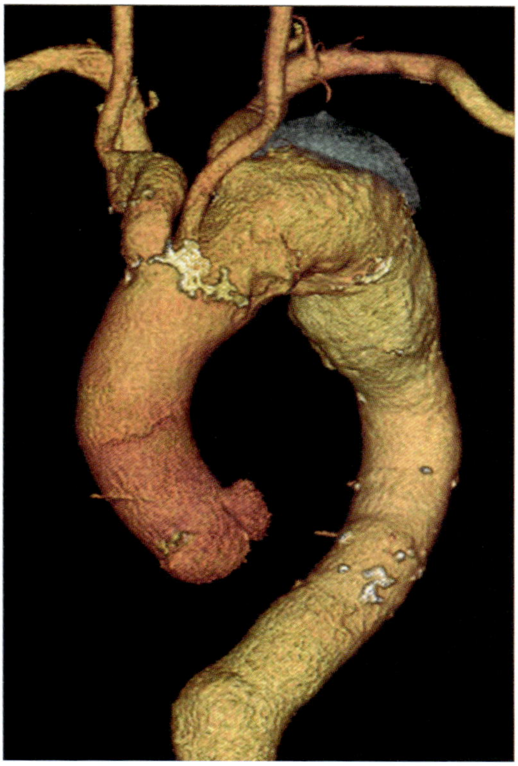

Fig. 4.1 Reconstructed 3D CT scan of the chest demonstrating a thoracic aortic aneurysm.

angiographic road map. At the time of deployment of the endoluminal graft, a systolic blood pressure of 90 mmHg is achieved to decrease the "windsock" effect in the thoracic aorta. We have not felt the need for adenosine-induced asystole. The device is deployed (Fig. 4.10a) and a Gore tri-lobe balloon (Fig. 4.10b) is used to perform post-deployment balloon angioplasty to both the proximal and distal segments of the graft for good fixation and any areas of overlap if more than one graft is deployed. A completion angiogram is then performed to confirm exclusion of the aneurysm and to determine if any endoleak is present (Fig. 4.11).

All wires and sheaths are removed from the right common femoral artery with the incision closed in a transverse fashion (Fig. 4.12). A 6 Fr angioseal vascular closure device (St. Jude Medical, St. Paul, MN) is deployed to the common femoral artery that was percutaneously accessed (Fig. 4.13). At the end of the procedure confirmation of the presence of bilateral peripheral pulses is performed, the patient is extubated prior to leaving the operating room, and is transferred to the recovery room. The blood pressure is kept elevated using a pressor agent if needed to keep the mean arterial pressure greater than 90 mmHg. A postoperative CT scan of the chest (Fig. 4.14) is

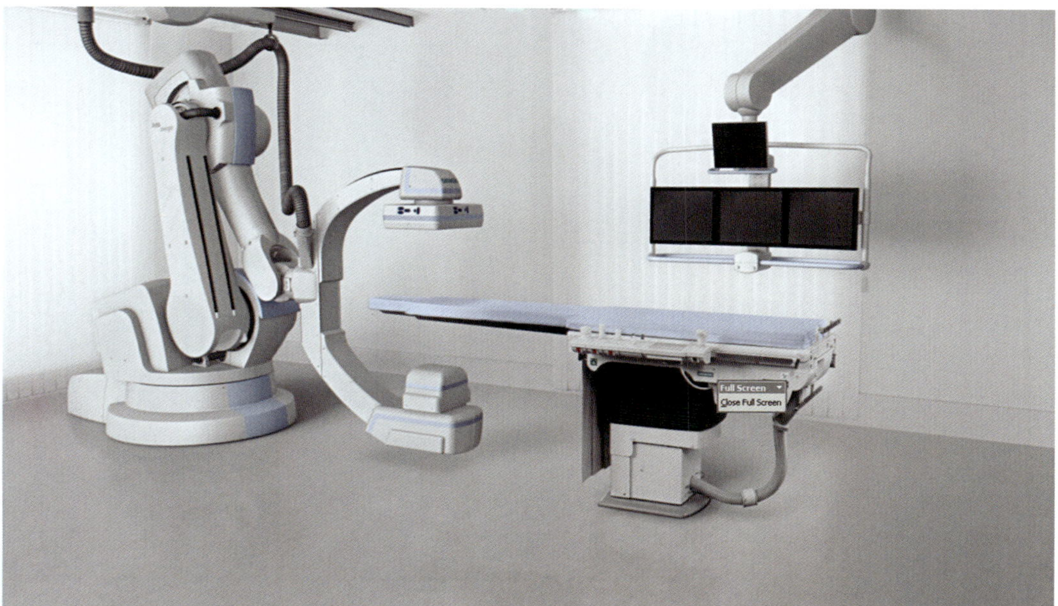

Fig. 4.2 A hybrid room with a fixed imaging system used for the endovascular management of thoracic aortic aneurysms.

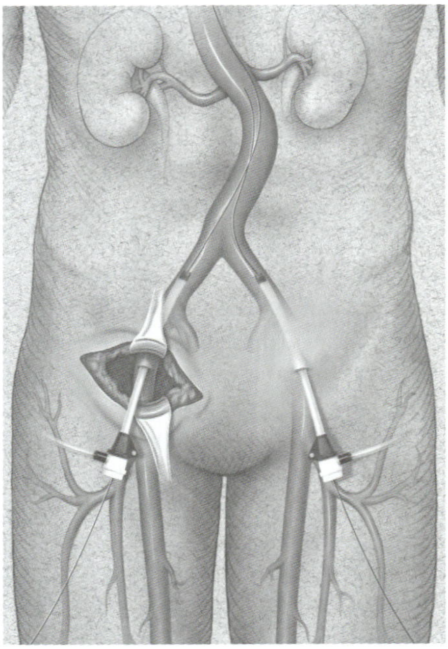

Fig. 4.3 Open retrograde cannulation of the right groin with an introducer sheath and a retrograde percutaneous access of the left common femoral artery using an 18 gauge needle.

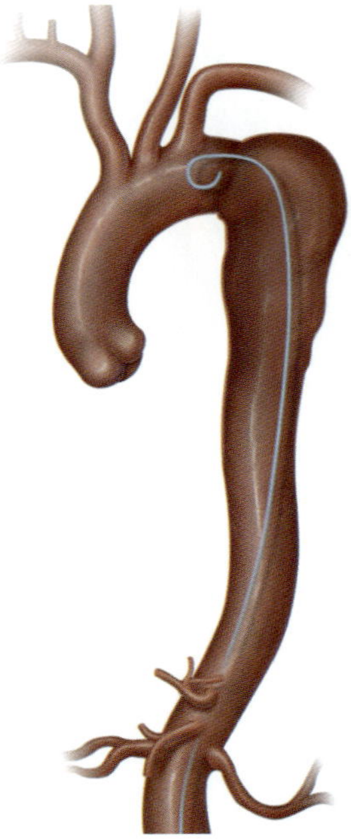

Fig. 4.5 Advancement of a pigtail angiographic catheter up the aortic arch for a thoracic aortogram.

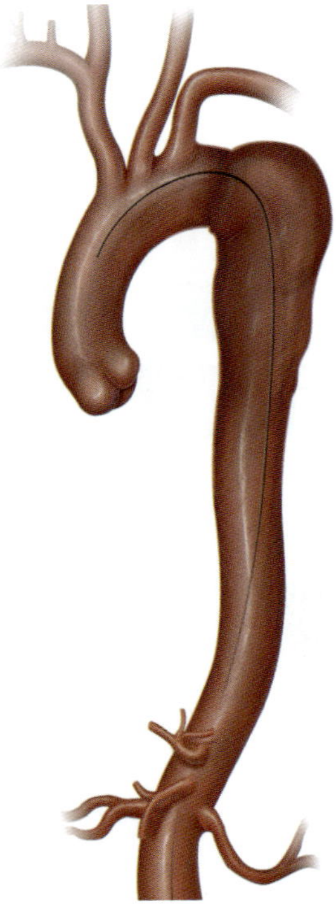

Fig. 4.4 Advancement of a glide wire up the aortic arch.

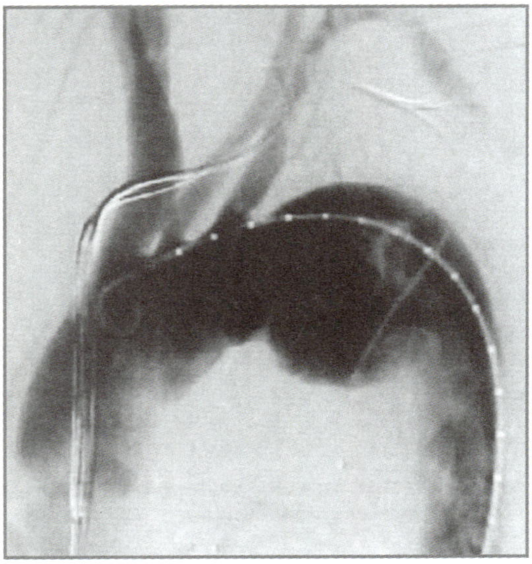

Fig. 4.6 Thoracic aortogram performed with an angiographic pigtail catheter.

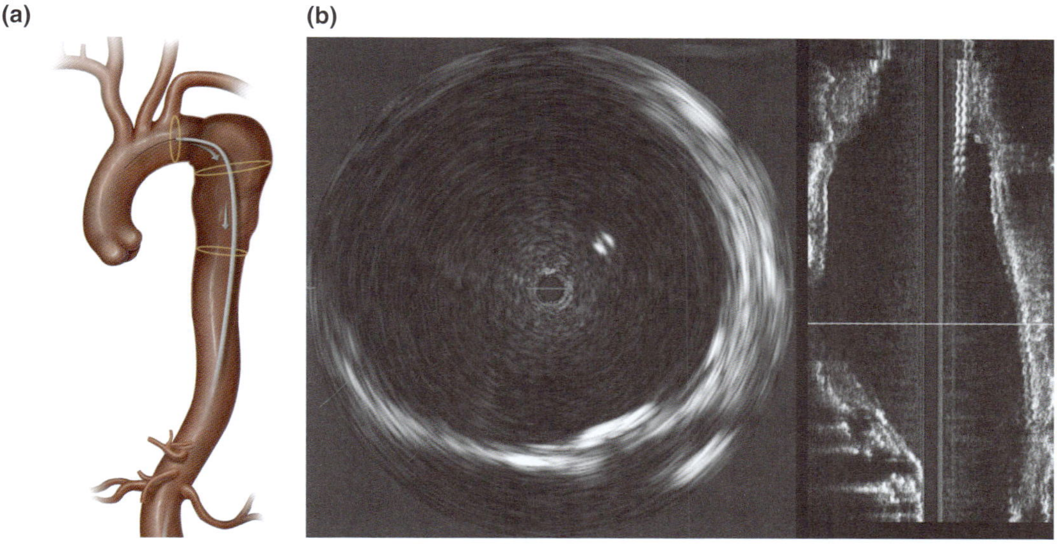

Fig. 4.7 (a) IVUS catheter advanced into the proximal thoracic aorta to determine the proximal and distal landing zone diameters, and diameter and length of the aneurysm. (b) IVUS image of a thoracic aneurysm.

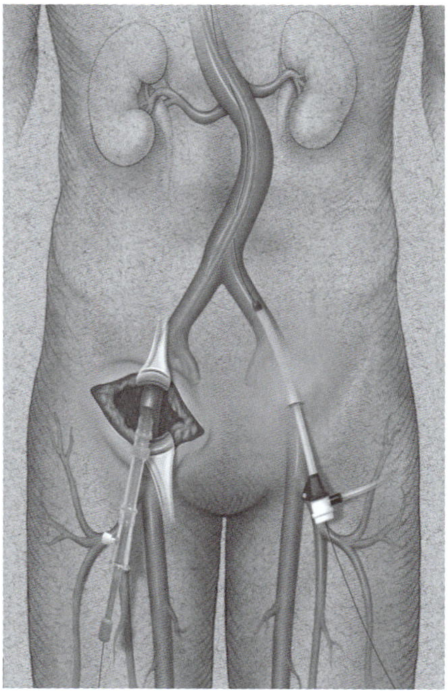

Fig. 4.8 Device sheath for an endograft advanced into the thoracic aorta.

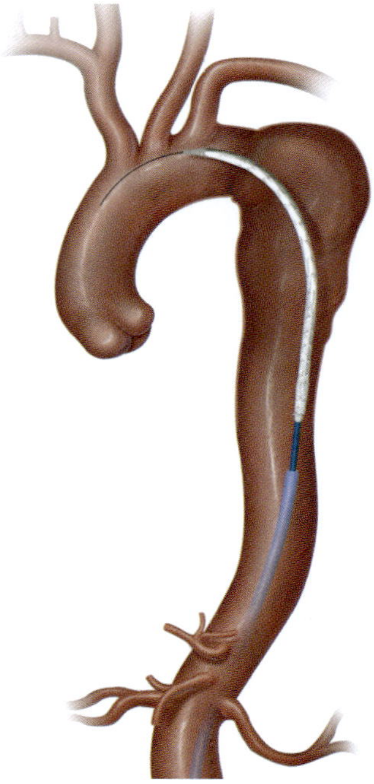

Fig. 4.9 Advancement of an endoluminal graft and its positioning for the exclusion of a thoracic aneurysm.

(a) (b)

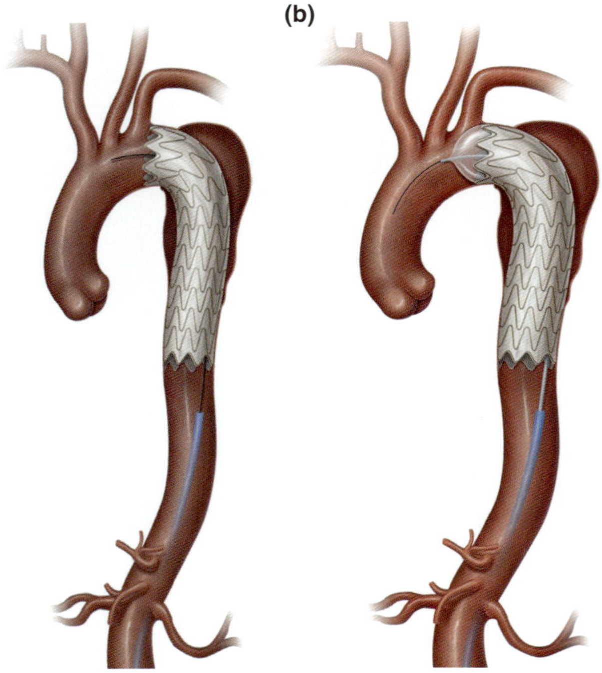

Fig. 4.10 (a) Deployment of an endoluminal graft to exclude a thoracic aneurysm. (b) Balloon angioplasty of the proximal end for adequate fixation to the aortic wall to prevent a type1 endoleak.

(a) (b)

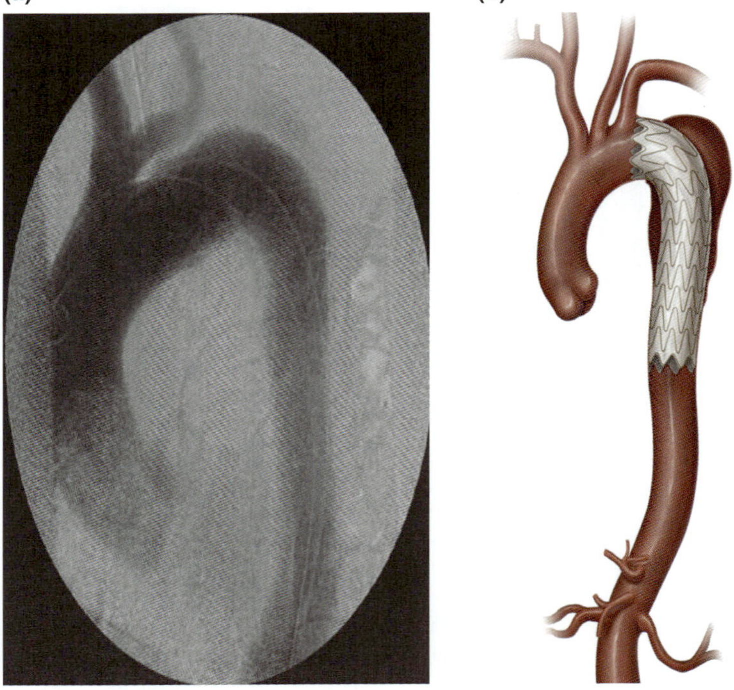

Fig. 4.11 (a) Completion angiogram and (b) illustration demonstrating an adequate position of an endograft with exclusion of an aneurysm.

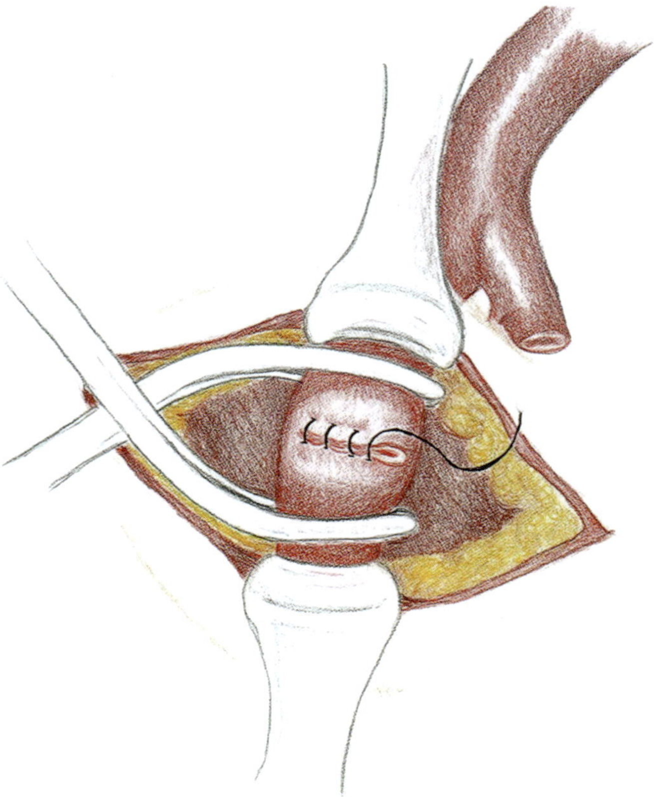

Fig. 4.12 Repair of a femoral arteriotomy used for device sheath introduction.

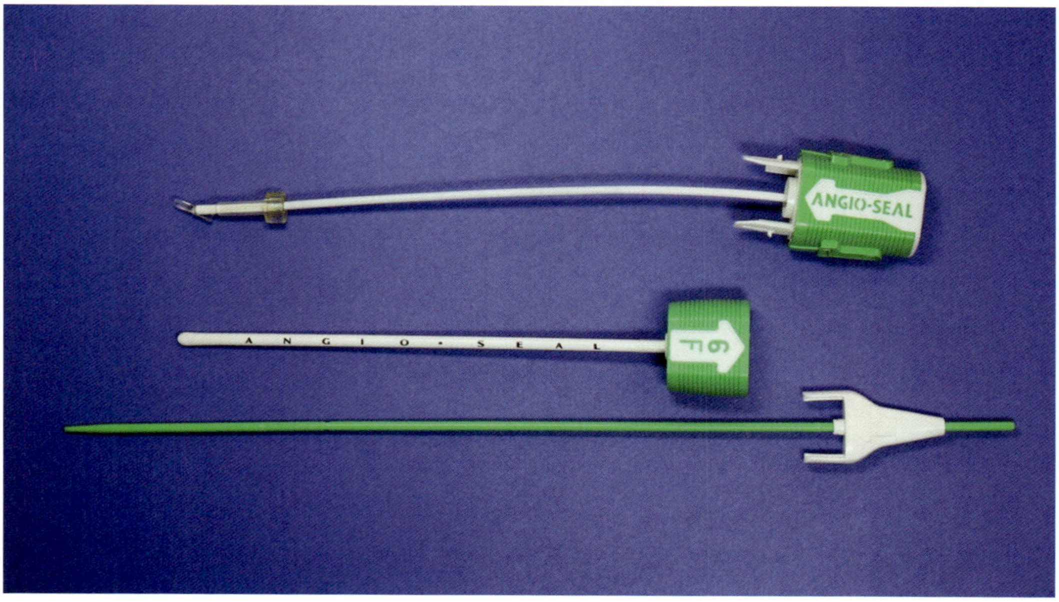

Fig. 4.13 Angioseal vascular devices used to achieve hemostasis of a percutaneous retrograde puncture.

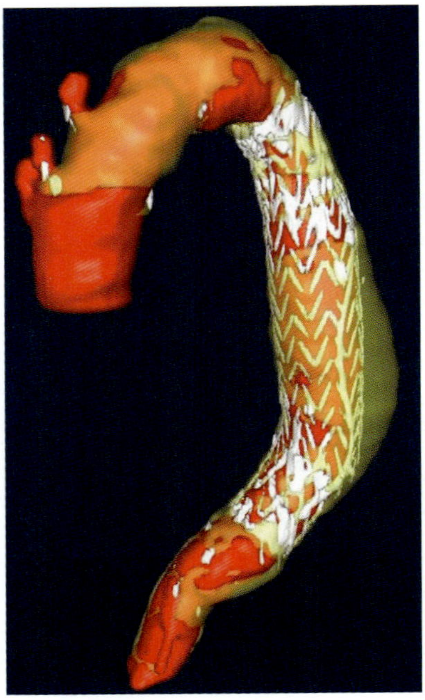

Fig. 4.14 Reconstructed 3D CT scan demonstrating the satisfactory exclusion of a thoracic aortic aneurysm with no endoleak.

performed prior to discharge to confirm exclusion of the thoracic aortic aneurysm and to identify any endoleaks that may have been missed on operative angiograms.

Appendix: preference card

EQUIPMENT:

- 18 GAUGE ACESS NEEDLE
- INDEFLATOR FOR THERAPEUTIC BALLOONING OF ILIAC ARTERIES
- 60CC SYRINGE FOR PROFILE BALLOONING OF AORTA AND GRAFT JUNCTIONS
- GUIDEWIRE .035 180CM ANGLED GLIDEWIRE / 260CM ANGLED FOR (THORACIC)
- GUIDEWIRE .035 260CM COOK LUNDERQUIST ({x2} ABDOMINAL) / LUNDERQUIST(LES3) FOR (THORACIC {x1})
- SHEATH 5FR, 6FR OR 9FR 11CM CORDIS BRITE-TIP FOR PERCUTANEOUS CONTRA
- SHEATH 12FR OR 14FR FOR POST ENDOLUMINAL GRAFT BALLOONING
- FLUSH CATHETER 5FR OR 6FR 100CM TR FLUSH / PIGTAIL / OR MARKER PIGTAIL
- BALLOON CORDIS OPTA-PRO 80CM OR ABBOTT FOX PTA 75CM (FOR LESIONSOF THE ILIAC VESSELS / TO ALLOW DELIVERY OF THE ELG)(SIZE TO BE DETERMINED BY PHYSICIAN)
- BALLOON CORDIS MAXI-LD 14,15,16,18, 20,22,25X4CM FOR GRAFT JUNCTION (SIZE TO BE DETERMINED BY PHYSICIAN)
- BALLOON COOK CODA 32MM OR 40MM (SIZE TO BE DETERMINED BY PHYSICIAN)
- ENDOLUMINAL GRAFT (SIZE TO BE DETERMINED BY PHYSICIAN)

PROCEDURE PEARLS:

- PATIENT PLACED SUPINE
- EKG LEADS AND EKG WIRES ARE POSITIONED SO THEY DO NOT APPEARON THE FLOUROSCOPIC IMAGES
- POSSIBLY PREP THE PATIENT ARM OUT FOR BRACHIAL FEMORAL WIRE (USEDFOR DIFFICULT ACCESS ANATOMY SUCH AS EXTREMELY TORTUOUS ILIACS)

1 OBLIQUE INCISION TO EXPOSE CFA (THORACIC / ENDOLOGIX {x1 SIDE CUT DOWN}) (ANEURX / EXCLUDER / ZENITH {x2 SIDE CUT DOWN})

2 PUNCTURE BOTH CFA WITH 18 GA. NEEDLE

3 PLACE .035 ANGLED GLIDEWIRE THROUGH NEEDLE LUMEN; UNDER FLOURO- SCOPIC GUIDANCE ADVANCE INTO DISTAL AORTA; **(PERCUTANEOUS)** MAKE A SMALL INCISION AT THE PUNCTURE SITE WITH A SCALPEL; LEAVE GUIDEWIRE IN PLACE AND REMOVE THE NEEDLE; WHILE LEAVING THE GUIDEWIRE IN PLACE; DILATE THE TRACT WITH A MOSQUITO HEMOSTAT

4 PLACE THE 5FR, 6FR OR 9FR(IVUS) 11CM BRITE-TIP SHEATH OVER THE GUIDEWIRE AND ADVANCE WELL INTO THE VESSEL; REMOVE THE OBTURATOR OF THE SHEATH LEAVING THE SHEATH AND GUIDEWIRE IN PLACE; FLUSH SHEATH WITH HEPARANIZED SALINE; HAVE ANESTHIOLOGIST / CRNA ADMINISTER 3000–5000 UNITS OF HEPARIN I.V.

– *IF SHEATH IS NOT ABLE TO BE ADVANCED; PLACE A CORDIS 4FR DILATOR OVER THE WIRE AND EXCHANGE THE WIRE FOR A STIFFER .035 GUIDEWIRE (E.G..035 75CM AMPLATZ); REMOVE THE DILATOR KEEPING THE WIRE IN PLACE; THEN PLACE SHEATH OVER THE STIFF GUIDEWIRE AND ADVANCE WELL INTO THE VESSEL; REPLACE THE STIFF GUIDEWIRE WITH THE ORIGINAL GLIDEWIRE*

5 UNDER FLOUROSCOPIC GUIDANCE ADVANCE THE GLIDEWIRE INTO THORACIC AORTA

6 PLACE 5FR OR 6FR FLUSH CATHETER OVER THE GUIDEWIRE AND ADVANCE INTO THE PROXIMAL ABDOMINAL AORTA AT THE LEVEL OF (L1-L2 VERTEBRAL SPACE FOR RENAL ARTERY VISUALIZATION (ABD): ADVANCE INTO ASCENDING THORACIC AORTA TO VISUALIZE THE GREAT VESSELS (THORACIC))

7 POSITION IMAGE INTENSIFIER FOR IMAGING (ABD) AP WITH A 10–15 DEGREE CRANIAL ANGULATION (THORACIC) 40–60 DEGREE LAO ANGUULATION

8 SHOOT AN AORTAGRAM TO DETERMINE IF YOU HAVE ADEQUATE LENGTH LANDING ZONE **(ROADMAP FOR IVUS MEASUREMENTS)**

9 PLACE THE LUNDERQUIST GUIDEWIRE INTO FLUSH CATHETER AND REMOVE FLUSH CATHETER LEAVING THE LUNDERQUIST IN PLACE

10 PLACE 8.2FR PV IVUS PROBE OVER THE WIRE AND PERFORM IVUS EXAMINATION (TAKE DIAMETER MEASUREMENTS/ EVALUATE PLAQUE AND THROMBUS BURDENS / PERFORM LONGITUDINAL PULL THROUGH / TAKE LENGTH MEASUREMENT)

11 REMOVE IVUS PROBE LEAVING THE LUNDERQUIST WIRE IN PLACE

12 SHOOT A RETROGRADE ANGIOGRAM THROUGH THE SHEATH TO EVALUATE THE ACCESS VESSELS (IF NEEDED PERFORM ANGIOPLASTY)

13 THROUGH CONTRALATERAL SHEATH PLACE FLUSH CATHETER IN POSITION TO PERFORM AORTAGRAM PRIOR TO ELG DEPLOYMENT

14 CHOOSE THE APPROPRIATE SIZED ELG

15 INTRODUCE ELG DELIVERY SHEATH OR ELG DELIVERY DEVICE INTO THE CFA OVER THE LUNDERQUIST WIRE (FOLLOW THE SHEATH/DELIVERY SYSTEM AS IT PASSES THROUGH THE AORTA AND ILIAC VESSELS

16 ROTATE THE C-ARM TO APPROPRIATE ANGLE FOR AORTAGRAM (SEE #7)

17 SHOOT AORTAGRAM (ROADMAP) TO DEPLOY THE ELG

18 PLACE A NEEDLE AT THE PROXIMAL LANDING ZONE

19 DEPLOY THE ELG (SMALL PUFFS OF CONTRAST THROUGH THE FLUSH CATHETER AID IN ACCURATE DEPLOYMENT)

20 FOLLOW THE IFU FOR EACH SPECIFIC DEVICE DEPLOYMENT STEPS

21 AFTER ELG IS DEPLOYED REMOVED THE FLUSH CATHETER FROM BEHIND THE ELG BY PLACING THE ANGLED GLIDEWIRE THROUGH THE CATHETER

22 IF THE ELG IS A BIFURCATED ABDOMINAL ELG; CANNULATE THE CONTRA-LATERAL GATE; SELECT THE APPROPRIATE LIMB AND DEPLOY ACCORDING TO THE DEVICE SPECIFIC IFU

23 PROFILE BALLOON THE LANDING ZONES AND OVERLAPPING AREAS WITH MAXI-LD BALLOON(S) OR CODA BALLOON

24 REINTRODUCE THE FLUSH CATHETER AND CHECK FOR ENDOLEAKS

25 PERFORM RETROGRADE ANGIOGRAM THROUGH THE SHEATHS TO CHECK FOR DISTAL SEAL OF THE ELG

26 DEPLOYMENT OF CLOSURE DEVICE IN ACESS VESSELS WITH SHEATHS LESS THAN 12FR. REPAIR OF ACCESS VESSELS WITH SHEATH SIZE LARGER THAN 12 FR

Reference

1 Diethrich EB, Ramaiah VG, Kpodonu J, et al. Endovascular and Hybrid Management of the Thoracic Aorta. A case-based approach, 1st edn. Oxford: Wiley-Blackwell. 2008.

5

CHAPTER 5

Axillary/subclavian access for endovascular management of ascending and descending aortic pathologies

Eduardo Keller Saadi

Federal University of Rio Grande do Sul, Hospital de Clinicas de Porto Alegre; Center for Aortic Diseases, Hospital Mae de Deus, Porto Alegre, Brazil

Introduction

Endovascular approaches are being increasingly utilized to treat a variety of thoracic aortic diseases (TADs), including aneurysms, pseudoaneurysms, dissections, penetrating aortic ulcers, traumatic aortic rupture, and coarctation. The treatment of descending aorta pathologies is well established but it is also possible to treat the arch and, more recently, the ascending aorta as the last frontier. Adequate vascular access is crucial to obtain good results. Thoracic endovascular aortic repair (TEVAR) is usually done through the femoral arteries. Transfemoral access can be achieved by direct surgical cut-down and surgical suture closure of the artery, percutaneous puncture with surgical suture closure, or percutaneous puncture with percutaneous closure of the femoral artery. Although there has been a dramatic improvement in device profiles and navigability with external hydrophilic coating in commercially available devices, the diameter of devices remains sizeable.

Sometimes access is impossible or not recommended because of the small size of the vessels, obstruction, calcification, dissection, or extreme tortuosity. Vascular access complications such as dissection, iliac rupture, and thrombosis are still frequent. Achieving safe and successful endovascular access for introduction and deployment of the stent-graft device is an important and often challenging step during TEVAR. Currently available thoracic endografts still have a large profile. In 10–30% of the patients suitable for TEVAR, inadequate femoral artery access anatomy will be found. Alternative access sites are important. The axillary/subclavian artery approach is a viable alternative in cases where the femoral arteries are not appropriate.

Vascular access evaluation

Complete anatomic evaluation of the thoracic aortic pathology and the access vessels are key to success. Preoperative meticulous planning is fundamental. Physical examination with pulse palpation and echo Doppler can be used as an initial screening. Currently, helical computed tomographic angiography (CTA) is the most useful imaging modality for detailed assessment of access arterial anatomy, overtaking axial computed tomography (CT) and digital subtraction angiography

Endovascular and Hybrid Therapies for Structural Heart and Aortic Disease, First Edition.
Edited by Jacques Kpodonu and Raoul Bonan.

(DSA) (Fig. 5.1). CTA demonstrates with sharp precision the course and appearance of all vessels of interest and provides the necessary tools for sizing and measurements of the devices and helps to determine the most appropriate access site (Fig. 5.2).

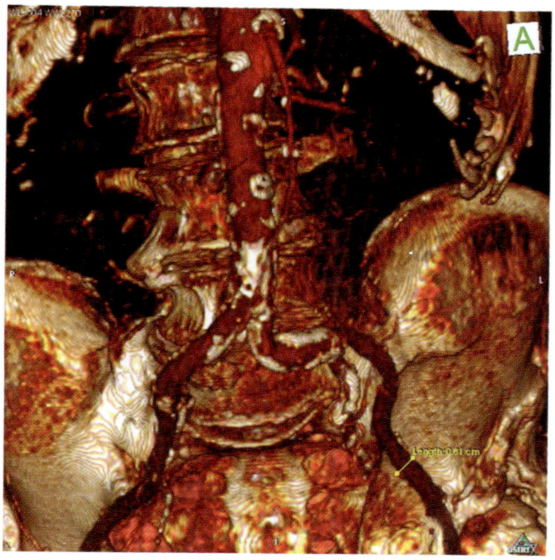

Fig. 5.1 CT with 3D reconstruction of the abdominal aorta and iliac and femoral arteries to evaluate groin access. Note the calcification in the distal aorta and left iliac artery but without obstruction, stenosis, or extreme tortuosity, with good size vessels (>8 mm).

Technique

Under general or local anesthesia the axillary artery is exposed through an incision in the delto-pectoral groove. The pectoralis major muscle is divided in the direction of its fibers and the insertion of the pectoralis minor divided. The axillary artery is easily seen superior to the axillary vein and dissected. The arterial wall is thin and usually free from atherosclerosis (Fig. 5.3). Care should be taken to avoid any injury to the brachial plexus. Following the administration of heparin (1 mg/kg) a side biting clamp is applied and an anastomosis constructed with an 8 or 10 mm Dacron tube with a running suture of 6-0 prolene (Fig. 5.4). The tube is brought from the same incision or, in cases when the artery is too deep, through a new small stab incision and left long and parallel to the artery (Fig. 5.5). The tube is left at least 25 cm long, away from the artery. A 7 Fr sheath is snared to the extremity of the Dacron tube to avoid bleeding and facilitate the manipulation of wires and catheters, and the insertion of the device (Fig. 5.6; Video 5.1).

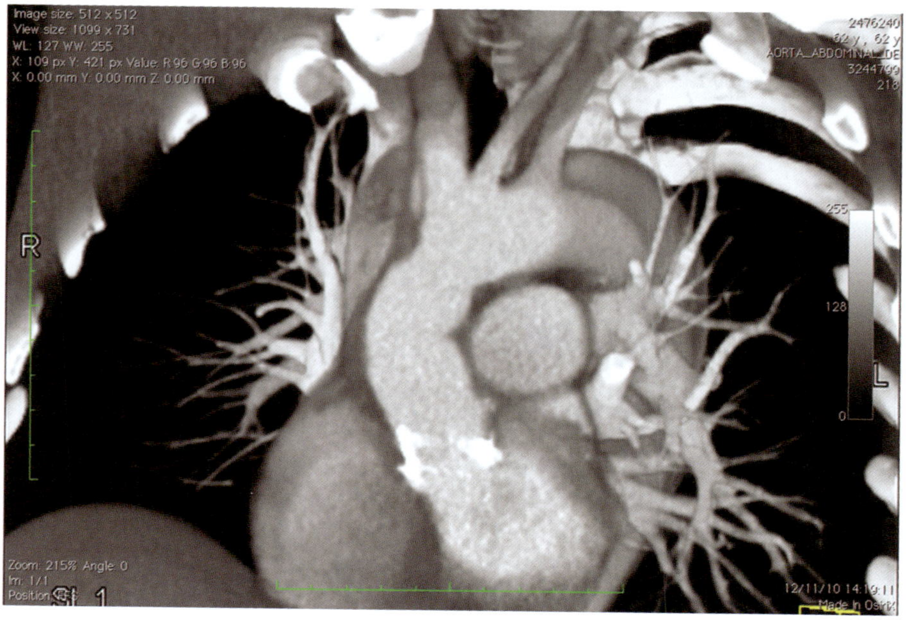

Fig. 5.2 CT with 3D reconstruction of the aortic arch showing a type B dissection involving the left subclavian artery and a bovine arch with a good angulation to access the descending aorta. In this patient the right axillary artery would be the preferred access.

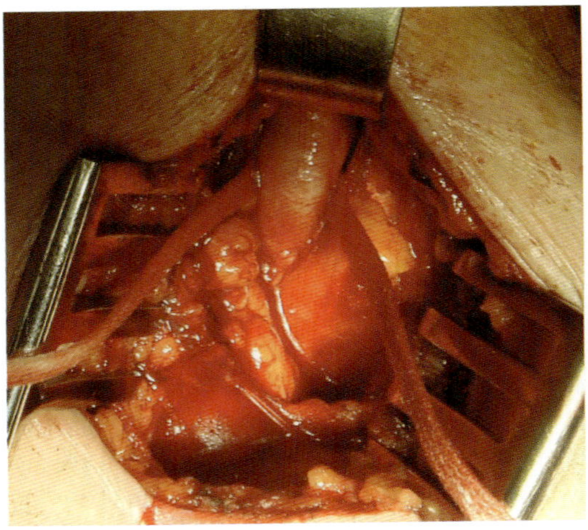

Fig. 5.3 Right axillary artery exposed and repaired with tapes.

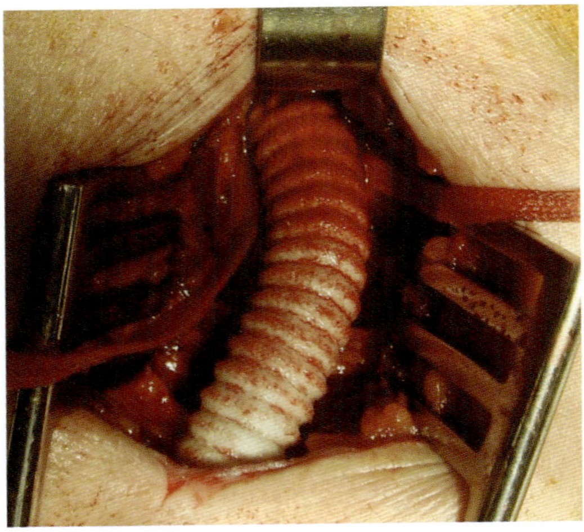

Fig. 5.4 An 8 mm Dacron tube anastomosed to the right axillary artery with 6-0 prolene.

The endoprosthesis is introduced by the distal end with or without the sheath, depending on the device selected, through the Dacron graft and on an extra stiff Landerquist 260 cm long guide wire (Cook Medical, Bloomington, IN) (Fig. 5.7; Video 5.2). If there is not another access the Dacron tube can be punctured more proximally and another 5 or 6 Fr sheath inserted (Figs 5.8 and 5.9). Catheters and the rigid guide wire, as well as the endoprosthesis, can be inserted after enlarging the hole with an 11 blade, while keeping the distal end of the graft for angiographic control (Fig. 5.10). An aortography is done with a pigtail introduced

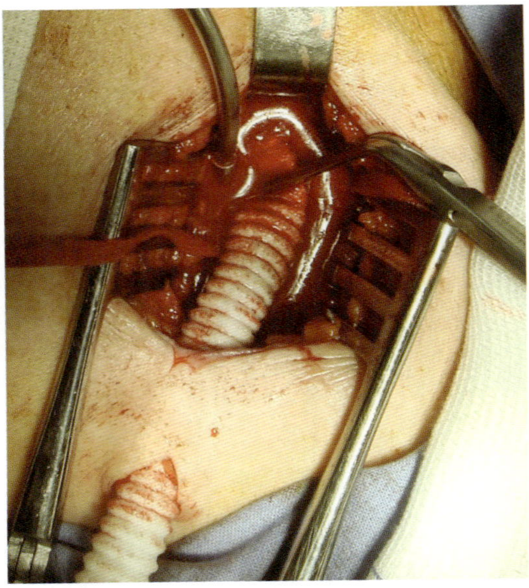

Fig. 5.5 Alternatively, a stab incision in the skin is used to exteriorize the Dacron tube parallel to the axillary artery.

from the same graft, the contralateral arm, or from the groin for diagnostic landmarks and before opening the device (Video 5.3). The endoprosthesis is then deployed (Video 5.4). Balloon accommodation is performed in the usual fashion through the axillary access (Video 5.5). Final aortography is performed to check there are no endoleaks. The wires are removed and the Dacron tube ligated with two large clips 1 cm away from the axillary artery and reinforced with a running suture of 5-0 prolene. The incision is closed in layers and no drains left. At least one CT scan is done in the early postoperative period to confirm the correct position of the endograft and the absence of endoleaks (Fig. 5.11). Follow-up is maintained for the patient's lifetime.

Discussion

The feasibility of endovascular surgery depends on many anatomic factors, including the diameter and the disease state of the access vessels [1–4]. Stenosis, calcifications, tortuosity, small sizes, or dissection of both femoral and iliac arteries can make the introduction of a large sheath hazardous or impossible. Aorto-iliac artery stenosis and obstruction is not uncommon in elderly patients. Women and small patients often have femoral arteries that are not

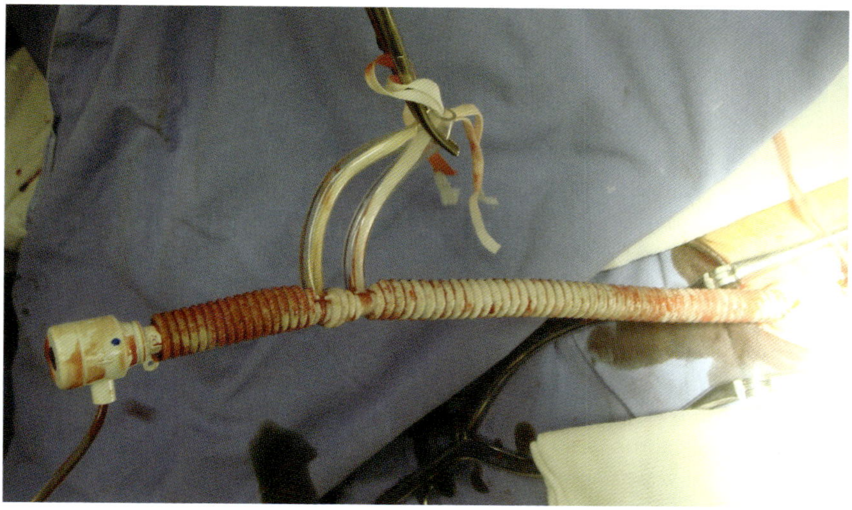

Fig. 5.6 Introducer snared to the distal end of the tube to avoid bleeding and allow manipulation of wires and catheters.

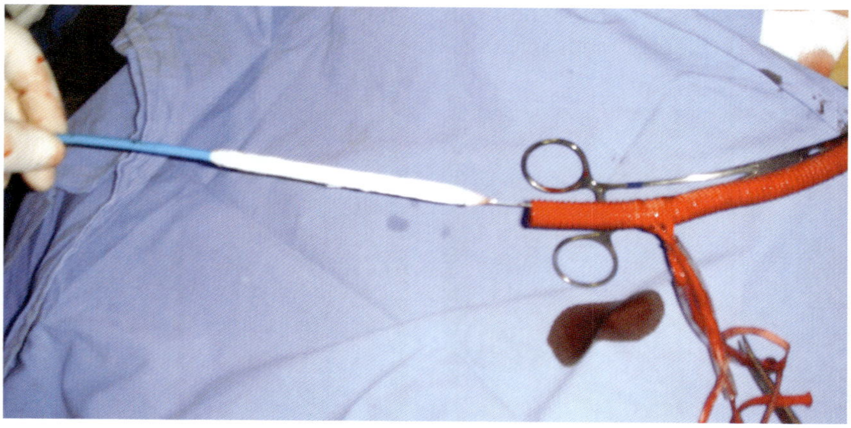

Fig. 5.7 Introducing the endoprosthesis through the distal end of the tube without the sheath.

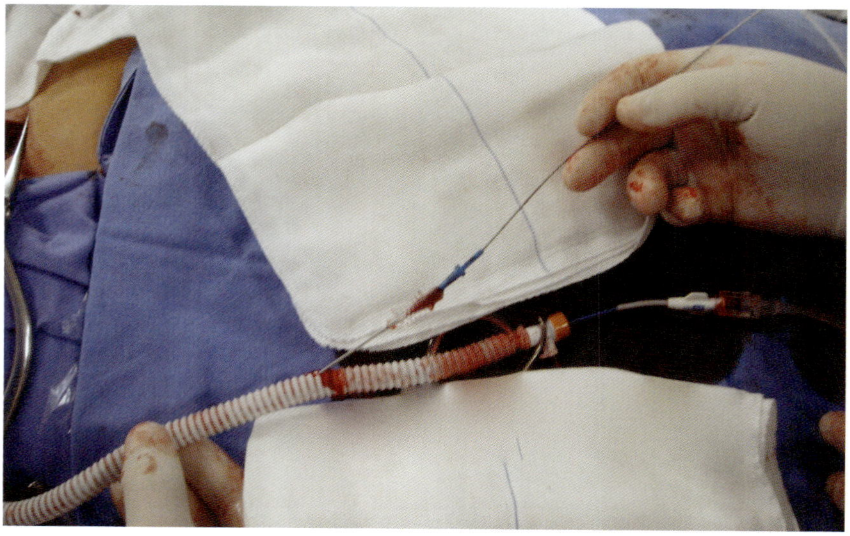

Fig. 5.8 Puncture in the Dacron graft in cases where there is no other access vessel.

compatible in size with large diameter sheaths and introducers needed to deploy thoracic endoprosthesis. A conduit anastomosed to the iliac artery is an option when the femoral arteries are not adequate [5]. Direct extraperitoneal access to the abdominal aorta with or without a conduit is also possible but is a big operation. An alternative to groin access is the axillary artery. The exposure of the axillary artery through a small infraclavicular incision is familiar to cardiovascular surgeons as arterial return in cardiopulmonary bypass in aortic arch surgery [6]. They are often good-sized vessels and usually free from atherosclerosis, even in patients with extensive aorto-iliac occlusive disease.

Both axillary arteries can be used. The decision of the side to use is made based on anatomic details and its angle detected in the preoperative multislice CT scan with 3D reconstruction. If both arteries are of good size and the angle in relation to the aortic arch is favorable, preference is given for the left subclavian artery. We believe there is less chance of debris embolization to the carotid artery when we avoid the brachiocephalic trunk. If the left subclavian artery is involved by dissection or aneurysm we use the right. Careful evaluation should be taken in patients with prior myocardial revascularization with the left internal mammary artery (LIMA), where the risk of left subclavian artery dissection or temporary occlusion of LIMA

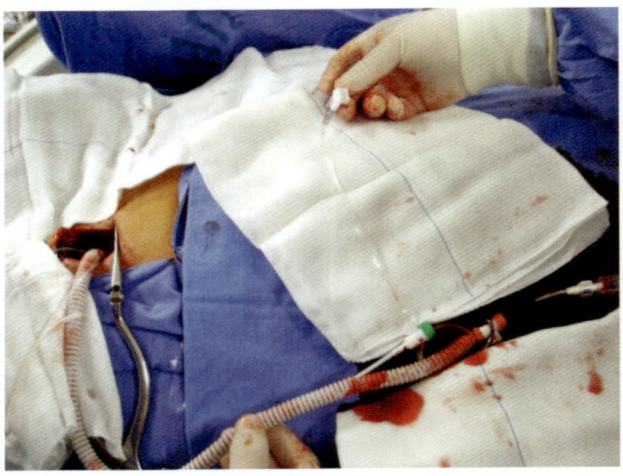

Fig. 5.9 Another introducer in place proximally in the tube while maintaining the distal end for angiographic control.

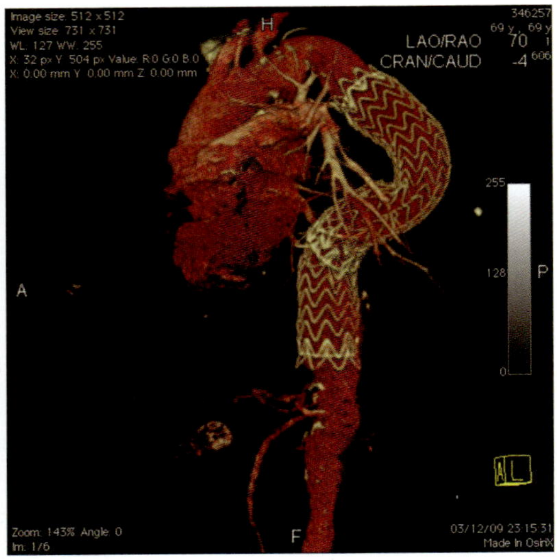

Fig. 5.11 Postoperative CT showing two grafts implanted in the descending aorta through the left axillary artery.

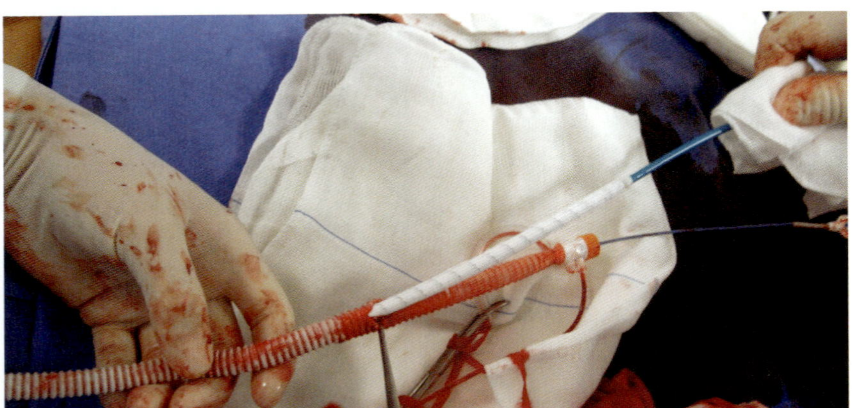

Fig. 5.10 Endoprosthesis introduced directly through the Dacron tube after enlarging the hole with an 11 blade and keeping the distal end to control deployment.

could be a relevant problem. In these cases the right axillary artery should be chosen if possible.

The infraclavicular incision to expose the axillary artery is very well tolerated with minimal pain or discomfort. The use of a side graft has been shown to reduce morbidity associated with axillary cannulation [6]. Direct cannulation is possible but can cause damage to the artery that sometimes is difficult to repair. The stab incision provides a smooth angle of entry when the artery is too deep and facilitates the introduction of large devices [5]. There are just a few case reports in the literature using the axillary artery to deploy endografts in the aorta [7]. If there is no other alternative the artery can be ligated without major consequences to the arm perfusion [8].

Major vascular injury remains a frequent complication of endovascular procedures in the aorta. We recently published a series of 255 patients submitted to endovascular treatment of thoracic aortic disease through the femoral artery with three (1%) experiencing major vascular access complications [9].

In an initial small series of five patients in which the axillary artery was used, technical success was achieved in all cases and there were no complications related to access or neurologic problems [10]. In four cases we used a Gore TAG (W.L. Gore & Associates, Flagstaff, AZ) thoracic endoprosthesis. In these patients we introduced the graft without a sheath through the Dacron tube and delivered it in an antegrade approach to the descending aorta. The advantage of the graft (Gore TAG) for antegrade insertion is that due to its design and configuration the same radial force is applied irrespective of the deployment site, which differentiates it from other stent-grafts commercially available. This is a promising approach to treat acute complicated type B aortic dissection because the subclavian and axillary arteries are rarely compromised by dissection and the antegrade deployment of the device facilitates its introduction in the true lumen without crossing several re-entry sites in the abdominal or descending thoracic aorta. When the true lumen is very compressed by the false lumen, axillary access is also easier and safer. Retrograde type A dissection after endovascular repair of type B dissection is a concern and has been reported [11].

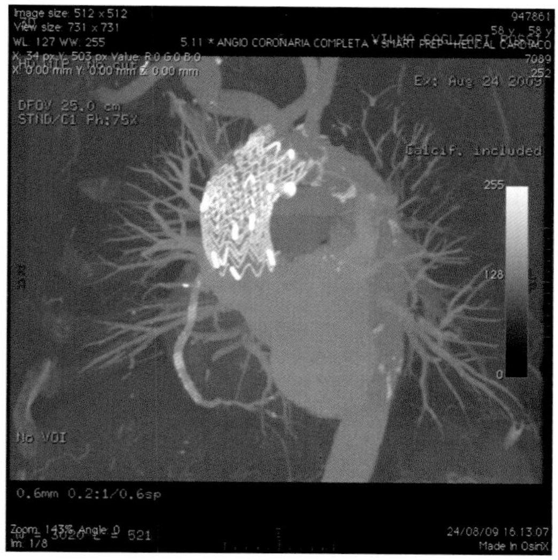

Fig. 5.12 Postoperative CT scan showing two abdominal extension cuffs deployed by the right axillary artery in the ascending aorta and percutaneous right coronary intervention in a patient with previous pseudoaneurysm.

Bird-beak configuration of the prosthesis in the aortic arch is a cause of type I endoleak and can compromise the results [12]. This problem has been addressed by industry recently.

In one of our cases of pseudoaneurysm of the ascending aorta we used two abdominal extension cuffs (aortic extender) through the right axillary artery (Fig. 5.12). This patient also had a right coronary artery stent implantation at the same time. The length of the delivery system, designed for the abdominal aorta, would not allow reaching the ascending aorta through the groin thereby making the axillary approach ideal for delivery of the graft. Currently available aortic endografts have limitations when used for ascending aorta and aortic arch pathologies. Endografts developed for the descending thoracic aorta are too long to be deployed between the coronary arteries and the brachiocephalic trunk and the delivery system, which is about 100 cm long, is usually too short to navigate to the ascending aorta from groin access. Also, the sharp nose cone of the majority of the endoprosthesis precludes its use in the ascending aorta because of the high risk of aortic valve damage and even left ventricular perforation. For that reason the Gore TAG device has an advantage since the nose is very short.

A complete understanding of the issues related to the vascular access and available technical solutions and materials should help to expand the indications as well as to prevent complications. We believe the technique in which the axillary artery is used to deliver the endograft is an important alternative for treatment of different thoracic aortic pathologies.

References

1 Melissano G, Bertoglio L, Civilini E, et al. Results of thoracic endovascular grafting in different aortic segments. J Endovasc Ther 2007; 14:150–7.

2 American College of Cardiology Foundation/American Heart Association Task Force on Practice Guidelines, American Association for Thoracic Surgery, American College of Radiology, American Stroke Association, Society of Cardiovascular Anesthesiologists, Society for Cardiovascular Angiography and Interventions, Society of Interventional Radiology, Society of Thoracic Surgeons, and Society for Vascular Medicine. Guidelines for the Diagnosis and Management of Patients with Thoracic Aortic Disease. Circulation 2010; 121:e266-e369.

3 Nienaber CA, Rousseau H, Eggebrecht H, et al. for the INSTEAD Trial. Randomized comparison of strategies for Type B aortic dissection. Circulation 2009; 120:2519–28.

4 Alric P, Canaud L, Branchereau P. et al. Preoperative assessment of anatomical suitability for thoracic endovascular aortic repair. Acta Chir Belg 2009; 109(4):458–64.

5 Criado FJ. Iliac arterial donduits for endovascular access: technical considerations. J Endovasc Ther 2007; 14: 347–51.

6 Sabik JF, Nemeh H, Lytle BW. et al. Cannulation of the axillary artery with a side graft reduces morbidity. Ann Thorac Surg 2004; 77:1315–20.

7 Probst C, Esmailzadeh B, Schiller W. et al. Emergent antegrade endovascular stent placement in a patient with perforated Stanford B dissection via right axillary artery. Eur J Cardiothorac Surg 2008; 33:1148–9.

8 Moore KL, Agur AMR. Essential clinical anatomy, 3rd edn. Philadelphia: Lippincott Williams & Wilkins, 2007, p. 428.

9 Almeida RM, Leal JC, Saadi EK. et al. Thoracic endovascular aortic repair – a Brazilian experience in 255 patients over a period of 112 months. Interact CardioVasc Thorac Surg 2009; 8:524–8.

10 Saadi EK, Dussin LH, Moura L. et al. The axillary artery – a new approach for endovascular treatment of thoracic aortic diseases. ICTVS 2010; 11:617–19.

11 Kpodonu J, Preventza O, Ramaiah VG, et al. Retrograde type A dissection after endovascular stenting of the descending thoracic aorta. Is the risk real? Eur J CardiothoracSurg 2008; 33(6):1014–18.

12 Ueda T, Fleischmann D. et al. Sze DY. Incomplete endograft apposition to the aortic arch: bird-beak configuration increases risk of endoleak formation after thoracic endovascular aortic repair. Radiology 2010; 255(2):645–52.

Videoclips

This chapter contains the following videoclips:

Video 5.1 Construction of an 8 mm Dacron conduit on the right axillary artery.

Video 5.2 Advancement of a thoracic aortic device through the axillary conduit.

Video 5.3 Positioning of a thoracic aortic device with contrast aortography.

Video 5.4 Deployment of a thoracic aortic device under fluoroscopic guidance.

Video 5.5 Balloon angioplasty of a thoracic aortic device.

They can be accessed at www.wiley.com/go/valverepair.

6

CHAPTER 6

Endovascular repair of thoraco-abdominal aortic aneurysms

Timothy A. M. Chuter
Division of Vascular Surgery, University of California San Francisco, San Francisco, CA, USA

Endovascular alternatives for thoraco-abdominal aortic aneurysm repair

The goal of endovascular aneurysm repair is to exclude the walls of the aneurysm from arterial flow and pressure. This goal becomes more elusive when the aneurysm has indispensable branches, in which case one has to provide an alternative source of inflow to the affected branches, either through bypass from a remote artery, or through branches of the stent-graft. The relative merits of these two approaches, hybrid surgical endovascular repair and branched endovascular repair, vary according to the aortic segment in question. The visceral branches of the thoraco-abdominal aorta lie in an inaccessible location where bypass entails a large operation with high complication rates. Multibranched repair is therefore the preferred option for thoraco-abdominal aortic aneurysm (TAAA) whenever the patient has suitable endovascular anatomy and the necessary equipment is available.

Principles of stent-graft design

All branched stent-grafts take one of two forms, unibody or modular, depending on the method of branch construction. Unibody stent-grafts are implanted whole and manipulated into position using a system of catheters. Modular stent-grafts are assembled in situ from multiple components.

The first branched stent-grafts were of the unibody design [1]. Even the simplest stent-grafts of this type (bifurcated), having only one branch, are more complicated to use than the multicomponent modular equivalents, but not prohibitively so, and they still have a role in the management of abdominal aortic aneurysm (AAA). However, every additional branch of a unibody stent-graft adds another level of complexity and another dimension to the matrix of potential failure modes. Unibody stent-grafts, having enough branches for use in the thoraco-abdominal aorta, will probably never achieve widespread use due to the irreducible complexity of stent-graft manufacture and implantation [2].

Modular stent-grafts are, by comparison, relatively easy to make and insert. They are also versatile. One can mix modular stent-graft components in an almost infinite variety of ways to match the needs of the patient's anatomy at the time of operation. In addition, modular design imparts an element of predictability to the performance of new devices because any component, or deployment technique, that works well in one part of the arterial tree will usually work well in another.

Endovascular and Hybrid Therapies for Structural Heart and Aortic Disease, First Edition.
Edited by Jacques Kpodonu and Raoul Bonan.

In essence, modular multibranched stent-grafts for arch aortic, thoraco-abdominal aortic and common iliac repair are variations on the same theme.

Like all members of the Zenith family (Cook Medical, Bloomington, IN), the typical modular multibranched stent-graft is made of woven polyester and z-stents. This central trunk is coupled with branches, consisting of various types of covered stents. The interface between components may be just a hole (fenestration) in the wall of the stent-graft [3], or a short branch (cuff) extending upwards, downwards, outwards, or in a helical configuration from the wall of the stent-graft [4]. As a rule, fenestrations are combined with balloon-expanded covered stents, whereas cuffs are combined with self-expanding covered stents. Each approach has its advantages, indications, and advocates [5–11]. At University of California San Francisco (UCSF), we prefer cuffed stent-grafts because we find them easier to plan, easier to insert, and more durable than fenestrated stent-grafts [12,13].

Basic insertion technique

Regardless of whether the primary stent-graft is fenestrated or cuffed, the basic approach to modular stent-graft assembly is the same. A catheter is directed from the lumen of the deployed stent-graft through a fenestration or cuff into the perigraft space, and through the perigraft space into the target artery. This bridging catheter is then exchanged for a bridging covered stent. In most cases the branches of a fenestrated stent-graft radiate straight out at right angles to the long axis of the aorta, whereas the branches of a cuffed stent-graft start in the same axial orientation as the cuffs and curve outwards as they traverse the perigraft space.

At UCSF, most of our multibranched stent-grafts have caudally oriented cuffs (Fig. 6.1), which open proximally to the lumen of the stent-graft and distally to the perigraft space. These cuffs are accessible only from above through a transbrachial access site. The details of multibranched stent-graft insertion vary, but the basic steps are always the same.

Overlapping aortic stent-grafts are inserted through surgically exposed femoral arteries, starting with the most proximal. The cuff-bearing thoraco-abdominal stent-graft is positioned relative to a selective catheter within one of the visceral arteries. We try to avoid aortic flush injections to minimize contrast load. Once all the aortic stent-grafts are in place, the primary access site is repaired and flow through the femoral artery restored. The contralateral femoral access is maintained as the exit site of a brachio-femoral wire. Constant tension in this wire stabilizes the position of a 10 or 12 Fr left brachial sheath (Fig. 6.2). The brachio-femoral wire occupies the center of the valve on the brachial sheath. A catheter (100 cm vertebral) is introduced through a puncture site in the periphery of this valve, directed through one of

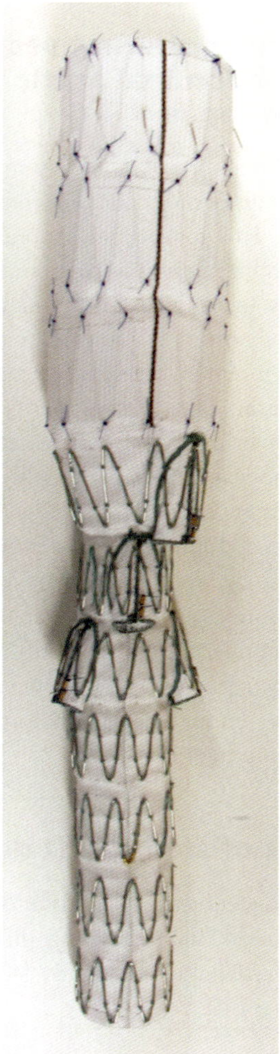

Fig. 6.1 Standard cuffed thoraco-abdominal aortic stent-graft.

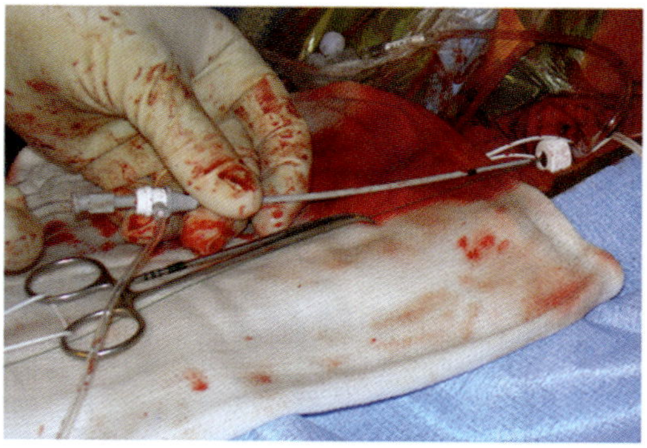

Fig. 6.2 Tensioned 14 inch coronary wire and a 5 Fr sheath both exiting the valve of a left brachial sheath.

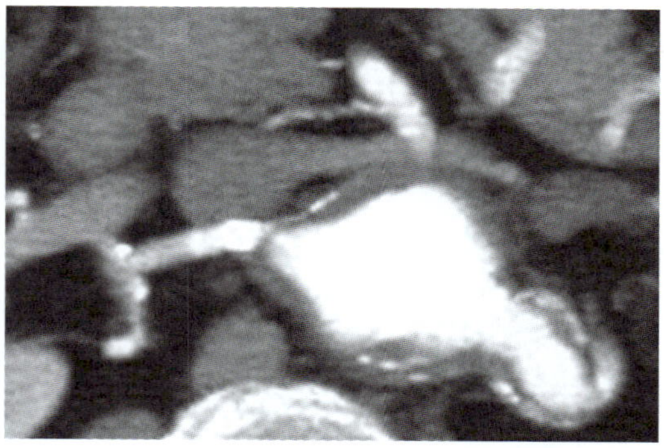

Fig. 6.3 Preoperative CT showing renal aneurysm, angulation, and stenosis.

the cuffs, across the perigraft space and into the corresponding branch artery, and exchanged over a stiff (0.035 inch Rosen) guide wire for the covered stent delivery system. The deployment of four covered stents, each with a lining of uncovered stent (usually a Wallstent) completes the procedure.

Patient selection

The current inclusion criteria at UCSF are: an aortic aneurysm wider than 60 mm in men and 55 mm in women, a life expectancy longer than 2 years, estimated mortality rate for conventional repair of over 20%, and suitable arterial anatomy. Our definition of suitable anatomy has evolved over the past 5 years. We have learned how to overcome a wide variety of anatomic obstacles, including: stenosis of the renal, superior mesenteric, celiac and iliac arteries; aneurysm of the renal and iliac arteries (Fig. 6.3); tortuosity of the iliac arteries (Fig. 6.4), the renal arteries and the aorta (Fig. 6.5); duplication of the renal arteries; dissection of the thoraco-abdominal aorta (Fig. 6.6); and aneurysm of the aortic arch (Fig. 6.7). In most cases, we chose to stage the repair by performing necessary corrective interventions two or more weeks before stent-graft implantation.

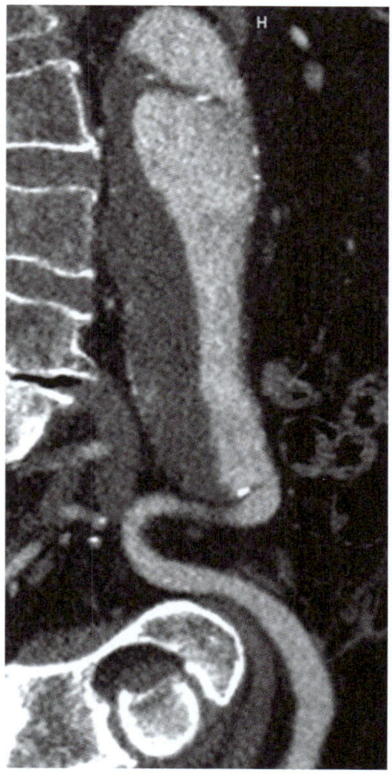

Fig. 6.4 Preoperative CT showing a common iliac aneurysm above a very tortuous external iliac artery. The other side was just the same.

Few patients are excluded solely on anatomic grounds. However, there are some anatomic obstacles we cannot overcome. For example, we cannot create a route of access around a densely calcified stenotic aortic bifurcation when the rest of the infrarenal aorta is aneurysmal, we cannot implant branches in duplicated renal arteries when both are smaller than 4 mm in diameter, and we cannot implant a branch in an aneurysmal proximal superior mesenteric artery when the aneurysmal segment gives rise to a replaced right hepatic artery.

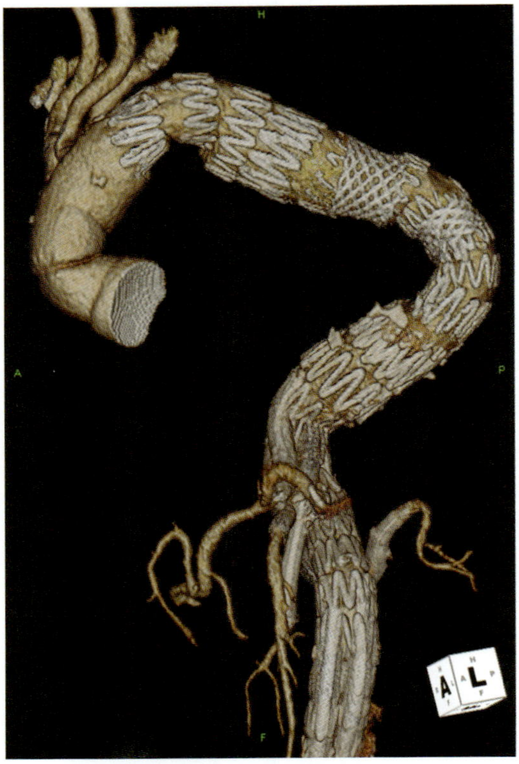

Fig. 6.5 Postoperative computed tomographic angiography (CTA) showing a very long tortuous thoracic aorta.

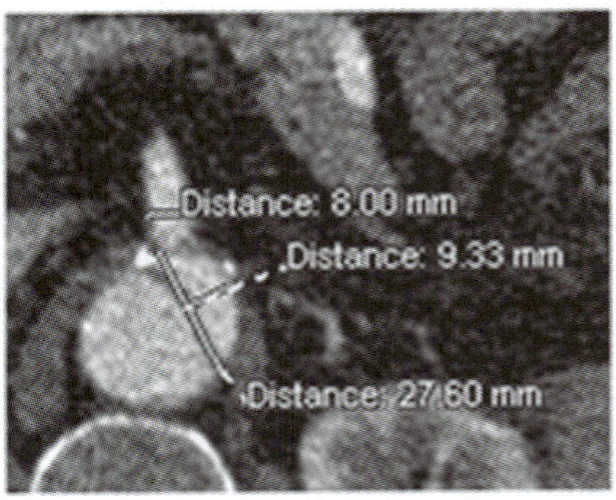

Fig. 6.6 Preoperative CT showing the small true lumen at the level of the superior mesenteric artery.

The presence of a perigraft space is an essential prerequisite for successful branch placement, and one might think that a non-dilated aorta at the level of the visceral or renal arteries would preclude

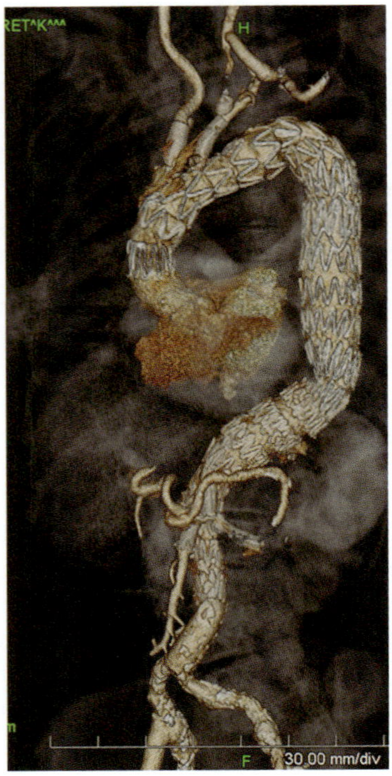

Fig. 6.7 Postoperative CTA showing a recent multibranched arch repair above a prior multibranched TAAA repair.

repair using a cuffed stent-graft. However, the trunk of the stent-graft tapers to 18 mm so that a luminal diameter of 25 mm provides more than enough perigraft space for the branches. The true lumen of a dissected aorta can be even smaller than this because the relatively robust branches will shoulder the septum aside (see Fig. 6.6).

Preoperative preparation

By the time a patient presents for possible endovascular TAAA repair, someone has already decided he or she is unfit for conventional repair. Most patients have already undergone an extensive cardiac and pulmonary work-up, many have been found to have uncorrectable coronary insufficiency, and most are on statins, angiotensin-converting enzyme (ACE) inhibitors and beta-blockers. There is not much more that one can to do optimize the patient's physiology. Instead, we try to optimize the patient's arterial anatomy through various preliminary interventions, including: the creation of a suitable route of transfemoral access around the external iliac arteries, which are frequently too small to accommodate a 22 Fr delivery system, especially in women; and the creation of a suitable implantation site in the renal arteries, which are frequently stenotic.

Because the procedure is staged, we prefer a formal ilio-femoral artery bypass to a blind-ended conduit. The proximal anastomosis is performed in an end-to-end fashion to the transected, endarterectomized proximal common iliac artery. The distal anastomosis is performed in an end-to-side fashion to either the distal external iliac artery or the distal common femoral artery. At the second operation, access is through a new surgical field to minimize the risk of wound complications. If the bypass graft ends on the distal external iliac artery, we subsequently expose the distal common femoral artery through a groin incision. If the bypass graft ends on the common femoral artery, we subsequently expose the graft limb, and only the graft limb, through a transverse incision at the inguinal ligament.

The stenotic renal artery is treated by implanting a short (15 mm), wide (6–7 mm), balloon-expanded stent through transbrachial access. We take great care to ensure that the proximal end of the stent does not protrude into the lumen of the aorta. The resulting orifice is wide, radiopaque and caudally oriented for easy catheterization through the caudally oriented cuff of a thoraco-abdominal stent-graft.

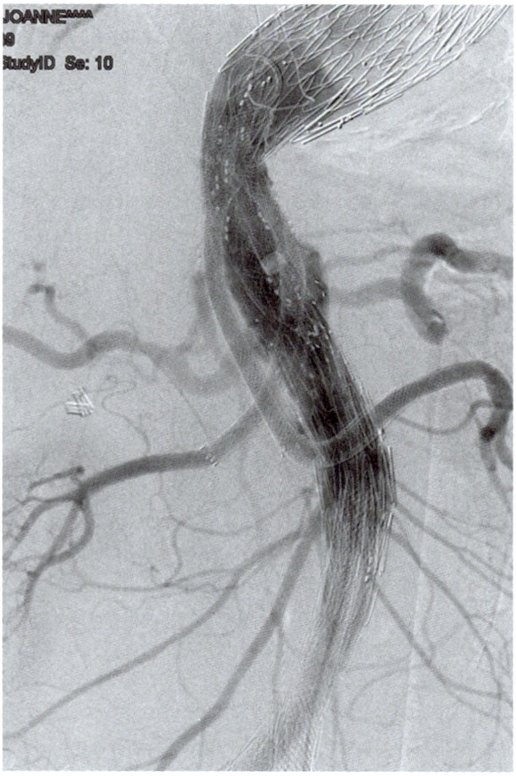

Fig. 6.8 Intraoperative angiography showing the right renal branch originating from the left renal cuff, and vice versa.

Evolution of the device

The first operation of this type was performed more than decade ago [4]. Although the essential features remain the same, the stent-graft has evolved to eliminate potential causes of failure. For example, a full stent exoskeleton was added to maintain the relative positions of the cuffs and prevent kinking. Our current IDE G000265 protocol was established in 2005, using fenestrated and cuffed stent-grafts, custom-made by Cook Medical, Australia to match individual patient anatomy. We soon discovered that cuffs made better attachment sites than fenestrations and caudally oriented cuffs were easier to plan, easier to insert, and more likely to remain patent than cranially oriented cuffs.

The branches of a cuffed thoraco-abdominal stent-graft bend anteriorly or posteriorly, to the right or to the left, depending on the relative axial orientation of the cuff and target artery orifice. Not only do the branches vary in shape, they also vary in length, depending on the relative longitudinal positions of the cuff and target artery orifice. These degrees of freedom make the technique forgiving. Errors in stent-graft position affect the shape and length of the branches, but not the chances of successful branch implantation. In the past 5 years we have treated 54 patients using four-branch cuffed stent-grafts with more than 250 branches, all of which were deployed successfully, despite wide-ranging disparities in the relative positions of the cuffs and their corresponding arterial orifices (Fig. 6.8).

The ability to vary branch morphology constitutes a form of intraoperative customization whereby a single stent-graft with uniform cuff distribution is used to treat patients with non-uniform visceral arterial anatomy. This was evidenced by the findings of a retrospective review of 3D computed tomography (CT) scans [14], which showed that 44/50 consecutive TAAA patients could have been treated using a standard four-cuff design with no branch lengths >5 cm, or branch angles >45°.

These observations prompted us to substitute a standard stent-graft, bearing four caudally oriented cuffs (see Fig. 6.3), for custom-made stent-grafts in a steadily increasing proportion of cases. We used the standard system in 10% of cases treated in 2008, 75% in 2009, and 100% treated so far in 2010. The standard cuffed component tapers from 34 mm proximally to 18 mm distally. The proximal stent is barbed, but covered, like the proximal end of a TX2 thoracic stent-graft. Each cuff is 18 mm long. The celiac and superior mesenteric cuffs are 8 mm wide, whereas the renal cuffs are 6 mm wide.

A variety of proximal and distal extensions accommodate variations in the longitudinal extent of the aneurysm. Some are commercially available – such as the TX2 and Zenith stent-grafts – and some are designed specifically for use in TAAA repair. This specialized inventory includes two tapered proximal extensions of different lengths, and two distal extensions. One distal extension is a simple flared tube for cases of prior infrarenal aneurysm repair, the other is bifurcated. Most of our branches consist of Fluency covered stents, measuring 6–10 mm in diameter and 40–80 mm in length, in combination with vascular Wallstents, measuring 6–10 mm in diameter and 36–39 mm in length.

Lessons of experience

Short-term lessons

In the 4 years from 2005 through 2009 the mean operative time fell from 8 hours to 4 as the lessons of experience were incorporated into device design, operative planning, and insertion technique. We learned to identify and correct challenging anatomic features, such as iliac stenosis or renal stenosis, before heading to the operating room for the definitive repair. We also learned a number of helpful little tricks. For example, it is important to stabilize the access sheath in the aortic arch where it takes a sharp angle out of the left subclavian artery. Otherwise looping in the arch causes uncontrolled back-and-forth movements of wires and catheters (push-back) whenever they encounter resistance to insertion. The resulting lack of control lengthened the operation, increased the blood loss, and occasionally resulted in renal artery injury. Dual sheaths (9 Fr inside 12 Fr) and kink-resistant sheaths (Flexor) help, but the greatest contribution is made by the tension in a brachio-femoral buddy wire.

Standardization of device design and insertion technique contributed to better outcomes. To date we have treated 54 patients using stent-grafts having four caudally oriented cuffs. There have been only two cases of perioperative death and two cases of paraplegia, all of which were in the 12 women in the series. There was not a single instance of perioperative death or paraplegia among the 42 men.

That is not to say only two patients had lower extremity weakness, but that lower extremity weakness was usually partial and treatable following endovascular aneurysm repair, even TAAA repair. In most cases, symptoms develop 4–8 hours after operation. The most important measure is cerebrospinal fluid (CSF) drainage. Blood pressure support may also play a role. In the absence of any information on the vasomotor control of spinal perfusion, measures directed at improving cardiac output (such as blood transfusion) are probably better than measures directed at increasing vasomotor tone (such as phenylephrine infusion). The key to a successful outcome is prompt recognition. We leave a CSF drain in place for 2 days, during which time the patient is monitored closely in the intensive care unit. We do not attempt to control CSF pressure, but prefer to titrate drainage to symptoms.

The primary endoleak rate is low. Type I endoleaks are usually the result of inadequate overlap between the distal end of the branch and the target artery. It is rare for leakage to occur at the aortic, or iliac, implantation sites. Type II endoleak is far less common following endovascular repair of a thoracic aneurysm or TAAA than AAA. Type III endoleaks occasionally occur at sites of overlap between aortic components, but never between cuffs and branches.

Long-term lessons

Cuffed multibranched stent-grafts have proven to be remarkably stable. In a series of more than 60 cases, spanning 5 years, we have seen changes in the structure, shape, position, or function of a stent-graft only twice. In one, a spicule of aortic calcium eroded the underlying stent-graft. In the other, the end of the stent-graft migrated upwards out of a short distal aortic implantation site. Both were treated using stent-graft extensions. There have been no other cases of secondary endoleak, and no cases of aneurysm dilation or rupture.

Renal artery occlusion is by far the commonest late complication. Seven (out of over 250) branches have occluded: six renal arteries and one celiac artery. Risk factors for occlusion include: early bifurcation, acute angulation, diameter <4 mm, and cranial orientation. These observations have led to several changes in patient selection, preoperative preparation, and implantation technique. For example, we have shortened the overlap between the renal artery and covered stent, and we try to leave a short (3–10 mm) segment of uncovered stent protruding through distal end of the covered stent into the renal artery. The goal is to avoid acute angulation of the renal artery at the distal end of the covered stent.

Conclusions

Endovascular repair of TAAA is safe, effective, durable, and versatile. The advantages over open repair [15,16], or open/endovascular hybrids [17], are particularly clear for male patients with severe cardiopulmonary disease and extensive aneurysms (types II and III). Standardization of device design has the potential to eliminate manufacturing delays. Staged intervention has the potential to eliminate most anatomic exclusions. Nevertheless, device cost and availability will remain major impediments to widespread application until a single manufacturer develops the capability to supply all the components as part of a uniform system that can be studied as a whole and sold for a fixed price.

References

1 Inoue K, Iwase T, Sato M, et al. Transluminal endovascular branched graft placement for a pseudoaneurysm: reconstruction of the descending thoracic aorta including the celiac axis. J Thorac Cardiovasc Surg 1997; 114:859–61.
2 Imai M, Kimura T, Toma M, et al. Inoue stent-graft implantation for thoracoabdominal aortic aneurysm involving the visceral arteries. Eur J Vasc Endovasc Surg 2008; 35:462–5.
3 Anderson JL, Berce M, Hartley DE. Endoluminal aortic grafting with renal and superior mesenteric artery incorporation by graft fenestration. J Endovasc Ther 2001; 8:3–15.
4 Chuter TAM, Gordon RL, Reilly LM, et al. An endovascular system for thoracoabdominal aortic aneurysm repair. J Endovasc Ther 2001; 8:25–33.
5 Greenberg RK. Aortic aneurysm, thoracoabdominal aneurysm, juxtrarenal aneurysm, fenestrated endografts, branched endografts and endovascular aneurysm repair. Ann NY Acad Sci 2006; 1085:187–96.
6 Bakoyiannis CN, Economopoulos KP, Georgopoulos S, et al. Fenestrated and branched endografts for the treatment of thoracoabdominal aortic aneurysms: a systematic review. J Endovasc Ther 2010; 17:201–9.
7 Verhoeven EL, Tielliu IF, Bos WT, et al. Present and future of branched stent-grafts in thoracoabdominal aortic aneurysm repair: single center experience. Eur J Vasc Endovasc Surg 2009; 38:155–61.
8 Greenberg RK, Lytle B. Endovascular repair of thoracoabdominal aneurysms. Circulation 2008; 117: 2288–92.
9 Chuter TA, Rapp JH, Hiramoto JS, et al. Endovascular treatment of thoracoabdominal aortic aneurysms. J Vasc Surg 2008; 47:6–16.
10 Ferreira M, Lanziotti L, Monteiro M. Branched devices for thoracoabdominal aneurysm repair: early experience. J Vasc Surg 2008; 48:30S–36S.
11 Ricotta JJ, 2nd. Commentary: fenestrated and branched stent-grafts for the treatment of thoracoabdominal aortic aneurysms: the future is now. J Endovasc Ther 2010; 17:212–15.
12 Eagleton MJ, Greenberg RK. Late complications after endovascular thoracoabdominal aneurysm repair. Semin Vasc Surg 2009; 22:87–92.
13 Resch T, Sonnesson B, Malina M. Incidence and management of complications after branched and fenestrated endografting. Cardiovasc Surg (Torino) 2009; 51:105–13.
14 Sweet MP, Hiramoto JS, Park KH. et al. A standardized multi-branched thoracoabdominal stent-graft for endovascular aneurysm repair. J Endovasc Ther 2009; 16:359–64.
15 Richards JM, Nimmo AF, Moores CR, et al. Contemporary results for open repair of suprarenal and type IV thoracoabdominal aortic aneurysms. Br J Surg 2010; 97(1):45–9.
16 Rigberg DA, McGory ML, Zinhgmond DS, et al. Thirty-day mortality statistics underestimate the risk of repair of thoracoabdominal aortic aneurysm: a statewide experience. J Vasc Surg 2006; 43:217–22.
17 Muehling BM, Bischoff G, Schelzig H, et al. Hybrid procedures for complex thoracoabdominal aortic aneurysms: early results and secondary interventions. Vasc Endovascular Surg 2010; 44(2):110–15.

7

CHAPTER 7

Hybrid endovascular aortic arch surgery

Bobby Yanagawa & Mark D. Peterson
Division of Cardiac Surgery, St. Michael's Hospital, University of Toronto, Toronto, Canada

Introduction

Pathology affecting the aortic arch continually challenges cardiovascular surgeons to develop novel therapeutic strategies with lower rates of morbidity and mortality. Contemporary surgical approaches to the aortic arch and proximal thoracic aorta have yielded both improved results and broadened the population of patients considered eligible for such operations, yet the operative morbidity and mortality remains high [1–4]. Since complex aortic arch reconstructions often require prolonged cardiopulmonary bypass (CPB) and deep hypothermic circulatory arrest (DHCA) times, even in the most experienced centers, many patients develop end-organ dysfunction, neurocognitive impairment, coagulopathy, and high rates of blood product transfusion [2,4]. Endovascular stent-graft therapy, initially developed for treating patients with pathology confined to the descending thoracic aorta, minimizes the surgical trauma and physiologic perturbations associated with open surgical replacement. Endovascular stenting offers an attractive alternative to conventional repair for high-risk patients due to advanced age or significant comorbidities such as coronary artery disease, renal failure, cerebrovascular disease, and chronic obstructive pulmonary disease, or otherwise inadequate physiologic reserves to survive an open operation. The avoidance of CPB and DHCA may have an even greater impact on patients with aortic arch pathology, leading many centers to extend the application of endovascular stenting, in combination with some form of extra-anatomic brachiocephalic vessel rerouting, to this population. A further advantage of endovascular repair is the ability to intervene rapidly for acute life-threatening pathologies such as traumatic aortic transection and contained aortic rupture.

Background

Endovascular stent-grafting using a homemade device was first performed by Dake and colleagues [5] for the treatment of thoracic aortic aneurysms and dissections. In 2005, the US Food and Drug Administration (FDA) approved the Gore TAG thoracic endoprosthesis for the treatment of degenerative aneurysms of the descending thoracic aorta [6]. The natural curvature of the aortic arch and the origin of the brachiocephalic vessels limited the proximal landing zone to the distal arch and the descending aorta. Many groups, eager to increase the subgroup of patients eligible for endovascular stenting, extended the proximal landing zone into the distal aortic arch by covering the origin of the left subclavian artery [7,8]. Currently, reported off-label applications of thoracic endovascular aortic repair (TEVAR) include aortic aneurysms and pseudoaneurysms [6], acute and chronic aortic dissections, intramural hematomas

Endovascular and Hybrid Therapies for Structural Heart and Aortic Disease, First Edition.
Edited by Jacques Kpodonu and Raoul Bonan.

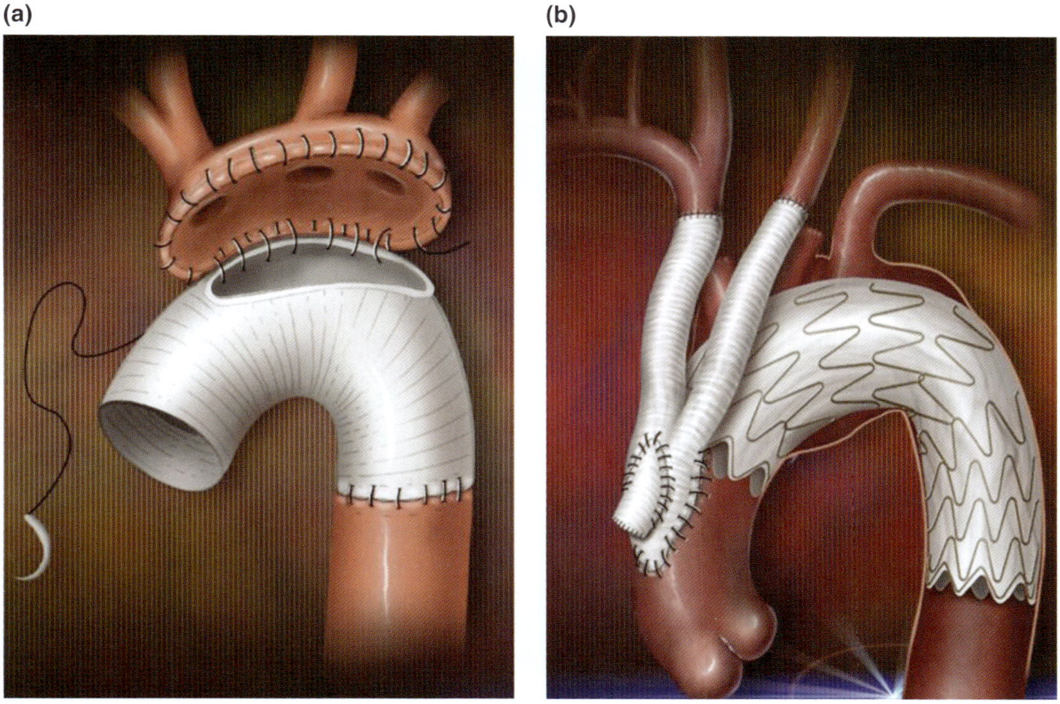

Fig. 7.1 Conventional versus hybrid TEVAR repair of an aortic arch aneurysm. (a) Conventional aortic arch reconstruction entails aorta-to-graft anastamoses with head vessel reattachment under deep hypothermic circulatory arrest. (b) Hybrid TEVAR involves rerouting the great vessels and stent-graft deployment.

and penetrating ulcers [9], aortic transections [10], aortic coarctation [11], and rarely, aorto-enteric or aorto-bronchial fistulas [12].

Recent promising mid-term outcomes suggest that this approach may be justified in a subset of patients who are poor surgical candidates [13]. However, there are no randomized clinical trials comparing endovascular to the gold standard approach, that being open repair. Thus, the decision to engage in this approach must be taken with the appreciation that long-term graft viability is still an open question.

A major limiting factor in the use of endovascular repairs is the adequacy of the proximal and distal landing zones to accommodate an endovascular stent without obstructing important major branches. Hybrid techniques have been developed to address this constraint.

Hybrid endovascular surgery

The term "hybrid" refers to the fusion of open surgical and stent-based approaches for repair of aortic pathology (Fig. 7.1). Although many groups simply overstent the left subclavian artery when extending the proximal landing zone into the distal arch, covering the left common carotid or innominate artery without prior extra-anatomic rerouting is not possible [7,8]. Thus hybrid strategies for aortic arch reconstruction usually combine partial or complete supra-aortic, extra-anatomic surgical debranching as an adjunct to stent-graft therapy [14–16]. The extent of aortic arch coverage is determined by the location of the pathology within either the proximal descending aorta or the arch itself, in order to obtain a sufficient proximal landing zone for adequate stent-graft fixation. Coverage of the entire aortic arch with a stent-graft mandates an intrathoracic rerouting strategy, whereby the inflow for the extra-anatomic bypasses originates from the proximal or mid-ascending aorta. If only partial arch coverage is required, extrathoracic methods of rerouting, such as a carotid–carotid–left subclavian bypass are performed.

Hybrid repairs may also be performed as part of a staged reconstruction for extensive ascending, arch and descending thoracic aneurysms [17–19]. The first stage addresses ascending and arch pathology with a conventional open arch reconstruction and elephant trunk, as well as any necessary proximal ascending or aortic root procedures. The second stage completes the repair by addressing the descending thoracic aortic pathology. A stent-graft is deployed into the previously placed elephant trunk graft, which serves as the proximal landing zone. The distal, non-aneurysmal, native thoracic aorta supports the stent-graft in the distal landing zone. Alternatively, "frozen elephant trunk" involves the use of a single-stage hybrid graft with a proximal conventional Dacron portion for surgical replacement of the aortic arch and proximal descending aorta, and a distal stented portion for deployment into the distal descending aorta.

Aortic transections and traumatic aortic ruptures are associated with roughly 20% operative mortality due to multiple related comorbidities [20]. These have also been successfully treated with an endovascular or hybrid endovascular repair [10,21]. TEVAR offers rapid revascularization and avoidance of sternotomy [22,23]. Left subclavian artery coverage is almost always necessary due to the location of the aortic tear at the insertion of the ligamentum arteriosus. If the subclavian artery requires revascularization, carotid-to-subclavian bypass may be necessary. Notably, these patients are usually young with small, angulated aortic arches that are at risk of graft kinking.

In this review, we discuss contemporary issues related to hybrid thoracic aortic repair, illustrating the principles with informative cases.

Personnel requirements

Hybrid procedures require a convergence of surgical and interventional skill sets which can only be obtained at an experienced endovascular center. This is usually accomplished in a collaborative manner between cardiovascular and vascular surgeons, cardiologists and radiologists. More specifically, the team should be adept at peripheral vascular exposure and retroperitoneal exposure of the iliac and distal aorta when the common femoral and external iliac arteries are of insufficient size to accommodate a large bore sheath. Importantly, the team should be experienced enough to convert to an open repair rapidly and under some degree of duress in the event of a catastrophic complication such as acute type A dissection or aortic rupture. A predefined protocol to deal with catastrophes such as iliac rupture may include having large aortic occlusion balloons and a range of covered stents.

Imaging requirements

Preoperative

High-quality preoperative imaging is critical for endovascular case planning to ensure a successful repair. Preoperative imaging is necessary for accurate and comprehensive evaluation of aortic pathology, as well as for assessing the size, length, and proximity to critical branches of the proximal and distal landing zones. This is necessary to determine optimal device type, diameter, length, anticipated number of stents required, primary and alternative vascular access sites, and the need for extra-anatomic bypass grafts due to coverage of critical aortic branches. All of our patients undergo computed tomography (CT), with a multislice scanner (64 slice), with multiplanar reconstruction and post-scan image processing performed on a dedicated TeraRecon (TeraRecon, San Mateo, CA) workstation. A preliminary endovascular plan may be formed from surveying the multiplanar reconstructions (MPRs) in axial, sagittal, and coronal planes; however, accurate selection of graft size and length is greatly improved with curved planar reconstructions (CPRs) and center line of flow analysis (Fig. 7.2). Center line of flow analysis is critical especially in the setting of tortuous vasculature where CT standard images alone may overestimate diameter and underestimate length. In a center line of flow analysis, a point is plotted in the center of a blood vessel in each axial cut and computer algorithms reconstruct the vessel in a straight line. The straightened vessel can be visualized in one image, and appropriate quantitative measurements performed.

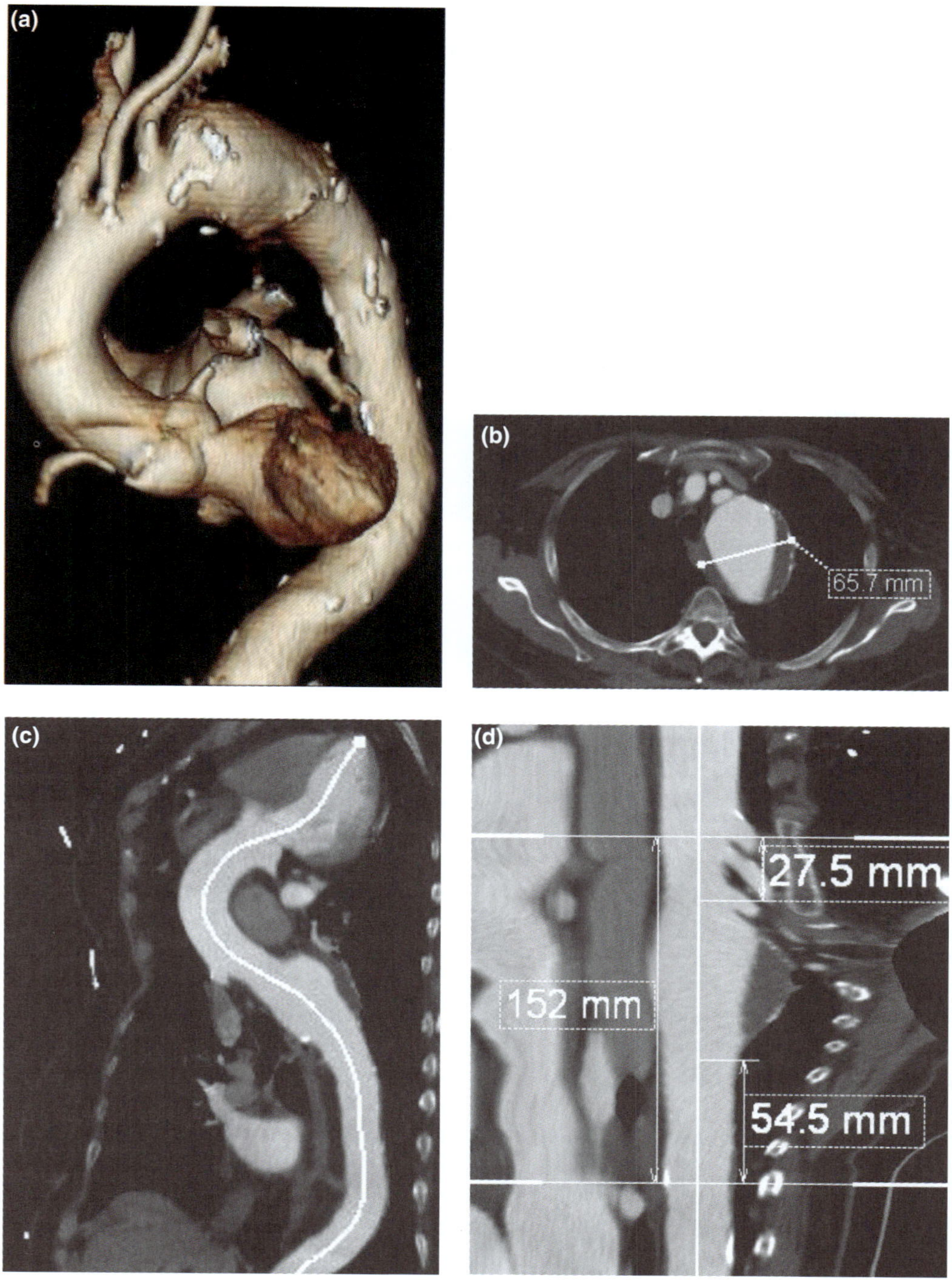

Fig. 7.2 Center of line flow analysis. (a) A 3D reconstruction of a patient with a large distal arch aneurysm and an axial cut through the arch (b). A line is plotted in the center of the aorta (c) and then the image is reprocessed into a straight line (d). This allows accurate measurement of the distance from the distal end of the innominate artery to the proximal aneurysm (27.5 mm), the length of the distal landing zone, as well as the total stent-graft length required to exclude the aneurysm, including adequate proximal and distal landing zones.

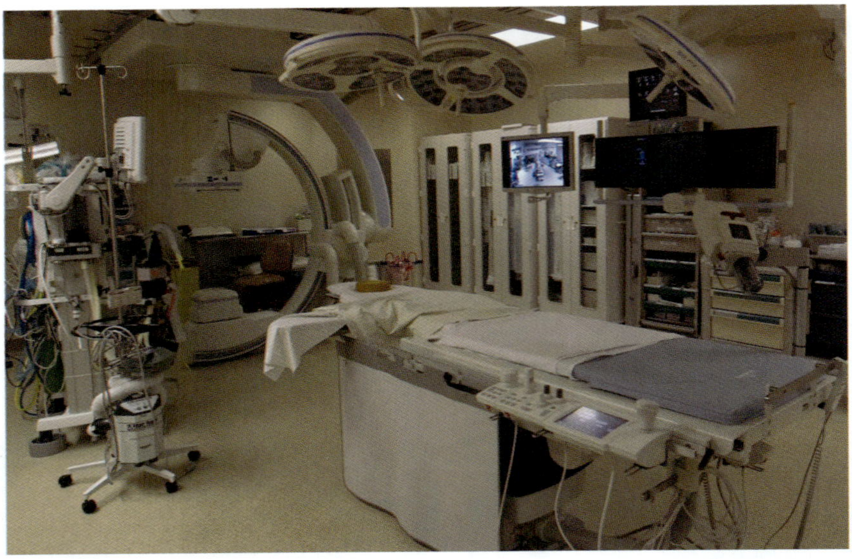

Fig. 7.3 Hybrid operating room at St. Michael's Hospital, Toronto. Hybrid operating rooms include a ceiling-mounted fixed image intensifier and C-arm (X-ray tube), imaging monitors, and necessary facilities to support conventional cardiovascular surgery.

Perioperative

In the past, endovascular surgery has been performed in either a standard operating room with a portable C-arm or in an interventional radiology suite. A hybrid operating room combines the advantages of both a traditional operating room and a high-tech interventional suite into one, multipurpose suite, which is the ideal location for complex hybrid procedures (Fig. 7.3). Important components of a hybrid operating room include adequate space (>650 square feet or 60 m^2), high-quality fixed imaging (i.e. ceiling or floor-mounted fixed image intensifier and C-arm), an adequate number of monitors, and equipment to support conventional surgical procedures such as cardiopulmonary bypass and transesophageal echocardiography (TEE). Additional imaging modalities such as integrated intravascular ultrasound (IVUS) and CT may be incorporated into a hybrid suite. The room dimensions should be sufficiently large to accommodate this equipment, as well as wall cabinets for vertical storage of a large numbers of endovascular stents, guide wires, and sheaths.

Access and device sizing

Patients are selected for potential endovascular repair based on CT evaluation. We routinely scan the chest, abdomen, and pelvis down to the level of the common femoral arteries in patients being considered for endovascular repair. This allows us to determine the size, tortuosity, and degree of calcification of the ilio-femoral vessels, thereby allowing accurate selection of the access site, which is usually the common femoral artery, and the access side. If the sizes of the femoral and iliac vessels are equal, we generally choose the side that provides a straighter line to the thoraco-abdominal aorta. Sheaths vary in diameter but generally the outer diameter is between 20 and 24 Fr (7.6–9.2 mm). Normal vessels are elastic and may accommodate a larger sheath, whereas atherosclerotic and calcified vessels are less likely to stretch during sheath insertion. Iliac rupture is a devastating and potentially life-threatening complication, therefore when the femoral and iliac arteries are judged too small to permit safe sheath insertion, we graft a 10 mm Dacron conduit directly to the common iliac artery or distal aorta.

Selecting an appropriate-sized endograft is determined by the diameter of the aorta in the proximal and distal landing zones. The seal is determined by the radial force of the graft against the aorta at the proximal and distal landing zones. To ensure optimal seal, 10–20% graft-to-aorta oversizing is

Table 7.1 Currently used stent-grafts.

	Gore TAG	*Cook Zenith TX2*	*Medtronic Talent*
Graft material	PTFE	Polyester	Polyester
Stent material	Nitinol	Stainless steel	Nitinol
FDA approval	2005	2009	2008
Aortic diameter	23–37 mm	24–38 mm	18–42 mm
Stent-graft diameter	26–40 mm	28–42 mm	22–46 mm
Seal zone length	>2.0 cm	>2.5 cm	>2.0 cm
Stent length	10, 15, 20 cm	12–21.6 cm	11.2–21.2cm
Proximal construction	Covered	Covered with barbs	Uncovered
Distal construction	Covered	Bare stent	Bare spring

FDA, US Food and Drug Administration.

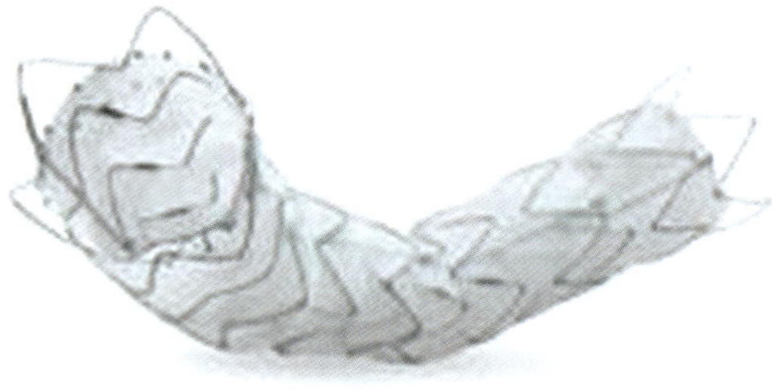

Medtronic talent

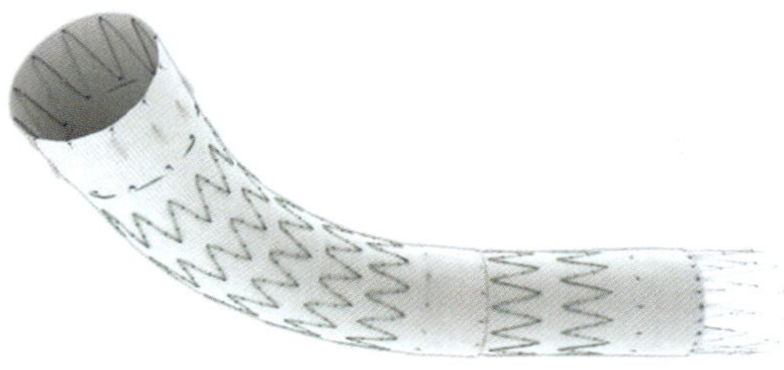

Cook zenith TX2

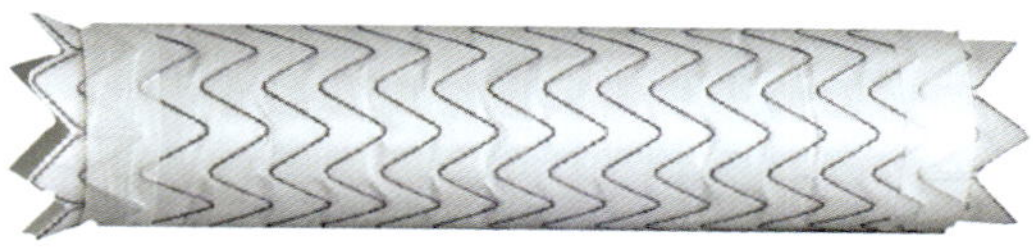

Gore TAG

Fig. 7.4 Thoracic endoprostheses: Medtronic Talent, Cook Zenith TX2, and Gore TAG.

recommended. Therefore the seal zone diameter for available non-customized grafts range from 20 to 38 mm (Table 7.1). Currently, Gore TAG (W.L. Gore & Associates, Flagstaff, AZ), Medtronic Talent (Medtronic, Minneapolis, MN), and Cook Zenith TX2 (Cook Medical, Bloomington, IN) thoracic endoprostheses are available for use (Fig. 7.4). Larger, custom-made grafts are available to treat patients with landing zone diameters up to 42 mm. The size of the native aorta in the proximal and distal landing zones often differs by more than 20%, therefore tapered grafts were developed to minimize oversizing in the distal landing zone. These tapered grafts available from Cook and Medtronic are 4 mm smaller at the distal compared with the proximal portion. Selecting two components of different sizes, one component matched for the proximal landing zone, and the other component matched for the distal landing zone, is an alternative method to deal with significant size discrepancies between the proximal and distal landing zones.

The appropriate endograft length is a balance between covering the pathology with adequate proximal and distal fixation and seal, and minimizing the risk of paraplegia (especially when long segments of the thoracic aorta need coverage) and need for extra-anatomic bypasses. The minimum length for adequate seal is 20–25 mm but a greater length may be necessary with non-linear aortic surfaces. We feel that 20 mm of proximal landing zone in the curving aortic arch is often insufficient for adequate seal therefore we will perform extra-anatomic bypasses as necessary to gain additional proximal landing zone. When graft length requirements necessitate two grafts, graft-to-graft overlap of 50 mm is recommended if the grafts are of equal size. When the proximal and distal landing zones differ by greater than 20%, grafts of different sizes may be necessary in which case 30 mm overlap is recommended.

Landing zone optimization

The landing zone map (Fig. 7.5), first published by Ishimaru et al. [24], serves as a guide for planning stent placement. As mentioned, generally an aortic

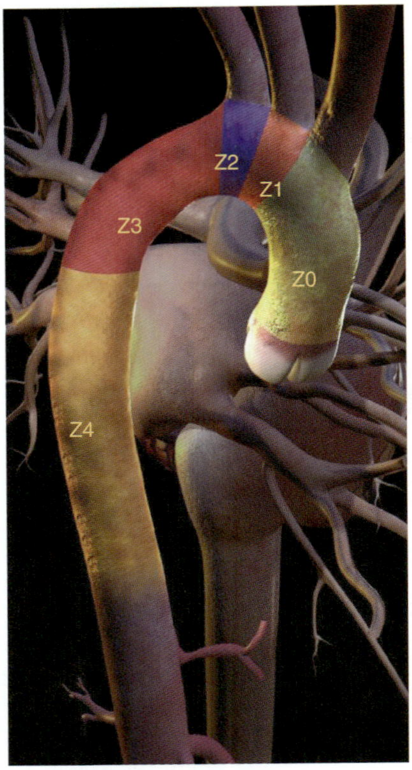

Fig. 7.5 Thoracic aorta landing zone map.

length >20 mm and diameter <38 mm is needed at the proximal and distal landing zones. The degree of supra-aortic rerouting of major aortic branches is based on the proposed landing zone.

Landing in zone 0 requires complete innominate and left carotid debranching and rerouting, usually with the use of a branched graft from the proximal ascending aorta (Fig. 7.6). This may be combined with an ascending aortic replacement (Fig. 7.7). Moreover, Szeto et al. [25] describe the use of a trifurcated Dacron graft (Vasculotek-Terumo, Ann Arbor, MI). Zone 0 landing and complete debranching can be performed either as a staged [16] or single-stage repair [26]. Furthermore, the endograft may be deployed in either a retrograde or an antegrade fashion [27]. Certain devices, such as the Gore TAG, may be deployed either retrograde or antegrade since the stent-graft is symmetric. Here the major advantage of a hybrid approach is the avoidance of DHCA. Furthermore, aortic debranching may be performed via an upper ministernotomy [27].

Zone I is anatomically complex and landing is associated with lower initial success compared with zone 0 and II landing [26]. This requires an extra-anatomic carotid-to-carotid bypass

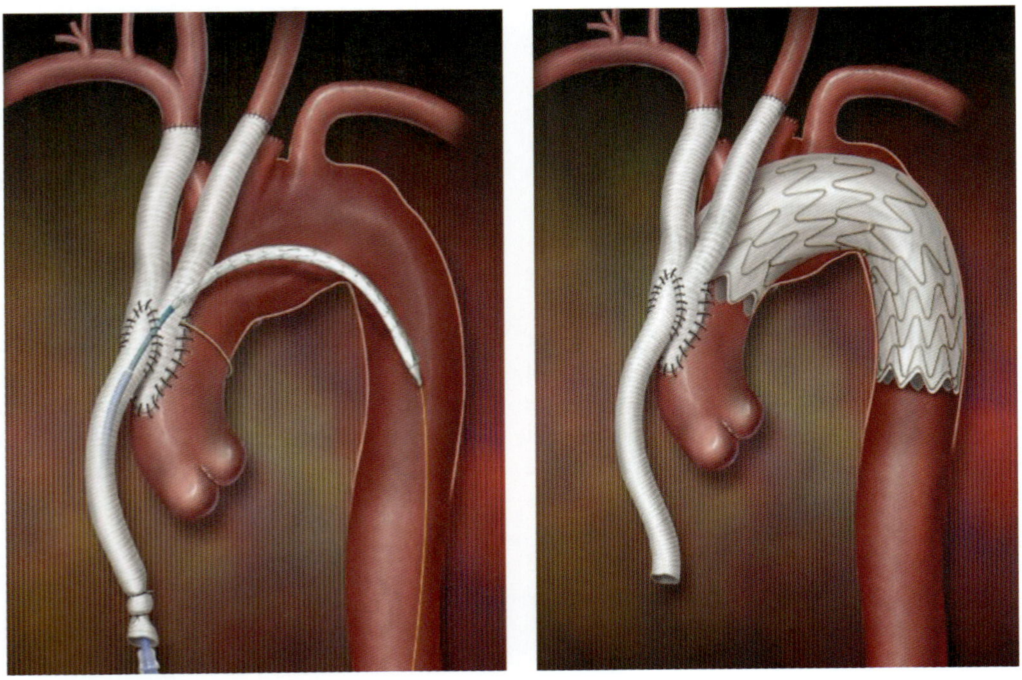

Fig. 7.6 Hybrid TEVAR for total arch repair stage 1: antegrade stent deployment.

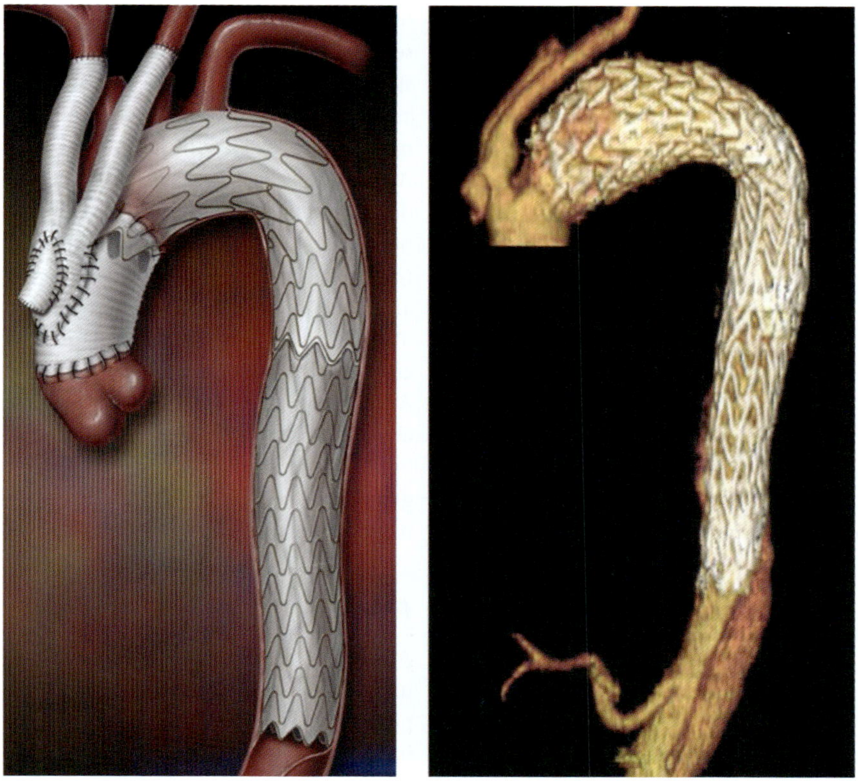

Fig. 7.7 Hybrid TEVAR for total arch repair stage 2: complete thoracic aorta stent coverage.

(Fig. 7.8). It is likely that the acute angulation of the proximal arch results in higher rates of type I endoleaks. As such, Melissano et al. [26] advocate >30 mm of proximal landing zone. Extrathoracic carotid-to-carotid bypass allows avoidance of a sternotomy. Left carotid-to-subclavian bypass may be necessary in some circumstances, or a simultaneous carotid–carotid–left subclavian bypass.

Zone II landing implies overstenting the left subclavian artery. Overstenting the left subclavian artery can be performed safely in most patients due to the presence of a rich collateral network, such as from the left internal mammary artery (LIMA) and vertebral artery [26,28]. A blood pressure gradient of approximately 50 mmHg may be observed but it is usually without clinical ramifications. However, an absolute contraindication to left subclavian artery coverage, without prior bypass, includes patients with previous coronary bypass surgery and a patent LIMA bypass graft, and patients with a functioning left-sided dialysis fistula. Relative contraindications to left subclavian coverage also include patients with an absent or hypoplastic contralateral vertebral artery (R vertebral), left-handed

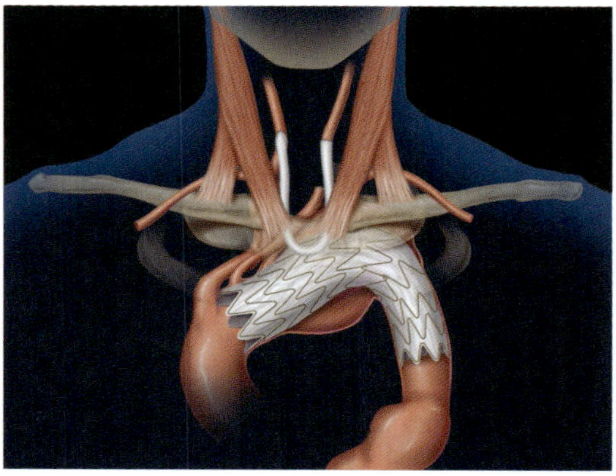

Fig. 7.8 Extrathoracic rerouting and endovascular repair of an arch aneurysm originating distal to the innominate artery. The illustration demonstrates endovascular exclusion of the arch aneurysm with a proximal landing zone distal to the origin of the innominate artery and a carotid-to-carotid bypass.

professionals, or in cases with previous abdominal aortic surgery. In such patients, prophylactic left carotid-to-subclavian artery bypass or left subclavian artery transposition should be considered [29–31].

Landing in zone III or IV are located distal to the left subclavian and as such do not require arch vessel debranching.

Hybrid procedures

Extensive thoracic aortic aneurysms may involve the ascending, arch and descending thoracic aorta which poses a considerable surgical challenge, particularly with regards to distal exposure. The evolution of surgical management of this complex pathology is reviewed by Karck and Kamiya [32]. Conventional repair is an open repair either with a two-staged elephant trunk technique or as a single-staged clamshell repair. From a median sternotomy, usually only the proximal third of the descending aorta is accessible. Surgeons initially developed a two-stage strategy to address the ascending aorta and arch in one stage, followed by a second operation 8–12 weeks later to replace the descending aorta. A two-staged approach may reduce the trauma associated with a single-stage repair via a clamshell incision. However, a significant proportion of patients die while awaiting the second stage or are lost to follow-up [33].

In 1983, the elephant trunk was developed by Borst et al. [34], which involves initial ascending aortic and arch replacement with a graft anchored to either the arch or proximal descending aorta, and the free end of the graft left suspended in the descending aorta. The second stage is performed through a separate lateral thoracotomy where the elephant trunk serves as the proximal anastamosis for the descending or thoraco-abdominal replacement. This is now considered the gold standard repair. However, this procedure involves two major surgical procedures and a significant risk of aortic rupture in the intervening time periods. Thirty-day mortality for this two-stage repair is 8.7% after the first stage and 9.7% after the second stage [35]. Overall, these repairs are still associated with significant morbidity and mortality [36]. This led to the development of a first-stage elephant trunk procedure and secondary endovascular completion. This strategy minimizes the surgical insult normally associated with an open second stage, and thus may be performed within days after the first stage. An even more aggressive strategy has been developed, namely the "frozen elephant trunk" procedure. This strategy allows for a single-stage repair, and involves the standard open ascending and arch replacement, combined with stenting of the descending thoracic aorta during the circulatory arrest phase of the operation [37–39]. A standard stent-graft can be deployed into an elephant trunk graft in an antegrade manner, or a hybrid stent-graft (the proximal part is a polyester graft fused with distal stent-graft component) may be used [40,41].

Anesthetic considerations

Although endovascular repair may be performed under local, spinal, or general anesthesia, hybrid procedures require general anesthesia. Standard intraoperative monitoring is employed, including multiple arterial monitoring lines. We do not routinely place cerebrospinal fluid (CSF) drains in patients undergoing hybrid aortic arch procedures, since the majority of stent-grafts do not cover the descending thoracic aorta beyond the proximal half. CSF drains are placed selectively in patients at high risk for paraplegia, such as those with a history of abdominal aortic aneurysm repair, planned coverage of the arch and entire thoracic aorta, or patients presenting with contained aortic rupture. If paraplegia or paraparesis develops postoperatively in patients who did not receive a CSF drain, we will insert a spinal drain and start a high-dose dexamethasone protocol. We also maintain a systolic blood pressure above 130–140 mmHg for the first 24 hours following stent deployment.

Procedural techniques

Extra-anatomic rerouting

Aortic debranching and revascularization of critical aortic branches is performed prior to aortic stenting. Although proximal landing zone lengths of 2–2.5 cm are considered acceptable, we believe that longer proximal landing zone lengths between 2.5 and 3.5 cm may be required for adequate proximal fixation, particularly in the curving aortic arch. We utilize an aggressive strategy to extend the proximal landing zone as necessary to obtain 2.5–3.0 cm routinely, with the use of simple or branched Dacron grafts ranging from 8 to 10 mm in size. For patients requiring complete aortic arch stenting with a Z0 landing, we have evolved our strategy from innominate and left common carotid bypasses to complete brachiocephalic rerouting. We formerly performed an ascending to innominate and left common carotid artery bypass with an inverted aorto-bifemoral graft (16 × 8 mm) through a median sternotomy (see Fig. 7.1), revascularizing the left subclavian only for a specific indication (see above). At present, all three brachiocephalic vessels are revascularized with a prefabricated polyester trifurcated graft (Vascutek, Inchinnan, Scotland) via a hemisternotomy. We extend the incision superiorly and laterally along the anterior border of the left sternocleidomastoid muscle as necessary to expose the left subclavian artery. Following exposure of the brachiocephalic vessels and heparinization with 100 U/kg, the proximal anastamosis is constructed off-pump with a partial occluding side-biting aortic clamp on the lateral and proximal half of the ascending aorta. Placing the inflow for the aortic debranching low on the ascending aorta is critical to ensure sufficient proximal landing zone in Z0. The innominate, left subclavian, and left common carotid arteries are bypassed sequential with the limbs of the trifurcated graft (typically 12 mm for the innominate, and 8 mm for the left carotid and subclavian arteries).

An extrathoracic revascularization strategy is employed when the proximal landing zone is in Z1. In these cases, the native innominate artery is not covered and provides the inflow for the extra-anatomic bypasses via the right common carotid artery (see Case 1). In preparation for a right-to-left carotid–carotid–subclavian bypass, we expose the base of the common carotid arteries through an incision made 2.5 cm above the sternal notch, from the anterior border of the right sternocleidomastoid muscle extending transversely across the base of the neck and superiorly over the left clavicle. This lateral extension allows exposure of the left subclavian artery for revascularization. Once the right and left common carotid arteries, as well as the left subclavian arteries, are exposed and controlled, we anastamose an 8 mm woven polyester graft to the anterior and medial aspect of the right common carotid artery and tunnel the graft behind the strap muscles, but not retropharyngeal, to the left common carotid artery. We transect and oversew the proximal left common carotid, and anastamose the distal left common carotid into the side of the 8 mm graft. Finally, the same graft is tunneled to the left subclavian artery where it is anastamosed in an end-to-side fashion with the left subclavian artery.

Stent-graft deployment

Arterial vascular access is normally achieved by exposing the common femoral artery and placing two pursestring sutures in the anterior wall of the vessel. If alternative arterial access is required, a 10 mm graft is sewn to the common iliac artery or distal abdominal aorta via a retroperitoneal approach. The contralateral femoral artery is cannulated percutaneously with a 6 Fr sheath to allow insertion of a marker pigtail or straight flush catheter. Patients are heparinized with 100 U/kg of IV heparin, to achieve an activated clotting time (ACT) of >250 seconds. We cannulate the exposed common femoral artery with a 9 Fr catheter to allow insertion of a regular stiffness, 0.035 inch, 260 cm guide wire which is advanced into the ascending aorta. Following a wire exchange to a double-curved, stiff Lunderquist wire (LES3, Cook Medical, Bloomington, IN), we insert the prepared stent-graft and advance it into position in the arch prior to performing aortography. We prefer this sequence to minimize contrast use. A digital subtraction aortogram is performed and the proximal landing zone is marked on the monitor. Prior to deployment, the systolic blood pressure is lowered to 100 mmHg and the endoprosthesis is deployed. If we are deploying a Cook Zenith stent-graft, we deploy the first segment of the graft and then perform an additional aortogram to confirm positioning. At this point, the Cook Zenith device may be advanced proximally, but it cannot be withdrawn since the proximal portion of the graft contains fixation barbs that insert into the aortic wall. Once the position of the graft is confirmed, we deploy the remainder of the device, retrieve the straight flush catheter over a wire and reposition it in the stent-graft. A secondary graft is deployed if necessary and a completion aortogram is performed to confirm the adequacy of seal at the proximal and distal landing zones. Type I endoleaks observed in the operating room are treated by profile ballooning at the proximal or distal landing zone, and type III endoleaks are treated by ballooning the overlap between stent-grafts. In cases where the sheath insertion was met with higher than normal resistance, we leave the ipsilateral wire in situ when removing the sheath, and perform a distal aorto-iliac arteriogram. Once all of the hardware and wires are removed, we reverse the heparin with protamine and the patient is observed overnight in our cardiovascular intensive care.

In select cases, the stent-graft may be placed antegradely rather than retrogradely. Antegrade stent-graft placement in the ascending aorta has the advantage of avoiding a separate incision and is particularly useful when distal access is marginal [27]. A side graft may be sewn to the proximal inflow graft to facilitate antegrade stent deployment (see Fig. 7.6).

Routine four-view chest X-rays (CXRs) (posteroanterior, lateral, 45° right anterior oblique, and 45° left anterior oblique) and non-contrast-enhanced and contrast-enhanced CTs are performed prior to discharge and at 1, 6, and 12 months postop and annually thereafter.

Staged hybrid procedures

The elephant trunk was developed as an adjunct to an open proximal ascending and arch replacement in patients with extensive aortic aneurysms or dissections. We perform the first stage via a standard median sternotomy, and CPB is achieved with a single two-stage venous cannula and arterial perfusion through the right axillary artery. We begin the arch reconstruction at 18 °C while antegrade cerebral protection is provided via the right axillary cannula at 10–15 ml/kg. We revascularize the innominate, left subclavian, and left common carotid arteries with a trifurcated graft as described by Spielvogel and colleagues [1,42] and then move the clamp from the innominate to the trifurcated graft to perfuse the upper body while the elephant trunk anastamosis is completed. Landmarking for second-stage endovascular completion can be facilitated by placing three large stainless steel clips at 120° apart (see Case 3). We leave a long elephant trunk of 8–10 cm to facilitate cannulation during the endovascular stage, as well as to provide as much proximal fixation as possible. The trifurcated graft is then anastamosed to the ascending/arch graft, the proximal ascending graft is clamped, and the patient rewarmed. Additional proximal procedures are completed during rewarming.

The second-stage endovascular procedure is completed within 4–6 weeks, depending on patient recovery from the first procedure. Access for the second stage is obtained as described above. The right arm is exposed and prepped in case brachial artery cannulation is required. Once the elephant trunk is cannulated, we confirm positioning with a pigtail catheter and perform an aortogram. If cannulation from the distal aorta is difficult, we pass a long wire through the right brachial artery and guide it down the elephant trunk and descending thoracic aorta. The wire is then snared from below and externalized through the common femoral artery. The stent-graft is positioned into the elephant trunk and advanced proximally up to the distal curve of the arch without committing the graft to the curve of the arch. This allows ample stent to elephant trunk overlap (Fig. 7.9; see Case 3).

The frozen elephant trunk or "open stent-grafting" has also been reported as a single-stage repair for similar clinical scenarios [19,39,43]. The advantage of a single-stage repair is less chance of interstage rupture, but this is achieved at the expense of a more complex and prolonged first stage [33]. This procedure has been described elsewhere [32]. Briefly, the frozen elephant trunk involves conventional surgical repair of the aortic arch. For the descending aorta, a hybrid graft is utilized with a proximal portion composed of a Dacron sleeve which is sutured into the arch repair itself. The distal stented portion is then deployed into the descending aorta, covering the aneurysm.

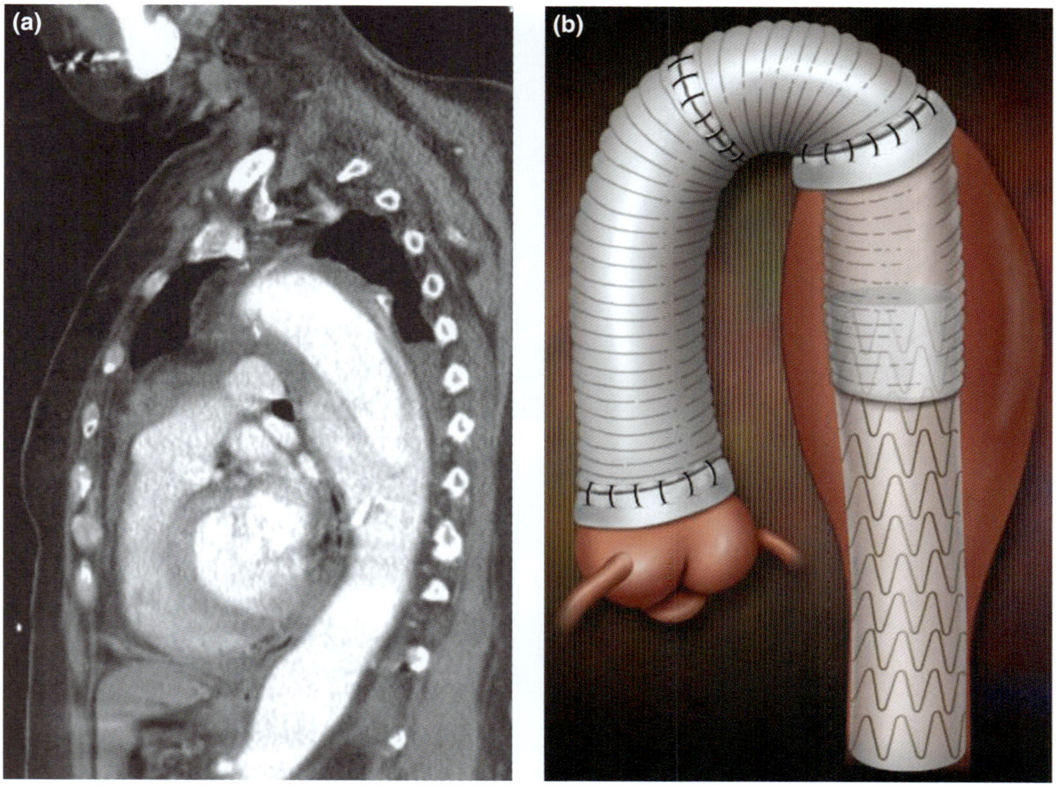

Fig. 7.9 Aortic arch repair using an elephant trunk with endovascular completion for total aortic aneurysm. (a) The CT scan demonstrates the elephant trunk with surrounding thrombus proximally and contrast material distally. (b) The illustration shows endovascular exclusion of the descending aneurysm with the stent-graft deployed into the elephant trunk proximally. The stent-graft is deployed distally in a non-aneurysmal segment of the aorta.

Cases

Case 1 – Z1 landing for distal aortic arch aneurysm repair: extrathoracic carotid–carotid–left subclavian bypass

A 79-year-old female presented with progressive exertional dyspnea. Past medical history included hypertension, atrial fibrillation, diabetes type II, obesity, factor V Leiden deficiency with pulmonary embolism, a spinal cord compression fracture, and she was an ex-smoker.

Imaging demonstrated a distal aortic arch aneurysm. Chest X-ray on presentation showed a large left mediastinal mass (Fig. 7.10a). A CT scan demonstrated a 6.5 × 6.7 cm saccular aneurysm beginning at the distal portion of the left subclavian artery (Fig. 7.10b,c). High-quality 3D reconstructions and curved planar reconstructions demonstrated that coverage of the left common carotid origin would be required for an adequate proximal landing zone.

She underwent a single-stage carotid–carotid bypass (Fig. 7.11, arrows), and left common carotid–left subclavian bypass (Fig. 7.11, arrowheads; as described above), and insertion of a thoracic stent-graft. The postoperative course was significant for a transient mild Horner's syndrome including mild ptosis and meiosis of the left eye, but no other neurologic sequelae. She was discharged home on day 4 and follow-up CT scans demonstrated good seal with no evidence of endoleaks.

Case 2 – Z0 landing for aortic arch aneurysm repair: thoracic rerouting of the innominate, right carotid, and left carotid using a trifurcated graft

A 39-year-old male sustained multiple injuries in a high-velocity motor vehicle accident serving in the Middle East 20 years ago. He presented with increasing dyspnea and a decrease in exercise tolerance. Examination revealed a massive

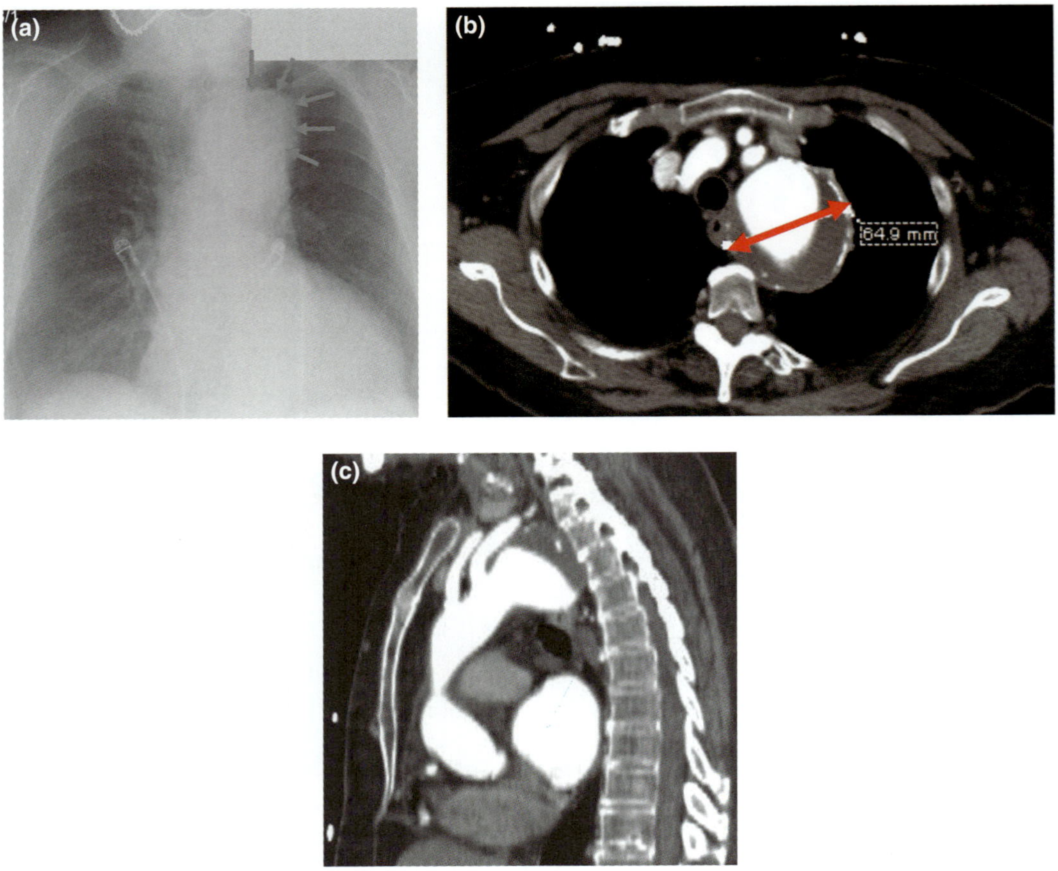

Fig. 7.10 Case 1: preoperative imaging. (a) Preoperative CXR with arrows highlighting the left mediastinal mass. (b, c) Preoperative CT demonstrating an aortic arch and descending aortic aneurysm with intraluminal thrombus.

diaphragmatic hernia with the intra-abdominal contents shifted into the left chest cavity and complete collapse of the left lung (Fig. 7.12). The diaphragmatic hernia was repaired through a thoraco-abdominal incison by reconstructing the left hemidiaphragm.

At the time of the initial trauma, the patient likely suffered an aortic transection that went unrecognized, as he also had a large aortic pseudoaneurysm measuring 4.6 cm at the level of the ligamentum arteriosum (Fig. 7.13). As previous thoracic surgery was undertaken, he underwent a hybrid endovascular repair strategy to avoid a redo thoracotomy. A hemisternotomy and complete supra-aortic rerouting procedure was performed, followed immediately by endovascular exclusion of the pseudoaneurysm. The proximity of the pseudoaneurysm to the arch vessels mandated complete coverage of the aortic arch vessels, as well as the proximal descending thoracic aorta (Fig. 7.14). The patient recovered uneventfully and was discharged at day 7. Notably, follow-up CT demonstrated complete exclusion of the pseudoaneurysm with thrombosis of the aneurysm sac and no evidence of endoleaks (Fig. 7.15).

Case 3 – Staged hybrid repair for extensive ascending, arch and descending aortic aneuyrsmal disease

A 60-year-old female presented with progressive dyspnea. Past medical history was significant for hypertension and included a 20-pack-year smoking history. A CXR revealed massive enlargement of the aortic silhouette (Fig. 7.16a). CT revealed a 10 cm ascending aneurysm, 7 cm arch aneurysm, and a 6 cm descending thoracic aneurysm (Fig. 7.16b,c), which was confirmed intraoperatively (Fig. 7.17). She underwent a

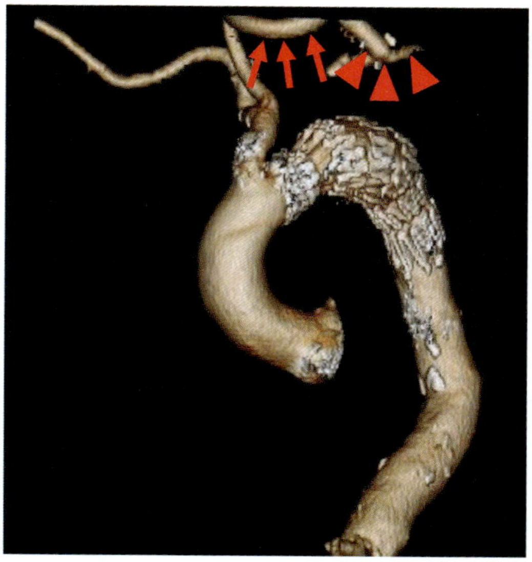

Fig. 7.11 Case 1: postoperative imaging. 3D CT reconstruction demonstrating the stent-graft with proximal aspect just distal to the innominate artery and extending to the proximal descending aorta. The carotid-to-carotid (arrows) and carotid-to-left subclavian artery (arrowheads) bypasses are shown.

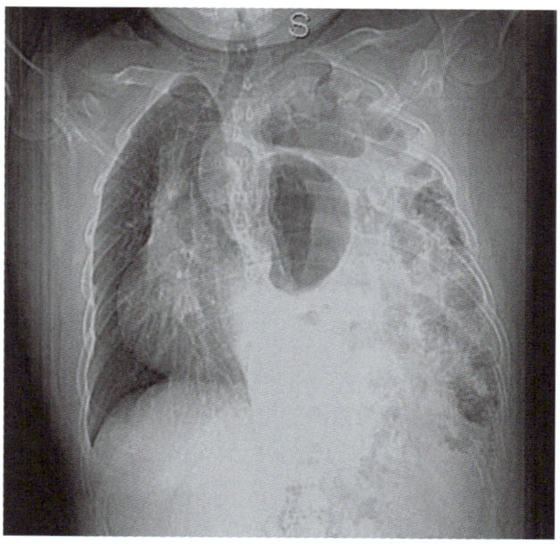

Fig. 7.12 Case 2: initial CXR. Initial imaging demonstrating the abdominal contents in the left thoracic cavity, significant tracheal deviation, complete left lung collapse, and mediastinal shift into the right thorax.

Bentall and total aortic arch reconstruction with an elephant trunk (Fig. 7.18). This was followed approximately 2 months later by a retrograde deployment of a thoracic stent-graft into her elephant trunk (Fig. 7.19). The maximum transverse diameter of the descending thoracic aorta was 65 mm and the distal landing zone above the celiac was about 32–36 mm in a funnel shape but with several centimeters of landing zone above the celiac artery. She did well for the first year after surgery but serial CTs eventually revealed a type Ib (distal) endoleak secondary to aortic dilation at the distal landing zone (Fig. 7.19, left panel, arrows). This had previously not been aneurysmal. The distal descending thoracic aorta was funnel shaped to the point of the celiac artery, but 1.5–2 cm above it was relatively non-aneurysmal. She successfully underwent a secondary endovascular procedure to extend the distal landing zone with a covered stent down to the level of the celiac (Figs 7.20 and 7.21).

Outcomes

As with conventional thoracic endovascular aortic surgery, there are no prospective clinical trials comparing hybrid endovascular aortic with contemporary open repairs. The safety and efficacy of the hybrid approach has been demonstrated by several small case series from single expert centers. Although hybrid repairs are technically feasible and offer potential advantages over conventional open repairs, the collective experience has yet to definitively demonstrate superiority.

Table 7.2 summarizes the outcomes from recent series of staged hybrid repairs and two-stage and frozen elephant trunk repairs. Overall, technical success is approximately 100%. Thirty-day mortality ranges from 0% to 20% for both aortic debranching and staged hybrid procedures. The rates of myocardial infarction, stroke, and paraplegia are lower than those for reported for open repair.

Endovascular repair is associated with fewer procedure-related complications such as blood transfusions, neurologic complications, and shorter postoperative hospital stays, compared with open repair [7]. Whether the same is true for hybrid repairs remains an open question. Hughes et al. [44] report no incidence of death or stroke, however one patient developed permanent paralysis (4%) at 30 days post-hybrid repair for arch

(a)

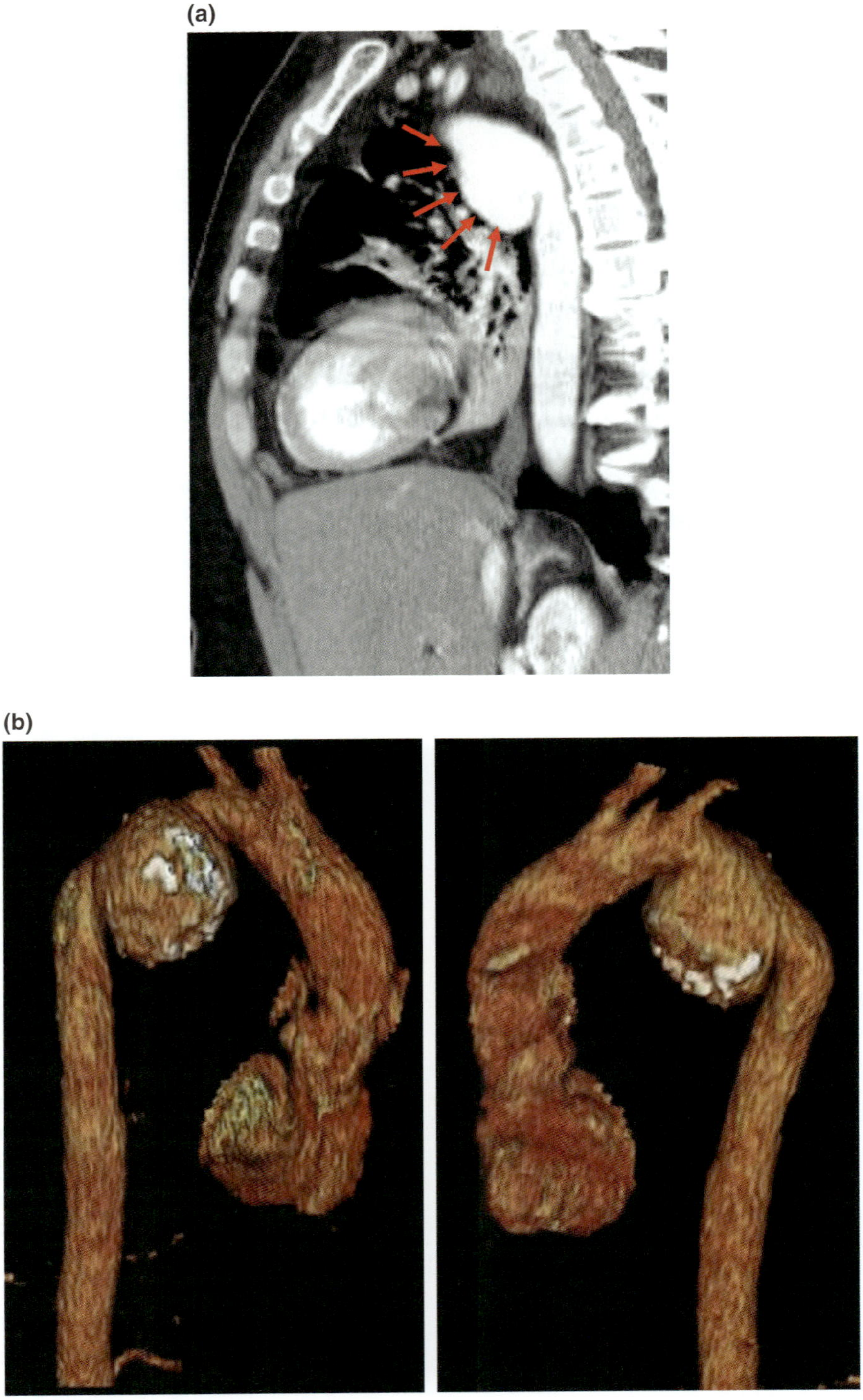

Fig. 7.13 Case 2: preoperative imaging. (a) On CT, arrows highlight a 4.6 cm aortic pseudoaneurysm. (b) 3D reconstruction demonstrating a discrete aortic pseudoaneurysm seen opposite the left subclavian artery at the level of the ligamentum arteriosum (left-sided view).

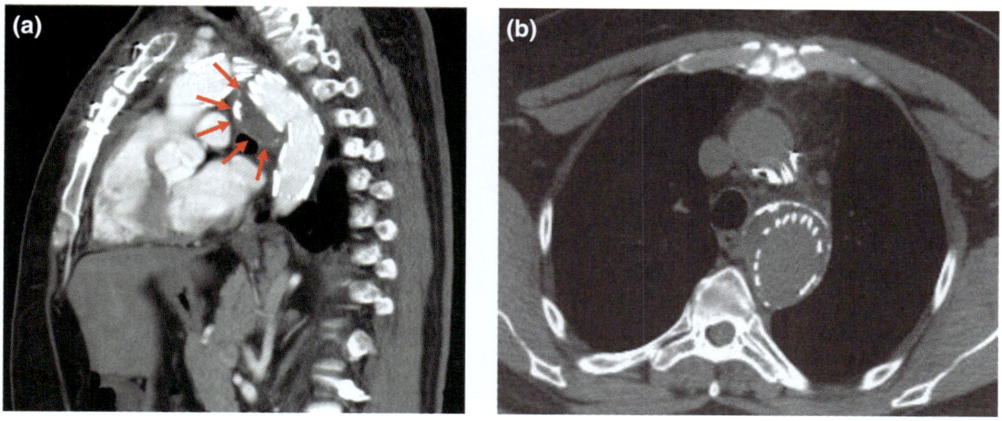

Fig. 7.14 Case 2: postoperative imaging. Complete stent-graft coverage of the pseudoaneurysm is confirmed by CT.

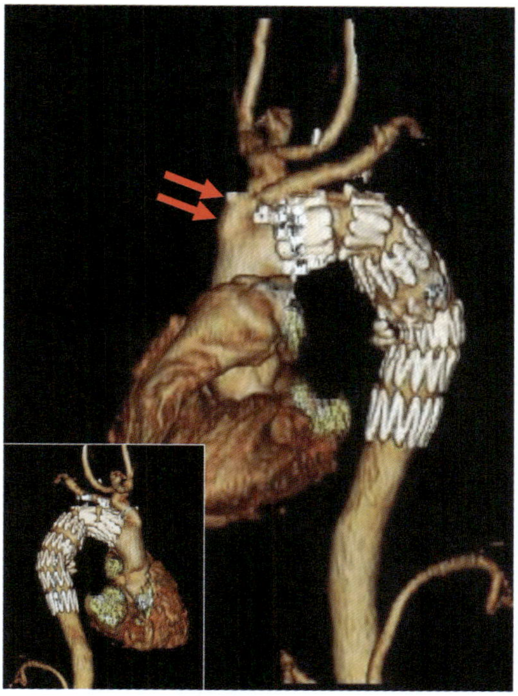

Fig. 7.15 Case 2: follow-up imaging. 3D reconstruction demonstrating a stent-graft in the correct location with bypass from the ascending aorta to bilateral carotid and subclavian arteries (arrows) and almost complete resolution of the pseudoaneurysm.

aneurysm. Xydas et al. [45] report shorter bypass and cross-clamp times and lack of need for DHCA with hybrid repair using a branched aortic graft and carotid–subclavian bypass for total arch replacement. Murphy et al. [46] show fewer days on mechanical ventilation, likely owing to lower sternotomy rates. In a series of 44 high-risk endovascular cases, of which 34 underwent debranching, the survival at 30 months was 70% [10].

Outcomes following staged and frozen elephant trunk repair from single center experiences demonstrates acceptable early and midterm outcomes. Karck and Kamiya [32] reviewed eight series with 215 patients and reported an overall 7% mortality, which is comparable to the gold standard repair. In a large single center experience, Uchida et al. [37] performed frozen elephant trunk repairs in 156 patients and found 1-, 5- and 10-year mortalities of 99.3%, 86.5% and 74.9%, respectively. Greenberg et al. [47] reported a 30-day mortality of 4.5% in a small series. Kim et al. [33] reported 18 patients who underwent second-stage TEVAR completion with no differences in mortality and, as expected, TEVAR patients had lower second-stage hospital stays, lower rates of transfusion, and lower renal impairment. Similarly, a series of 34 patients demonstrated 6% in-hospital mortality and spinal cord ischemia in 9% of patients [48]. Kawaharada et al. [49] demonstrated 6.4% and 26.7% mortality for frozen elephant trunk repair at 1 and 60 months, respectively.

Complications

Despite the excitement surrounding endovascular repair and hybrid endovascular repair for thoracic

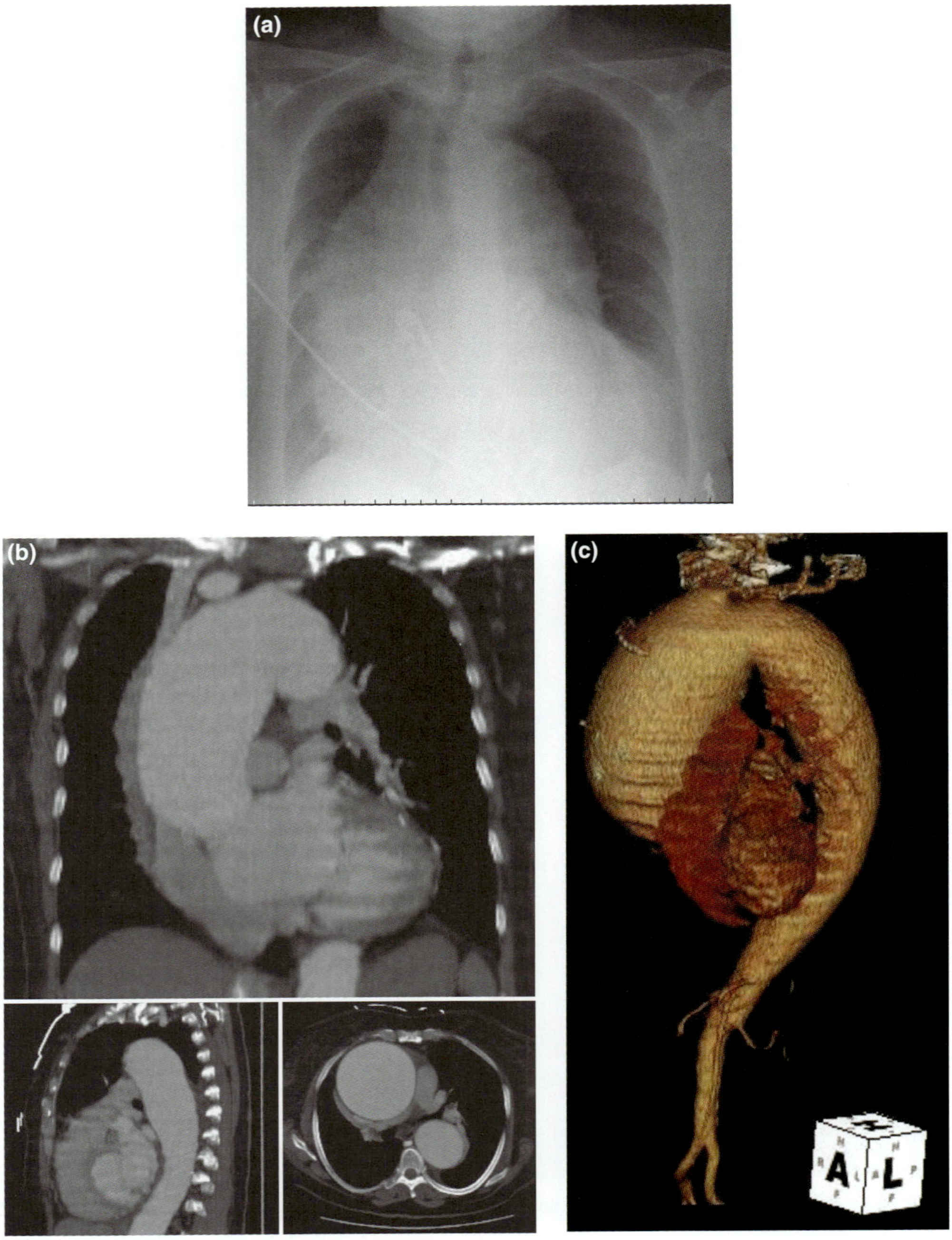

Fig. 7.16 Case 3: preoperative imaging. (a) CXR demonstrating a grossly enlarged aortic silhouette. (b) CT views demonstrating a total thoracic arch aneurysm with a 10 cm massive ascending segment. (c) Preoperative 3D reconstruction showing the complete view of a total thoracic arch aneurysm.

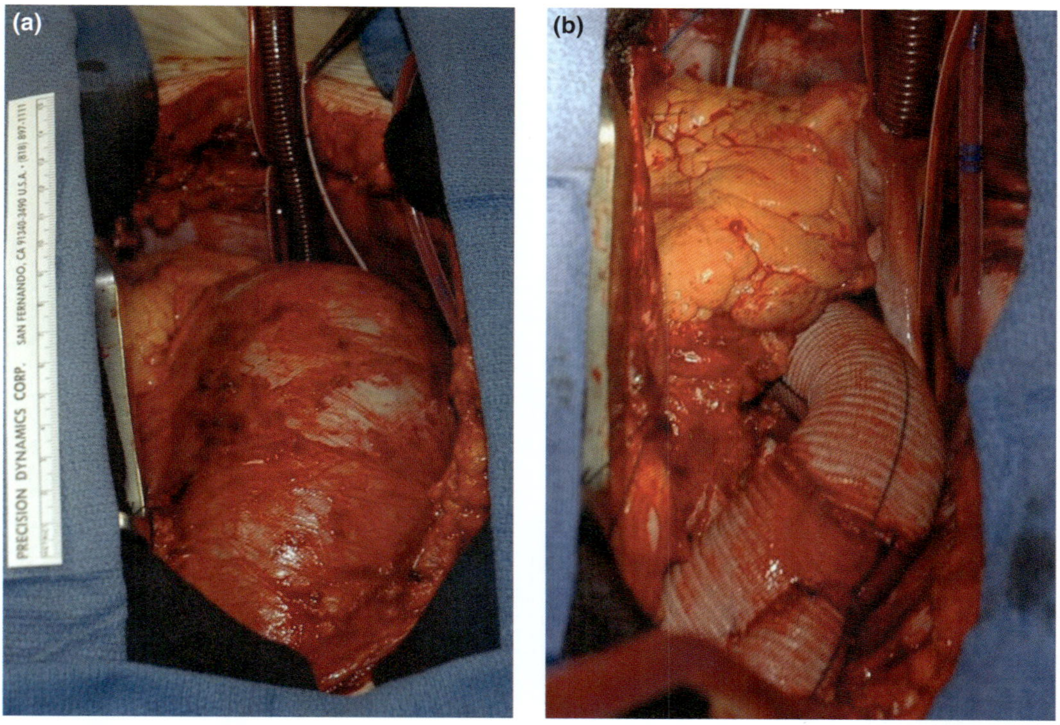

Fig. 7.17 Case 3: intraoperative images. Massive ascending aorta (a) and aortic arch replacement (b).

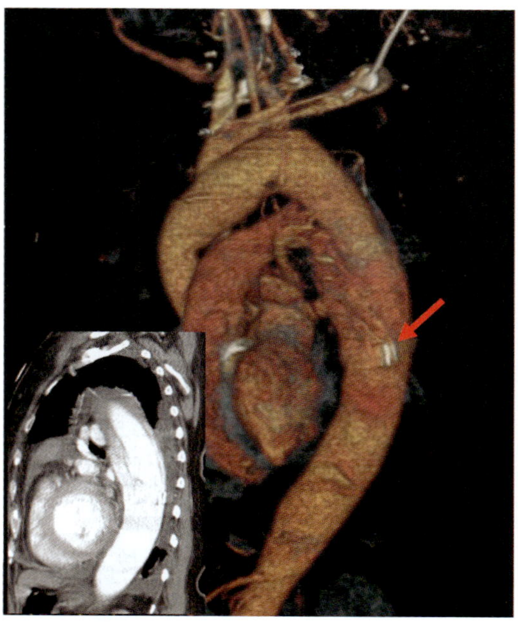

Fig. 7.18 Case 3: post aortic arch replacement with elephant trunk. CT and 3D reconstruction of the aortic arch and elephant trunk graft with clips marking the distal end (arrow).

Box 7.1 Complications from endovascular and hybrid endovascular repair of thoracic aortic disease

- Endoleaks I–IV
- Graft collapse
- Graft migration
- Retrograde aortic dissection
- Aortic rupture (stent strut)
- Access complications:
  - iliac rupture
  - iliac dissection
- Reintervention
- Branch vessel complications:
  - occlusion
  - injury
  - malperfusion

aortic pathology, this new technology is beset with a new set of complications (Box 7.1). A few important complications deserve brief mention here.

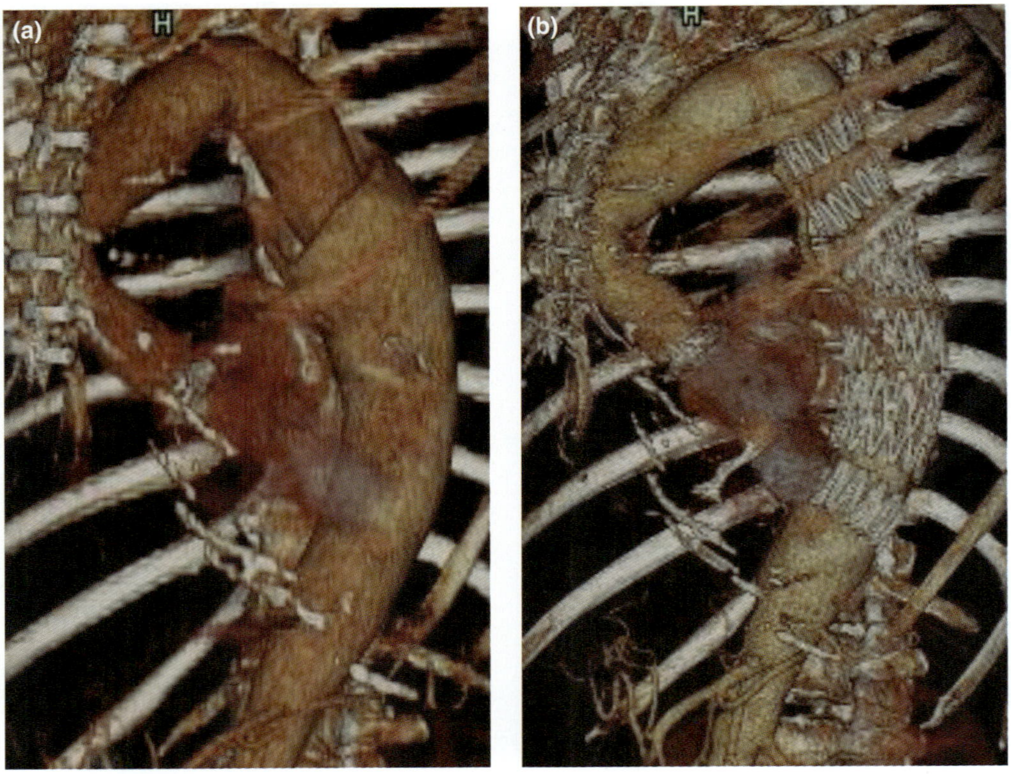

Fig. 7.19 Case 3: 3D reconstruction of pre (a) and post (b) endovascular completion by stent-graft deployment into the elephant trunk.

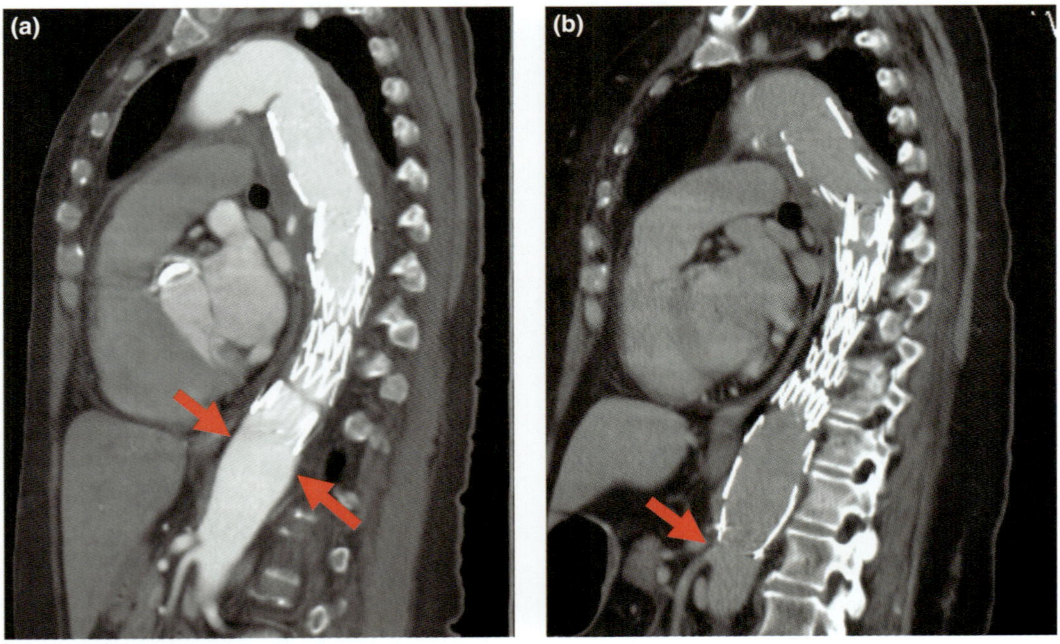

Fig. 7.20 Case 3: post staged elephant trunk repair. (a) CT imaging demonstrating an enlarged descending aorta distal to the endovascular graft (arrows) with a type Ib endoleak (endoleak not shown). (b) Additional stent deployment just proximal to the celiac artery (arrow).

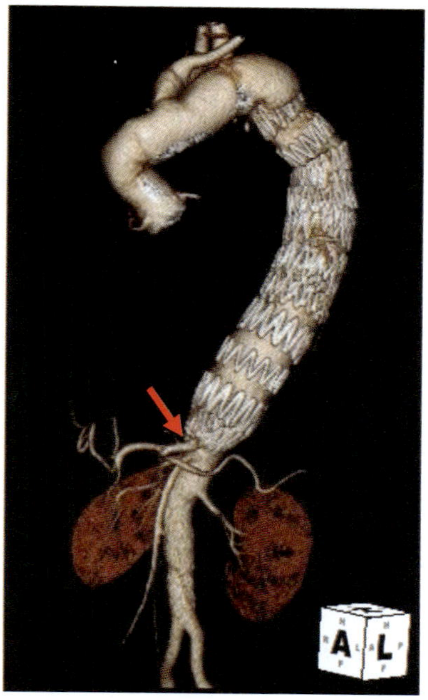

Fig. 7.21 Case 3: final imaging. 3D reconstruction demonstrating aortic arch reconstruction, elephant trunk, and endovascular completion using two grafts, just proximal to the celiac artery (arrow).

Endoleaks

Endoleaks are defined as persistent blood flow into the aneurysmal sac around the graft from patent collateral arteries, graft tears or at sites of graft-to-graft overlap [50,51]. Endoleaks may result from poor graft placement or sizing, graft fatigue, displacement, distortion or dilation of the native aorta at either the proximal or distal landing zones. Endoleaks are primarily diagnosed radiolographically. They are classified into types I–IV, depending on the underlying cause. Types I and II are the most commonly observed endoleaks. Canaud et al. [10] observed seven cases of endoleak in 44 (16%) endovascular cases, six of which were types I and II.

Untreated type I endoleaks are associated with adverse outcomes and generally require a secondary procedure, either open or endovascular to prevent aortic rupture [28]. This results from incomplete seal at the proximal (Ia) or distal (Ib) landing zones. Early filling of the aneurysm sac at the proximal or distal sites may be diagnosed by aortography during the initial procedure, however most are diagnosed by follow-up CT. Type I endoleaks may be treated conservatively, percutaneously, or with open

Table 7.2 Review of outcomes of hybrid thoracic endovascular repairs.

Debranching	*Author*	*Year*	*N*	*Technical success, N (%)*	*30-day mortality*	*MI, N (%)*	*TIA/CVA, N (%)*
	Younes et al. [31]	2010	35	35 (100%)	2 (5%)	1 (9%)	8 (23%)
	Canaud et al. [10]	2010	44	43 (98%)	9 (20%)	1 (2%)	3 (7%)
	Hughes et al. [44]	2009	21	21 (100%)	0 (0%)	0 (0%)	1 (4%)
	Szeto et al. [25]	2007	8	8 (100%)	1 (13%)	1 (%)	2 (%)
	Czerny et al. [15]	2006	11	11 (100%)	0 (0%)	0 (0%)	0 (0%)
	Bergeron et al. [16]	2006	25	25 (100%)	2 (8%)	0 (0%)	1 (4%)
Two-stage and frozen elephant trunk	*Author*	*Year*	*N*	*Technical success, N (%)*	*30-day mortality*	*Paraplegia, N (%)*	*TIA/CVA, N (%)*
	Uchida et al. [37]	2010	156	58 (100%)	0 (0%)	3 (2.0%)	4 (2.6%)
	Di Bartolemeo et al. [48]	2009	34	34 (100%)	1 (3%)	3 (9%)	0 (0%)
	Kim et al. [33]	2009	24	24 (100%)	4 (17%)	1 (4%)	2 (8%)
	Kawaharada et al. [49]	2009	31	31 (100%)	1 (3%)	2 (7%)	1 (3%)
	Baraki et al. [53]	2007	39	38 (97%)	5 (13%)	0 (0%)	5 (13%)
	Liu et al. [54]	2006	60	57 (95%)	1 (2%)	1 (2%)	3 (6%)
	Flores et al. [55]	2006	25	25 (100%)	3 (12%)	6 (24%)	4 (16%)
	Greenberg et al. [47]	2005	22	22 (100%)	1 (5%)	0 (0%)	0 (0%)

CVA, cerebrovascular accident; MI, myocardial infarction; TIA, transient ischemic attack.

revision. Several authors have reported resolution of type I endoleaks by 6 months with conservative management and serial imaging [15,16,26,27]. Persistent type I endoleaks may be initially treated by profile ballooning with a semi-compliant balloon to ensure complete apposition of the stent-graft with the aortic wall. If this is unsuccessful, the proximal or distal landing zone may be extended with additional stent-grafts. In some cases, extra-anatomic bypasses may be required to achieve the necessary additional landing zone.

Type II endoleaks occur secondary to retrograde filling from branch vessels. On CT, the aneurysm sac fills but does not communicate with either the proximal or distal graft edge. In some cases, it may be very difficult to distinguish between a type I or type II endoleak. Type II endoleaks are associated with a more benign natural history compared with type I endoleaks, and may initially be managed conservatively with close CT follow-up. If progressive aneurysm sac dilation occurs during follow-up, we would advise treatment to occlude the feeding artery. In the case of a type II endoleak from a patent left subclavian artery, embolization coils or an Amplatzer occluder (AGA Medical Corp., Plymouth, MN) may be deployed at the origin of the artery.

Types III and IV are less common and represent graft leaks as a result of graft disruption or in the absence of obvious disruption, respectively. Type IIIa and IIIb result from a disruption or hole in the graft, respectively, and are of concern as they may result in an acute increase in aneurysm pressure. They may be treated with coverage using another stent-graft. Type IV endoleaks are mostly historical in nature. It occurs due to porosity of early graft material and is treated conservatively.

Paraplegia

Endovascular repair may be associated with higher levels of spinal cord ischemia and paraplegia due to exclusion of the spinal arteries. CSF drainage likely lowers the incidence of this complication. The overall incidence is about 3.3% according to a review of published reports [32]. Recent reports with staged and frozen elephant trunk procedures, where paraplegia rates are higher due to the long segment of thoracic aorta covered, report an incidence between 0% and 9%, with one series reporting up to a 24% incidence (see Table 7.2).

Stroke

Cerebrovascular accident rates are generally acceptable with hybrid TEVAR, however the incidence reported in the literature varies widely at 0–23% in recent series (see Table 7.2).

Contrast-enhanced imaging

Post-hybrid endovascular repair requires regular contrast-enhanced imaging. Despite renal protection strategies such as the use of hydration, mannitol, or sodium bicarbonate, the liberal use of contrast dye may lead to renal injury. Those with pre-existing renal insufficiency or diabetes are at particular risk.

Other complications

Other complications include retrograde aortic dissections which occur in about 1–2% of proximal hybrid repairs as a result of aortic injury during stent deployment [52].

On the horizon

The success of hybrid thoracic aortic procedures has catapulted enthusiasm for further device development, that may ultimately provide for a fully endovascular solution to these challenging clinical problems. Custom-designed branched grafts that may preclude the need for branch vessel rerouting are currently being developed and tested (Fig. 7.22). Cook has developed several branched grafts for the aortic arch. The first generation included a bifurcated first component that was inserted through a side graft sewn onto the innominate artery, with one limb extending into the innominate artery, and a second shorter and wider limb in the mid-arch; the proximal portion of this graft landed in the proximal to mid ascending aorta (Fig. 7.23). The second component consisted of a proximal Zenith TX2 stent-graft that docked with the shorter limb of the first graft to complete the arch replacement. This type of hybrid arch replacement also required a pre-procedural carotid-to-carotid bypass; however it obviated

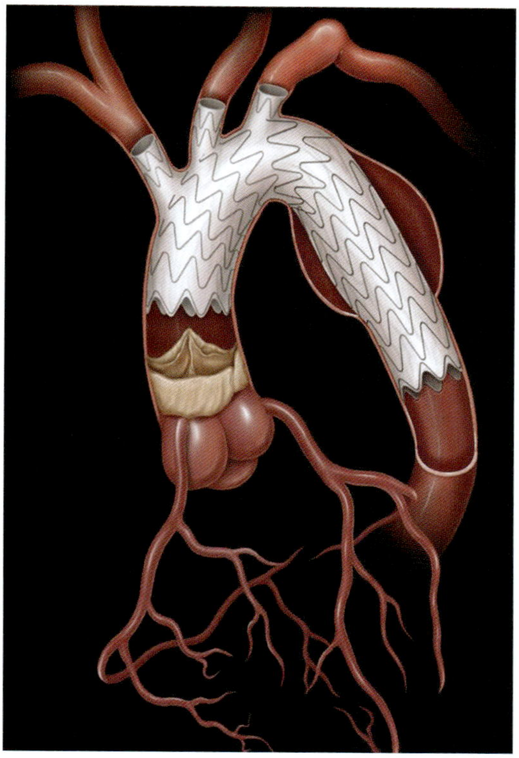

Figure 7.22 Branched arch endograft for exclusion of arch aneurysms.

the need for a sternotomy. Cook has subsequently developed several second and third generation arch grafts, with the latest iteration containing several internal branches designed to support covered stents that extend into the innominate and left carotid arteries and do not require extensive extra-anatomic bypasses, with the exception of a left carotid–subclavian bypass.

Conclusions

Since the deployment of the first endovascular stent-graft in 1994, the field of hybrid thoracic aortic surgery has made great strides forward and is rapidly becoming part of the surgical mainstream [5]. Pioneering endovascular teams around the world have advanced the application of this technology beyond the initial indications to an array of thoracic aortic pathologies. Several clinical series demonstrate impressive support of the therapeutic promise of hybrid TEVAR. These encouraging early results, as well as advances in stent-graft design, promise to expand the application of complex hybrid endovascular therapies for patients with challenging aortic arch pathology.

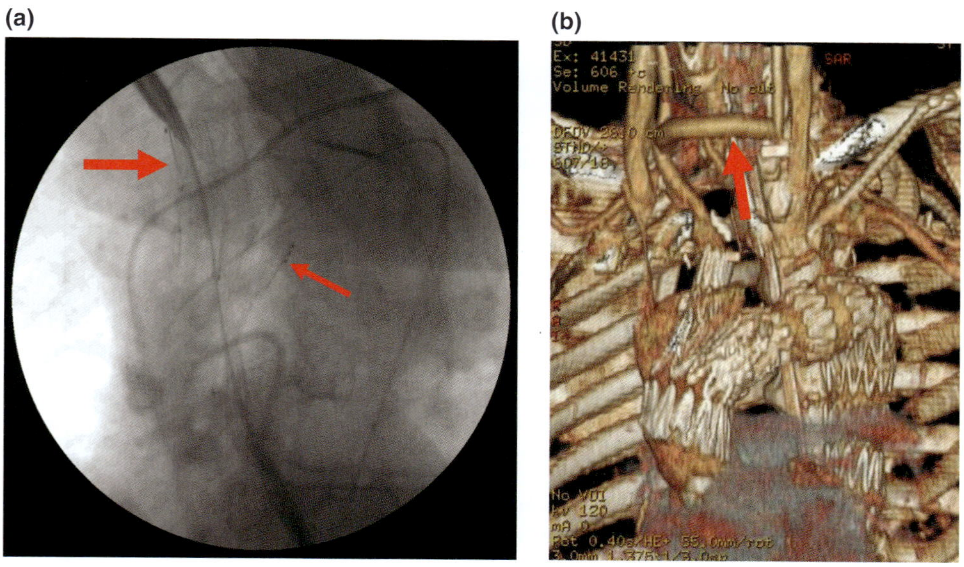

Figure 7.23 (a) Fluoroscopic image demonstrating the proximal portion of a branched ascending and arch graft with a wire from the innominate artery through the innominate limb of the graft (heavy arrow), as well as from the femoral artery through the short, wide mid-arch limb of the graft (thin arrow). (b) Postoperative 3D reconstruction demonstrating the ascending and arch graft with a limb into the innominate artery, as well as a carotid–carotid bypass (arrow).

References

1 Spielvogel D, Etz CD, Silovitz D, et al. Aortic arch replacement with a trifurcated graft. Ann Thorac Surg 2007;83(2):S791–5; discussion S824–31.

2 Coselli JS, Bozinovski J, LeMaire SA. Open surgical repair of 2286 thoracoabdominal aortic aneurysms. Ann Thorac Surg 2007;83(2):S862–4; discussion S90–2.

3 Estrera AL, Miller CC, 3rd, Madisetty J, et al. Ascending and transverse aortic arch repair: the impact of glomerular filtration rate on mortality. Ann Surg 2008;247(3):524–9.

4 Kazui T, Yamashita K, Washiyama N, et al. Aortic arch replacement using selective cerebral perfusion. Ann Thorac Surg 2007; 83(2):S796–8; discussion S824–31.

5 Dake MD, Miller DC, Semba CP, et al. Transluminal placement of endovascular stent-grafts for the treatment of descending thoracic aortic aneurysms. N Engl J Med 1994;331(26):1729–34.

6 Makaroun MS, Dillavou ED, Kee ST, et al. Endovascular treatment of thoracic aortic aneurysms: results of the phase II multicenter trial of the GORE TAG thoracic endoprosthesis. J Vasc Surg 2005;41(1):1–9.

7 Bavaria JE, Appoo JJ, Makaroun MS, et al. Endovascular stent grafting versus open surgical repair of descending thoracic aortic aneurysms in low-risk patients: a multicenter comparative trial. J Thorac Cardiovasc Surg 2007;133(2):369–77.

8 Peterson MD, Wheatley GH, 3rd, Kpodonu J, et al. Treatment of type II endoleaks associated with left subclavian artery coverage during thoracic aortic stent grafting. J Thorac Cardiovasc Surg 2008;136(5): 1193–9.

9 Stone DH, Brewster DC, Kwolek CJ, et al. Stent-graft versus open-surgical repair of the thoracic aorta: mid-term results. J Vasc Surg 2006;44(6):1188–97.

10 Canaud L, Hireche K, Berthet JP, et al. Endovascular repair of aortic arch lesions in high-risk patients or after previous aortic surgery: midterm results. J Thorac Cardiovasc Surg 2010;140(1):52–8.

11 Wheatley GH, 3rd, Koullias GJ, Rodriguez-Lopez JA, et al. Is endovascular repair the new gold standard for primary adult coarctation? Eur J Cardiothorac Surg 2010;38(3):305–10.

12 Jonker FH, Heijmen R, Trimarchi S, et al. Acute management of aortobronchial and aortoesophageal fistulas using thoracic endovascular aortic repair. J Vasc Surg 2009;50(5):999–1004.

13 Cheng D, Martin J, Shennib H, et al. Endovascular aortic repair versus open surgical repair for descending thoracic aortic disease a systematic review and meta-analysis of comparative studies. J Am Coll Cardiol 2010;55(10):986–1001.

14 Gottardi R, Lammer J, Grimm M, et al. Entire rerouting of the supraaortic branches for endovascular stent-graft placement of an aortic arch aneurysm. Eur J Cardiothorac Surg 2006;29(2):258–60.

15 Czerny M, Gottardi R, Zimpfer D, et al. Transposition of the supraaortic branches for extended endovascular arch repair. Eur J Cardiothorac Surg 2006;29(5):709–13.

16 Bergeron P, Mangialardi N, Costa P, et al. Great vessel management for endovascular exclusion of aortic arch aneurysms and dissections. Eur J Vasc Endovasc Surg 2006;32(1):38–45.

17 Kato M, Ohnishi K, Kaneko M, et al. New graft-implanting method for thoracic aortic aneurysm or dissection with a stented graft. Circulation 1996;94(9 Suppl):II188–93.

18 Usui A, Fujimoto K, Ishiguchi T, et al. Cerebrospinal dysfunction after endovascular stent-grafting via a median sternotomy: the frozen elephant trunk procedure. Ann Thorac Surg 2002;74(5):S1821–4; discussion S5–32.

19 Suto Y, Yasuda K, Shiiya N, et al. Stented elephant trunk procedure for an extensive aneurysm involving distal aortic arch and descending aorta. J Thorac Cardiovasc Surg 1996;112(5):1389–90.

20 Rousseau H, Dambrin C, Marcheix B, et al. Acute traumatic aortic rupture: a comparison of surgical and stent-graft repair. J Thorac Cardiovasc Surg 2005;129(5):1050–5.

21 Ryu YG, Choo SJ, Lim JY, et al. Hybrid procedure for a traumatic aortic rupture consisting of endovascular repair and minimally invasive arch vessel transposition without sternotomy. J Korean Med Sci 2010;25(1):142–4.

22 Morgan R, Loosemore T, Belli AM. Endovascular repair of contained rupture of the thoracic aorta. Cardiovasc Intervent Radiol 2002;25(4):291–4.

23 Wellons ED, Milner R, Solis M, et al. Stent-graft repair of traumatic thoracic aortic disruptions. J Vasc Surg 2004;40(6):1095–100.

24 Ishimaru S. Endografting of the aortic arch. J Endovasc Ther 2004;11(Suppl 2):II62–71.

25 Szeto WY, Bavaria JE, Bowen FW, et al. The hybrid total arch repair: brachiocephalic bypass and concomitant endovascular aortic arch stent graft placement. J Card Surg 2007;22(2):97–102; discussion 3–4.

26 Melissano G, Civilini E, Bertoglio L, et al. Results of endografting of the aortic arch in different landing zones. Eur J Vasc Endovasc Surg 2007; 33(5):561–6.

27 Zhou W, Reardon M, Peden EK, et al. Hybrid approach to complex thoracic aortic aneurysms in high-risk patients: surgical challenges and clinical outcomes. J Vasc Surg 2006;44(4):688–93.

28 Criado FJ, Abul-Khoudoud OR, Domer GS, et al. Endovascular repair of the thoracic aorta: lessons learned. Ann Thorac Surg 2005;80(3):857–63; discussion 63.

29 Peterson BG, Eskandari MK, Gleason TG, et al. Utility of left subclavian artery revascularization in association with endoluminal repair of acute and chronic thoracic aortic pathology. J Vasc Surg 2006;43(3):433–9.

30 Gorich J, Asquan Y, Seifarth H, et al. Initial experience with intentional stent-graft coverage of the subclavian artery during endovascular thoracic aortic repairs. J Endovasc Ther 2002;9(Suppl 2):II39–43.

31 Younes HK, Davies MG, Bismuth J, et al. Hybrid thoracic endovascular aortic repair: pushing the envelope. J Vasc Surg 2010;51(1):259–66.

32 Karck M, Kamiya H. Progress of the treatment for extended aortic aneurysms; is the frozen elephant trunk technique the next standard in the treatment of complex aortic disease including the arch? Eur J Cardiothorac Surg 2008;33(6):1007–13.

33 Kim T, Martin TD, Lee WA, et al. Evolution in the management of the total thoracic aorta. J Thorac Cardiovasc Surg 2009;137(3):627–34.

34 Borst HG, Walterbusch G, Schaps D. Extensive aortic replacement using "elephant trunk" prosthesis. Thorac Cardiovasc Surg 1983;31(1):37–40.

35 Safi HJ, Miller CC, 3rd, Estrera AL, et al. Staged repair of extensive aortic aneurysms: long-term experience with the elephant trunk technique. Ann Surg 2004;240(4):677–84; discussion 84–5.

36 Estrera AL, Miller CC, 3rd, Porat EE, et al. Staged repair of extensive aortic aneurysms. Ann Thorac Surg 2002;74(5):S1803–5; discussion S25–32.

37 Uchida N, Katayama A, Tamura K, et al. Long-term results of the frozen elephant trunk technique for extended aortic arch disease. Eur J Cardiothorac Surg 2010;37(6):1338–45.

38 Usui A, Ueda Y, Watanabe T, et al. Clinical results of implantation of an endovascular covered stent-graft via midsternotomy for distal aortic arch aneurysm. Cardiovasc Surg 2000;8(7):545–9.

39 Karck M, Chavan A, Hagl C, et al. The frozen elephant trunk technique: a new treatment for thoracic aortic aneurysms. J Thorac Cardiovasc Surg 2003; 125(6):1550–3.

40 Jakob H, Tsagakis K, Leyh R, et al. Development of an integrated stent graft-dacron prosthesis for intended one-stage repair in complex thoracic aortic disease. Herz 2005;30(8):766–8.

41 Schoenhoff FS, Schmidli J, Eckstein FS, et al. The frozen elephant trunk: an interesting hybrid endovascular-surgical technique to treat complex pathologies of the thoracic aorta. J Vasc Surg 2007; 45(3):597–9.

42 Spielvogel D, Strauch JT, Minanov OP, et al. Aortic arch replacement using a trifurcated graft and selective cerebral antegrade perfusion. Ann Thorac Surg 2002; 74(5):S1810–14; discussion S25–32.

43 Usui A, Tajima K, Nishikimi N, et al. Implantation of an endovascular covered stent-graft for distal aortic arch aneurysm via midsternotomy under pigtail catheter guidance. Eur J Cardiothorac Surg 1999;16(3):356–8.

44 Hughes GC, Daneshmand MA, Balsara KR, et al. "Hybrid" repair of aneurysms of the transverse aortic arch: midterm results. Ann Thorac Surg 2009;88(6):1882–7; discussion 7–8.

45 Xydas S, Wei B, Takayama H, et al. Use of carotid-subclavian arterial bypass and thoracic endovascular aortic repair to minimize cerebral ischemia in total aortic arch reconstruction. J Thorac Cardiovasc Surg 2010;139(3): 717–22; discussion 22.

46 Murphy EH, Beck AW, Clagett GP, et al. Combined aortic debranching and thoracic endovascular aneurysm repair (TEVAR) effective but at a cost. Arch Surg 2009;144(3):222–7.

47 Greenberg RK, Haddad F, Svensson L, et al. Hybrid approaches to thoracic aortic aneurysms: the role of endovascular elephant trunk completion. Circulation 2005;112(17):2619–26.

48 Di Bartolomeo R, Di Marco L, Armaro A, et al. Treatment of complex disease of the thoracic aorta: the frozen elephant trunk technique with the E-vita open prosthesis. Eur J Cardiothorac Surg 2009;35(4):671–5; discussion 5–6.

49 Kawaharada N, Kurimoto Y, Ito T, et al. Hybrid treatment for aortic arch and proximal descending thoracic aneurysm: experience with stent grafting for second-stage elephant trunk repair. Eur J Cardiothorac Surg 2009;36(6):956–61.

50 White GH, Yu W, May J. Endoleak – a proposed new terminology to describe incomplete aneurysm exclusion by an endoluminal graft. J Endovasc Surg 1996;3(1):124–5.

51 Pamler RS, Kotsis T, Gorich J, et al. Complications after endovascular repair of type B aortic dissection. J Endovasc Ther 2002;9(6):822–8.

52 Kpodonu J, Preventza O, Ramaiah VG, et al. Retrograde type A dissection after endovascular stenting of the descending thoracic aorta. Is the risk real? Eur J Cardiothorac Surg 2008;33(6):1014–18.

53 Baraki H, Hagl C, Khaladj N, et al. The frozen elephant trunk technique for treatment of thoracic aortic aneurysms. Ann Thorac Surg 2007;83(2):S819–23; discussion S24–31.

54 Liu ZG, Sun LZ, Chang Q, et al. Should the "elephant trunk" be skeletonized? Total arch replacement combined with stented elephant trunk implantation for Stanford type A aortic dissection. J Thorac Cardiovasc Surg 2006;131(1):107–13.

55 Flores J, Kunihara T, Shiiya N, et al. Extensive deployment of the stented elephant trunk is associated with an increased risk of spinal cord injury. J Thorac Cardiovasc Surg 2006;131(2):336–42.

8

CHAPTER 8

Acute aortic dissection

Ricardo Aun
Universidade de São Paulo, Hospital Albert Einstein, São Paulo, Brazil

Introduction

Acute aortic dissection, aortic intramural hematoma, and penetrating aortic ulcer are components of acute aortic syndrome. These events have similar clinical and epidemiologic aspects, and may also represent different stages of the same pathologic process [1].

Aortic dissection results from a tear in the intimal lining of the aortic wall, followed by blood entering between the intima and the media, usually taking a distal course resulting in a new lumen in the aorta. The true lumen is circumscribed by the intimal layer. The false lumen is circumscribed by both the intima and the media layers. Ordinarily, the blood flow is slower in the false lumen than in the true lumen [2,3].

Usually, aortic dissection extends until it reaches an important arterial branch, whether it affects it or not. As the blood flows, another intimal tear can occur and communicate within the two lumen ("re-entry"). Aortic dissection generally starts at certain points:

- Ascending aorta
- 2–3 cm above coronary artery ostia (65% of all cases).
- Descending aorta
- immediately after the left subclavian artery emergence (25%).
- Aortic arch and abdominal aorta (5–10% of all cases).

Aortic dissection frequently assumes a spiral aspect and the false lumen is wider than the true lumen.

Classification

Acute aortic dissections are defined as dissections that have been diagnosed up to 2 weeks after onset of symptoms. When diagnosed after a 2-weeks period they are called chronic dissections. Despite being arbitrary, this is the period when immediate and life-threatening complications happen [2–4]. The two most accepted classifications are those of De Bakey and Stanford [3,4].

According to De Bakey's system, aortic dissections are separated in to:

- Type I: originates in the ascending aorta, and propagates to the aortic arch and descending aorta.
- Type II: confined to the ascending aorta.
- Type III: originates in and is confined to the descending aorta.

Stanford's classification is easier and more popular. It is divided in two groups:

- Type A: affects the ascending aorta, and may or not affect the rest of the aorta.
- Type B: does not affect the ascending aorta (Fig. 8.1).

Epidemiology

Aortic dissections are the most common emergencies related to the aorta. It occurs two or three times more frequently than aortic aneurysm rupture. Actual incidence of aortic dissections is hard to predict, mainly because of high mortality before patients could get to a hospital. Some population

Endovascular and Hybrid Therapies for Structural Heart and Aortic Disease, First Edition.
Edited by Jacques Kpodonu and Raoul Bonan.

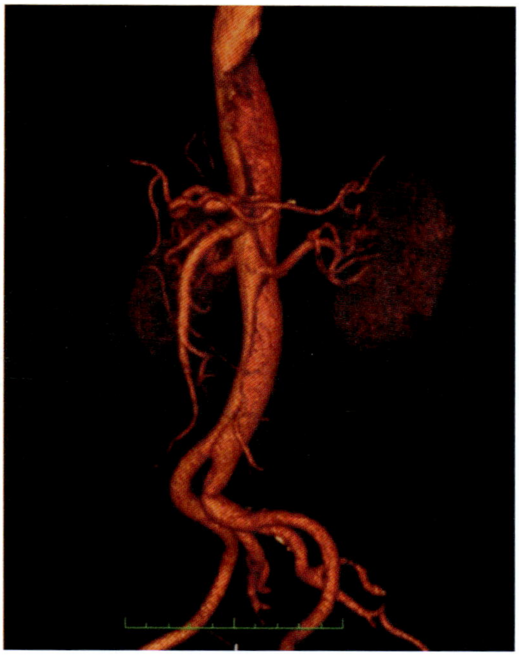

Fig. 8.1 Acute dissection with thrombosis of a proximal false lumen with sternosis of the true lumen causing abdominal distention, pain, and renal failure.

studies estimate the incidence at 0.5–3.5 cases per 100,000 individuals per year [2,5,6].

Aortic dissections occur more frequently in people of African descent than in Caucasians and are much rarer in Asians; 75% of cases are in people aged between 40 and 70 years. There is a peak of incidence of type A dissections from 50 to 60 years, and for type B dissections from 60 to 70 years of age. It is also more common in men (2–5 times). Affected men are usually younger than women (median age of 63 for men and 69 for women). Type A dissections represent 60% of all cases [6].

Morbidity and mortality

Aortic dissection has an extremely high lethality rate. According to population studies, 21% of patients with aortic dissection died before being admitted to a hospital. When admitted to a hospital, without treatment, the mortality rate is 22.7% in the first 6 hours, 50% in 24 hours, and 68% during the first week [1,6,7].

Once the ascending aorta is involved the mortality is related to complications like cardiac tamponade, acute aortic insufficiency, and involvement of the ostia of coronary arteries. If there is no involvement of the ascending aorta, the main causes of death are visceral artery obstruction, iliac artery obstruction, and aortic rupture [8].

An analysis of the results of current therapy has been given in the International Registry of Acute Aortic Dissection (IRAD) study. Looking at 464 patients in 12 centers between 1996 and 1998, global mortality was 27.4%. In patients with type A dissections, submitted to surgical treatment, the mortality rate was 26% against 58% in clinically treated patients, and aortic rupture was the main cause of death (41.5%). Patients with type B dissections and clinical treatment had a mortality rate of 10.7%. A mortality rate of 31.4% was found in complicated type B dissections when surgical treatment was needed [6].

Pathogenesis

Despite the extensive literature on aortic dissection, its etiology, for various reasons, remains poorly understood [9]. Histologic changes found in dissected aortas show a correlation with age and may represent the normal aging process for the aorta. The same histologic pattern found in the aorta of normal elderly subjects showed that none of the histologic changes observed can be considered as a specific structural change responsible for the development of aortic dissection [10]. These changes are: fragmentation of elastin, fibrosis, defined as an increase in collagen, and necrosis of the middle layer, defined as areas with apparent loss of nuclei. They are identified in histologic studies of the dilated aorta, in dissected and even in normal aortas of the elderly [11,12].

All mechanisms of weakening of the aortic media layer through microapoplexia of the vessel wall seem to lead to more stress, which can induce aortic dilation and aneurysm formation or an acute aortic syndrome. Therefore, it seems to be that histologic changes are not specific, but are due to general hemodynamic events occurring within the aorta [1].

In this context, individuals with a dilated ascending aorta, with a known altered hemodynamic profile, were compared with aortic dissection and subjects with Marfan's syndrome, a condition that predisposes to aortic dissection. Only quantitative histologic differences were found between the normal aorta of "aging" and the abnormal aorta. In this reading, the dissection is understood as part of a *spectrum* of lesions that have as a common denominator the process of wound repair. Thus, histologic characteristics of the dissected aorta in this context would represent the morphological substrate of this process [13].

Morphological studies of aortic dissection provide another etiology mechanism of thoracic aortic dissection. These studies have noted that the location of points in the aortic intimal injury match: (i) the entry of the false lumen, (ii) the arteries affected by the progression of the dissection through their ostia, (iii) the points of re-entry into the true lumen, (iv) the extent of dissection, and (v) rupture points of false light and multiple re-entries [14].

Poullis et al., using mathematical models to assess the shape of curvature of the aortic arch in the ascending aorta, demonstrated that the conformation of curvature is an independent risk factor in the etiology of type A dissection and aneurysm of the ascending aorta [15]. There are no morphological studies devoted to studying the association between type B dissection and morphology of the aortic arch.

Autopsy studies aiming to describe morphological features of the dissected aorta, due to advances and improvement in imaging resolution, have been replaced by studies such as angiotomography [16], transesophageal echo Doppler [17] and magnetic resonance imaging (MRI) [18].

Knowing the biomechanical aspects of each component of the arterial wall is essential for a better understanding of growth and vascular remodeling, and for the development of vascular substitutes (prosthetics, endoprothesis, stents). The stress in the aortic wall and the structural changes arising from it are the target of biomechanical studies of the aorta. The biomechanical analysis of aortic dissection takes as its premise that changes related to flow and how this interacts with the wall of the aorta are the etiology of dissection. Biomechanical studies from computer models of the aorta [19] and bovine carotid arteries [20] show that the variation of stress through the thickness of the aortic wall is not homogeneous and that stress is greater in the middle layer. These results could explain the location of the dissection in the aortic media. Other biomechanical studies using models from computed tomography (CT) scans confirm the control of risk factors traditionally associated with aortic diseases such as hypertension [21] with increased blood pressure leading to an increase in stress in the aortic wall.

Other studies in the aorta of pigs [22,23] and rats [24] were used to better understand the biomechanical aspects of the aorta, using destructive tests. Although rare in human models, such methods have been employed in some biomechanical studies of the aorta. The following tests were performed to determine the strength of aortic tissue: uniaxial tension test in the radial [25], axial and circumferential [26,27] direction, breaking stress test in circular samples of aorta and balloon inflation in the intact artery [28]. Only a few of these techniques have been employed to investigate the aortic dissection [29]. Sommer et al. propose a new method for the specific destructive biomechanical study of aortic dissection, using segments of infrarenal aorta, a segment where dissection is rare [14], and not affected by atherosclerosis, a risk factor traditionally associated with aortic dissection [30].

Uniaxial destructive biomechanical tests in aortic tissue have limitations due to the nature of the forces acting on the aorta during the cardiac cycle (radial strain, circumferential and longitudinal). However, they are easy to understand, are widely used in the field of engineering material, and allow characterization of the material. Otherwise the large number of variables makes the mathematical models and constitutive equations extremely complex, complicating the interpretation of results [31].

In a study not yet published in our Biomechanics Laboratory (Department of Vascular Surgery, University of São Paulo Medical School), we demonstrated the different behavior between the thoracic and abdominal aorta in biomechanical characteristics (Table 8.1). A detailed knowledge of aortic tissue pbtained by analyzing biomechanical, histologic, and morphological characteristics can contribute to a better understanding of aortic dissection and the development and refinement of possible vascular substitutes.

Table 8.1 Comparison between the average values of strength, tension and stress needed to break the tissue, maximum deformation, and thickness of the fragments of the thoracic and abdominal aorta.

	Thoracic aorta			*Abdominal aorta*			*T*	*P*	*P-value*
	N	*Media*	*dp*	*N*	*Media*	*dp*			
Stregth (newtons)	86	6.2746	2.024	59	4.7918	2.0696	4.29	0.000032	0.9807
Tension (newtons/mm)	86	2.0708	0.9316	59	1.4448	0.7360	4.32	0.000029	0.9816
Stress (newtons/mm$^{2)}$	86	1.7731	1.1121	59	1.3584	0.9881	2.31	0.022527	0.6170
Deformation (strain)	86	0.6823	0.3209	59	0.4750	0.2430	4.20	0.000046	0.9768
Thickness (mm)	86	1.6960	0.4824	59	1.4332	0.3571	3.56	0.000495	0.9260

While studies help describe the natural history of aortic dissection, important advances have occurred in their treatment, especially with the advent of endovascular surgery. Thus studies with medium-term follow-up demonstrate that the use of endoprotheses for the treatment of uncomplicated and complicated diseases of the descending aorta is safe, less invasive, and low risk when compared to traditional surgical approach [32–35].

Considering that the fixation of the endoprothesis is based on the graft–aortic wall, with different aspects of this interaction in early and late implantation, great attention was given to the mechanism of attachment of the stent, with improving technology of these devices (oversize, self-expanding or balloon-expandable stents, hooks, free-flow stents) [36]. The evolution of materials composing the endografts caused difficulties in understanding the behavior of a specific device model in the long term. Issues such as integration between the prosthesis and the aortic wall, morphological remodeling of aneurysms, and dissection of the aorta and endograft migration have always been highlighted as a limitation of this therapy [37].

Studies of the aortic wall in patients with aortic dissection have failed to point out the interaction between the histologic, morphological, and biomechanical aspects in etiology of aortic dissection and its implications for surgical treatment of this disease.

Box 8.1 Risk factors for acute aortic dissection.

Hypertension
- Smoking, dyslipidemia, cocaine/crack

Connective tissue diseases
- Marfan's syndrome
- Ehlers–Danlos syndrome

Hereditary vascular diseases
- Bicuspid aortic valve
- Aortic coarctation

Inflammatory diseases
- Giant cell arteritis
- Takayasu arteritis
- Behçet's disease
- Syphilis

Blunt chest trauma
Iatrogenic
- Diagnostic and therapeutic endovascular procedures
- After aortic or heart valves surgery

Risk factors

Hypertension is present in 70–80% of cases of aortic dissection, being the most prevalent risk factor for it (Box 8.1) [6,7]. Some aortic diseases are well-established risk factors: the presence of bicuspid aortic valves associated with aortic artery root dilation (7–14% of all dissections); coarctation; aortic annulus ectasia; chromosomal abnormalities (Turner's and Noonan's syndromes); hypoplasia aortic arch; arteritis; and connective tissue diseases (Marfan's and Ehlers–Danlos syndromes). Marfan's syndrome is responsible for most cases of aortic dissection in patients younger than 40 years. In women younger than 40 years, 50% of aortic dissections occur during pregnancy, generally when the diagnosis of Marfan's syndrome is established [2–4,6,9].

Intramural hematoma and penetrating aortic ulcer

The violation of the tunica intima of the aortic wall is a common feature between the aortic dissection, intramural hematoma, and penetrating aortic ulcer. Moreover, they present a similar clinical presentation to that of sudden chest pain in hypertensive patients. Both processes can be a precursor of classic dissection. Severe atherosclerotic changes are common in patients with these diseases, so that patients with a penetrating aortic ulcer tend to be older (mean age 77 years) than those with dissection [1,3].

An intramural hematoma of the thoracic aorta is characterized by an absence of intimal rupture, identifiable by radiographic means, and by the column of coagulated blood between the intima and media layers of the aortic wall, or variable length. Generally, they are more segmental that aortic dissections and do not cause occlusion of aortic branches. It postulates a rupture of the vasa vasorum or, more likely, the violation of the intima by an atherosclerotic ulcer, allowing that blood to penetrate the aortic wall [1,3,37].

Penetrating ulcers in a plaque of the aorta can cause intramural hematomas, aortic dissections, or perforation. Symptomatic atherosclerotic ulcers are deeper and involve a greater risk of rupture (up to 40% in some series); the prognosis is worse if they are located in the ascending aorta. The combination of an ulcer and intramural hematoma occurs in 90% of cases in the descending aorta. Despite the overall poor prognosis, the indication for surgery in aortic ulcers remains related to the aortic diameter, or clinical and radiologic signs of deterioration [1,3,38].

Malperfusion syndromes

Involvement of the branches of the aorta in a framework of aortic dissection can occur by different mechanisms and with varying severity, resulting in ischemia of target organs, named the malperfusion syndrome. Several studies characterize malperfusion syndromes as a complication of acute aortic dissection in approximately 25–40% of cases [8]. While carotid artery involvement is often associated with stroke, obstruction of the subclavian artery or arteries in the legs are generally well tolerated. In the IRAD study, mesenteric ischemia was responsible for 15% of deaths related to acute aortic dissection [6].

Occlusion of a branch can occur by propagation of the dissection into a branch artery, causing thrombosis or stenosis, and characterized as static obstructions. However, the main mechanism of interruption of flow in a branch artery in aortic dissection (80% of cases) is called dynamic obstruction, in which the true lumen is collapsed and unable to provide adequate volume of blood to the organs, or the flap of intimal dissection suffers prolapse into the ostium of the branch vessel. Generally, diagnostic tests and imaging are unable to quantify this type of obstruction, creating doubt and delaying diagnosis, especially in cases of visceral ischemia. The diagnosis must be established by the patient's clinical presentation, laboratory tests, and indirect signs such as the presence of a slit true lumen [8,39].

Clinical findings

The clinical manifestations of acute aortic dissections are diverse and overlap with a broad differential diagnosis, requiring a high index of suspicion to diagnose. The prevalence of coronary artery disease is 100–200 times more common then aortic dissection and its incidence in the emergency room is 0.3% in patients with chest pain [37,39]. Diagnosis of acute aortic dissections is missed on initial exam in up 38% of patients [37].

Severe chest pain is the commonest symptom in acute aortic dissection, and the majority of patients recall abrupt onset. Pain is described as "sharp," "tearing," or "ripping". Patients with type B dissection more often experience pain in the back or abdomen, although there is substantial overlap [2,40]. The localization and irradiation of pain can suggest extension of the dissection: anterior chest pain is associated with dissection of the ascending aorta; pain radiating to the neck is associated with dissection of the aortic arc; and pain to the shoulders or lumbar region relates to dissection of the descending aorta [2,40].

Syncope can complicate the clinical presentation of aortic dissection in 5–13% of cases, often indicating the development of complications such as cardiac tamponade or obstruction of cerebral vessels [6].

Hypertension is present in the initial physical examination in 70% of patients with type B dissection and in 25–35% of patients with type A, being refractory to the initial clinical therapy in more than 64% of cases [6].

A pulse deficit occurs in 30–50% of patients with involvement of the aortic arc, thoraco-abdominal segment, or both. The innominate artery is involved in 14.5% of patients, the left carotid artery in 6%, the left subclavian artery in 14.5%, and a femoral artery in 13% [6].

Symptoms of a malperfusion syndrome for the occlusion of branches of the aorta can be prominent in acute aortic dissection, but may also disguise other diagnoses: chest pain with myocardial ischemia (occlusion of coronary arteries); focal neurologic deficit or syncope (for involvement of the supra-aortic trunks); ischemia of a superior extremity; paraplegia (for occlusion of the spinal arteries); and abdominal pain (mesenteric ischemia) [6].

Peripheral nerve compression by the hematoma can rarely occur, causing Horner's syndrome, and/or dysphonia, by paresis of the left vocal cord related to compression of the recurrent laryngeal nerve.

The presence of sudden-onset chest pain, pulse deficits and mediastinal enlargement in an X-ray increases by 66 times the likelihood ratio of acute aortic dissection; however, this diagnostic triad is found in only 27% of patients. Given the polymorphism of symptoms, some population studies show that in only 28.8% of cases of aortic dissection was the diagnosis suspected on initial evaluation. Thus, a high index of suspicion and rational use of available diagnostic tests are essential for early diagnosis of aortic dissection [6].

Diagnostic tests and imaging studies

The initial evaluation of a patient with acute chest pain involves performing an electrocardiogram, which may show acute ischemic changes in about 20% of dissections of the ascending aorta. Laboratory tests are essential in the evaluation of malperfusion syndromes and associated organ dysfunction (myocardial ischemia, renal, mesenteric and limbs) and the blood loss associated with serious cases [6].

The diagnosis is confirmed by performing a CT scan with contrast or transesophageal echocardiography, depending on the ease of completion of each examination in the emergency room.

Chest X-ray

A chest X-ray can be readily obtained, and can to show some signs of acute aortic dissection: 60–90% of cases have an increased aortic silhouette [6]. The main findings are: mediastinal widening; a sign of double aortic arch; diffuse enlargement of the aorta with little definition and irregularity of contour; medial displacement of the calcified aortic ring of >10 mm; deviation of the trachea to the right; pleural effusion; increased cardiac area; and opacification of the left lung apex. However, these modifications are non-specific and no chest radiograph abnormality was noted in 10–15% of patients.[6]

Computed tomography

Used for three decades, this is the most commonly used imaging procedure for the detection and evaluation of aortic dissection, with a sensitivity of 83–95% and specificity of 87–100%, and showing some limitation in the evaluation of ascending aorta. With helical CT, the study can be done in less time, with high accuracy and a low amount of iodine contrast. It identifies the two lumens and the flap of intimal dissection, and, in 90% of cases, the false lumen is larger than the true. CT can determine the initial and final sites, visceral branches compromised, and possible points of re-entry of the false to true lumen. The CT scan also shows possible points of rupture and contrast extravasation to the pleura, or to the hollow viscera (esophagus, duodenum). The orientation of the concavity of the flap dissection toward the false lumen or the presence of a collapsed true lumen suggests low pressure in the true lumen and may correlate to the malperfusion syndrome of the kidneys, gut, or lower limb [16,41]. CT is less dependent on operator skill, and provides useful images about anatomic correlates to the surgical and endovascular procedures, obtaining reliable information for measurement and analysis.

Transesophageal echocardiography

Transesophageal echocardiography (TEE) has a sensitivity of 98% and specificity of 63–96%, and can be performed at the bedside or in an unstable patient with a suspected diagnosis. TEE has limitations in assessing the distal part of the ascending aorta and aortic arch because the trachea and left bronchus interfere in visualization of the infradiaphragmatic extent of dissection. Despite these limitations, it is extremely useful in assessing the ascending aorta, complementing the information provided by CT for planning surgical treatment [17].

Nuclear magnetic resonance

Although accurate (sensitivity and specificity 95–100%), nuclear magnetic resonance has little application compared with CT scans because of the longer time required for the exam and the difficulty of monitoring a critically ill patient during it [18].

Aortography

Aortography has gradually been replaced by helical imaging tests. With the need for rapid diagnosis, its limitation is clearly that of being an invasive procedure, time consuming, and expensive. It has no advantages in terms of sensitivity and specificity compared with CT and TEE. Currently, it is not performed before surgical repair of proximal dissections, although it can be performed in treatment of distal dissections as part of the endovascular repair.

Treatment

Successful treatment of aortic dissection depends on rapid diagnosis and correct assessment of the extent of the pathologic process. Clinical treatment seeks to reduce blood pressure, aiming to stabilize the extent of dissection and decrease the risk of rupture [42–44].

Clinical management

- Monitoring in the intensive care unit, oxygen, intravenous access, and blood sampling. Quickly evaluate the possibility of cardiac tamponade, avoiding pericardial puncture in favor of definitive treatment [42].
- Beta-blockers: the goal is to let the heart rate reduce to <60 beats/min, if tolerated. Prescribe metoprolol (5 mg) IV in 3–5 minutes, in case of dissection; this is the maximum dose. The reduction in heart rate and inotropism are essential in the management of acute dissection (if there is contraindication to beta-blockers, the patient may be prescribed IV verapamil or diltiazem) [42].
- Reduction in blood pressure: reduction to the lowest tolerated by the patient. If possible, leave the systolic blood pressure at 100–110 mmHg; for that, prescribe sodium nitroprusside starting at 0.3–0.5 mg/kg/min, with increases of 0.5 mg/kg/min every 3–5 minutes. Vasodilators should always be used in combination with beta-blockers and never alone, because of the risk of increasing the stress on the aortic wall with an increased ejection fraction [42].
- Morphine: give a dose of 2–4 mg IV to achieve adequate analgesia [42].

Type A dissection

The risk of rupture and complications related to aortic insufficiency, cardiac tamponade, or obstruction of the coronary ostia are associated with a hospital mortality of 60% with medical therapy, thus justifying immediate surgical treatment in all cases of type A aortic dissections [2,6]. In patients with type A dissection complicated by malperfusion, clinical treatment followed by endovascular fenestration can reduce risks and create the conditions needed for definitive surgical intervention [45].

Definitive treatment consists of resection of the dissected segment with interposition of a Dacron graft. Reimplantation of the coronary ostia or correction of aortic valve lesions may be needed. The mortality rate is 10–35% depending on comorbidities and associated conditions; the neurologic status at presentation is the main factor of poor prognosis [6].

High rates of surgical mortality related to visceral malperfusion (50–80% in patients with renal ischemia and 87% in those with mesenteric ischemia) in patients undergoing replacement of the ascending aorta, make some authors propose an open or endovascular fenestration of the distal aorta before definitive surgical repair of the ascending aorta. This increases the survival rate of

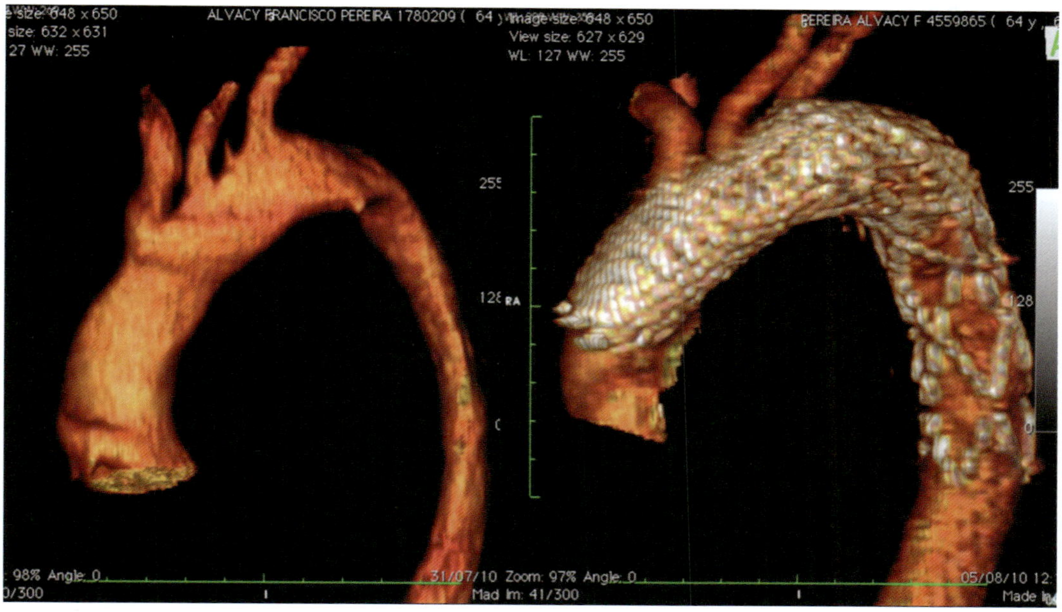

Fig. 8.2 Type B dissection with retrograde component involving the aortic root, after bare stent implantation into the aortic arch and endograft below the left subclavian artery.

aortic intervention to 75% with only 15% mortality before definitive surgery [2,45,46].

Thoracic endovascular aortic repair

Endovascular treatment of diseases of the ascending aorta and aortic arch is limited by their anatomic (aortic valve, coronary ostia, supra-aortic trunks) and hemodynamic characteristics. Reports of treatment of aneurysms or pseudoaneurysms of the aortic arch with an endograft and bypass of supra-aortic branches have been described [5]. The latest development of a percutaneous aortic valve [6] and stent implantation in type A dissection [47,48] has expanded the indications of endovascular approaches in the ascending aorta.

In some cases of aortic type A dissection, with a limited involvement of the ascending aorta, the open stent-graft (Z-stents such as the Zenith or Jotec E-XL) can be used to stabilize the flap of dissection in the aortic arch and prevent a progression of the dissection to the aortic valve or pericardium. Despite its limited application, the development of new technologies and the combination of endovascular treatment can reduce mortality related to conventional procedures on the ascending aorta.

The type B dissection may also extend proximally up to the aortic arch and ascending aorta. In these cases we may prevent rupture with a bare stent proximally (Fig. 8.2).

Type B dissection

In acute type B aortic dissection, the option is for medical management in most cases. Surgery is reserved for dissection complicated by ischemia of the brain, upper or lower limbs, kidney, gut, or spinal cord. Moreover, patients with persistent pain, with a progressive increase in the diameter of the false lumen, or with hemothorax are treated surgically [6,49].

The rupture evident or imminent in the proximal aorta, which occurs rarely (6% in the most recent case series, a result of improved clinical management), is the sole indication of replacement of the descending aorta by the graft. It is associated with significant technical challenges for friability of the aortic wall [6,49].

In malperfusion syndromes, patients should undergo a vascular intervention directed to each complication. In the presence of renal or mesenteric ischemia, the patient should be referred for fenestration of the distal aorta by endovascular or conventional methods. Some authors advocate that on suspicion of intestinal ischemia, open fenestration should be preferred to inspect the ischemic gut. In patients with severe lower limb ischemia, in addition to the fenestration, extra-anatomic bypasses like femoro-femoral or axillary–femoral, that have lower morbidity, may be the therapy of choice [39,50].

Thoracic endovascular aortic repair

In some trials, thoracic endovascular aortic repair (TEVAR) is used in stable cases of type B dissections and, as in case of Fig. 8.2, type A dissections (without valve and coronary compromise). A large bare stent may be used to stabilize the progression of the dissection by sealing the entry hole, promoting the thrombosis of the false lumen, reducing the incidence and severity of the malperfusion syndromes, and minimizing the risk of progression to aneurysmal degeneration of the false lumen [33–35,51–71].

Accepted goals for endovascular treatment of aortic dissections are closure of the primary intimal entry tear, depressurization and thrombosis of the false lumen, and expansion of the true lumen [54]. To achieve the latter end-points and avoid further aneurysmal evolution of the false lumen, stabilization of the intimal flap may play an important role [72]. The movements of the intimal flap and the continuous motion of the blood in the false lumen clearly contribute to preventing thrombosis. Based in a conceptual model of risk according to the status of the false lumen, there is an increased mortality in patients with partial thrombosis of the false lumen at 3 years, being a significant predictor of death and the need for supporting treatments that encourage remodeling of the false channel [73].

The INSTEAD trial included 140 patients with a stable clinical condition who were randomly subjected to elective stent-graft placement in addition to optimal medical therapy ($n = 72$) or to optimal medical therapy alone ($n = 68$). The trial found that the aorta-related death rate was not different in the two groups, and the risk for the combined end-point of aorta-related death (rupture) and progression (including conversion or additional endovascular or open surgery) was similar in patients receiving medical treatment only. Finally, aortic remodeling (with true lumen recovery and thoracic false lumen thrombosis) occurred in 91.3% of patients with TEVAR versus 19.4% of those who received medical treatment only ($P < 0.001$), suggesting ongoing aortic remodeling [62].

This strategy is considered useful by some authors, who believe that the re-entry points remain open, particularly those located close to the visceral arteries. Aiming to solve this problem, new types of uncoated stents have been developed for collapsing the false lumen at the time of emergence of the visceral arteries. This makes this technique promising for treatment of early complications and the prevention of aortic aneurysm degeneration in patients with aortic dissection type B.

Complications like retrograde type A dissection during or after an endoluminal graft can occur in 2–4% of cases [74]. Female gender, use of proximal uncovered stent-grafts for dissection, and possibly aggressive balloon angioplasty may play a role in the cause of retrograde type A dissection [74–76].

Coverage of the left subclavian artery can be used to extend the proximal seal zone for TEVAR without increasing the risk of spinal cord ischemia or stroke [67]. Ischemic symptoms in the left upper extremity can occur in 3–7.6% of cases and subclavian steal syndrome in another 3% [77,78]. Indications for revascularization include long segment aortic coverage, prior or concomitant infrarenal aortic replacement, and renal insufficiency. In addition, a hypoplastic right vertebral artery, a patent left internal mammary artery graft, and a functioning dialysis fistula in the left arm are also indications to perform revascularization [77,79].

Bird-beak configuration, defined as the incomplete apposition of the proximal endograft with a wedge-shaped gap between the device and the aortic wall, can occur with almost all thoracic endografts available, mainly in younger patients. Bird-beak configuration was correlated significantly with the risk of developing a type IA or IIa endoleak, with close to 21% incidence of stent-graft collapse or infolding [80].

Zenith dissection endovascular stent

Case reports of Z-stent use for the prevention of malperfusion complicating chronic dissection suggest its usefulness in aortic dissection [56,57]. In a series of 17 cases of patients with complicated type

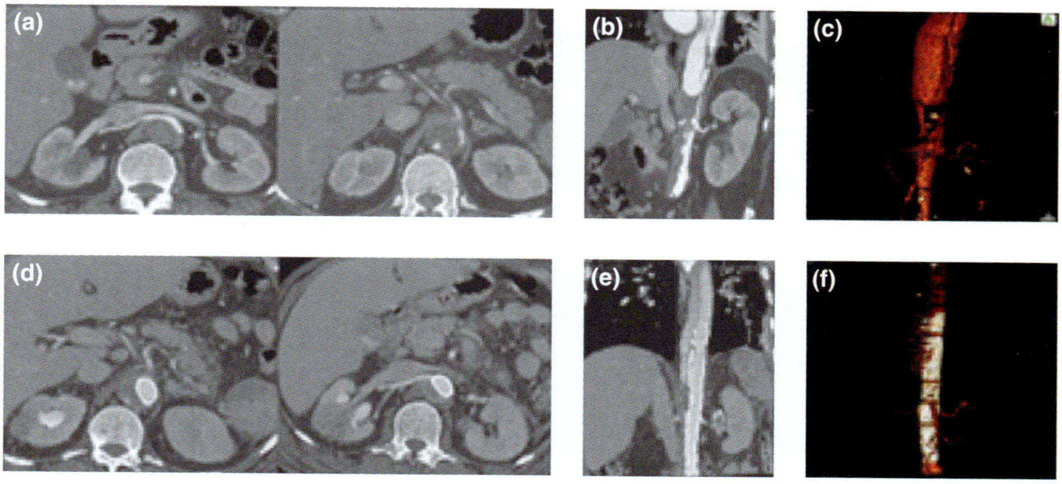

Fig. 8.3 (a, b) Severe true lumen collapse and (c) 3D image reconstruction. Correction with only deployment of the Zenith dissection endovascular stent at the visceral level 2 days after surgical procedures, with (d, e) true lumen opening and patency of the visceral trunks and (f) 3D image reconstruction.

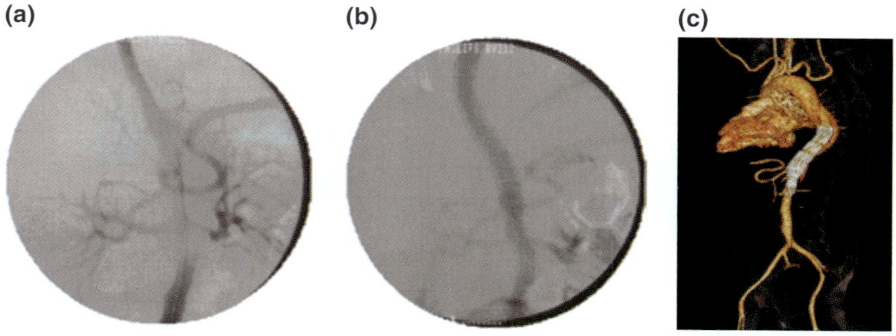

Fig. 8.4 Aortogram of a patient with true lumen collapse before (a) and after (b) Zenith dissection endovascular stent deployment. Note complete expansion of the true lumen. (c) Angiographic 3D reconstruction.

B dissection, we have found that bare metal stenting accelerates true lumen remodeling, reduces false lumen volume, and enhances branch vessel perfusion. All patients were treated endovascularly, with placement of Zenith dissection endovascular stents at the level of the visceral arteries. Fourteen patients also received a thoracic endograft to cover the entry site. Total or partial false lumen thrombosis was observed in all cases, and thoracic endografts were placed. In cases where only the Zenith dissection endovascular stent devices were employed and no thoracic endografts were used, the true lumen flow increased even with a false lumen maintaining flow. Bare metal stents only were used in two out of three patients due to acute dissection with severe visceral ischemia and true lumen collapse (Figs 8.3 and 8.4), with immediate true lumen expansion. Flow was obtained with ischemia reversal, renal function was regained, and hemodialysis stopped. Three deaths occurred within 30 days (17.6%).

The rationale of endovascular treatment for aortic dissection is based on the exclusion of the false lumen from the circulation. In chronic dissections, the graft does not immediately compress the dissection membrane against the aortic wall as in acute dissections, resulting in partial thrombosis of the false lumen and a higher mortality at 3 years. Collapse of the true lumen is a critical event in this disease. True lumen patency is very important for

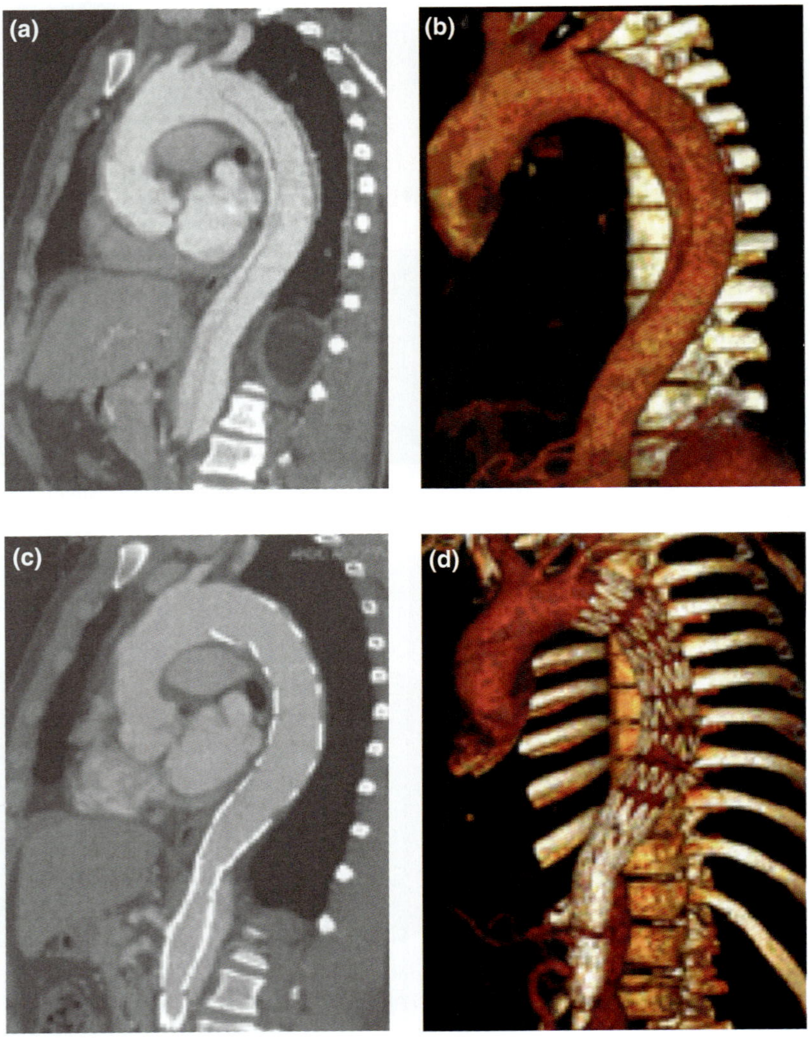

Fig. 8.5 Angio-CT showing (a, b) main fenestration in a patient with type B aortic dissection before management, and (c, d) fenestration closure, true lumen opening, and patency of the visceral trunks 4 months after endovascular procedures (proximal endografts and dissection).

treating these patients. Complete healing of a chronic dissection may be expected in only a fraction of cases; healing requires some time and has relevant prognostic consequences [73].

Accepted goals of the simple exclusion of proximal entry tears are decompression of the thoracic false lumen, promotion of proximal thrombosis, and remodeling of the false lumen (Fig. 8.5). However, the distal thoracic and abdominal dissected aortas fail to remodel in 50–80% of cases, probably due to distal communication sites between the true and false lumens and the flapping motion of the dissecting lamella, which prevents complete false lumen thrombosis [57,58].

In some acute dissections, it seems that true lumen patency is the mainstay of treatment. This may be achieved using bare metal Zenith dissection endovascular stents, as shown by Mossop et al. [59].

Precise knowledge of the individual aortic anatomy dissection is essential in deciding on the exact intervention. Ito et al. [56] reported a case of type B aortic dissection with malperfusion that was successfully treated with implantation of a Gianturco Z-stent (Cook Medical, Bloomington,

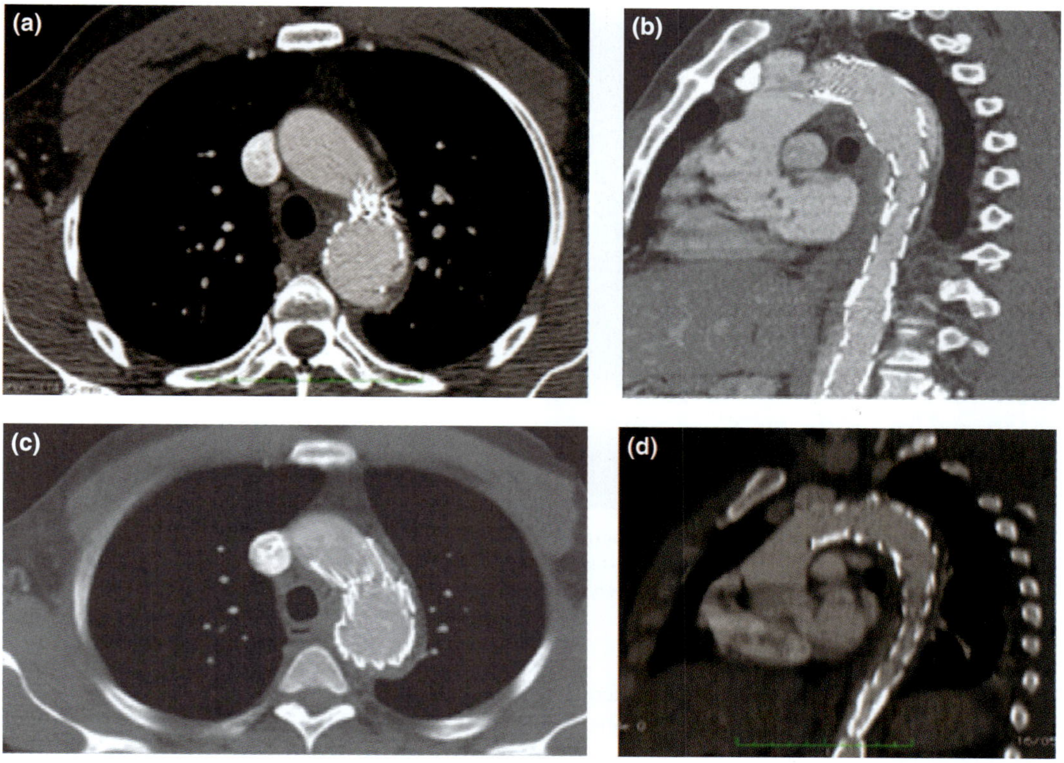

Fig. 8.6 Angio-CT showing (a, b) a type IA endoleak 10 days after surgical procedures, and (c, d) the endoleak correction after placement of a new endograft in zone 2.

IN) in the distal thoracic and abdominal aorta. Kato et al. [60] studied the long-term outcome for bare stent implantation in aortic dissection and reported that bare aortic stent implantation is likely to promote clot formation in the false lumen and reduce the size of the false lumen in the chronic phase. Clot formation in the false lumen was observed in 100% of patients. The size of the false lumen shrank within 6 months in 93%, and had completely disappeared in 64%. These findings are similar with our experience.

Mossop et al. [59] recently reported treatment of seven patients with type B acute aortic dissection with stent-graft (Zenith TX2 thoracic aortic aneurysm endovascular graft, Cook Medical) closure of the proximal entry tear and a bare metal Z-stent deployed in the residual delaminated aorta. Stent deployment in the thoracic aorta resulted in an immediate increase in the thoracic true lumen index (true lumen area/total aorta area) from 39 ± 15% to 71 ± 16% ($P = 0.001$), and was maintained at the 3-month follow-up (74 ± 17%). Average true lumen expansion was 141%. The mean abdominal aortic true lumen index increased from 41 ± 17% to 75 ± 14% ($P = 0.001$) after stenting, and was maintained at the 3-month follow-up (79 ± 16%). Mean immediate abdominal true lumen expansion was greater than 130%. Melissano et al. [57] used the complete Zenith dissection endovascular system in 11 patients. At follow-up they (just like us) observed a successful proximal thrombosis of the false lumen in all patients and enlargement at 12 months, despite exclusion of the false lumen in one patient (9%). No adverse events related to the Zenith dissection endovascular stents were observed. A median rate of re-expansion of the true lumen of the distal thoracic and abdominal aorta of 5 mm was detected. In our series, we obtained some degree of false lumen thrombosis and true lumen patency in all cases. These variations occur due to time of follow-up and type of dissections (acute versus chronic).

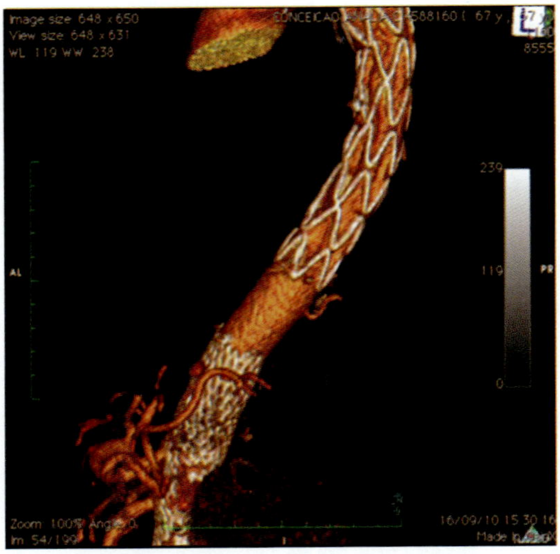

Fig. 8.7 Acute dissection of the aorta. A short endograft is placed proximally, preserving the Adamkiewicz artery. At the visceral atery level a bare stent is used to open the true lumen.

Despite short-term results, the treatment of complicated type B aortic dissections with the Zenith dissection endovascular system is feasible and safe. Further studies and longer follow-up are needed to confirm these data.

Recently we had opportunity to treat 16 patients with a new device (Jotec E-XL, Hechingen, Germany). This device is bone shaped, with extremities 4 mm larger than the body. It constitutes closed cells in the extremities and open cells in the body, to assure flexibility. The radial force is low and there are several sizes of diameter from 14 mm up to 36 mm and the extension is 13 cm for all samples. Sixteen type B dissection patients have been studied with the Jotec E-XL device: 10 patients had malperfusion syndrome, three had intractable lumbar pain, and two had retrograde dissections to the aortic arch and aortic root. All the patients in this series are alive and only two patients required reoperation (a femoro-femoral bypass graft) due to iliac artery occlusion in the early postoperative period. Another patient was reoperated on 10 days after the primary operation due to a type I proximal endoleak. A proximal extension was placed with good results (Fig. 8.6).

All patients are in follow-up protocol. The bare stent (E-XL) has a good conformability and the expansion rate of the true lumen seems to be the same as that of the Zenith dissection stent (Fig. 8.7).

Acute complicated dissections must be managed by covering the main entry with a short endograft, trying to maintain the patency of the Adamkiewicz artery as well as the maximum number of intercostal arteries possible. These endografts may not have more than 10–20% of oversizing. The bare stent is used to tack the aortic flap to ensure aortic remodeling and true lumen re-expansion.

Conclusions

With our experience of cases we have learnt some critical points to ensure good results and patient survival:

- Bare stents allow aortic remodeling.
- Flow redirection is fundamental in aortic remodeling.
- Flow redirection allows depressurization of the false lumen and decreases the likehood of expansion even when it remains patent.
- Balloon accommodation of the stent *should not* be done!
- Stent size should be the original aorta size: *do not oversize*!
- True lumen patency seems to be more important than fenestration occlusion.
- Proximal tear coverage should be with the shortest available graft, while a true lumen bare stent should be as long as needed.
- This procedure is intended to save lives in the acute period. Some patients will need reoperations. To date, we have had two reoperations to correct aortic dilation.

Acknowledgments

Thanks to Boulanger Miotto Neto, Erasmo Simão da Silva, Alex Lederman, Luciano Dias Nascimento, Fábio Rodrigues Espirito Santo, Daniel Augusto Benitti, and Grace Carvajal Mulatti.

References

1 Tsai TT, Nienaber CA, Eagle KA. Acute aortic syndromes. Circulation 2005;112:3802–13.

2 Pate JW, Richardson RL, Eastridge CE. Acute aortic dissections. Am Surg 1976;42:395–404.

3 Black JH, III, Cambria RP. Aortic dissection: perspectives for the vascular/endovascular surgeon. In: Rutherford RB. (ed.) Vascular Surgery, 6th edn. New York: Elsevier, 2007, pp. 1512–31.
4 Nienaber CA, Eagle KA. Aortic dissection: new frontiers in diagnosis and management, Part I: from etiology to diagnostic strategies. Circulation 2003;108:628–35.
5 Kouchoukos NT, Dougenis D. Surgery of the thoracic aorta. N Eng J Med. 2007;336:1876–88.
6 Hagan PG, Nienaber CA, Isselbacher EM, et al. The International Registry of Acute Aortic Dissection (IRAD): new insights into an old disease. JAMA 2000;283:897–903.
7 Suzuki T, Mehta RH, Ince H, et al. Clinical profiles and outcomes of acute type B aortic dissection in the current era: lessons from the International Registry of Aortic Dissection (IRAD). Circulation 2003;108(Suppl II):312–17.
8 Lauterbach SR, Cambria RP, Brewster DC, et al. Contemporary management of aortic branch compromise resulting from acute aortic dissection. J Vasc Surg 2001;33:1185–92.
9 Wilson SK, Hutchins GM. Aortic dissecting aneurysms: causative factors in 204 subjects. Arch Pathol Lab Med 1982;106(4):175–80.
10 Schlatmann TJ, Becker AE. Histologic changes in the normal aging aorta: implications for dissecting aortic aneurysm. Am J Cardiol 1977;39(1):13–20.
11 Kita Y, Nakamura K, Itoh H. Histologic and histometric study of the aortic media in dissecting aneurysm. Comparison with true aneurysm and age-matched controls. Acta Pathol Jpn 1990;40(6):408–16.
12 Hasleton PS, Leonard JC. Dissecting aortic aneurysms: a clinicopathological study. II. Histopathology of the aorta. Q J Med 1979;48(189):63–76.
13 Schlatmann TJ, Becker AE. Pathogenesis of dissecting aneurysm of aorta. Comparative histopathologic study of significance of medial changes. Am J Cardiol 1977;39(1):21–6.
14 Roberts WC, Bethesda. Aortic dissection: anatomy, consequences and cases. Am Heart J 1981;2:195–214.
15 Poullis MP, Warwick R, Oo A, et al. Ascending aortic curvature as an independent risk factor for type A dissection, and ascending aortic aneurysm formation: a mathematical model. Eur J Cardiothorac Surg 2008;33: 995–1001.
16 Quint LE, Platt JF, Sonnad SS, et al. Aortic intimal tears: detection with spiral computed tomography. J Endovasc Ther 2003;10(3):505–10.
17 Erbel R. Role of transesophageal echocardiography in dissection of the aorta and evaluation of degenerative aortic disease. Cardiol Clin 1993;11(3):461–73.
18 Longe TF, Lesser JR, Schwartz RS. Early aortic intimal tear without haematoma or dissection: early diagnosis by cardiac magnetic resonance imaging. Heart 2005;91(3):416.
19 Gao F, Watanabe M, Matsuzawa T. Stress analysis in a layered aortic arch model under pulsatile blood flow. Biomed Eng Online 2006;24:5–25.
20 Maltzahn WWV, Warriyar RG, Keitzer WF. Experimental measurements of elastic properties of media and adventitia of bovine carotid arteries. J Biomech 1984;17:839–48.
21 Truijers M, Pol JA, Schultzekool LJ, et al. Wall stress analysis in small asymptomatic, symptomatic and ruptured abdominal aortic aneurysms. et al. 2007;33(4):401–7.
22 Lillie MA, Gosline JM. Mechanical properties of elastin along the thoracic aorta in the pig. J Biomech 2007;40:2214–21.
23 Purslow PP. Positional variations in fracture toughness, stiffness and strength of descending thoracic pig aorta. J Biomech 1990;16:947–53.
24 Assoul N, Flaud P, Chaouat M, et al. Mechanical properties of rat thoracic and abdominal aortas. J Biomech 2008;41:2227–36.
25 MacLean NF, Dudek NL, Roach MR. The role of radial elastic properties in the development of aortic dissection. J Vasc Surg 1999;29:703–10.
26 Mohan D, Melvin JW. Failure properties of passive human aortic tissue. I. Uniaxial test. J Biomech 1982;15:887–902.
27 Vorp DA, Schiro BJ, Ehrlich MP, et al. Effect of aneurysm on the tensile strength and biomechanical behaviour of the ascending aorta. Ann Thorac Surg 2003;800:1210–14.
28 Groenink M, Langerak SE, Vanbavel E, et al. The influence of aging and aortic stiffness on permanent dilation and breaking stress of the thoracic descending aorta. Cardiovasc Res 1999;43:471–480.
29 Sommer G, Gasser TC, Regitnig P, et al. Dissection properties of the human aortic media: an experimental study. J Biomech Eng 2008;130:1–12.
30 Meszaros I, Morocz J, Szlavi J, et al. Epidemiology and clinicopathology of aortic dissection. Chest 2000; 117:1271–8.
31 Raghavan ML, Webster MW, Vorp DA. Ex vivo biomechanical behaviour of abdominal aortic aneurysm: assessment using a new mathematical model. Ann Biomed Eng 1996;24(5):573–82.
32 Tespili M, Banfi C, Valsecchi O, et al. Endovascular treatment of thoracic aortic disease: mid-term follow-up. Catheter Cardiovasc Interv 2007;70(4):595–601.
33 Duebener LF, Lorenzen P, Richardt G, et al. Emergency endovascular stent-grafting for life-threatening acute type B aortic dissections. Ann Thorac Surg 2004; 78(4):1261–6; discussion 1266–7.
34 Verhoye JP, Miller DC, Sze D, et al. Complicated acute type B aortic dissection: midterm results of emergency endovascular stent-grafting. J Thorac Cardiovasc Surg 2008;136(2):424–30.

35 Song TK, Donayre CE, Walot I, et al. Endograft exclusion of acute and chronic descending thoracic aortic dissections. J Vasc Surg 2006;43(2):247–58.

36 Cao P, Verzini F, De Rango P, et al. Different types of thoracic endografts. J Cardiovasc Surg (Torino) 2009;50(4):483–92.

37 Tsai T, Trimarchi S, Nienaber CA. Acute aortic dissection: perspectives from International Registry of Acute Aortic Dissection (IRAD). Eur J Vasc Surg 2009;37:149–59.

38 Eggebrecht H, Plicht B, Kahlert P, et al. Intramural hematoma and penetrating ulcers: indications to endovascular treatment. Eur J Vasc Endovasc Surg 2009;38(6):659–65.

39 Cambria RP, Brewster DC, Gertler J, et al. Vascular complications associated with spontaneous aortic dissection. J Vasc Surg 1988;7:199–209.

40 Spitell PC, Spitell J, Joyce JW. Clinical features and differential diagnosis of aortic dissection: experience with 236 cases. Mayo Clin Proc 1993;68:897–903.

41 McMahon MA, Squirrell CA. Multidetector CT of aortic dissection: a pictorial review. Radiographics 2010;30(2):445–60.

42 Mano R. Manuais de Cardiologia. Temas comuns da cardiologia para médicos de todas as especialidades – livro virtual. Available at http://www.manuaisdecardiologia.med.br/aorta/aorta.htm, February 10–20, 2009.

43 Feldman M, Shah M, Elefteriades JA. Medical management of acute type A aortic dissection. Ann Thorac Cardiovasc Surg 2009;15(5):286–93.

44 Niino T, Hata M, Sezai A, et al. Optimal clinical pathway for the patient with type B acute aortic dissection. Circ J 2009;73:264–8.

45 Slonim SM, Nyman URO, Semba CP, et al. Aortic dissection: percutaneous management of ischemic complications with endovascular stents and balloon fenestration. J Vasc Surg 1996;23:241–53.

46 Williams DM, Lee DY, Hamilton BH, et al. The dissected aorta: percutaneous treatment of ischemic complications – principles and results. J Vasc Intervent Radiol 1997; 8:605–25.

47 Jiang J, Ding X, Zhang G, et al. Endovascular stent-graft placement for retrograde type A aortic dissection. J Vasc Interv Radiol 2011;22(3):415–17.

48 Sueda T, Watari M, Orihashi K, et al. Open stent-graft repair for acute type A aortic dissection with an intimal tear in the descending aorta. Ann Thorac Cardiovasc Surg 1999;5(4):273–5.

49 Mackenzie KS, Le Guillan MP, Steinmetz OK, et al. Management trends and early mortality rates for acute type B aortic dissection: a 10-year single-institution experience. Ann Vasc Surg 2004;18:158–66.

50 Fann JI, Sarris GE, Mitchell RS, et al. Treatment of patients with aortic dissection presenting with peripheral vascular complications. Ann Surg 1990;212:705–13.

51 Dake MD, Kato N, Mitchell RS, et al. Endovascular stent graft placement for the treatment of acute aortic dissection. N Engl J Med 1999;340:1546–52.

52 Nienaber CA, Fattori R, Lund G, et al. Nonsurgical reconstruction of thoracic aortic dissection by stent-graft placement. N Engl J Med 1999;340:1539–45.

53 Palma JH, de Souza JA, Rodrigues Alves CM, et al. Self-expandable aortic stent-grafts for treatment of descending aortic dissections. Ann Thorac Surg 2002;73:1138–42.

54 Dake MD, Wang DS. Will stent-graft repair emerge as treatment of choice for acute type B dissection? Semin Vasc Surg 2006;19:40–7.

55 Gaxotte V, Thony F, Rousseau H, et al. Midterm results of aortic diameter outcomes after thoracic stent-graft implantation for aortic dissection: a multicenter study. J Endovasc Ther 2006;13:127–38.

56 Ito N, Tsunoda T, Nakamura M, et al. Percutaneous bare Z-stent implantation as an alternative to surgery for acute aortic dissection with visceral ischemia. Catheter Cardiovasc Interv 2003;58:95–100.

57 Melissano G, Bertoglio L, Kahlberg A, et al. Evaluation of a new disease-specific endovascular device for type B aortic dissection. J Thorac Cardiovasc Surg 2008; 136:1012–18.

58 Eggebrecht H, Nienaber CA, Neuhäuser M, et al. Endovascular stent-graft placement in aortic dissection: a meta-analysis. Eur Heart J 2006;27:489–98.

59 Mossop P, Nixon I, Oakes J, et al. Immediate "total" aortic true lumen expansion in type A and B acute aortic dissection after endovascular aortic endografting and GZSD bare stenting. J Thorac Cardiovasc Surg 2007;134:1360–2.

60 Kato M, Kaneko M, Kuratani T, et al. Outcomes of stent-grafts treatment of false lumen in aortic dissection. Circulation 1998;98:305–11.

61 Kahn SL, Dake MD. Stent graft management of stable, uncomplicated type B aortic dissection. Perspect Vasc Endovasc Ther 2007;19(2):162–69.

62 Nienaber CA, Rousseau H, Eggebrecht H, et al. Randomized comparison of strategies for type B aortic dissection: the INvestigation of STEnt Grafts in Aortic Dissection (INSTEAD) trial. Circulation 2009;120(25): 2519–28.

63 Cambria RP, Crawford RS, Cho JS, et al. A multicenter clinical trial of endovascular stent graft repair of acute catastrophes of the descending thoracic aorta. J Vasc Surg 2009;50(6):1255–64, e1–4.

64 Khoynezhad A, Gupta PK, Donayre CE, et al. Current status of endovascular management of complicated acute type B aortic dissection. Future Cardiol 2009; 5(6):581–8.

65 Khoynezhad A, Donayre CE, Omari BO, et al. Midterm results of endovascular treatment of complicated acute type B aortic dissection. J Thorac Cardiovasc Surg 2009;138(3):625–31.

66 Kische S, Ehrlich MP, Nienaber CA, et al. Endovascular treatment of acute and chronic aortic dissection: mid-term results from the Talent Thoracic Retrospective Registry. J Thorac Cardiovasc Surg 2009;138(1):115–24.
67 Guangqi C, Xiaoxi L, Wei C, et al. Endovascular repair of Stanford type B aortic dissection: early and mid-term outcomes of 121 cases. Eur J Vasc Endovasc Surg 2009;38(4):422–6.
68 Conrad MF, Crawford RS, Kwolek CJ, et al. Aortic remodeling after endovascular repair of acute complicated type B aortic dissection. J Vasc Surg 2009;50(3):510–17.
69 Lumsden AB, Reardon MJ. Once dissected always dissected! Can stent grafts change the natural history of type B dissections? A report from the International Registry of Acute Aortic Dissection. JACC Cardiovasc Interv 2008;1(4): 403–4.
70 Akin I, Kische S, Ince H, et al. Indication, timing and results of endovascular treatment of type B dissection. Eur J Vasc Endovasc Surg 2009;37(3):289–96.
71 Kpodonu J, Ramaiah VG, Diethrich EB. Successful management of a combined ruptured Stanford type B aortic dissection and malperfusion syndrome with an endoluminal graft. Interact Cardiovasc Thorac Surg 2008;7(2):339–41.
72 Nienaber CA, Kische S, Zeller T, et al. Provisional extension to induce complete attachment after stent graft placement in type B aortic dissection: the PETTICOAT concept. J Endovasc Ther 2006;13:738–46.
73 Tsai TT, Evangelista A, Nienaber CA, et al. Partial thrombosis of the false lumen in patients with acute type B aortic dissection. N Engl J Med 2007;357:349–59.
74 Kpodonu J, Preventza O, Ramaiah VG, et al. Retrograde type A dissection after endovascular stenting of the descending thoracic aorta. Is the risk real? Eur J Cardiothorac Surg 2008;33(6):1014–18.
75 Neuhauser B, Greiner A, Jaschke W, et al. Serious complications following endovascular thoracic aortic stent-graft repair for type B dissection. Eur J Cardiothorac Surg 2008;33:58–63.
76 Rubin S, Bayle A, Poncet A, et al. Retrograde aortic dissection after a stent graft repair of a type B dissection: how to improve the endovascular technique. Interact Cardiovasc Thorac Surg 2006;5:746–8.
77 Kotelis D, Geisbüsch P, Hinz U, et al. Short and midterm results after left subclavian artery coverage during endovascular repair of the thoracic aorta. J Vasc Surg 2009;50(6):1285–92.
78 Peterson MD, Wheatley GH, 3rd, Kpodonu J, et al. Treatment of type II endoleaks associated with left subclavian artery coverage during thoracic aortic stent grafting. J Thorac Cardiovasc Surg 2008;136(5):1193–9.
79 Gawenda M, Brunkwall J. When is safe to cover the left subclavian and celiac arteries. Part I: Left subclavian artery. J Cardiovasc Surg (Torino). 2008;49(4):471–7.
80 Ueda T, Fleischmann D, Dake MD, et al. Incomplete endograft apposition to the aortic arch: bird-beak configuration increases risk of endoleak formation after thoracic endovascular aortic repair. Radiology 2010;255(2):645–52.

9

CHAPTER 9

Complications of endovascular aneurysm repair

Babak J. Orandi[1] *& James H. Black, III*[2]

[1] Department of Surgery, Johns Hopkins Hospital, Baltimore, MA, USA

[2] Division of Vascular Surgery and Endovascular Therapy, Johns Hopkins University School of Medicine, Baltimore, MA, USA

Introduction

The treatment of abdominal aortic aneurysms (AAAs) has been transformed since the first endovascular aortic repair (EVAR) in 1991 [1]. EVAR offers shorter hospitalizations and improved short-term morbidity and mortality rates than traditional open surgical repair (OSR), particularly in the elderly [2]. EVAR has also been shown to decrease aneurysm-related mortality compared to no intervention in patients deemed too ill to undergo OSR [3]. Despite some of the advantages, however, EVAR does have a number of known complications, some that are particular to the endovascular approach and some that are shared with OSR, especially in a patient population frequently afflicted with a heavy comorbidity burden. These complications encompass the entire spectrum, from transient, minor problems to those that threaten life and limb.

Complications

Endoleak

Endoleak, a complication unique to endovascular aneurysm repair, is defined as persistent blood entry into the aneurysm sac following EVAR. This all too common complication results in continued pressurization of the aneurysm sac, placing the patient at risk for continued aneurysm growth and rupture. Endoleaks are classified into five categories (Fig. 9.1), types I through IV and endotension (sometimes referred to as type V endoleak); the category aids in determining the appropriate treatment and its urgency. Endoleaks can be seen at the time of device delivery and at any time thereafter. Endoleak rates as high as 50% at 2 years have been reported [4]. Because of these concerns, patients require routine surveillance. While the optimal surveillance regimen is still debated, there is mounting evidence that ultrasonography may be able to supplant to some degree computerized tomography (CT), the current gold-standard, to minimize intravenous contrast and radiation exposures. A meta-analysis of studies comparing the imaging modalities found that duplex ultrasound is only 77% sensitive and 94% specific compared to CT, but that non-nephrotoxic contrast-enhanced ultrasound is 98% sensitive and 88% specific in detecting endoleak [5].

Type I endoleak

Type I endoleak occurs when there is an incomplete seal between the stent-graft device and the native vessel, either at the proximal (type Ia) or distal (type Ib) attachment site, resulting in continued blood flow into the aneurysm sac and concomitant sac growth (Fig. 9.2). Type I endoleaks typically are encountered at the time of EVAR

Endovascular and Hybrid Therapies for Structural Heart and Aortic Disease, First Edition.
Edited by Jacques Kpodonu and Raoul Bonan.

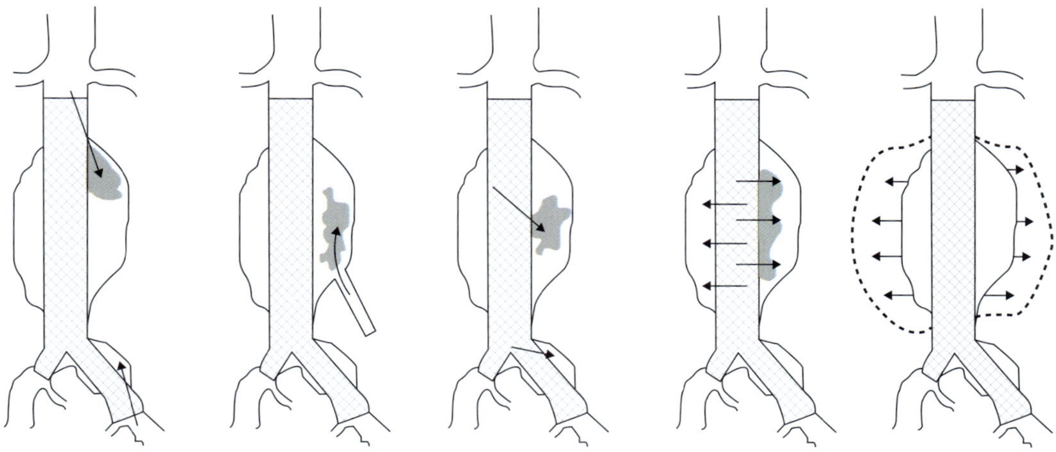

Fig. 9.1 Classification system of endoleaks, as applied to EVAR. Thoracic endovascular aortic repair (TEVAR) also uses the same classification scheme, although a type II endoleak after TEVAR would be attributed to sac reperfusion via the intercostals or the left subclavian artery. Reproduced from Pelberg and Wojciech [49].

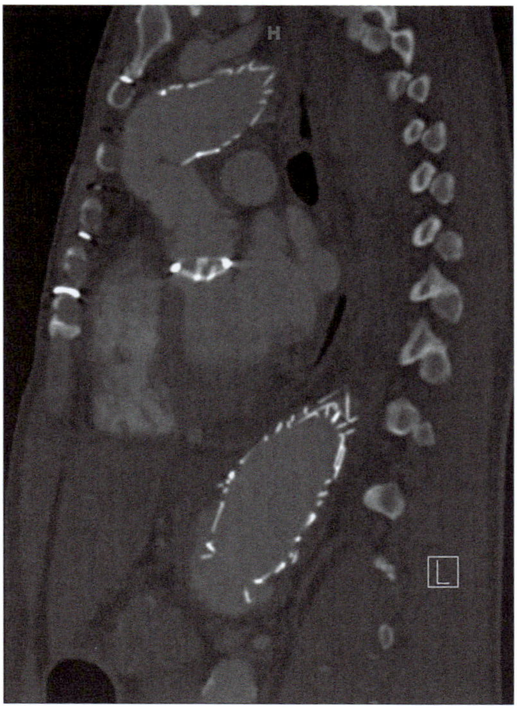

Fig. 9.2 Distal type I endoleak (IB) after TEVAR. The proximal stent-graft is deployed with proximal fixation in a descending thoracic aorta graft ("elephant trunk"). A blush of contrast is appreciated in the distal stent-graft fixation zone from an inadequate seal.

placement and in the early post-procedure period, though they can develop later. They represent a continued risk for aneurysm rupture and treatment is generally mandated. Initial treatment of either type Ia or Ib endoleaks usually consists of balloon angioplasty to approximate more fully the device to the vessel in an attempt to exclude the aneurysm from blood flow. If that fails, type Ia endoleaks can be treated with a Palmaz stent placement (Cordis Corporation, Miami Lakes, FL) and Ib endoleaks can be remedied by deploying an extension aortic cuff or iliac limb.

Type II endoleak

Type II endoleak results from persistent retrograde blood flow into the aneurysm sac secondary to collateral vessels, usually the inferior mesenteric artery or patent lumbar arteries (Fig. 9.3). These can present at any point after EVAR, and the optimal management remains controversial. The clinical equipoise on this subject is important because up to 30% of EVAR patients will have a type II endoleak [6]. Steinmetz and colleagues have advocated a conservative approach to the management as over 60% of these endoleaks will resolve spontaneously, only 1% are associated with aneurysm sac enlargement, and the presence of a type II endoleak does not alter survival at 48

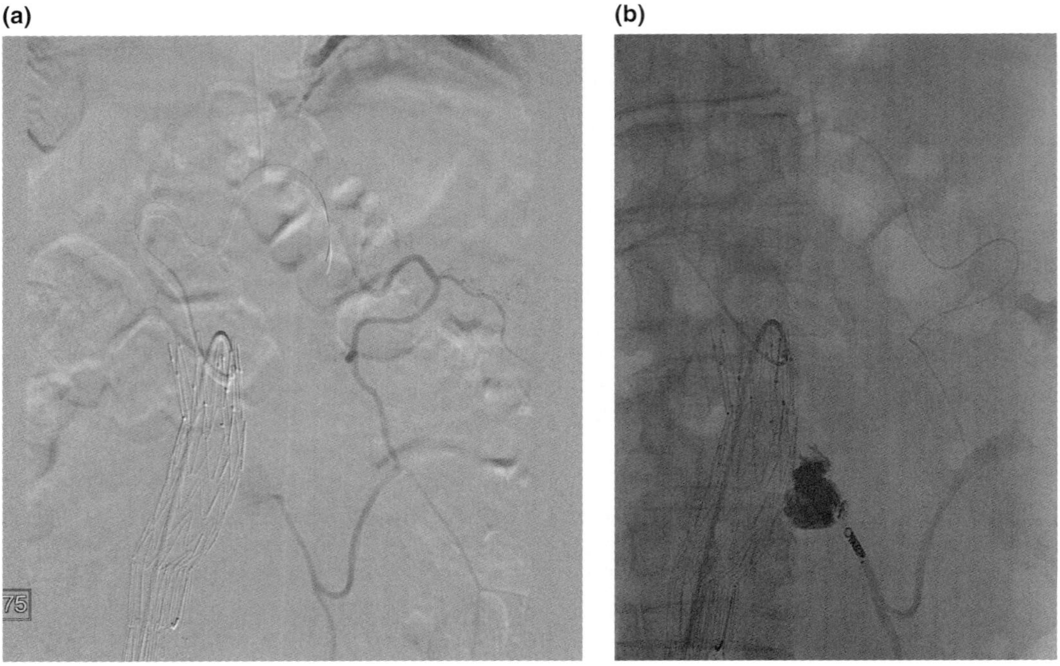

Fig. 9.3 Type II endoleak into the aneurysm sac. (a) The inferior mesenteric artery is collateralized from the superior mesenteric artery to reperfuse the aneurysm sac. (b) The endoleak nidus is thrombosed with Onyx glue and the inflow through the inferior mesenteric artery is occluded with coils.

months [7]. For those type II endoleaks that are apparent immediately at the time of the procedure, the discontinuation of anticoagulation at the end of the procedure will frequently cause a spontaneous resolution of the leak. Others have reported spontaneous and permanent resolution rates as high as 80% [8]. However, persistent type II endoleaks, defined as those lasting for more than 6 months, may require reintervention as they are associated with a significantly higher rate of sac expansion and are a significant predictor of rupture. In addition, treatment is indicated for symptoms (abdominal or back pain) or in the setting of continued aneurysm growth. Interventions range from embolization to laparoscopic ligation of the culprit vessel.

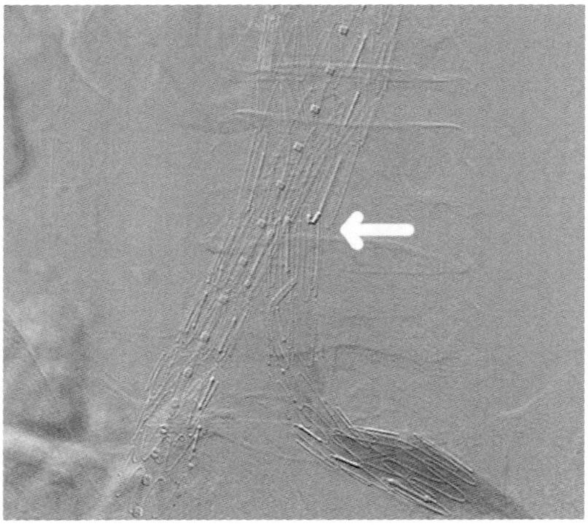

Fig. 9.4 Type III endoleak arising at the overlap of the main body and the left iliac limb (arrow). In this patient the limb had migrated in his massive (11 cm) aneurysm sac to open the leak, and was resolved with a new stent-graft limb to secure the overlap.

Type III endoleak

Blood flow through a tear or rupture in the fabric of the graft or flow between separated components of the graft is a type III endoleak (Fig. 9.4). The natural history of continued aneurysm sac growth and increased risk of rupture is similar to that of a type I endoleak, necessitating an intervention. Treatment entails the placement of a cuff or redeployment of a stent within the stent to

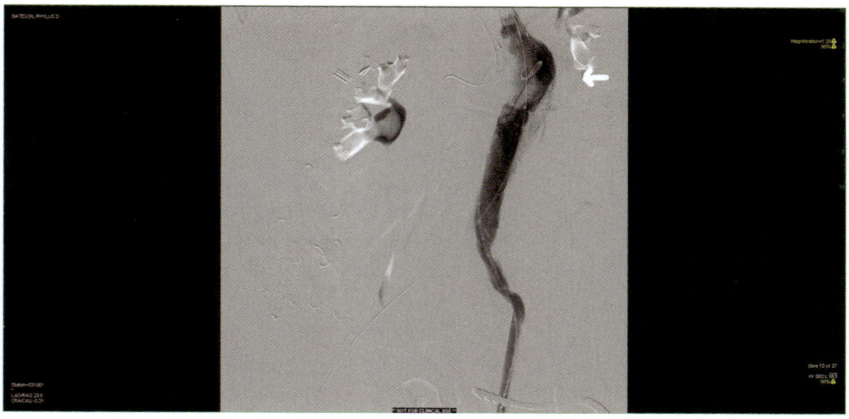

Fig. 9.5 Type IV endoleak seen in the original graft deployment (arrow). Type IV leaks rarely persist after surgery and reversal of anticoagulation, but in early generation devices with significant porosity they could engender aneurysm growth.

cover the tear in the fabric. Component separation is best appreciated using multiple plain view radiographs.

Type IV endoleak

Type IV endoleak, a rather rare finding, especially in contemporary stent-graft devices, is the passage of blood through the graft fabric and is related to the graft's porosity (Fig. 9.5). It is most apparent in fully anticoagulated patients and, as with type II endoleak, will often resolve once the anticoagulation has been discontinued [9]. Type IV endoleak was mostly seen in the high-porosity Excluder device (W.L. Gore & Associates, Flagstaff, AZ).

Type V endoleak (endotension)

Type V endoleak, more commonly called endotension, refers to persistently elevated intra-aneurysmal sac pressure in the absence of an endoleak on delayed contrast CT scan (Fig. 9.6). A number of theories exist to explain the etiology of endotension, which underscores the uncertainty surrounding this phenomenon and the appropriate methods of diagnosing and treating it. For example, it has been proposed that endotension results from endoleak that is so slow in nature as to be invisible to current radiographic techniques [10]. Others advocate that the aneurysm growth results from pressure transmitted across thrombus, whether the thrombus is within occluded vessels that communicate with the sac or clot that sits between the aortic wall and the stent-graft [11], though other theories abound.

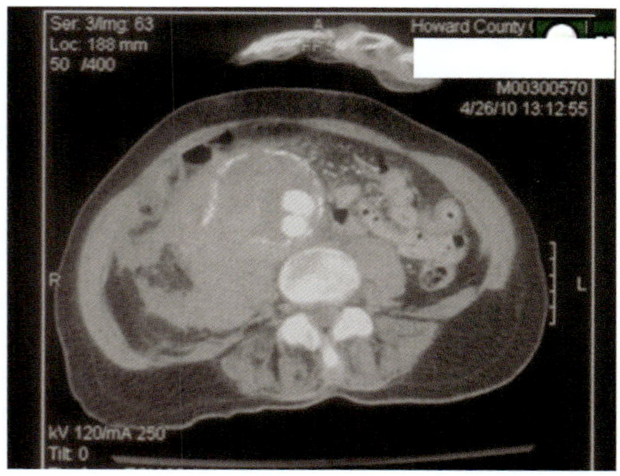

Fig. 9.6 Type V endoleak – no discernible leak. CT reveals rupture of the AAA sac years after device placement. The patient was hemodynamically stable and reported a 3-week history of flank pain. At open conversion there was no abnormality found.

The classification scheme proposed by the Society for Vascular Surgery/American Association for Vascular Surgery for endoleak and endotension [12] has more recently been augmented by an international consensus conference (Box 9.1) [13]. This updated classification system breaks endotension down into four types, A through D; however, an open

Box 9.1 Classification scheme for endoleaks and endotension. Reproduced from Veith et al. [13]

*Endoleak type**	*Description(source of perigraft flow)*
I	Attachment site leaks†
A	Proximal end of endograft
B	Distal end of endograft
C	Iliac occluder (plug)
II	Branch leaks‡ (without attachment site connection)
A	Simple or to-and-fro (from only one patent branch)
B	Complex or flow through (with two or more patent branches)
III	Graft defect†
A	Junctional leak or modular disconnect
B	Fabric disruption (midgraft hole)
	Minor (<2 mm; e.g. suture holes)
	Major (≥2 mm)
IV	Graft wall (fabric) porosity (<30 days after graft placement)
Endotension type§	
A	With no endoleak
B	With sealed endoleak (virtual endoleak)
C	With type I or type III leak‖
D	With type II leak‖

*Endoleaks also can be classified on the basis of the time of first detection as: *perioperative*, within 24 hours of endovascular aortic repair (EVAR); *early*, 1–90 days after EVAR; and *late*, after 90 days. In addition, they can be described as: *primary*, from the time of EVAR; *secondary*, appearing only after not being present at time of EVAR; and *delayed*, occurring after prior negative computed tomography (CT) scan results. Endoleaks also can be described as: *persistent, transient* or *sealed, recurrent, treated successfully*, or *treated unsuccessfully*. Endoleaks and endotension may be associated with abdominal aortic aneurysm (AAA) enlargement, stability, or shrinkage.

†Some type I and type III leaks may also have patent branches opening from the AAA sac and providing an outflow for the leak.

‡From lumbar, inferior mesenteric, hypogastric, renal, or other arteries.

§Endotension (*strict* definition) is defined here as increased intrasac pressure after EVAR without visualized endoleak on delayed contrast CT scans. In the *generic* sense, endotension is any elevation of intrasac pressure and occurs with type I, type III, and most type II leaks and endotension in the strict sense.

‖Detectable only on opening the aneurysm sac.

operation is required for definitive classification of endotension based on this system. In type A endotension, there exists persistent sac pressurization without radiographic findings of an endoleak and no gross endoleak visualized at the time of open operation. Type B endotension refers to an endoleak that has clotted or sealed off but still permits transmission of pressure across the clot. The leak becomes apparent at the time of surgery when the clot is removed. Type I and/or type III endoleak that is not visualized radiographically but results in high sac pressure is considered to be type C endotension. An analogous situation with type II endoleak defines type D endotension. As with types A and B, endotension types C and D become apparent at the time of OSR.

Endotension affects 5.4% of EVAR patients [14], and is usually asymptomatic, though it can occasionally present with symptoms of mass effect, such as abdominal pain and constipation. While rupture is rare, rapid aneurysm growth and/or symptoms attributable to the enlarged sac are indications for intervention. A variety of repair methods have been described, including OSR and relining the stent-graft with another stent-graft via an endovascular approach.

Graft occlusion

Stent-graft occlusion, whether by limb thrombosis or kinking of the stent, typically results in claudication symptoms, which can vary in severity. Affected patients may have claudication with exertion, particularly in the buttocks, rest pain, or acute ischemia. Occasionally, graft kinking or occlusion will present as an incidental radiographic finding on routine follow-up [15].

According to one prospective series conducted over 10 years, limb occlusion occurred in 3.1% of EVAR cases [16]. This study looked exclusively at supported stent-grafts, though the incidence of limb occlusion is known to be significantly higher, as high as 44%, in unsupported grafts [15,17]. Most of these events occur in the intra- and early postoperative period, though graft kinking and thrombosis can occur years after EVAR. The fact that many of these problems were observed and subsequently managed at the time of the procedure serves to underscore the importance of completion angiography to ensure limb patency to avoid a return to the endovascular suite and/or operating room in the postoperative period. Another study found that 31% of patients had either a perceived or measurable decrease in the flow of blood to the lower extremity after EVAR [18]. Of those patients, 89% required an intervention, and 22% had thrombosis of the stent-graft.

Contributing factors include: pre-existing iliac artery stenosis, heavily angulated vessels, and tortuous anatomy. Small iliac arteries have also shown to predispose to limb occlusion, which may explain why women are at an increased risk for this complication. Other known risk factors include the use of an unsupported graft and maldeployment at the time of the procedure resulting in stent twisting.

As with many of the complications of this emerging technology, no consensus exists as to the optimal treatment for stent-graft limb occlusion or thrombosis. A variety of approaches have been used, including further stent placement to provide support to the iliac limbs, chemical thrombolysis, and angioplasty. Surgical approaches include femoro-femoral bypass, axillary–femoral bypass, axillary–bifemoral bypass, or surgical thrombectomy. Thrombectomy, whether done in an open or endovascular manner, may result in damage to the stent-graft, component separation, or stent-graft migration, and due diligence is required to avoid these complications.

Ischemic complications

The known ischemic complications of EVAR can result from one or a combination of several possible mechanisms: direct vessel occlusion by the stent-graft or occlusion of the stent-graft itself, atheroembolic events during catheter manipulation and/or device deployment, inadequate collateralization of the mesenteric circulation, and somewhat controversially, hypogastric artery embolization or exclusion via a covered stent. Interestingly, the early EVAR experience was notable for a higher rate of ischemic complications, partially due to the learning curve, but also because the Ancure device (Guidant, Menlo Park, CA) had a higher rate of ischemic complications. It was subsequently been removed from the market in 2003 [19]. Maldonado and colleagues reported a 9% rate of ischemic complications between 1994 and 2003, but only a 1.7% rate between 2003 and 2005 ($P < 0.01$) [20].

Pelvic ischemia

Pelvic ischemia broadly refers to a range of possible ischemic complications: sexual dysfunction, buttock claudication and/or necrosis, and colon ischemia and/or infarction. These complicate 2–3% of endovascular aneurysm repairs [19,21]. A great deal of controversy exists as to the exact etiology of pelvic ischemia – some argue that iliac or hypogastric artery coil embolization predisposes patients to these complications, while others implicate atheroembolic events in the pathogenesis.

Sexual dysfunction, likely an underreported complication of EVAR, has been reported to be as high as 82% following EVAR (from a preoperative baseline incidence of 74%); however, this is not different from OSR, and both groups tended to return to their baseline after approximately 3 months [22]. A large, multicenter, randomized controlled trial demonstrated equivalent outcomes in terms of sexual function at baseline, 1, and 2 years of follow-up [23]. The new incidence of sexual dysfunction in patients following EVAR with unilateral or bilateral hypogastric artery embolization can be over 40%, with patients who have bilateral hypogastric artery embolization demonstrating significant reductions in pre- and postoperative penile–brachial indices [24]. Some have advocated internal iliac artery revascularization in conjunction with EVAR to prevent sexual dysfunction and other symptoms of pelvic ischemia [25]; however, many patients undergoing EVAR do so because they are poor operative candidates and this approach ought to be used very selectively and reserved only for patients most at risk for pelvic ischemia.

Buttock ischemia can present as claudication or frank necrosis of the skin and muscle. Claudication can occur in as many as one-third of patients who have internal iliac artery occlusion during EVAR. Typically, this is managed conservatively, as most cases improve with time [26]. Necrosis occurs less frequently and requires aggressive surgical debridement. Because of the risk of myoglobinuria secondary to necrosis, pre-existing renal insufficiency, and a contrast load from EVAR, these patients are at high risk of acute renal failure and renal protective measures should be instituted.

In the DREAM trial that randomized patients to either EVAR or OSR, colon ischemia was a rare event in both groups (0.6% and 1.1%, respectively), with no significant difference between the two approaches [27]. The severity can range from ischemic colitis to bowel infarction. The former can be managed with bowel rest and broad-spectrum antibiotics, while the latter requires colectomy. Patients may present with diarrhea, rectal bleeding, leukocytosis, hypotension, fever, sepsis, and/or multisystem organ failure. Because the mortality rate is exceedingly high (>50%) [28], any suspicion of colon ischemia mandates early endoscopic evaluation, close monitoring, serial laboratory testing and abdominal examinations, and a low threshold for aggressive operative intervention.

Spinal cord ischemia

Spinal cord ischemia, which can result in paraplegia, is a dreaded complication of aortic aneurysm repair. Patients can present with a variety of neurologic symptoms, from urinary and/or fecal incontinence, to sensory or motor deficits, to frank paralysis. Proposed etiologies include intra- and post-procedural hypotension, prolonged deployment that causes temporary aortic occlusion, poor collateral blood flow of the spinal cord, disruption of the pelvic circulation, and embolic events. Open surgical repair is associated with a 0.25% rate of paraplegia [29], and analysis of the Eurostar database of patients undergoing EVAR reveals a comparable rate of 0.21% [30].

Stent-graft deployment in the thoracic aorta has a higher rate of spinal cord ischemia (4–10%), with older age, longer procedure times, more extensive stent-graft coverage, and perioperative hypotension, defined as a mean arterial pressure less than 70 mmHg, and prior aortic surgery being significant risk factors for the development of this complication [31,32].

A variety of strategies have been employed to prevent and/or treat spinal cord ischemia: hypothermic techniques, steroids, naloxone, the use of somatosensory evoked potentials, and perhaps most commonly, arterial blood pressure augmentation using vasoactive medications and/or cerebrospinal fluid (CSF) drainage [33]. These latter two strategies increase the perfusion pressure of the spinal cord. Mean arterial pressure goals of 90mmHg or above are common, and are more easily achieved in endovascular aneurysm repair because there is no concern about increased stress placed on the new vascular anastamoses, as there is in open aneurysm repair. CSF drains are often set to maintain pressure of less than 10mmHg. While these methods are often used to treat post-procedure neurologic deficits in EVAR, they tend to be used as prophylaxis in cases involving the thoracic aorta.

Postoperative renal insufficiency and renal artery occlusion

Postoperative renal insufficiency is a common complication of OSR, occurring in over 10% of cases according to one large population-based study [2]. Postoperative renal insufficiency is a problem that plagues EVAR as well. Greenberg and colleagues reported that patients undergoing EVAR using suprarenal fixation of the graft had an attenuated rise in serum creatinine at the time of discharge compared to OSR patients. However following those patients to 12 months revealed no difference in serum creatinine based on the operative approach undertaken [34]. The goal of suprarenal stent-graft fixation is to increase the length of the proximal neck coverage and to improve the fit of the stent-graft. It also makes more patients eligible for EVAR. Some have posited that suprarenal fixation causes a decrement in renal function, through a variety of mechanisms, including blockage or narrowing of the renal ostia; however, several studies have demonstrated equal declines in renal function, irrespective of supra- or infrarenal fixation [35,36]. Regardless of the fixation point, there tends to be a 10% decline in creatinine clearance at 1 year post EVAR. The exact etiology of this finding is unknown, but it has prompted some to recommend minimization of pre- and post-procedure contrast-enhanced radiographic studies, alternative radiographic studies that do not utilize contrast when feasible, the institution of measures to mitigate contrast-induced nephropathy, and utilizing the minimum amount of contrast necessary during EVAR [34].

Renal artery occlusion by the stent-graft at the time of the operation is a technical error and ought to be caught at the latest by the end of the operation when a completion angiogram is performed (Fig. 9.7); however, a more nuanced discussion is warranted in the case of accessory renal arteries and late renal artery occlusion. Accessory renal arteries are a frequent anatomic variant, being present in over 15% of the population [37]. Some clinicians are reluctant to offer EVAR to patients with accessory renal arteries for fear of causing segmental renal infarction and a subsequent decline in renal function, as well as creating a possible source of endoleak. It would be unfortunate to deny such a large subset of the population the benefits of EVAR, but the long-term effects of excluding these accessory arteries are not known. Karmacharya and colleagues reviewed their experience with EVAR in this patient population and found that an accessory renal artery was not implicated in any of their endoleaks [38]. In follow-up, 20% of the patients who had accessory renal arteries had renal infarcts found on CT imaging; however, they did not observe any long-term effect on patients' blood pressure, serum creatinine, or creatinine clearance. The mean follow-up for these patients was 16 months. These findings suggest that patients with this normal variant can still be candidates for EVAR. However, these results must be interpreted with caution given the known decline in renal function as part of the normal aging process, the relatively frequent use of contrast-enhanced imaging for surveillance in these patients, and the lack of follow-up on the order of years.

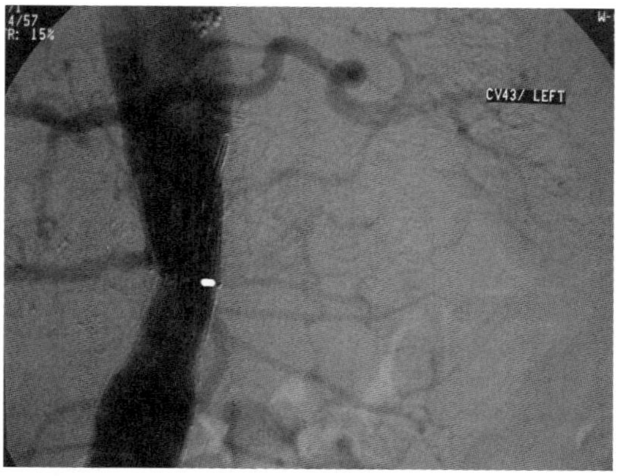

Fig. 9.7 Inadvertent left renal occlusion during EVAR. The left renal artery (white mark) fills slowly and its origin is covered by the stent-graft. The angiogram reveals a common source for such operator error with the overlying jejunal branches of the superior mesenteric artery mimicking the course of a renal artery as they travel leftward in the mesentery.

Damage to the device

Most often an incidental finding on abdominal radiographs, stent-graft fractures have been found to occur in 0–5.8 of cases [39,40]. The concern is that fractures of the graft could lead to type III endoleak, though this appears to be mostly a theoretical concern. Barb separation, also a rare finding, occurring in only 1.7% of patients, is of concern because the barbs aid in fixing the stent-graft in place proximally. Early versions of the Zenith stent graft system (Cook Medical, Bloomington, IN) had relatively few barbs and separation of one or several barbs caused migration and type I endoleak in some patients. Subsequent versions of the device increased the number of barbs significantly such that separation of one or a few barbs is generally without clinical consequence [39].

Conversion to open repair and secondary surgical intervention

Conversion of EVAR to OSR at the time of stent-graft deployment is a relatively rare event, occurring in just over 1% of cases [41,42]. Conversion can occur because of technically difficult anatomy – particularly narrow, tortuous iliac vessels – that prevents successful advancement of the device. Earlier generation devices suffered from maldeployment more commonly than the newer generations.

Late open repair has a mortality rate of 24%, significantly higher than the 4.7% mortality rate associated with OSR as the primary intervention in the absence of EVAR [41,43]. Risk factors for late open conversion are type I, II, and III endoleak, stent-graft migration and kinking, and large aneurysm size [44]. Because of this significant mortality rate, OSR following EVAR should only be done in patients at exceptionally high risk of aneurysm rupture, and a thorough conversation with the patient about the risks of such an undertaking is necessary.

Aside from conversion to OSR, there are a variety of other conditions that can occur after EVAR that may require a secondary surgical intervention. As mentioned previously, a variety of surgical bypass options exist for graft limb occlusion that cannot be managed utilizing an endovascular approach. Clinically significant renal artery narrowing, whether by graft migration or atherosclerotic disease, may require aortorenal or ileorenal bypass, though the need for this is relatively uncommon.

Late rupture

Because the most important objective of aortic aneurysm repair is the prevention of sac rupture, late rupture of the aneurysm, defined as rupture at least 30 days after EVAR, represents absolute treatment failure. The prospectively collected Eurostar Registry demonstrated a 1% per year rate of late rupture, with a nearly 60% associated mortality rate [41]. Type I and type III endoleaks are significant risk factors for late rupture, underscoring the importance of expeditiously treating these findings. Stent-graft migration and endograft kinking are also risk factors. Late rupture occurs at a median of 20 months post EVAR [45]. The most common presenting symptoms are abdominal or back pain, hypovolemia/hypotension, syncope, and/or shock.

Infectious complications

Infections involving aortic stent-grafts are not well described in the literature, and fortunately occur fairly rarely. Vogel and colleagues reported 2-year rates of graft infection of 0.2%, irrespective of an open or endovascular approach to aneurysm repair based on data from a large administrative database [46]. A different group reported an incidence of graft-related sepsis in EVAR of 6.2 per 1000 person-years [47]. Implicated species in stent-graft infections include *Staphylococcus*, *Streptococcus*, *Propionibacterium*, and *Enterobacter*, with the former two being the most common in OSR graft infection. Advanced age and an immunocompromised state from any number of conditions, including diabetes mellitus, chronic steroid use, and HIV positivity, are likely risk factors. An additional possible risk factor for aortic stent-graft infection that is quite relevant to the EVAR population is the need for secondary endovascular interventions, such as coil embolization, which, as mentioned earlier, is rather common. Each subsequent intervention allows for another opportunity for the introduction of a bacterial inoculum that could set the stage for a stent-graft infection.

Presentations of stent-graft infection can vary and may range from fever of unknown origin, constitutional symptoms, abdominal pain, or frank sepsis. Imaging of the graft may demonstrate perigraft abscess, fluid collections, and/or gas (Fig. 9.8). The diagnosis can often be made on the basis of blood cultures and CT imaging, though

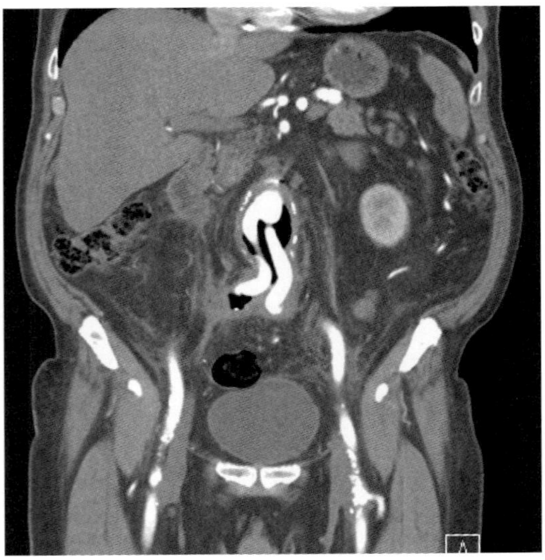

Fig. 9.8 Aortic sac–colon fistula after EVAR. The patient reported night sweats only and was successfully converted to a surgical graft with omental wrapping.

occasionally a tagged white blood cell scan may be necessary. No consensus exists as to the optimal treatment for these patients, though the options include removal of the infected graft with extra-anatomic bypass, replacement of the stent-graft with an in situ homograft, or medical therapy. The decision is often made based on the patient's condition and likelihood of surviving a major open operation. All three approaches are associated with a high mortality and, regardless of the approach taken, patients are typically placed on long-term intravenous antibiotics and subsequent lifelong oral antibiotic suppressive therapy.

A specific subtype of aortic stent-graft infection bears mentioning – aortoenteric fistula (AEF). Classically, these patients present with upper gastrointestinal bleeding, and the presence of AEF can often be confirmed with esophagogastroduodenoscopy. A number of mechanisms for this fistulization process have been proposed: continued aneurysm growth secondary to endoleak, inflammatory aortic aneurysm, inflammatory bowel disease, graft migration or erosion, and injury to the bowel from fixation hooks [48]. As with other forms of aortic stent-graft infection, AEF occurs infrequently enough to preclude a consensus as to the best treatment approach, though the options are generally the same; however, repair of the fistula is required.

Conclusions

The treatment of aneurysmal disease of the aorta has been revolutionized with the advent of endovascular technologies; however, certain complications of aortic aneurysm repair remain problematic, such as ischemic and infectious complications. Other complications, such as endoleak and graft migration, are novel and exclusive to EVAR. Accordingly, there is clinical equipoise as to how best to treat some of these complications. As long-term clinical experience grows with endovascular stent-grafts, and a better understanding of the natural history of some of these complications develops, surveillance and treatment algorithms will become better defined to improve outcomes for patients with aortic aneurysms.

References

1 Parodi JC, Palmaz JC, Barone HD. Transfemoral intraluminal graft implantation for abdominal aortic aneurysms. Ann Vasc Surg 1991; 5(6):491–9.

2 Schermerhorn ML, O'Malley AJ, Jhaveri A, et al. Endovascular vs. open repair of abdominal aortic aneurysms in the Medicare population. N Engl J Med 2008; 358(5):464–74.

3 Greenhalgh RM, Brown LC, Powell JT, et al. Endovascular repair of aortic aneurysm in patients physically ineligible for open repair. N Engl J Med 2010; 362(20): 1872–80.

4 Parent FN, Meier GH, Godziachvili V, et al. The incidence and natural history of type I and II endoleak: a 5-year follow-up assessment with color duplex ultrasound scan. J Vasc Surg 2002; 35(3):474–81.

5 Mirza TA, Karthikesalingam A, Jackson D, et al. Duplex ultrasound and contrast-enhanced ultrasound versus computed tomography for the detection of endoleak after EVAR: systematic review and bivariate meta-analysis. Eur J Vasc Endovasc Surg 2010; 39(4):418–28.

6 van Marrewijk CJ, Fransen G, Laheij RJ, et al. Is a type II endoleak after EVAR a harbinger of risk? Causes and outcome of open conversion and aneurysm rupture during follow-up. Eur J Vasc Endovasc Surg 2004; 27(2):128–37.

7 Steinmetz E, Rubin BG, Sanchez LA, et al. Type II endoleak after endovascular abdominal aortic aneurysm repair: a conservative approach with selective intervention is safe and cost-effective. J Vasc Surg 2004; 39(2):306–13.

8 Jones JE, Atkins MD, Brewster DC, et al. Persistent type 2 endoleak after endovascular repair of abdominal aortic aneurysm is associated with adverse late outcomes. J Vasc Surg 2007; 46(1):1–8.

9 Liaw JV, Clark M, Gibbs R, et al. Update: complications and management of infrarenal EVAR. Eur J Radiol 2009; 71(3):541–51.

10 Heikkinen MA, Arko FR, Zarins CK. What is the significance of endoleaks and endotension. Surg Clin North Am 2004; 84(5):1337–52, vii.

11 Toya N, Fujita T, Kanaoka Y, et al. Endotension following endovascular aneurysm repair. Vasc Med 2008; 13(4):305–11.

12 Chaikof EL, Blankensteijn JD, Harris PL, et al. Reporting standards for endovascular aortic aneurysm repair. J Vasc Surg 2002; 35(5):1048–60.

13 Veith FJ, Baum RA, Ohki T, et al. Nature and significance of endoleaks and endotension: summary of opinions expressed at an international conference. J Vasc Surg 2002; 35(5):1029–35.

14 Buth J, Harris PL, van Marrewijk C, et al. The significance and management of different types of endoleaks. Semin Vasc Surg 2003; 16(2):95–102.

15 Erzurum VZ, Sampram ES, Sarac TP, et al. Initial management and outcome of aortic endograft limb occlusion. J Vasc Surg 2004; 40(3):419–23.
16 Maleux G, Koolen M, Heye S, et al. Limb occlusion after endovascular repair of abdominal aortic aneurysms with supported endografts. J Vasc Interv Radiol 2008; 19(10):1409–12.
17 Baum RA, Shetty SK, Carpenter JP, et al. Limb kinking in supported and unsupported abdominal aortic stent-grafts. J Vasc Interv Radiol 2000; 11(9):1165–71.
18 Fairman RM, Baum RA, Carpenter JP, et al. Velazquez OC. Limb interventions in patients undergoing treatment with an unsupported bifurcated aortic endograft system: a review of the Phase II EVT Trial. J Vasc Surg 2002; 36(1):118–26.
19 Maldonado TS, Rockman CB, Riles E, et al. Ischemic complications after endovascular abdominal aortic aneurysm repair. J Vasc Surg. 2004 Oct;40(4):703–9; discussion 9–10.
20 Maldonado TS, Ranson ME, Rockman CB, et al. Decreased ischemic complications after endovascular aortic aneurysm repair with newer devices. Vasc Endovasc Surg 2007; 41(3):192–9.
21 Dadian N, Ohki T, Veith FJ, et al. Overt colon ischemia after endovascular aneurysm repair: the importance of microembolization as an etiology. J Vasc Surg 2001; 34(6):986–96.
22 Prinssen M, Buskens E, Nolthenius RP, et al. Sexual dysfunction after conventional and endovascular AAA repair: results of the DREAM trial. J Endovasc Ther 2004; 11(6):613–20.
23 Lederle FA, Freischlag JA, Kyriakides TC, et al. Outcomes following endovascular vs open repair of abdominal aortic aneurysm: a randomized trial. JAMA 2009; 302(14):1535–42.
24 Lin PH, Bush RL, Chaikof EL, et al. A prospective evaluation of hypogastric artery embolization in endovascular aortoiliac aneurysm repair. J Vasc Surg 2002; 36(3):500–6.
25 Faries PL, Morrissey N, Burks JA, et al. Internal iliac artery revascularization as an adjunct to endovascular repair of aortoiliac aneurysms. J Vasc Surg 2001; 34(5):892–9.
26 Karch LA, Hodgson KJ, Mattos MA, et al. Adverse consequences of internal iliac artery occlusion during endovascular repair of abdominal aortic aneurysms. J Vasc Surg 2000; 32(4):676–83.
27 Prinssen M, Verhoeven EL, Buth J, et al. A randomized trial comparing conventional and endovascular repair of abdominal aortic aneurysms. N Engl J Med 2004; 351(16):1607–18.
28 Becquemin JP, Majewski M, Fermani N, et al. Colon ischemia following abdominal aortic aneurysm repair in the era of endovascular abdominal aortic repair. J Vasc Surg 2008; 47(2):258–63; discussion 63.
29 Szilagyi DE. A second look at the etiology of spinal cord damage in surgery of the abdominal aorta. J Vasc Surg 1993; 17(6):1111–13.
30 Berg P, Kaufmann D, van Marrewijk CJ, et al. Spinal cord ischaemia after stent-graft treatment for infra-renal abdominal aortic aneurysms. Analysis of the Eurostar database. Eur J Vasc Endovasc Surg 2001; 22(4):342–7.
31 Chiesa R, Melissano G, Marrocco-Trischitta MM, et al. Spinal cord ischemia after elective stent-graft repair of the thoracic aorta. J Vasc Surg 2005; 42(1):11–17.
32 Feezor RJ, Martin TD, Hess PJ, Jr, et al. Extent of aortic coverage and incidence of spinal cord ischemia after thoracic endovascular aneurysm repair. Ann Thorac Surg 2008; 86(6):1809–14; discussion 14.
33 McGarvey ML, Mullen MT, Woo EY, et al. The treatment of spinal cord ischemia following thoracic endovascular aortic repair. Neurocrit Care 2007; 6(1):35–9.
34 Greenberg RK, Chuter TA, Lawrence-Brown M, et al. Analysis of renal function after aneurysm repair with a device using suprarenal fixation (Zenith AAA Endovascular Graft) in contrast to open surgical repair. J Vasc Surg 2004; 39(6):1219–28.
35 Alsac JM, Zarins CK, Heikkinen MA, et al. The impact of aortic endografts on renal function. J Vasc Surg 2005; 41(6):926–30.
36 Cayne NS, Rhee SJ, Veith FJ, et al. Does transrenal fixation of aortic endografts impair renal function? J Vasc Surg 2003; 38(4):639–44.
37 Bude RO, Forauer AR, Caoili EM, et al. Is it necessary to study accessory arteries when screening the renal arteries for renovascular hypertension? Radiology 2003; 226(2):411–16.
38 Karmacharya J, Parmer SS, Antezana JN, et al. Outcomes of accessory renal artery occlusion during endovascular aneurysm repair. J Vasc Surg 2006; 43(1):8–13.
39 Greenberg RK, Chuter TA, Sternbergh WC, 3rd, et al. Zenith AAA endovascular graft: intermediate-term results of the US multicenter trial. J Vasc Surg 2004; 39(6):1209–18.
40 Criado FJ, Fairman RM, Becker GJ. Talent LPS AAA stent graft: results of a pivotal clinical trial. J Vasc Surg 2003; 37(4):709–15.
41 Harris PL, Vallabhaneni SR, Desgranges P, et al. Incidence and risk factors of late rupture, conversion, and death after endovascular repair of infrarenal aortic aneurysms: the EUROSTAR experience. European Collaborators on Stent/graft techniques for aortic aneurysm repair. J Vasc Surg 2000; 32(4):739–49.
42 Elkouri S, Gloviczki P, McKusick MA, et al. Perioperative complications and early outcome after endovascular and open surgical repair of abdominal aortic aneurysms. J Vasc Surg 2004; 39(3):497–505.
43 Greenhalgh RM, Brown LC, Kwong GP, et al. Comparison of endovascular aneurysm repair with open repair in patients with abdominal aortic aneurysm (EVAR trial 1), 30-day operative mortality results: randomised controlled trial. Lancet 2004; 364(9437):843–8.

44 Becquemin JP, Allaire E, Desgranges P, et al. Delayed complications following EVAR. Tech Vasc Interv Radiol 2005; 8(1):30–40.

45 Schlosser FJ, Gusberg RJ, Dardik A, et al. Aneurysm rupture after EVAR: can the ultimate failure be predicted? Eur J Vasc Endovasc Surg 2009; 37(1):15–22.

46 Vogel TR, Symons R, Flum DR. The incidence and factors associated with graft infection after aortic aneurysm repair. J Vasc Surg 2008; 47(2):264–9.

47 Sharif MA, Lee B, Lau LL, et al. Prosthetic stent graft infection after endovascular abdominal aortic aneurysm repair. J Vasc Surg 2007; 46(3):442–8.

48 Ruby BJ, Cogbill TH. Aortoduodenal fistula 5 years after endovascular abdominal aortic aneurysm repair with the Ancure stent graft. J Vasc Surg 2007; 45(4):834–6.

49 Pelberg RA, Wojciech M. Vascular CT Angiography Manual. Springer, 2011. DOI: 10.1007/978-1-84996-260-5_7.

10

CHAPTER 10

Complications of thoracic aortic endografting

Jacques Kpodonu
University of California Irvine,
Cardiovascular Hybrid Interventions, Hoag Heart and Vascular Institute, Newport Beach, CA, USA

Introduction

Endoleaks are defined as blood flow outside the lumen of the stent-graft but within the aneurysm sac. The endoleak rate after endovascular thoracic aortic aneurysm repair ranges from 5% to 25%. Eighty percent of endoleaks are classified as type I and III endoleaks; type II endoleaks are less frequent. Risk factors for developing thoracic aortic endoleaks include an aortic implantation zone of less than 2 cm from the left subclavian artery (LSA) and the existence of an entry tear at the lesser curvature of the arch aorta. Type III endoleaks occur when there is structural failure with the stent-graft including holes in the stent-graft fabric, stent-graft fractures, and junctional separations that occur with modular devices. Type IV endoleaks are detected at the time of implantation when patients are fully anticoagulated and are caused by stent-graft porosity and usually resolve by reversal of anticoagulation. Type V endoleak refer to expansion of an aneurysm sac without the presence of an identifiable endoleak. Causes may include an undiagnosed endoleak, ultrafiltration, or thrombus which provides an ineffective barrier to pressure transmission.

Postoperative image surveillance for endoleaks

The goal of postoperative image surveillance is to evaluate for aneurysm expansion or shrinkage, to detect stent-graft migration or fracture, and to detect endoleaks. Thin-section triple-phase computer tomographic angiography (CTA) images obtained before, during, and after contrast administration is a highly accurate study. The time-resolved nature of the triple-phase imaging gives important information as to when contrast enters or exits the aorta. Finding a collection of contrast outside the stent-graft lumen and inside the aneurysm sac defines an endoleak. Other useful imaging studies include intravascular ultrasound (IVUS) and magnetic resonance angiography (MRA), which can both be used in patients with renal failure or iodine contrast allergy.

Type I endoleak

Type I endoleaks have flow that originates from either the proximal or distal stent-graft attachment site (Fig. 10.1). Separation between the stent-graft and the native arterial wall creates a direct communication with the systemic arterial circulation. Development of a type I endoleak after thoracic aortic aneurysm

Endovascular and Hybrid Therapies for Structural Heart and Aortic Disease, First Edition.
Edited by Jacques Kpodonu and Raoul Bonan.

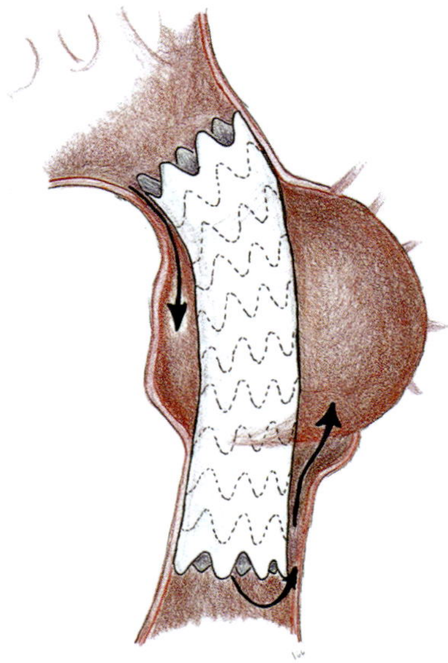

Fig. 10.1 Complications in endografting: type I endoleaks (arrows)

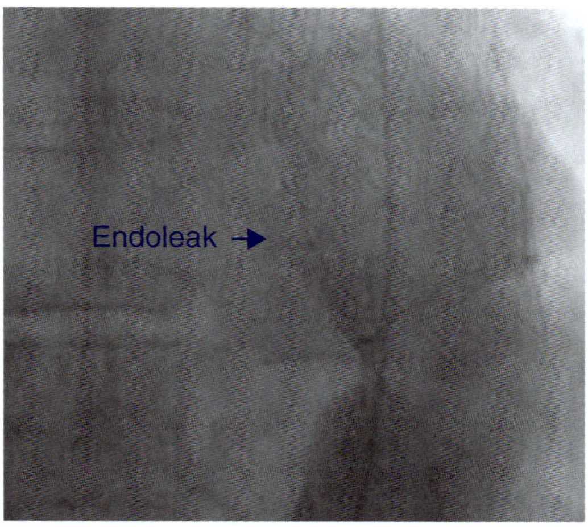

Fig. 10.2 Digital substraction angiography demonstrating a type I endoleak.

repair is associated with aneurysmal sac expansion and a potential rupture of the sac. Endoleaks are detected commonly intraoperatively using angiography or electively using CTA (Figs 10.2 and 10.3).

Management of a type I endoleak

Balloon angioplasty

Balloon angioplasty is the first line of treatment of a type I endoleak. Balloon angioplasty at the end of the endoluminal graft is performed using a non-compliant balloon to ensure appropriate apposition of the graft to the aortic wall (Fig. 10.4).

Placement of a proximal or distal cuff

An endoluminal graft cuff to extend the proximal or distal landing can be placed with or without balloon angioplasty. The presence of a short proximal landing zone may require a left carotid-to-left subclavian artery transposition or a transposition of the left subclavian artery to the left carotid artery (Fig. 10.5) in addition to deployment of a proximal cuff to extend the proximal landing zone for an appropriate seal and resolution of the endoleak.

Coil emboilization

Embolization coils can be used to thrombose flow that is feeding the aneurysm sac by assessing the aneurysm sac with the help of a guiding catheter (Fig. 10.6).

Open conversion

Failure to resolve a type I endoleak by an endovascular approach with an increase in aneurysm sac size is an indication for open conversion with removal of the endoluminal graft and a repair using a tube graft (Fig. 10.7).

Management of a distal type I endoleak

Management of a distal type I endoleak can also be managed by balloon angioplasty and the extension of the distal landing zone with a cuff. The presence of a short distal landing zone (<2.0 cm) requires coverage of the celiac trunk or a celiac/superior mesenteric bypass to lengthen the distal landing zone.

Retrograde type I endoleak associated with the treatment of type B aortic dissections

Retrograde type I endoleak post endoluminal graft for type B dissections mostly represents some form of false lumen flow and the majority develop progressive thrombosis with time. The presence of a retrograde type I endoleak in the absence of any incremental increase in the false lumen sac size can be managed conservatively.

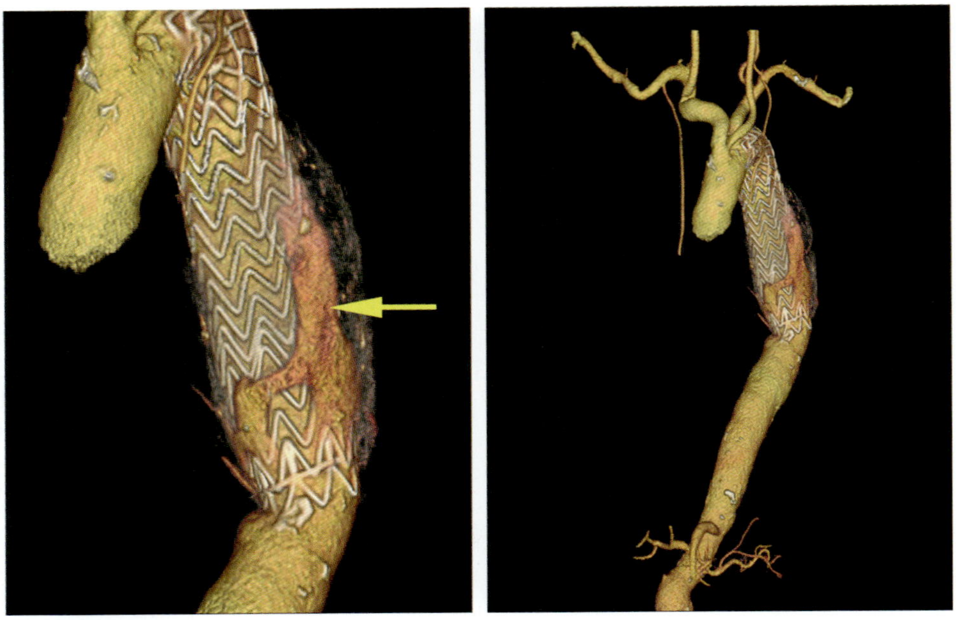

Fig. 10.3 Sixty-four-slice CT scan demonstrating a distal type I endoleak (arrow) post stent-graft.

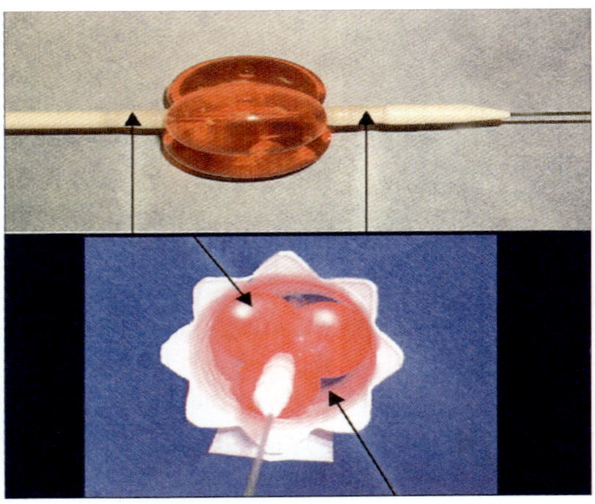

Fig. 10.4 Gore trilobed balloon used for balloon angioplasty of an endograft for management of type1 endoleaks.

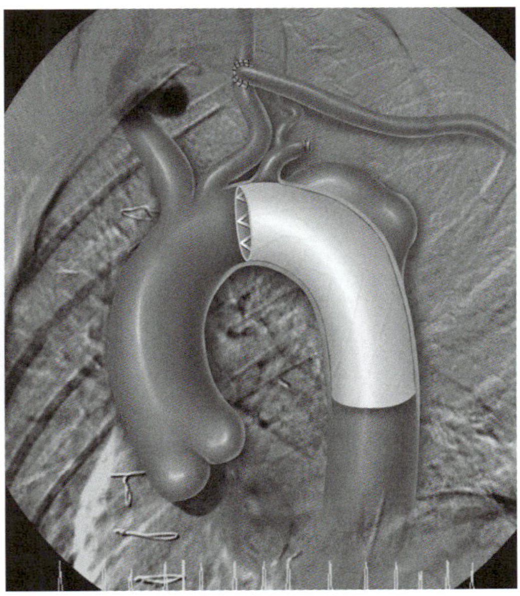

Fig. 10.5 Transposition of the left subclavian artery with extension of the proximal landing zone >2.0 cm to prevent a type I endoleak.

Type II endoleaks

Type II endoleaks can result from retrograde flow from a covered artery (e.g. the left subclavian artery into the aneurysm sac) or when blood travels through branches from the non-stented portion of the aorta through anastomotic connections into vessels with a direct communication with the aneurysm sac. They are more usual from an intercostal or covered subclavian artery. Most type II endoleaks will thrombose (Figs 10.8 and 10.9).

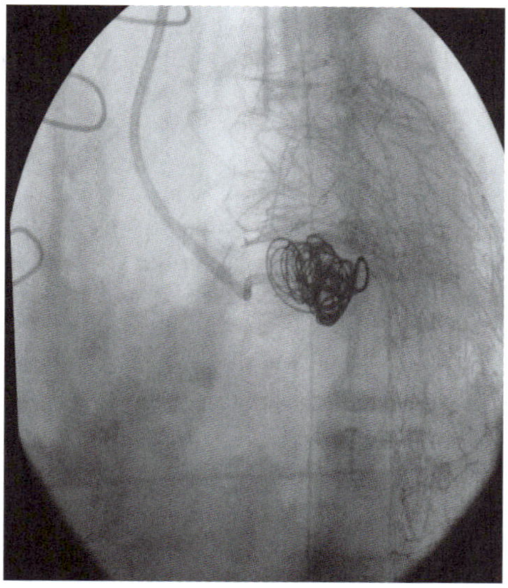

Fig. 10.6 Coil embolization of an endoleak.

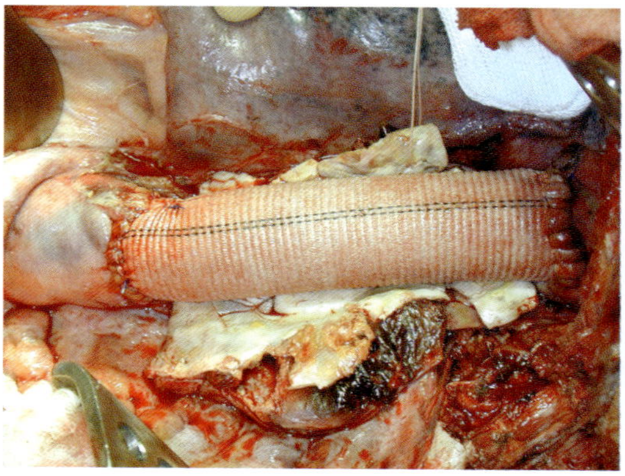

Fig. 10.7 Management of a type I endoleak by open conversion.

A small percentage of type II endoleaks transmit sufficient pressure to cause sac enlargement. Management: includes: (i) doil embolization of the subclavian artery by the retrograde approach; (ii) coil embolization of the aneurysm sac; (iii) injection of thrombin in to the sac; and (iv) thoracoscopic ligation of the intercostal artery.

Management of a type II endoleak by coil embolization

The technique of coil embolization to manage a type II endoleak involves placing bilateral radial arterial lines to confirm there is no gradient between both arms. The patient is subsequently placed under

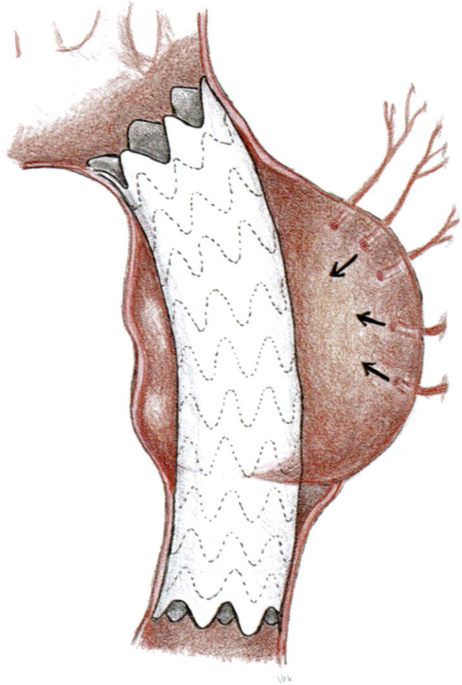

Fig. 10.8 Complications in endografting: type II endoleaks.

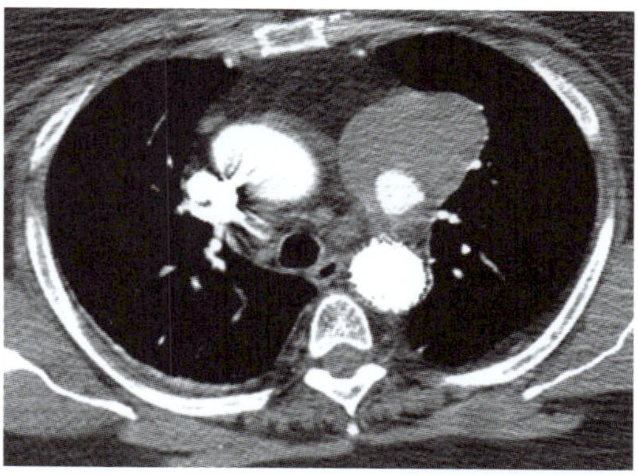

Fig. 10.9 CT scan demonstrating a type II endoleak.

general anesthesia. A left percutaneous retrograde approach is used to cannulate the left brachial artery with a 35 cm 6 Fr sheath. Heparin is given to achieve an activated time greater than 200 seconds. A 5 Fr pigtail catheter is advanced over a 180 cm angled soft-tip glide wire through the left brachial sheath and a selective left subclavian artery arch angiogram is performed to confirm the type II endoleak (Fig. 10.10). A Bereinstein catheter is exchanged for the 5 Fr angiographic pigtail catheter and a

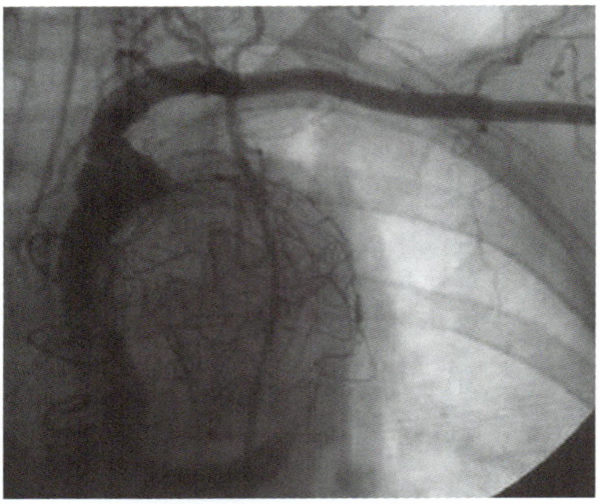

Fig. 10.10 Selective left subclavian artery angiogram demonstrating a type II endoleak.

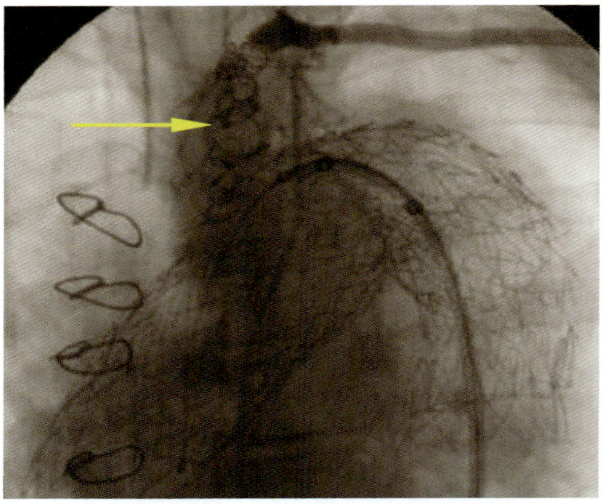

Fig. 10.11 Angiogram taken after coil embolization of the left subclavian artery with resolution of a type II endoleak.

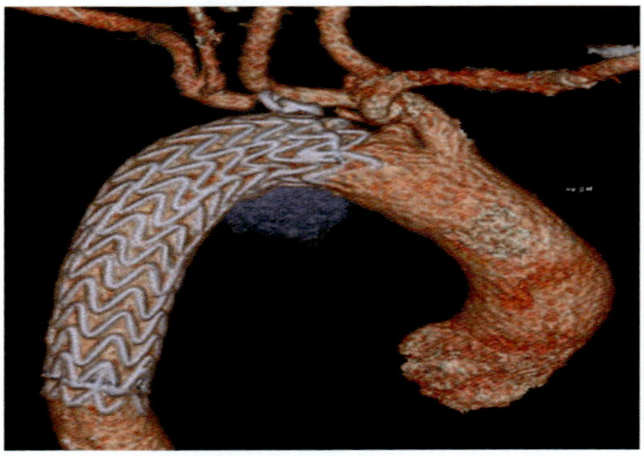

Fig. 10.12 Postoperative CT scan with coils demonstrated in the left subclavian artery, with resolution of a type II endoleak.

couple of 15 mm × 15 cm Cook embolization coils (Bloomington, IN) are deployed in the ostium of the left subclavian artery with care not to coil embolize the left vertebral artery in the process. Upon embolization, there should be a noticeable drop in the left radial arterial line pressure with flattening of the pressure wave form. A completion angiogram performed post embolization is performed to confirm satisfactory repair of the type II endoleak from the left subclavian artery origin (Fig. 10.11). A postoperative computed tomography (CT) scan is performed to confirm satisfactory results (Fig. 10.12).

Management of a type II endoleak by injection of thrombin in the sac

Similarly, an angiographic catheter can be used to perform an angiogram to confirm the type II endoleak. A guiding catheter is used to go behind the thoracic endograft to access the aneurysm sac. Thrombin can subsequently be injected into the sac. The dose of thrombin varies from 1 ml (500 IU) to 3 ml (1500 IU).

Thoracoscopic ligation of the intercostal artery

Thoracoscopic ligation of the intercostals vessel feeding the aneurysm sac can be performed to interrupt flow to the aneurysm sac when the endovascular approach fails.

Type III endoleaks

Type III endoleaks, whether from disconnecting parts or fabric damage, are associated with an increased risk of aneurysm rupture. Most type III endoleaks appear during medium-term follow-up and are thought to be caused by late endograft disintegration. Treatment consists of placement of an extra piece of graft (Figs 10.13 and 10.14).

Complications

Retrograde type B dissection after endovascular management of type B dissection

Retrograde type B dissection following stent-graft placement for the treatment of type B dissection is a rare but fatal complication associated with a high mortality [1–7]. Once ascending aortic dissection

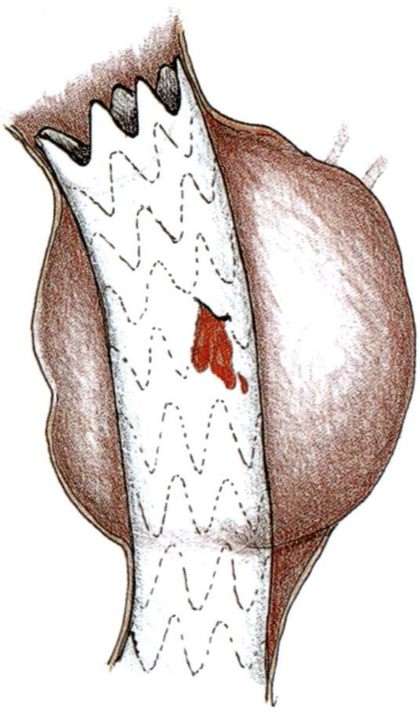

Fig. 10.13 Complications in endografting: type III endoleaks.

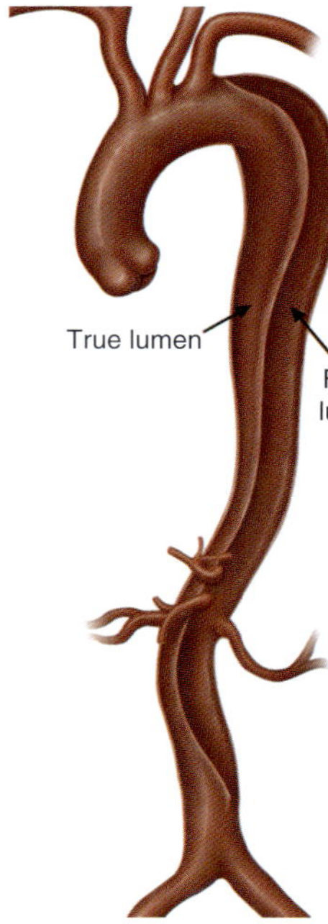

Fig. 10.15 Type B dissection.

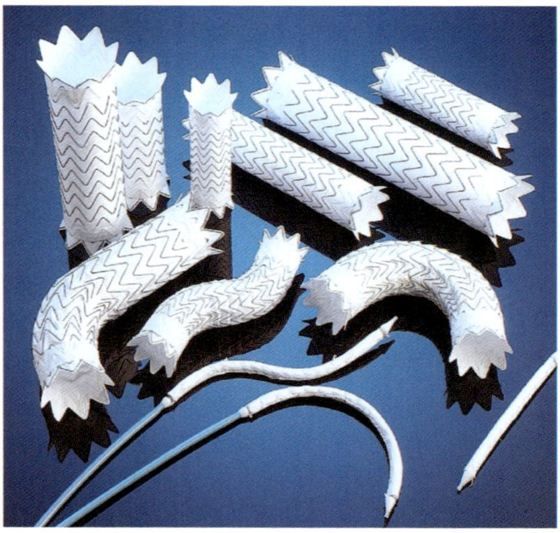

Fig. 10.14 Components of the endoluminal graft available to treat endoleaks as a result of late endograft disintegration from a type III endoleak.

occurs, emergent surgical treatment should be performed as soon as possible [8]. Despite the minimal invasive nature of stent-graft implantation, sometimes fatal complications may arise from its deployment, with retrograde ascending aortic dissection being one of the most severe types (Fig. 10.15).

Between 1998 and 2007 a total of 512 patients with a thoracic aortic stent-graft for various aortic pathologies were treated at the Arizona Heart Institute. The Gore TAG excluder device (W.L. Gore & Associates, Flagstaff, AZ) was used in 400 patients with eight patients developing a retrograde type A dissection (2.0%). There were three males and five females, with the diagnosis made at a median of 116 days; 50% of the patients were identified during the perioperative period. Retrograde type B dissection was diagnosed within the perioperative period in three patients with 100% mortality [9,10]. Of the eight patients who developed a retrograde type A dissection one patient was previously treated for a thoracic aortic aneurysm, one patient for a penetrating aortic ulcer, and six patients for a type B dissection (75%). There were 97 patients treated for type B dissection during that time period, resulting in a 6/97 (6.2%) incidence of a retrograde type dissection in that group category. The mortality rate for a retrograde type B dissection was 5/8 (62.5%), mostly as a result of complications with three deaths within the perioperative period. The three surviving patients were diagnosed at 1, 7, and 19 months respectively, and all had an ascending aorta replacement with a tube graft.

Table 10.1 Initial seven patients who developed a retrograde type A dissection following stent-graft therapy for various thoracic aortic pathologies.

Patient	*Age (years)*	*Sex*	*Etiology*	*Graft used % oversize*	*Time to discovery*	*Result*
1	83	F	Dissection	11.1	POD no. 1	Death
2	78	F	Dissection	8.1	POD no. 10	Death
3	53	M	Dissection	21.2	1 month	Tube graft
4	78	F	Aneurysm	27.6	7 months	Tube graft
5	67	M	Dissection	21.2	19 months	Tube graft
6	60	M	Dissection	19.4	21 months	Death
7	74	F	Dissection	17.2	30 months	Death

Table 10.1 shows data on the initial seven patients. Possible etiologies for retrograde type A dissection that we knew of were possibly related to oversizing by more than 20% of the indication for use. The larger the stent-graft, the greater the radial force it gives to the aortic wall, resulting in good apposition to the aortic wall. Occasionally, oversizing has resulted in intimal injuries especially in fragile aortas. In the treatment of two patients oversizing of the aorta was responsible for retrograde type A dissection, with one patient receiving an endograft that had been oversized by 27.4%. Incomplete seal of the entry tear of a type B dissection occurred in one patient, with progression of disease of the aorta responsible in one patient diagnosed at 19 months before stent-graft placement for a type B dissection. Other possible etiologies could have been related to balloon dilation of endografts to achieve good wall apposition, resulting in aortic intimal injury, and the tips of the guide wire and the delivery system could cause damage to the aortic intima. In our report we did not use any stent-grafts with uncovered struts, which have been known to cause intimal injuries at the proximal and distal fixation points.

Stent related maldeployment

Failure to land the endograft in the correct location usually requires placement of an additional device, either an additional endograft or a cuff. A supply of these should be available for use if required to prevent procedural failure. Maldeployment is avoided by not hurrying during deployment. Perform check angiograms during deployment in the appropriate obliquity.

Complications related to vascular access

This may consist of iliac artery rupture because of trauma caused by the large endograft delivery system. This is best treated by insertion of a covered stent. A supply of these should always be kept in stock.

General complications

- *Stroke*: Increased by excessive manipulations in the aortic arch, by covering the left subclavian artery without bypass, and in the presence of atheroma in the aortic arch.
- *Paraplegia*: Increased by endografting long lengths of aorta; long areas of aortic stent-grafting in patients with previous abdominal aortic repair should be treated by spinal drainage.
- *Fever*: May occur as a result of thrombosis of the aneurysmal sac or the false lumen.

References

1 Totaro M, Miraldi F, Fanelli F. et al. Emergency surgery for retrograde extension of type B dissection after endovascular stent graft repair. Eur J Cardiothorac Surg 2001;20:1057–8.
2 Fanelli F, Salvatori FM, Marcelli G, et al. Type A aortic dissection developing during endovascular repair of an acute type B dissection. J Endovasc Ther 2003;10:254–9.
3 Nienaber CA, Eagle KA. Aortic dissection: new frontiers in diagnosis and management. Part II: therapeutic management and follow-up. Circulation 2003;108:772–8.
4 Pasic M, Bergs P, Knollmann F, et al. Delayed retrograde aortic dissection after endovascular stenting of the descending thoracic aorta. J Vasc Surg 2002;36:184–6.
5 Grabenwoger M, Fleck T, Ehrlich M, et al. Secondary surgical interventions after endovascular stent-grafting of

the thoracic aorta. Eur J Cardiothorac Surg 2004;26: 608–13.

6 Bethuyne N, Bove T, Van den Brande P, et al. Acute retrograde aortic dissection during endovascular repair of a thoracic aortic aneurysm. Ann Thorac Surg 2003;75:1967–9.

7 Misfeld M, Notzold A, Geist V, et al. Retrograde type A dissection after endovascular stent grafting of type B dissection [in German]. Z Kardiol 2002;91:274–7.

8 Totaro M, Miraldi F, Fanelli F, et al. Emergency surgery for retrograde extension of type B dissection after endovascular stent graft repair. Eur J Cardiothorac Surg 2001;20:1057–8.

9 Kpodonu J, Preventza O, Ramaiah VG, et al. Retrograde type A dissection after endovascular stenting of the descending thoracic aorta. Is the risk real? Eur J Cardiothorac Surg 2008;33(6):1014–18.

10 Diethrich EB, Ramaiah VG, Kpodonu J, et al. Endovascular and Hybrid Management of the Thoracic Aorta. A case-based approach, 1st edn. Oxford: Wiley Blackwell, 2008.

11

CHAPTER 11

Endovascular robotics for complex aortic intervention

Celia V. Riga, Colin D. Bicknell, Mohamad S. Hamady & Nicholas J. W. Cheshire

Regional Vascular Unit, St. Mary's Hospital, Imperial College, London, UK

Introduction

Vascular surgery is a rapidly evolving speciality driven largely by new advances in technology and a desire to perform less invasive procedures for patients that have significant comorbidities. The number of minimally invasive endovascular procedures has steadily risen as a result of increased operator experience, availability of more sophisticated and versatile endovascular tools, and advances in imaging modalities. Endovascular intervention, however, is not applicable to all. The mainstay of image guidance in most endovascular suites remains two-dimensional fluoroscopy, with its attendant radiation exposure to patients and staff and need for nephrotoxic contrast agents. Anatomic factors such as short landing zones, arch and visceral vessel involvement, tortuosity, and angulation as well as poor visualization of key aortic regions may therefore limit its uptake. Complex endovascular procedures can be time consuming and require a high degree of technical performance and long training pathways as their success is determined largely by operator skill.

New-generation custom-made fenestrated and branched devices were designed to extend the proximal sealing zone from the infrarenal segment to the suprarenal and thoraco-abdominal aorta by incorporating the visceral and supra-aortic vessels. In selected patients, fenestrated and branched stent-grafting appears to be a safe and effective alternative to open and hybrid surgery for juxtarenal and thoraco-abdominal aortic aneurysms (TAAAs), with encouraging short- and intermediate-term results [1–6]. However, even with accurate custom-made device designs in patients with straightforward anatomy, the process of cannulating branch vessels can be extremely challenging. Aortic angulation and iliac tortuosity leading to graft rotation can pose significant problems with stent deployment, and even small degrees of misalignment at the fenestration/target vessel ostium interface can hinder safe and efficient target vessel access. Conventional catheters have a relatively small repertoire of shapes and sizes and, more importantly, lack active maneuvrability of the tip and stability when passing stiff wires and other endovascular tools. The delivery of torque at the distal end is also impeded by the unanticipated contact friction between the catheter and the access vessel at the proximal end. Access vessels can be tortuous and angulated; non-compliant rigid arteries increase the risk of iatrogenic vessel damage whilst making catheter control more challenging. Repeated instrumentation, especially in the presence of vessel thrombus or calcification, increases the risk of vessel dissection, perforation, and distal embolization. A high

Endovascular and Hybrid Therapies for Structural Heart and Aortic Disease, First Edition.
Edited by Jacques Kpodonu and Raoul Bonan.

degree of finesse by the operator is therefore required in order to safely position the catheter tip and maintain stability at target sites, necessitating frequent catheter changes, which can threaten the stable positioning of guide wires and result in loss of vessel access and significantly prolonged overall procedure and fluoroscopic times.

Advanced catheter technology

There are commercially available endovascular catheters with manually "shapeable" tips and steerable sheaths. These devices have been developed in an attempt to overcome the limitations of standard endovascular technology outlined above. However, these are heavily dependent upon operator skill to manually shape the catheter tip via pull-wires to achieve the appropriate tip curvature. This manual control has limitations, and the amount of fine maneuvrability and stability over the catheter tip is often insufficient for performing complex vessel cannulation and other therapeutic procedures.

Robot-assisted surgery, also known as surgical telemanipulation or computer-assisted surgery, is being developed to overcome human limitations and eliminate impediments associated with conventional surgical and interventional tools. Robotic technologies are increasingly being used by surgical disciplines to facilitate and improve performance of minimally invasive intervention and have been shown in many fields to significantly improve outcomes [7,8]. The Da Vinci robot (Intuitive Surgical, Sunnyvale, CA) used in cardiac, gastrointestinal, and urologic surgery allows for greater precision of movement through an intuitive hand-operated console which is able to translate fine hand movements into target tissue contact. The Da Vinci system has been in use at many institutions for the last decade, however as yet does not offer a suitable platform for endovascular procedures.

Emerging endovascular robotic technologies utilizing magnetic fields offer the ability to remotely control the catheter tip. These include the NIOBE (Stereotaxis, St. Louis, MO). In this system, which is currently used for the ablation of arrhythmogenic cardiac pathways, two permanent magnets, whose location can be controlled by a central computer, generate a magnetic field of around 0.08 T around the patient's chest. The distal tip of the mapping or ablation catheter contains three magnets, which automatically align with the direction of the external magnetic field, thereby steering the catheter. Such a magnetic navigation system has been reported in the treatment of human peripheral arterial disease [9]. The disadvantages of this system include the cumbersome nature of the magnets and the time delay between instruction and movement of the catheter tip; the magnetic field produced also requires a purpose-built angiography suite.

A second system that has the ability to remotely control and steer endovascular catheters is the Hansen Sensei system (Hansen Medical, Mountain View, CA), currently being used to great effect in patients undergoing ablation of abnormal heart rhythms, a clinical use that has been pioneered by the cardiac unit in our institution [10]. The Hansen robot is a steerable endovascular catheter system designed to facilitate the physicians' ability to position and manipulate catheters within the vascular tree. This control is provided via a "master – slave" electromechanical system that controls a guide catheter and sheath (Artisan catheter) from a remote workstation away from the radiation source (Fig. 11.1). This intuitive technology replicates the hand movement of the operator delivering control in three dimensions and with 7 degrees of freedom via a 3D hand-operated joystick at the workstation console (Fig. 11.2). An

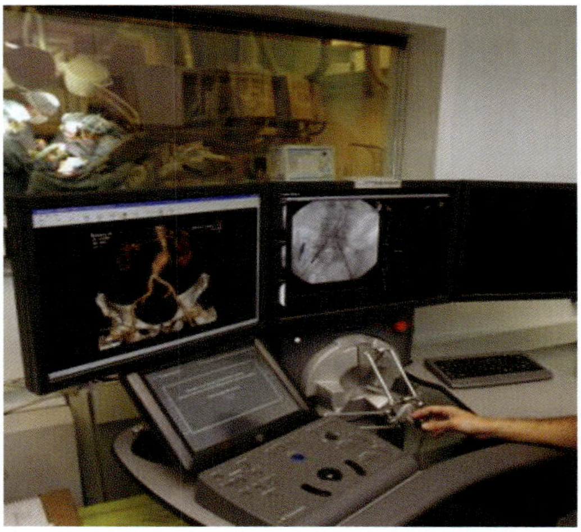

Fig. 11.1 Hansen robotic catheter system. The workstation is located outside the operating theater suite and away from the radiation source.

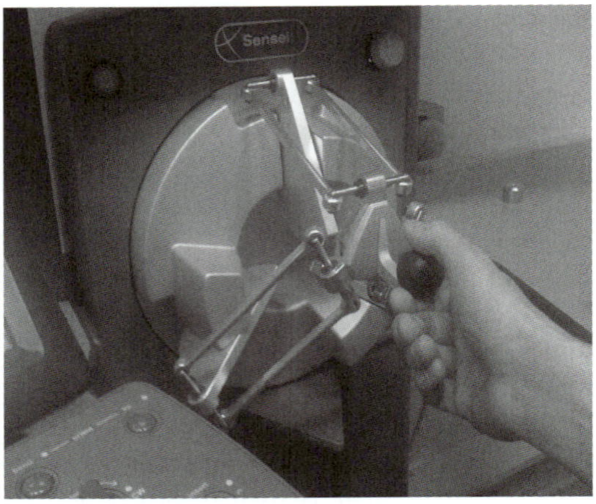

Fig. 11.2 The robotic catheter is controlled via a 3D hand-operated joystick with 7 degrees of freedom.

endovascular robotic catheter system has advantages over conventional catheterization in that it allows accurate cannulation of vessels and stable positioning for the introduction of diagnostic and therapeutic endovascular tools. A limitation of other remote catheter control systems is the lack of mechanical feedback that the operator receives from manual catheter manipulation and hence the ability to assess the amount of force that is being applied to the target tissues. However, visual feedback of force applied to the catheter tip can be obtained (Intellisens Fine Force Technology, Hansen Medical, Mountain View, CA) using the robotic system; damage or perforation of the vessel wall can be avoided improving therefore the safety of the device. Recognizing the need and potential

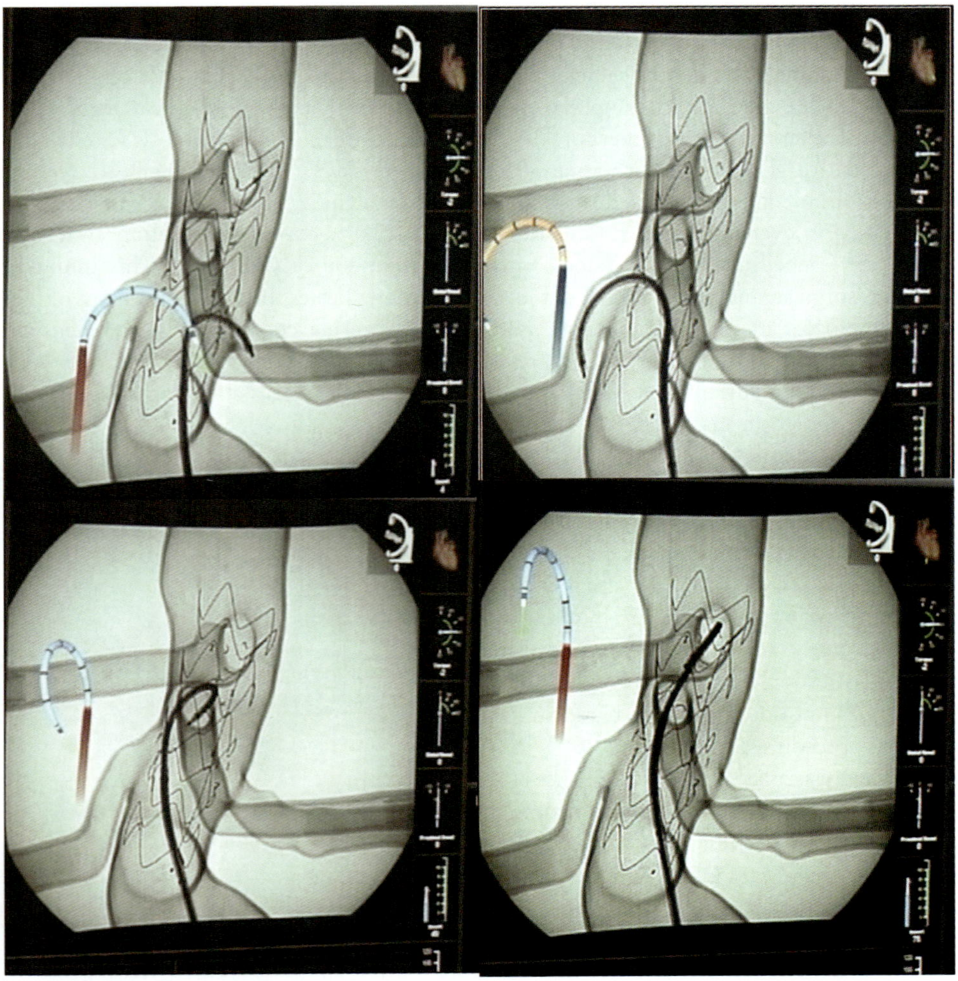

Fig. 11.3 Robotic cannulation of the target vessels in a fenestrated stent model.

for more advanced catheter technology in complex endovascular intervention, we have installed and investigated the use of this robotic system within our interventional endovascular suite – the first system of its kind worldwide, dedicated for use in the aorta and its branches.

Robotic assistance for fenestrated stent-grafting

We have tested the applicability of the Hansen system in vitro and in vivo. Our early studies have shown no advantage with robotic technology during simple endovascular tasks [11]. A pre-clinical study in our institution involving 15 endovascular specialists, demonstrated clear advantages using robotic catheterization techniques for target vessel cannulation and effectiveness in reducing procedure times during fenestrated stent-grafting, with greater accuracy and minimal contact with the vessel wall [12]. Robotic cannulation was significantly faster than standard cannulation using conventional endovascular catheters for all target vessels, namely the renal, celiac, and superior mesenteric arteries (Fig. 11.3). The reduction in time to cannulate all four vessels was from 15–20 minutes for most operators using conventional catheters to less than 5 minutes using the robotic steerable catheter (Fig. 11.4). The number of movements at the catheter tip required to complete successful target vessel cannulation was also significantly reduced (Fig. 11.5). This is likely a result of a greater range of motion with the robotic catheter and increased 3D control at the catheter tip. With conventional catheters the operator is required to make a series of movements, adjusting the amount of manual torque in order to reach a given target.

Mere target vessel catheterization does not necessarily reflect technical success in complex endovascular intervention. Equally important is the ability to advance stiff guide wires and other endovascular tools whilst maintaining stability at target sites. The robotic system is effectively a steerable sheath supporting a more flexible inner guide. Consequently, the catheter resists the tendency to herniate back into the aorta as wires and other endovascular tools are being advanced through its lumen. In 216 stiff guide wire exchanges studied, robotic endovascular catheters maintained stability at target sites with zero deflection during stiff guide wire exchanges, independent of the distance the catheter was introduced into the target vessel and with no loss of access. In contrast, conventional catheters required positioning at least 2 cm into the target vessel in order to avoid catheter deflection and subsequent loss of access. Robotic catheters, demonstrated increased stability at the target vessel ostium; this may prove useful when tackling angulated aortic arches, aneurysm necks, and tortuous branches.

Investigating the system further, we have demonstrated an overall improvement in operator performance whilst attempting complex endovascular tasks. We have developed a procedure-specific rating scale (the Imperial College Complex Cannulation Scoring Tool IC3ST) for the assessment of procedure skill. Studies of different groups of operators, determined by experience, have shown that the degree of operator skill can be assessed accurately using video assessment and procedure-specific scoring, as evidenced by a stepwise increase in score for conventional catheterization of vessels as experience increases. For robotic catheterization, groups with varying experience in conventional endovascular procedures obtained equal scores, indicating that skill using conventional catheters does not translate to robotic competence. However, the scores obtained using the robotic catheter were similar to those of highly experienced operators using the conventional approach, despite only a short training period on the robotic system (Fig. 11.6). These data raise the question of whether training to proficiency is faster using novel robotic endovascular catheters and may have important implications in terms of training and assessment in the future.

Experience with the robot has allowed our group to perform early clinical cases and design a trial to study the use of this catheter for branch vessel cannulation in fenestrated stent-grafting (Video 11.1). Following standardized training with this robotic system and after rehearsing the procedure in a laboratory environment, in August 2008, we were able to undertake the first human case of robotically assisted endovascular infrarenal aneurysm repair

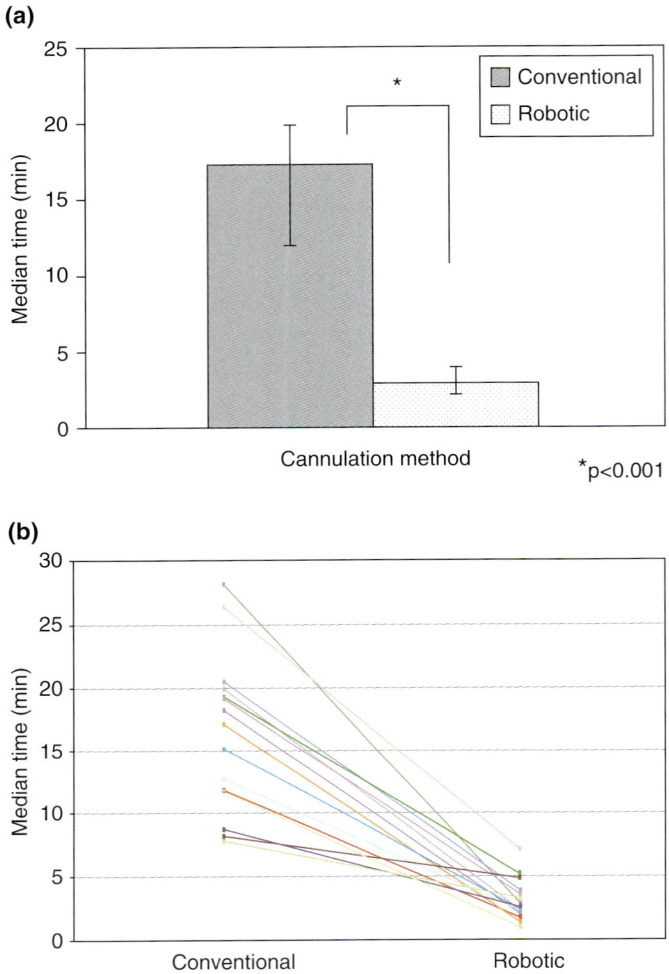

Fig. 11.4 Overall procedure times. (a) Bar chart representing whole procedure time (minutes) with conventional versus robotic catheters. Median procedure times are shown on the *y*-axis. The error bars represent the interquartile ranges (Wilcoxon signed rank test). (b) Line chart illustration of the data showing reductions in median procedure time with the robotic system versus conventional techniques, for each individual operator. Each operator is represented as a marker on either side of the plot area.

(Figs 11.1 and 11.7) to assess the feasibility of using this novel and innovative approach in a clinical setting [13]; its role, however, clearly lies in more complex endovascular procedures. Refining this procedure using in vivo and in vitro models and studying outcomes as part of our ongoing clinical trial, we aim to further evaluate the clinical use of this robotic system in complex aneurysm repair, significantly reduce procedure times, and improve overall clinical outcomes.

Future applications

Endovascular robotic technology could also assist in achieving in situ fenestration of aortic stent-grafts, which would obviate the need for expensive, bespoke fenestrated stents that can take weeks to manufacture. The technique of robot-assisted in situ fenestration may offer the option of total endovascular aneurysm repair to many patients who are either anatomically unsuitable for custom endovascular fenestrated stent-grafting, or who require the procedure on an urgent basis. To date, we have achieved antegrade, in situ fenestration in a porcine model using the Hansen system [14], 3D rotational angiography, and intravascular ultrasound (Fig. 11.8). Accurate positioning of the catheter tip within the main aortic body, and adjacent to the vessel ostia, is crucial in this procedure. Its position must also be stable, so as to allow precise puncture of the stent-graft and subsequent target

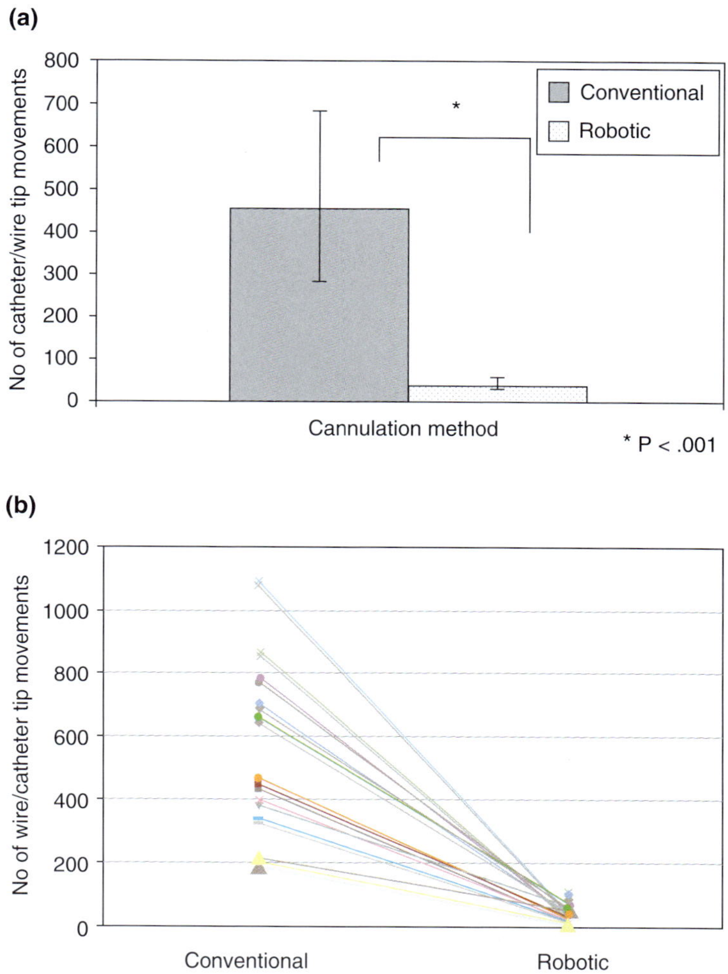

Fig. 11.5 Overall procedure movements. (a) Bar chart representing whole procedure movements at the wire/catheter tip with conventional versus robotic catheters. The median number of movements is shown on the *y*-axis. The error bars represent the interquartile ranges (Wilcoxon signed rank test). (b) Line chart illustration of the data showing reductions in median number of wire/catheter movements with the robotic system versus conventional techniques, for each individual operator. Each operator is represented as a marker on either side of the plot area.

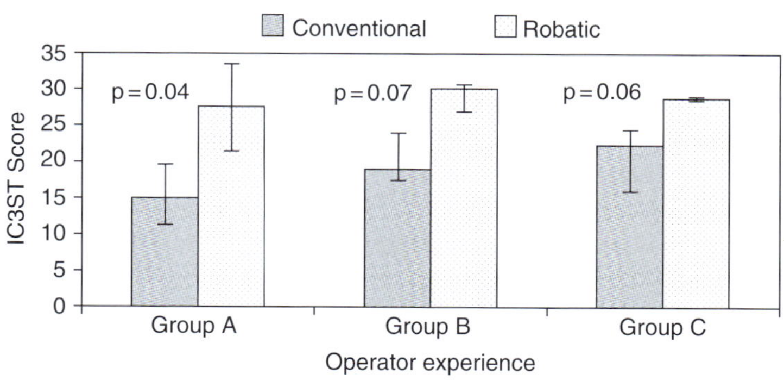

Fig. 11.6 Performance scores according to endovascular experience. Bar chart representing operator performance scores between groups A (low-volume intervention), B (medium-volume intervention), and C (high-volume intervention) using conventional and robotic techniques (Wilcoxon signed rank test).

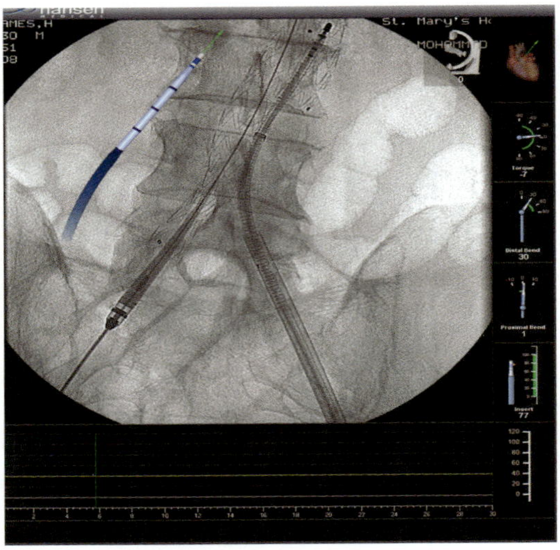

Fig. 11.7 Robotic cannulation of the contralateral limb of a bifurcated stent-graft for endovascular exclusion of an infrarenal abdominal aortic aneurysm.

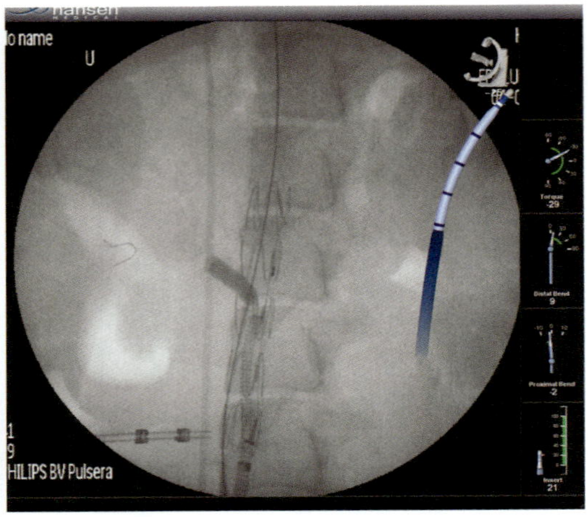

Fig. 11.8 Successful antegrade in situ fenestration of an aortic stent-graft (16 mm iliac extension covered stent; Valiant, Medtronic, Minneapolis, MN) with subsequent stenting of the right renal artery in a porcine model. The robotic catheter can be seen in position, adjacent to the orifice of the left renal artery.

vessel cannulation, serial balloon dilations, and stenting. This procedure may be further enhanced by 3D navigation technology; the Hansen system is compatible with existing non-fluoroscopic mapping systems such as NavX (St. Jude Medical, St. Paul, MN) [15]. Integration of robotics with 3D navigation technology may further improve the accuracy of catheter positioning and manipulation, which is of paramount importance in complex endovascular intervention.

Conclusions

Complex endovascular procedures can be time consuming and require a high degree of technical performance and long training pathways as their success is determined largely by operator skill. Despite recent advances in device technology for catheter-based peripheral arterial revascularization procedures, the inadequacy of conventional catheters for the variable and often unpredictable anatomy of patients with complex arterial disease implies that alternative catheter designs are essential. Integration of robotic technology into clinical practice may lead to improved catheter accuracy, stability, and safety in comparison with conventional techniques whilst minimizing radiation exposure. By maximizing the use of existing technologies while developing new approaches to treating these challenging cases, we are hoping to improve overall clinical outcomes and reduce the high mortality and morbidity rates associated with aortic disease. With experience, we hope to maximize the applicability of minimally invasive endovascular technology to a larger cohort of patients with improved overall clinical outcomes and a high degree of staff and patient safety.

References

1 Sun Z, Mwipatayi BP, Semmens JB, et al. Short to midterm outcomes of fenestrated endovascular grafts in the treatment of abdominal aortic aneurysms: a systematic review. J Endovasc Ther 2006;13:747–53.

2 O'Neill S, Greenberg RK, Haddad F, et al. A prospective analysis of fenestrated endovascular grafting: intermediate-term outcomes. Eur J Vasc Endovasc Surg 2006;32:115–23.

3 Muhs BE, Verhoeven EL, Zeebregts CJ, et al. Mid-term results of endovascular aneurysm repair with branched and fenestrated endografts. J Vasc Surg 2006;44:9–15.

4 Greenberg RK, Lytle B. Endovascular repair of thoracoabdominal aneurysms. Circulation 2008;117:2288–96.

5 Bicknell CD, Cheshire NJ, Riga CV, et al. Treatment of complex aneurysmal disease with fenestrated and branched grafts. Eur J Vasc Endovasc Surg 2009;37:175–81.

6 Chuter TA, Rapp JH, Hiramoto JS, et al. Endovascular treatment of thoracoabdominal aortic aneurysms. J Vasc Surg 2008;47(1):6–16.
7 Howe RD, Matsuoka Y. Robotics for surgery. Annu Rev Biomed Eng 1999;1:211–40.
8 Lanfranco AR, Castellanos AE, Desai JP, et al. Robotic surgery: a current perspective. Ann Surg 2004; 239(1):14–21.
9 Iyengar S, Gray WA. Use of magnetic guidewire navigation in the treatment of lower extremity peripheral vascular disease: report of the first human clinical experience. Catheter Cardiovasc Interv 2009;73(6): 739–44.
10 Kanagaratnam P, Koa-Wing M, Wallace DT, et al. Experience of robotic catheter ablation in humans using a novel remotely steerable catheter sheath. J Interv Cardiol Electrophysiol 2008;21(1):19–26.
11 Riga CV, Cheshire NJW, Hamady M, et al. Robotic endovascular catheters improve accuracy, reduce time and minimize radiation exposure in complex vascular procedures. Br J Surg 2009;96:S1.
12 Riga CV, Cheshire NJ, Hamady MS, et al. The role of robotic endovascular catheters in fenestrated stent grafting. J Vasc Surg 2010;51(4):810–19; discussion 819–20.
13 Riga C, Bicknell C, Cheshire N, et al. Initial clinical application of a robotically steerable catheter system in endovascular aneurysm repair. J Endovasc Ther 2009;16(2):149–53.
14 Riga CV, Bicknell CD, Wallace D, et al. Robot-assisted antegrade in-situ fenestrated stent grafting. Cardiovasc Intervent Radiol 2009;32(3):522–4.
15 Dickfeld T, Calkins H, Zviman M, et al. Anatomic stereotactic catheter ablation on three-dimensional magnetic resonance images in real time. Circulation 2003;108:2407–13.

Videoclip

This chapter contains the following videoclip:

Video 11.1 Video demonstration of vascular robotic cannulation of fenestration in an in vivo model.

It can be accessed at www.wiley.com/go/valverepair.

PART II

Structural heart disease

12

CHAPTER 12

Cardiovascular hybrid operating rooms

Georg Nollert[1,2], *Sabine Wich*[1], *Thomas Hartkens*[1] *& Anne Figel*[1]

[1] Siemens AG Healthcare Sector, Angiography, Fluoroscopic and Radiographic Systems, Forchheim
[2] Clinic of Cardiac Surgery, University of Munich, Munich, Germany

Introduction

Recent developments in vascular and cardiac care have led to new therapies integrating transcatheter techniques into surgery. To allow these procedures to be performed, operating rooms with integrated X-ray imaging capabilities have to be installed. These hybrid operating rooms need, as well as surgical equipment, high-end imaging equipment equivalent to the angiography devices used in interventional radiography and cardiology. Imaging devices have been used in operating rooms (ORs) for a long time. Mobile C-arms, ultrasound, and endoscopy are standard for many operations. The idea of hybrid operating rooms has a tradition of approximately 20 years and was introduced shortly after the start of endovascular procedures [1]. However, new devices, more complex transcatheter techniques, and longer procedures demand high-powered equipment to visualize thin guide wires, quantify small vessel diameters, evaluate delicate anastomoses, and detect endoleaks in the operating room. Because of their size and complexity these integrated endovascular suites or hybrid ORs require special considerations, planning, and design as well as new skills to be learned by the team. Guidelines on hybrid ORs are currently missing, but are under development by multidisciplinary teams.

Use of a hybrid operating room

Before a hybrid OR is planned, all stakeholders in the hospital should be identified and a detailed plan of room usage developed. These high tech rooms cost approximately double the investment and maintenance of conventional ORs and are 90% more costly than a cardiac cath lab mainly due to higher space and equipment requirements [2]. Therefore, flexible concepts for room usage have to be introduced, including conventional surgery and interventions. Even though the high investment for such ORs is only justified if the planning focuses on hybrid procedures, experience with existing installations has shown that initial planning underestimates the actual demand for such a facility, because of growing indications and increased referrals once the system is installed [3]. For instance, the cardiac surgery team of Vanderbilt University was able to nearly triple the number of coronary artery bypass graft (CABG) patients and identified their hybrid OR as one of the reasons [4].

Pediatric hybrid operations, hybrid coronary revascularization, transcatheter valve replacement and repair, and endovascular aortic repair are just some of the new developments that are ideally performed in a hybrid OR. Currently the strongest drivers for hybrid therapies are complex

Endovascular and Hybrid Therapies for Structural Heart and Aortic Disease, First Edition.
Edited by Jacques Kpodonu and Raoul Bonan.

endovascular aortic repair and transcatheter replacement of the stenotic aortic valve.

Hybrid therapy for congenital heart disease

Although surgery remains the treatment of choice for many congenital cardiac malformations, interventional cardiology approaches are increasingly being used in simple and even complex lesions. The percutaneous approach can be challenging due to low patient weight or poor vascular access, induced rhythm disturbances, and hemodynamic compromise [5]. Difficult and complex anatomy as in double-outlet right ventricle or transposition of the great arteries, or acute turns or kinks in the pulmonary arteries of tetralogy of Fallot patients, can make percutaneous procedures challenging if not impossible [6]. On the other hand, surgery also has its limitations. Examples are operative closure of multiple apical muscular ventricular septal defects, the collection of multiple major aorto-pulmonary collateral arteries (MAPCAs), adequate and lasting relief of peripheral pulmonic stenosis, or management of a previously implanted stenotic stent. Combining interventions and surgery into a single therapeutic procedure leads to reduction of complexity, cardiopulmonary bypass time, risk, and improved outcomes [7]. The hybrid approach to hypoplastic left heart syndrome serves as a role model of the concept (Fig. 12.1) [8,9].

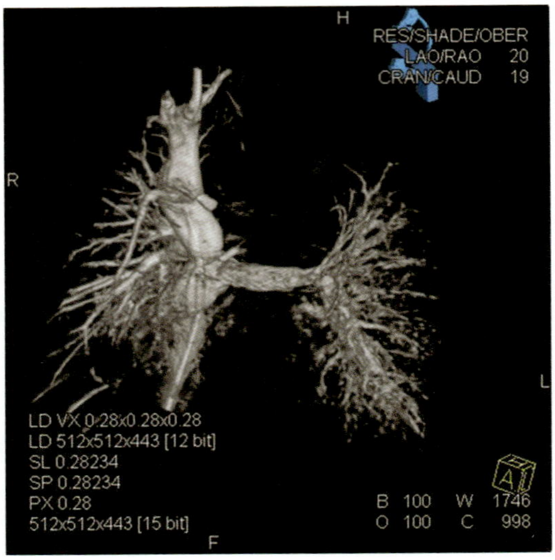

Fig. 12.1 Hypoplastic left heart syndrome: intraoperative post-Fontan evaluation of the superior and inferior venae cavae and the stented pulmonary arteries. Courtesy of Professor Berger and Dr. Ewert, Deutsches Herzzentrum, Berlin. Copyright: Siemens AG HIM AX, Forchheim, Germany

Hybrid therapy for valve disease

Transcatheter valve therapies are currently developed for the commonest valve diseases: mitral valve regurgitation, aortic stenosis, and – in children – pulmonary valve disease. For the repair of mitral regurgitation, more than 30 devices are currently under investigation and await US Food and Drug Administration (FDA) approval. Experimentally, prostheses for mitral und tricuspid valve replacement are under development and will certainly be available within the next few years. Aortic stenosis is the most frequent acquired heart valve lesion currently treated by surgery in developed countries. Conventional aortic valve replacement for aortic stenosis is based upon standardized guidelines with excellent outcomes, particularly in younger patients at relatively low risk. It will remain the gold standard for aortic valve replacement in the upcoming years. However, transcatheter techniques have developed as valid alternatives in high-risk patients where conventional surgical techniques are considered too invasive and risky [10]. Joint recommendations of the European Society of Cardiology and the European Society of Cardiac Surgery consider the hybrid OR to be the optimal environment for these new therapeutic options [11].

Coronary artery disease

Routine evaluation of bypass grafts is the first indication for imaging needs in coronary artery bypass grafting. Several groups reported a considerable number of technical bypass graft failures in the range of 13–20% that could be diagnosed intraoperatively by angiography and immediately repaired [12,13]. Surgical bypass grafting and percutaneous coronary artery revascularization are traditionally considered isolated options. A simultaneous hybrid approach may allow an opportunity to match the best strategy for a particular anatomic lesion. Revascularization of the left anterior descending artery with the left internal mammary artery is by far the best treatment option in terms of long-term results. Integrating this therapy with percutaneous coronary angioplasty (hybrid procedure) offers multivessel revascularization through a minithoracotomy. Particularly in high-risk patients, morbidity

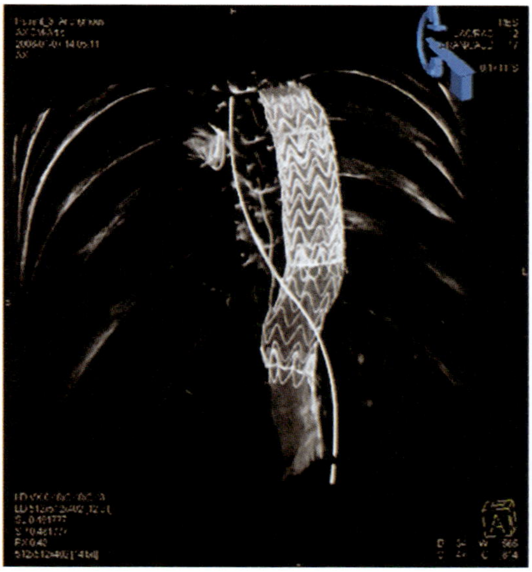

Fig. 12.2 Aortic stent graft visualized with 3D CT-like imaging. Courtesy of Professor Fosse, Rikshospitalet, Oslo. Copyright: Siemens AG HIM AX, Forchheim, Germany

and mortality decreases in comparison to conventional surgery [14,15].

Heart rhythm disturbances

The combination of the surgical epicardial approach with the interventional endocardial approach for the treatment of rhythm disturbances in particular atrial fibrillation offers theoretically advantages over conventional therapy. First reports emphasize the potential benefits [16].

Endovascular aortic repair

Endovascular aortic repair (EVAR) for the abdominal aorta in chronic aneurysms has become a valid alternative to open repair with superior survival [17]. EVAR is also increasingly used for the thoracic aorta (Fig. 12.2). In selected cases EVAR in combination with open surgery is even used for pathologies of the aortic arch and distal ascending aorta [18]. Endoleaks are common complications of EVAR and may be missed by angiographic evaluation. Computed tomography (CT) like imaging with the angiographic C-arm enables the surgeon to diagnose this complication intraoperatively and correct it, if it is deemed necessary [19].

Pacemaker and implantable cardioverter defibrillator implantation

Pacemakers and implantable cardioverter defibrillators (ICDs), particularly biventricular systems, may be optimally implanted in a hybrid OR environment. This is because the hybrid OR offers the required superior angulation and imaging capabilities in comparison to mobile C-arms and the higher hygienic standards compared to cath labs.

Interdisciplinary use

The need for hybrid operating theaters is not restricted to cardiovascular disease. Vascular and neuro specialists have equally developed hybrid procedures necessitating angiography systems in a surgical environment. Imaging needs, hygienic requirements, and room set up – particularly for neuro interventions – may be considerably different. Other surgical disciplines may want to introduce navigation systems, magnetic resonance imaging, endoscopy, biplane angiography systems, or a lateral position of anesthesia equipment. However, the hybrid ORs are more commonly shared between vascular cardiac surgeons, interventionalists including cardiologists, interventional radiologists, electrophysiologists, neuroradiologists, and pediatric cardiologists. Their specific needs have to be carefully considered and weighted when planning the hybrid theater.

Basics of the hybrid room

Location

The hybrid room is used by an interdisciplinary team of surgeons, interventional cardiologists, anesthesiologists, and others and it is good practice to involve all stakeholders deeply in the planning and keeping of such a facility. Ideally, the hybrid OR is located next to interventional suites and operating rooms in order to keep logistics simple. However, if the ORs are separated from the interventional cath labs it is recommended to establish the hybrid OR next to the other operating rooms [20], because all OR equipment and personnel (e.g. heart–lung machine and perfusionists) are immediately ready and anesthesia and intensive care are available.

Room size and preparation

Interventional rooms have excellent imaging capabilities but frequently lack the prerequisites, size, and equipment required for formal ORs. Operating rooms meet those required standards,

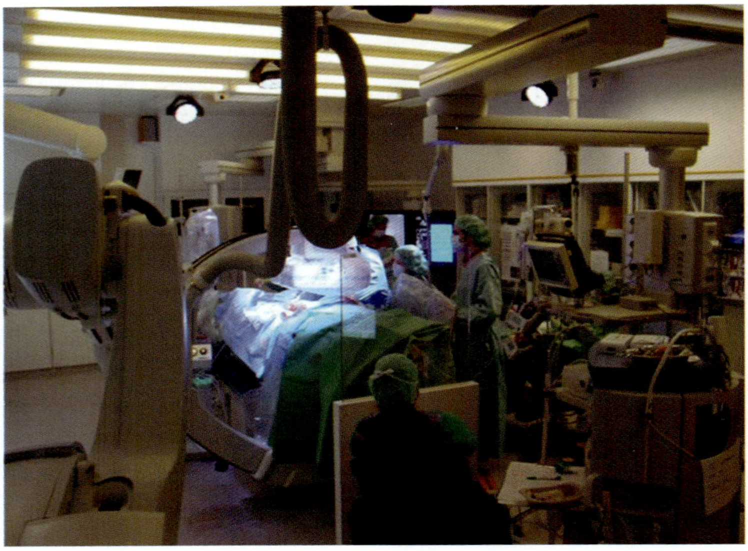

Fig. 12.3 Set-up of a hybrid OR at Rikshospitalet in Oslo, Norway. The robotic multi-axis system offers high flexibility and advanced 3D imaging capabilities in the operating theater. Anesthesia space is maximized in the park position when the system is not needed. Courtesy of Professor Fosse, Rikshospitalet, Oslo. Copyright: Siemens AG HIM AX, Forchheim, Germany

but usually lack high-level imaging capabilities. A hybrid suite should be larger than a standard OR and the basic principle for planning is the larger the better, because not only the imaging equipment needs sufficient space. Staff calculations have shown that in hybrid procedures 8–20 people are needed in the team including anesthesiologists, surgeons, nurses, technicians, perfusionists, experts from device companies, and so forth [21]. Expert opinions recommend for newly built ORs at least 70 m^2 [22]. Additional space for a control room and a technical room is mandatory, which along with washing and prep rooms, total approximately 150 m^2 for the whole area. If a fixed C-arm system is considered, an OR size of 45 m^2 is the absolute lower limit. Rebuilding in terms of lead shielding (2–3 mm) will be needed. Depending on the system it may be necessary to enforce the ceiling or the floor to hold the weight of the stand (c. 650–1800 kg).

Planning

Planning of the hybrid room is truly an interdisciplinary task. Clinicians and technicians of all involved disciplines should define their requirements and form a responsible planning team. The concrete planning is refined in several steps by specialized architects and vendors of OR equipment and imaging systems in a close feedback loop with the planning team. Virtual visualization of the room, visits of established hybrid rooms, and information exchange with experienced users help tremendously during the planning process. In the recent literature a number of case studies are published for planning guidance [23–26].

Lights, monitors, and other devices

In general, all members of the team need access to all important information. Therefore, multiple moveable and flexible booms need to be installed in the hybrid OR. If there are two booms, one boom on each side of the table will best serve the team. Collision of the ceiling-mounted displays with operating lights or other ceiling-mounted equipment should be avoided. Large displays are now available capable of showing multiple video inputs in various sizes, decreasing the need for multiple screens. A dedicated ceiling plan with all ceiling-mounted components including air conditioning should be drawn up to ensure the function and usability of all devices.

Conventional surgical lights may collide with the imaging equipment, particularly with ceiling-mounted systems. If a laminar air flow is present in combination with a ceiling-mounted system, light pendants need very long arms, making them cumbersome to handle. An alternative may be new light concepts with ceiling-integrated multiple theater lights, as developed at the Interventional Centre at Rikshospitalet in Oslo, which solve the problem of collision with the imaging equipment. A remote control offers the possibility of focusing light where it is needed (www.lightor.com, accessed 2 November 2012) (Fig. 12.3).

Hygiene

Hygienic requirements differ from country to country and even among surgical disciplines, with the highest standards in orthopedic surgery. In order to guarantee highest flexibility in room usage, hospitals tend to equip all ORs according to the highest standards and that includes a laminar air flow ceiling. Some hospitals even require skirts around the laminar air flow field and this set up may preclude ceiling-mounted systems. Ceiling-mounted systems with running parts above the operating field, which are difficult to clean and interfere with the air flow by causing turbulences, are not recommended from a hygienic standpoint [20].

Imaging equipment

Mobile and fixed systems

Mobile C-arms have been commonly used in vascular and cardiac surgery and they are readily available in every department, e.g. for pacemaker implantation. Mobile C-arms may depict larger stents or catheters well. However, their technical specifications do not meet the recommendations of the cardiology societies [27]. The power (2–25 kW versus 80–100 kW recommendation) and frame rate (up to 25 frames/s 50 Hz or 30 frames/s 60 Hz versus 30–60 frames/s 50 Hz recommendation) are below the standards of the American College of Cardiology (ACC). The cardiology recommendations need to be met, because cardiology or neuroradiology interventions are an integral part of the hybrid procedure. Thin guide wires (0.2 mm) and stents must be visualized even in obese patients and stenoses of small vessels have to be quantified, which requires adequate power. Mobile C-arms generally have a heat storage capacity of up to 300,000 heat units (HU) (except rare water-cooled systems). A heat storage capacity of more than 1 million HU is recommended by cardiology societies for cath labs to avoid overheating and a dangerous shutdown during complex procedures, which may occur in mobile C-arms for example during complex EVAR procedures. For these reasons expert consensus recommends the use of fixed C-arms [20]. A semi-mobile system with a fixed generator (80 kW; AXIOM Artis U, Siemens AG, Forchheim, Germany) may accommodate high-power imaging demands even in average-sized ORs too small to house a fixed C-arm (<45 m^2).

Image intensifier and flat panel detector systems

Modern fixed C-arm systems are equipped with a flat panel detector. Contrast resolution is far higher compared with image intensifier systems, leading to a higher image quality in detector systems. Additionally in image intensifier systems the image is slightly distorted at the edges compared with the center. As a consequence image intensifier systems are not capable of 3D imaging with soft tissue contrast resolution.

Ceiling- and floor-mounted systems

Expert consensus recommends floor-mounted systems for hygienic reasons. In fact, some hospitals do not allow running parts immediately above the operative field, because dust may fall down and cause infections. Despite these facts, a large number of hospitals decide to have ceiling-mounted systems as these cover the whole body with more flexibility and – most importantly – without moving the table, which is a sometimes difficult and dangerous undertaking during surgery because many lines and catheters have to be moved too. Some ceiling-mounted systems are capable of 3D imaging from a surgical position, perpendicular to Lthe patient from both the right and left table side. Moving from a parking to a working position during surgery, however, is easier with a flexible floor-mounted system, because the C-arms just turn in from the side without interference with the anesthesiologist, whereas ceiling-mounted systems can hardly move during hybrid procedures in the park position at the head side without colliding with the anesthesia equipment.

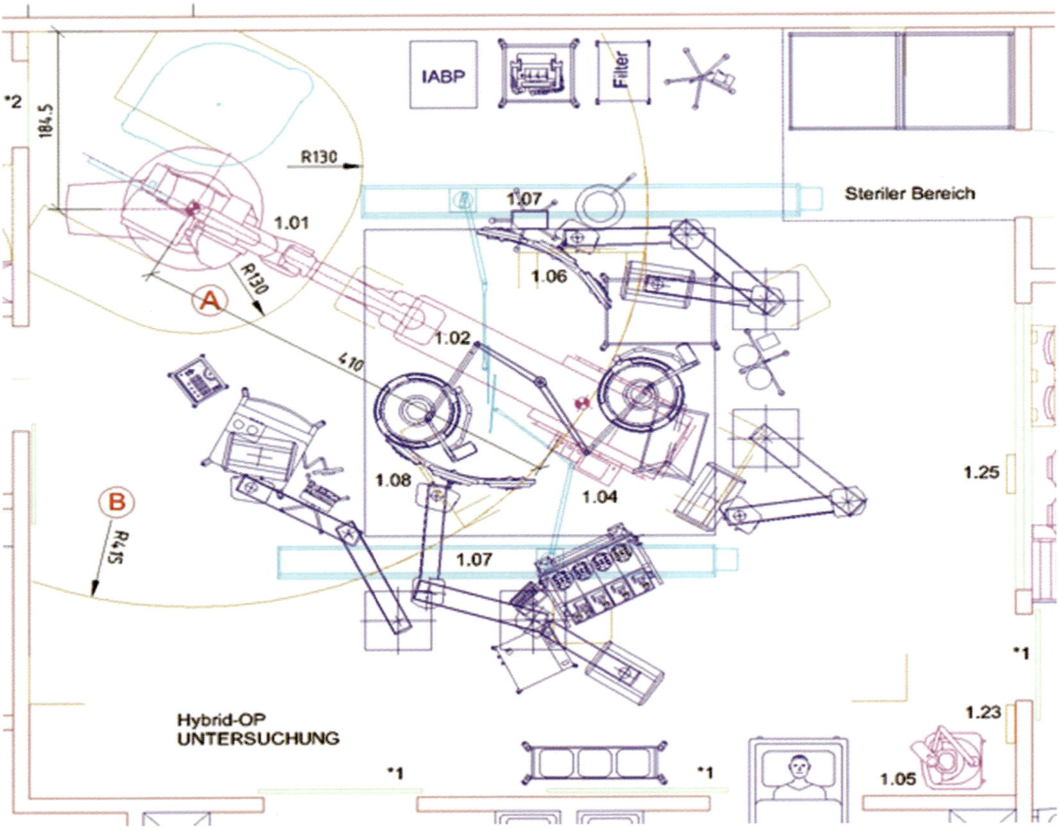

Fig. 12.4 Example of a room plan with a robotic floor-mounted imaging system. A room size of 70 m² or larger is recommended for hybrid ORs because of the large amount of equipment and people needed. Copyright: Siemens AG HIM AX, Forchheim, Germany

Monoplane and biplane systems

In an overcrowded environment like a hybrid suite, biplane systems add to the complexity and interfere with anesthesia except for neurosurgery, where anesthesia is not at the head side. Monoplane systems (Fig. 12.4) are therefore clearly recommended for rooms mainly used for vascular, cardiac, and orthopedic procedures. There are exceptions; if pediatric cardiologists, electrophysiologists, or neuroradiologists are important stakeholders in room usage, a biplane system may also be considered.

Table considerations

The operating table should meet the expectations of both surgeons and interventionalists. This is in fact a special challenge, because the expectations may be mutually exclusive. Surgeons expect a table with a breakable tabletop. For imaging reasons the table has to be radiolucent and should allow coverage of the patient over a wide range. Therefore carbon-fiber tabletops are used that are not breakable. Cardiovascular surgeons in general do not have very sophisticated positioning needs and are used to having fully motorized movements of the table and the tabletop. For the positioning of the patients, inflatable cushions are sometimes used for positioning if a breakable table is not available. Interventionalists require a floating tabletop to allow fast and precise movements during angiography, and in some countries floating tabletops are among the technical requirements for performing coronary angiographies or are at least highly recommended by expert consensus [28]. Floating tabletops are not available with conventional OR tables. The radiolucent area of the OR table only meet the needs in pediatric cases – complete coverage of an adult can not be achieved with today's systems.

As a compromise, tables with a floating tabletop and vertical and lateral tilt are recommended [21]. Special rails for mounting special surgical equipment such as retractors or camera holders should be available on the table. Placing the operating table in a diagonal position in the hybrid suite may gain space. A crucial element when selecting the imaging system and table is the possibility of having access to the patient from all sides and being able to tilt the table both head up and down and sidewise. In order to perform 3D imaging with the operating table, the C-arm has to be fully integrated with the table because a fast and precise rotation around the patient lying in the isocenter is necessary. Breakable OR tables are currently not fully integrated and therefore 3D CT-like imaging on these tables is impossible.

Imaging methods and technologies

Fluoroscopy and acquisition are the basic and most important imaging modes and are offered by all systems. Since fluoroscopy needs much less radiation dose, brilliant fluoroscopy images are the predominantly used images during the procedure. However, modern angiography systems offer advanced imaging and post-processing capabilities including image fusion with any type of previously acquired 3D volumes (e.g. CT, magnetic resonance (MR), positron emission tomography (PET), single-photon emission computed tomography (SPECT) images), guidance, or 3D imaging.

Computer tomography-like 3D imaging with the angiography system

Surgery very much depends on 3D visualization of the anatomy and therefore 3D CT-like imaging with the angiography system is an important feature, because it enables the surgeon to navigate in real time in 3D volumes. In principle, CT-like imaging of the heart is performed by one or two sweeps of up to 220° of the C-arm around the patient. During the rotation several hundred images are acquired and then reconstructed as a 3D volume. If the acquisition is gated by an electrocardiogram (ECG) 3D volumes over time can be generated to depict the beating heart. Radiation dose with new protocols is approximately

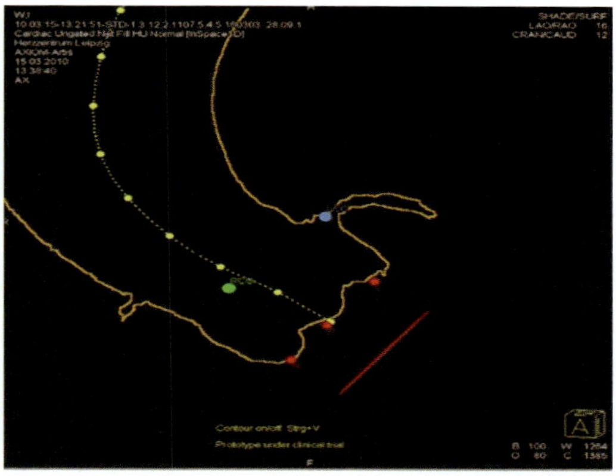

Fig. 12.5 Deployment of an Edwards Sapien valve with 3D guidance. 3D images are acquired at the start of the procedure with the patient lying on the OR table within 5 seconds. The 3D volume of the aortic valve and ascending aorta are automatically reconstructed and segmented in less than 1 minute. The coronaries are automatically detected and marked with coloured dots. A red ring is reconstructed 1 cm below the sinuses. On the workstation the 3D volume can be rotated so that the ring becomes a line. Once this is achieved the projection is perpendicular to the aortic annulus. Through the push of a button the C-arm moves into a position to give the surgeon exactly the projection shown on the workstation. The volume is then overlaid over the live two-dimensional fluoroscopy images and supports precise placement of the aortic valve under rapid pacing. Courtesy of the Heart Center, Leipzig; prototype software under clinical trial. Copyright: Siemens AG HIM AX, Forchheim, Germany.

one-third that of a conventional multislice CT. The OR staff can move out of the OR completely during a CT-like run, because it lasts in most cases 5 seconds. Reconstruction is performed within 1 minute. Accurate information of the cardiac anatomy in the OR supports planning of complex procedures like redo operations, surgery for complex congenital heart disease, and transcatheter valve replacement. Segmentation of anatomic structures and overlay of the 3D volumes over live fluoroscopy (3D roadmap) enables the surgeon to virtually navigate in 3D anatomy (Fig. 12.5). First investigations demonstrate the value of this new technology in transcatheter aortic valve replacement (Video 12.1) [29], particularly with anatomic adjustable valve prosthesis such as the Medtronic Engager valves (Medtronic, Minneapolis, MN). In pulmonary valve replacement the 3D valve anatomy in relation to the coronary artery anatomy is of great importance inorder to avoid obstruction. In EVAR [19]

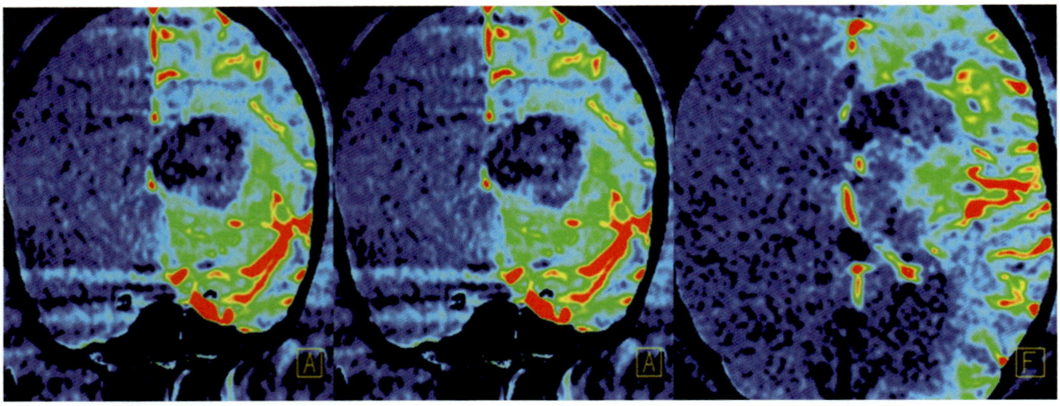

Fig. 12.6 Functional imaging will be a future application in a hybrid OR. Angiography systems will be capable of acquiring blood pool and perfusion-related parameters by DynaCT imaging. The image shown depicts the parenchymal blood volume in a 70-year-old patient with a non-vascularized tumour. Courtesy of Dr. Mawad, Houston, TX. Copyright: Siemens AG HIM AX, Forchheim, Germany

endoleaks can be evaluated in the OR and corrected, if deemed necessary.

Future trends in hybrid operating rooms

The wider use of hybrid ORs started recently and the first dedicated surgical applications and systems aiming to support specific workflows are currently being developed. There are some specifics in surgery that need to be addressed further. Extensive training for surgeons to operate systems is difficult, because these complex systems are not their foremost specialty. Therefore specific software applications for surgical procedures are necessary that are easy to operate with little or no interaction with the surgeons. A first such prototype software is demonstrated in Video 12.1. Surgeons are used to 3D anatomy and not so much to two-dimensional images. Acquisition and reconstruction of 3D volumes with DynaCT and their live display during fluoroscopy will become standard as fluoroscopy is today (Video 12.2). The combination of robotic endovascular navigation with 3D imaging will allow completely new technologies such as complete endovascular stenting of the aorta and in vivo construction of fenestrated branched grafts (Video 12.3). Functional imaging will gain importance since the functional not the anatomic result of the surgical intervention determines patient outcomes. First steps have been made with the imaging of tissue blood volume (Fig. 12.6).

Conclusions

The hybrid OR facilitates a whole new spectrum of cardiovascular therapies and will therefore become an essential resource of every cardiovascular center. The trend towards hybrid techniques is more a revolution than an evolution due to the rapid integration into the surgical techniques. All areas of cardiac therapies – procedures for ischemic, structural, and rhythm heart disease – are deeply affected. Fluoroscopy represents the basic imaging mode. Furthermore, image fusion, 3D/4D imaging, soft tissue visualization, modeling, and navigation allow very advanced surgical applications. The hybrid operating suite itself represents an extremely complex working environment that demands careful planning by all stakeholders. Bundling of clinical, technical, and architectural expertise as well as a realistic view of what is achievable is key for a successful hybrid OR project. Due to wide variations in utilization, generic recommendations are only of limited use for these highly individual rooms and certainly cannot replace the diligent work of the project team. However, once the room is successfully established it really transforms surgical techniques and paves the way for revolutionary new minimally invasive therapies.

References

1 Fogarty, AM. Angioscopy. New developments in vascular surgery. AORN J 1991;53(3):725–8.
2 Neumann FJ. EuroPCR (abstracts book) 2009.

3 Sternbergh WC, 3rd, Tierney WA, Money SR. Importance of access to fixed-imaging fluoroscopy: practice implications for the vascular surgeon. J Endovasc Ther 2004;11:404–10.
4 Greelish JP. Routine angiography after bypass. Paper presented at the Trans Catheter Therapeutics Meeting, Washington, October 12–15, 2008.
5 Bacha EA, Marshall AC, McElhinney DB, et al. Expanding the hybrid concept in congenital heart surgery. Semin Thorac Cardiovasc Surg Pediatr Cardiol Surg Annu 2007;146–50.
6 Sivakumar K, Krishnan P, Pieris R, et al. Hybrid approach to surgical correction of tetralogy of Fallot in all patients with functioning Blalock Taussig shunts. Catheter Cardiovasc Interv 2007;70:256–64.
7 Li SJ, Hu SS, Zhang H, et al. One-stop hybrid cardiac surgery for neonates and young children with congenital heart disease. Zhonghua Xin Xue Guan Bing Za Zhi 2009;37:986–9.
8 Bacha EA, Daves S, Hardin J, et al. Single-ventricle palliation for high-risk neonates: the emergence of an alternative hybrid stage I strategy. J Thorac Cardiovasc Surg 2006;131:163–71.e2.
9 Gutgesell HP, Lim DS. Hybrid palliation in hypoplastic left heart syndrome. Curr Opin Cardiol 2007;22:55–9.
10 Walther T, Chu MW, Mohr FW. Transcatheter aortic valve implantation: time to expand? Curr Opin Cardiol 2008;23:111–16.
11 Vahanian A, Alfieri OR, Al-Attar N, et al. Transcatheter valve implantation for patients with aortic stenosis: a position statement from the European Association of Cardio-Thoracic Surgery (EACTS) and the European Society of Cardiology (ESC), in collaboration with the European Association of Percutaneous Cardiovascular Interventions (EAPCI). Eur J Cardiothorac Surg 2008;34(1):1–8.
12 Mack MJ. Intraoperative coronary graft assessment. Curr Opin Cardiol 2008;23:568–72.
13 Zhao DX, Leacche M, Balaguer JM, et al. Routine intraoperative completion angiography after coronary artery bypass grafting and 1-stop hybrid revascularization results from a fully integrated hybrid catheterization laboratory/operating room. J Am Coll Cardiol 2009;53(3):232–41.
14 Bonatti J, Schachner T, Bonaros N, et al. Simultaneous hybrid coronary revascularization using totally endoscopic left internal mammary artery bypass grafting and placement of rapamycin eluting stents in the same interventional session. The COMBINATION pilot study. Cardiology 2008;110:92–5.
15 Reicher B, Poston RS, Mehra MR, et al. Simultaneous "hybrid" percutaneous coronary intervention and minimally invasive surgical bypass grafting: feasibility, safety, and clinical outcomes. Am Heart J 2008;155:661–7.
16 Bisleri G. Combined surgical and interventional electrphysiology approaches to atrial fibrillation: the hybrid ablation procedure. Paper presented at the Trans Catheter Therapeutics Meeting, Washington, October 12–15, 2008.
17 Schermerhorn ML, O'Malley AJ, Jhaveri A, et al. Pomposelli F, Landon BE. Endovascular vs. open repair of abdominal aortic aneurysms in the Medicare population. N Engl J Med 2008;358:464–74.
18 Walsh SR, Tang TY, Sadat U, et al. Endovascular stenting versus open surgery for thoracic aortic disease: systematic review and meta-analysis of perioperative results. J Vasc Surg 2008;47:1094–8.
19 Biasi L, Ali T, Ratnam LA, et al. Intra-operative DynaCT improves technical success of endovascular repair of abdominal aortic aneurysms. J Vasc Surg 2008;Nov 26.
20 Bonatti J, Vassiliades T, Nifong W, et al. How to build a cath-lab operating room. Heart Surg Forum 2007;10:E344–8.
21 ten Cate G, Fosse E, Hol PK, et al. Integrating surgery and radiology in one suite: a multicenter study. J Vasc Surg 2004;40(3):494–9.
22 Benjamin ME. Building a modern endovascular suite. Endovasc Today 2008;3:71–8.
23 Eagleton, MJ, Schaffer, JL. The vascular surgery operating room. Endovasc Today 2007;8:25–30.
24 Hirsch R. The hybrid cardiac catheterization laboratory for congenital heart disease: from conception to completion. Catheter Cardiovasc Interv 2008;71:418–28.
25 Peeters P, Verbist J, Deloose K, et al. The catheterization lab of the future. Endovasc Today 2008;3:94–6.
26 Sikkink CJ, Reijnen MM, Zeebregts CJ. The creation of the optimal dedicated endovascular suite. Eur J Vasc Endovasc Surg 2008;35:198–204.
27 Bashore TM, Bates ER, Berger PB, et al., American College of Cardiology, Task Force on Clinical Expert Consensus Documents, American College of Cardiology/Society for Cardiac Angiography and Interventions Clinical Expert Consensus Document on cardiac catheterization laboratory standards. A report of the American College of Cardiology Task Force on clinical expert consensus documents. J Am Coll Cardiol 2001;37:2170–214.
28 Hamm CW, Bösenberg H, Brennecke R, et al., German Society of Cardiology-Heart and Cardiovascular Research. Guidelines for equipping and managing heart catheter rooms (1st revision). Issued by the governing body of the German Society of Cardiology-Heart and Cardiovascular Research. Revised by order of the Committee of Clinical Cardiology [in German] Z Kardiol 2001;90:367–76.
29 Kapadia SR. Role of CT angiography to evaluate patient eligibility and guide transcatheter aortic valve eligibility. Paper presented at the Trans Catheter Therapeutics Meeting, Washington, October 12–15, 2008.

Videoclips

This chapter contains the following videoclips:

Video 12.1 Aortic valve replacement with the help of intraoperative DynaCT imaging and overlay of reconstructed 3D volumes on live fluoroscopy. The video is described comprehensively in the legend of Fig. 12.3. Courtesy of the Heart Center, Leipzig; prototype software under clinical trial.

Video 12.2 The abdominal aortic aneurysm was diagnosed with multislice CT. The rendered 3D volume of the aorta was registered with an intraoperatively obtained DynaCT volume. Contours of the 3D volume are then overlayed on live fluoroscopy and are automatically adjusted by changes of projection, table position, zoom factor, etc. Courtesy of St. Olav's Hospital, Trondheim; prototype software under clinical trial.

Video 12.3 Intraoperative DynaCT of a fenestrated stent-graft for the repair of a complex abdominal aneurysm. Courtesy of Dr. Roy Greenberg, Cleveland Clinic Foundation, Cleveland, OH.

They can be accessed at www.wiley.com/go/valverepair.

13

CHAPTER 13

Access techniques for transcatheter aortic valves

Jacques Kpodonu
University of California Irvine,
Cardiovascular Hybrid Interventions, Hoag Heart and Vascular Institute, Newport Beach, CA, USA

Introduction

Aortic stenosis is a common valvular degenerative process in the adult population, with increased prevalence in advanced age. It is estimated that 300,000 patients have severe aortic stenosis in the USA, and approximately 60,000 undergo aortic valve replacement (AVR) every year. Within 3 years of the onset of angina, syncope, or congestive heart failure, 75% of patients die (2% per month mortality) unless treated with aortic valve replacement. The 3-year survival rates have been reported to be 87% and 21% for operated and non-operated patients, respectively [1]. Even in apparently asymptomatic patients, when the valve area is 0.8 cm^2 or less, the mortality rate is high without AVR [2]. The mortality rate for AVR is approximately 3–4% in the USA, but it increases with higher baseline risk factors, reaching 20–50% in the highest risk groups [3]. Patients in the highest risk group are considered inoperable. High surgical risk can be defined as a logistic EuroScore calculated risk of mortality ≥15%, the Society of Thoracic Surgeons' score risk of mortality ≥10%, or the presence of other comorbidities rendering conventional aortic valve surgery difficult, such as a porcelain aorta, previous cardiac surgery with the presence of patent grafts, or severe adhesions, previous radiation therapy, liver cirrhosis, need to avoid sternotomy due to patient immobilization, or marked patient frailty. The introduction of a transcatheter option for AVR [4–6] may provide a potential alternative solution for patients considered high risk for aortic valve replacement.

Patient selection

The selection of patients for transcatheter AVR requires a thorough assessment of the access vessel sites [7]. Safe performance of transcatheter aortic valve procedures and other complex endovascular procedures for structural heart disease requires zero tolerance for major access-related complications. Thorough preoperative planning, understanding the pathology of aorto-iliac occlusive disease, advanced endovascular skills, and ability to use alternate access sites (including being able to perform an iliac conduit via a retroperitoneal approach) are necessary to achieve excellent results. Furthermore, deliverability of large sheath devices through tortuous anatomy or old graft material may be improved by more proximal access provided by an iliac conduit [1]. An evaluation of the iliac and common femoral arteries is important to make certain that these vessels will allow the delivery of sheaths ranging from 18 to 25 Fr. A minimum diameter of 9 mm (3 Fr ≈ 1 mm) may be necessary

Endovascular and Hybrid Therapies for Structural Heart and Aortic Disease, First Edition.
Edited by Jacques Kpodonu and Raoul Bonan.

for safe access via the common femoral arteries. A detailed quantitative angiogram and computed tomography (CT) are performed and analyzed for diameter, tortuosity, and calcification; occasionally intravascular ultrasound of these vessels is performed for further clarification. Expect knowledge of the devices, access techniques, and bail-out maneuvers are necessary for a successful transcatheter aortic valve program.

Transcatheter aortic valve devices

The two front runners seeking to bring transcatheter aortic valves to the market in the USA include Carpentier-Edwards Lifesciences (Irvine, CA; the Sapien transcatheter aortic valve) and CoreValve Inc. (Irvine, CA; the revalving device). A thorough knowledge of both devices and their deployment characteristics are essential for successful deployment of transcatheter aortic valves.

The CoreValve prosthesis consists of a trileaflet, bioprosthetic, porcine, pericardial tissue valve, which is mounted and sutured in a self-expanding nitinol stent (Fig. 13.1). The prosthetic frame/stent is manufactured by a laser cutting tool and has an overall length of 50 mm. The lower portion of the prosthesis has high radial force to expand against the calcified leaflets and to avoid recoil. The middle portion carries the valve and is constrained and narrower to avoid the coronary arteries, while the upper portion is flared to center and fix the stent firmly in the ascending aorta and to provide longitudinal stability. The device is deployed via a delivery system into which the valve is loaded shortly before implantation. The CoreValve transcatheter valve is manufactured in two sizes, with the smaller prosthesis generally used for aortic annulus sizes ≤23 mm; the larger valve fits annulus sizes up to 27 mm in diameter. The sizes of the CoreValve delivery systems have been gradually reduced over time to allow easier deployment. Generally, a femoral artery is chosen for device placement due to the 18 Fr profile of the catheter, however alternative access sites – including the axillary artery with a cutdown procedure – are possible in cases of inadequate femoral access.

The Sapien transcatheter aortic valve is composed of a balloon-expandable, stainless steel frame with an integrated trileaflet, bovine, pericardial valve (Fig. 13.2). The pericardial leaflet material is treated with a similar process to the one used for the surgical Carpentier-Edwards Perimount Magna pericardial valves (thermafix anticalcification treatment, leaflet deflection testing for matched elasticity, and proprietary tissue processing). The valve is available in two sizes (23 and 26 mm) to achieve optimal matching with the aortic annulus dimensions. The valve is crimped on a balloon just before implantation

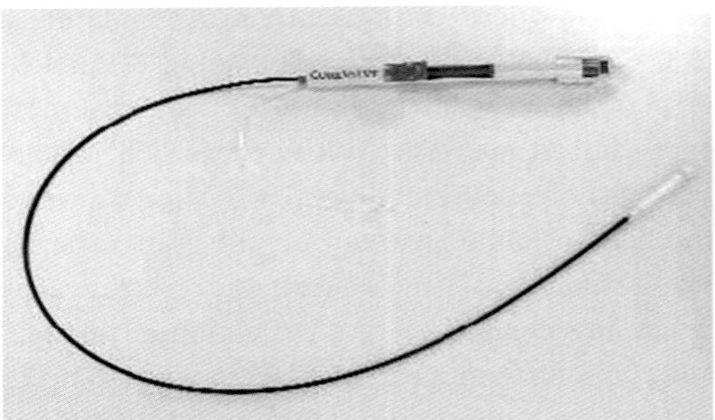

Fig. 13.1 The CoreValve transcatheter aortic valve system consists of pericardial leaflets attached to a self-expanding nitinol frame. In the deployed state, the flared distal end assists in anchoring in the ascending aorta. The stent covers the coronary ostia, but cell size is designed to allow coronary artery perfusion and later coronary catheterization.

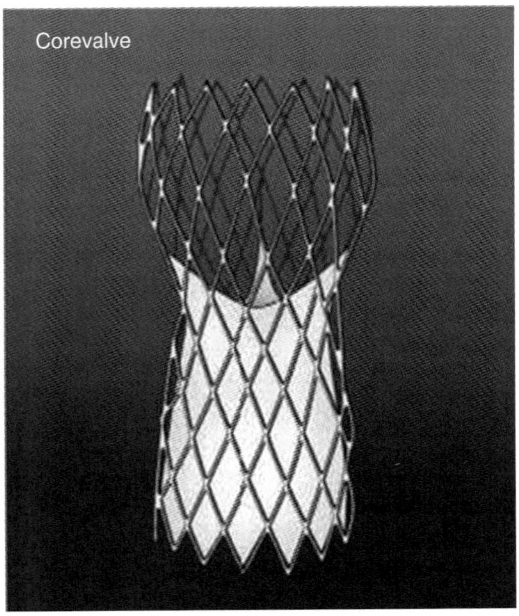

Fig. 13.2 The Carpentier-Edwards Sapien aortic valve.

with a specially designed mechanical crimper to achieve a symmetric low profile and to ensure retention onto the delivery system. The RetroFlex catheter delivery system has an 18 Fr shaft that increases at the distal end to 22 or 24 Fr for the 23 and 26 mm valves, respectively.

Femoral access techniques

The most common percutaneous access sites for transcatheter aortic valve approaches are the femoral arteries. When choosing which site to use to access the vascular tree, one must not only consider the intended procedure but also the size of the sheath and distance to the pathology. The goal for percutaneous access is to create the smallest incision that provides safe and effective entry, without creating vascular trauma. Sheaths up to 12 Fr (4.0 mm) can be safely placed percutaneously. Larger sheaths require a cutdown to ensure vascular hemostasis and minimize traumatic injury.

Percutaneous retrograde femoral artery access

Most right-handed physicians will prefer the patient's right groin for femoral access, although both groins should be prepped in case of inaccessibility. After the pulse is identified, the inguinal ligament is found by tracing a line between the anterior iliac spine and the pubic tubercle. Often, especially in obese individuals, the inguinal crease is inferior to this landmark. Access should be made below the inguinal ligament corresponding to the common femoral artery. If access is made too high, corresponding with the external iliac artery, hemostasis is difficult to achieve with manual pressure. In this situation, hemorrhage can occur after removal of devices and a retroperitoneal hematoma can develop, which is often insidious in onset. In addition, the risk of pseudoaneurysm formation is higher in an external iliac stick, again because direct manual pressure cannot be applied this superiorly.

A properly equipped endovascular suite will allow fluoroscopic imaging of the groin to identify all anatomic landmarks. In addition to surface landmarks, most physicians use the medial half of the femoral head to guide femoral artery access; this ensures common femoral artery entry and avoids the complications of a higher stick. It is also useful in the pulseless femoral artery. Most vascular access kits include an 18 gauge straight angiographic entry needle. This is inserted using the dominant hand at a 45° angle, while using the non-dominant hand for guidance using a Seldinger technique. Percutaneous arterial femoral access is usually obtained by the Seldinger technique. A careful palpation of the femoral pulse is performed and a beveled needle (usually 18 gauge) is introduced through the arterial wall. The needle is slowly withdrawn until the return of arterial blood is achieved, signifying the intraluminal position of the needle. The presence of poor blood flow signifies that the tip is misplaced or the needle is too close to the arterial wall. A soft-tip angled 0.035 inch guide wire is then introduced through the central lumen of the needle under fluoroscopic guidance. Progress of the guide wire intraluminally should be monitored with fluoroscopy to avoid diversion into branched vessels and dissection of the vessel. The presence of resistance in passing a guide wire signifies possible misdirection or dissection of the vessel wall. In instances where the vessel may be small, calcified, or tortuous, a smaller access needle may be desirable. A micropuncture kit (Cook Medical, Bloomington, IN) exists which includes a 21 gauge needle for initial access. Once access is achieved a small nick is made in the skin with a no. 11 blade and a dilator, and an introducer sheath is then advanced over the glide wire with the dilator preceding the introducer sheath by a few inches – again under fluoroscopic visualization. Once the introducer sheath is positioned the dilator is removed .A hemostatic valve at the end of the introducer sheath prevents leakage of blood. The introducer sheath permits various guide wires, balloons, and stents to be introduced safely within the arterial lumen. The introducer sheath can subsequently be upgraded to a larger delivery sheath for the deployment of an endograft. In patients with a femoral-to-femoral graft, percutaneous access can be performed either through the inflow limb of the femoral–femoral graft or above the inflow limb.

Open retrograde femoral access

The common femoral artery is usually exposed for retrograde cannulation and the introduction of various large-sized introducer sheaths, balloons, self-expandable and balloon-expandable stents,

(a) (b)

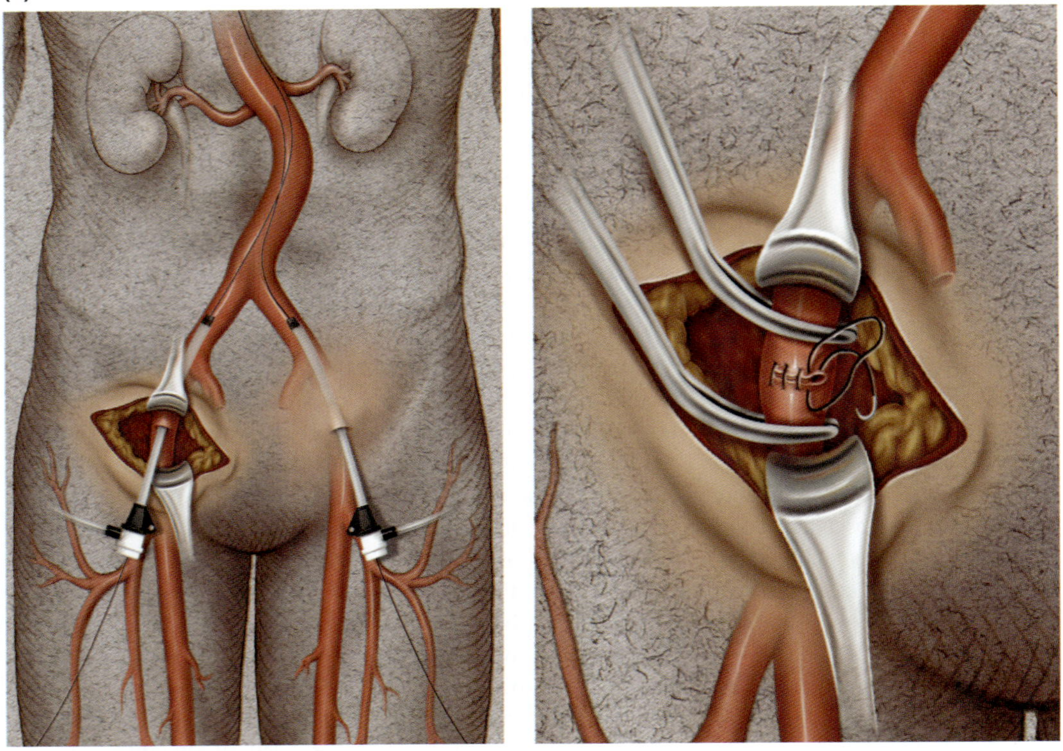

Fig. 13.3 (a) Open retrograde cannulation of the right common femoral artery and percutaneous retrograde access of the left common femoral artery. (b) Closure of the common femoral artery with a prolene stitch.

and endoluminal grafts. In an open retrograde approach a curvilinear incision is made two fingerbreaths above the groin crease and over the palpable femoral pulse. The incision is carried down to the femoral sheath. Retraction is performed with a Gelpe retractor or a Wietlander retractor. The femoral sheath is incised to expose the common femoral artery. Heavy silk sutures are passed circumferentially round the various side branches. Adequate mobilization of the common femoral artery is achieved in order to allow adequate proximal and distal control of the vessel. A Rummel tourniquet is applied to the common femoral artery to serve as a proximal control. The fluoroscopic C-arm is then positioned over the exposed femoral artery. Retrograde cannulation of the common femoral artery is performed with a beveled needle (18 gauge) until pulsatile blood flow is visualized. A soft-tip angled guide wire is then advanced in the vessels under fluoroscopy. The needle is exchanged for a selected size dilator and introducer sheath. The dilator is then removed and the sheath flushed with heparinized saline. Open cannulation or retrograde percutaneous access can be similarly performed in the contralateral common femoral artery (Fig. 13.3a). Once the procedure is completed all wires and sheaths are removed under fluoroscopic guidance to ensure no injury is caused to the vessel wall. The arteriotomy is closed with a 5-0 prolene suture after proximal and distal control is achieved (Fig. 13.3b).

Complications

Rupture

Attempts to introduce a delivery sheath in a small, tortuous, calcified artery or an artery with a combination of any of these factors will lead to rupture of the access vessel, typically at the junction of the external and internal iliac artery or at the aorto-iliac bifurcation. Rupture of an access vessel should be suspected if there is a drop in the blood pressure during advancement or removal of the delivery

(a)

(b)

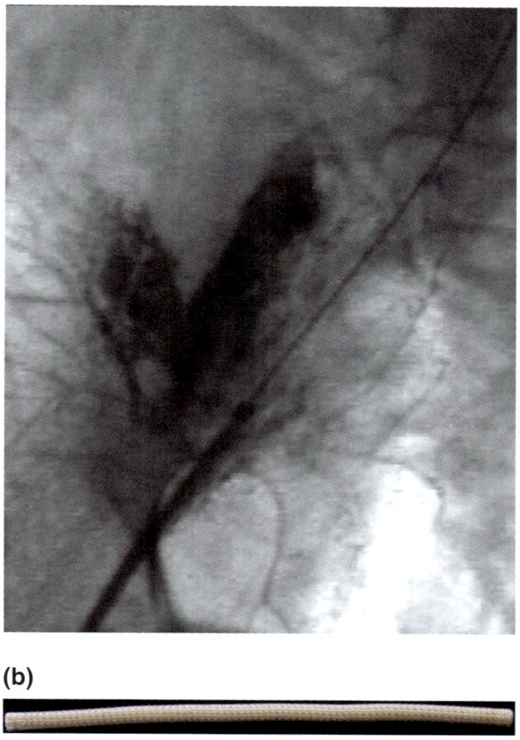

Fig. 13.4 (a) Iliac angiogram of a patient demonstrating the rupture of the right external iliac artery. (b) A covered stent-graft used to exclude the site of rupture.

sheath. The guide wire should be maintained at all times prior to removal of a delivery sheath and an iliac angiogram performed prior to removal of introducer sheaths to confirm extravasation of contrast (Fig. 13.4). Once rupture is confirmed, an appropriate covered stent length and diameter should be chosen and deployed across the area of rupture (Fig. 134b). In most instances coverage of the hypogastric artery is required.

Dissections

The introduction of guide wires and introduction and delivery sheaths may result in dissection of the access vessels. Similarly, balloon angioplasty of calcified access vessels may also result in a dissection flap of the resulting access vessels. Once a dissection is identified on angiogram, gentle balloon angioplasty may be performed to seal the dissecting septum or a covered or uncovered balloon-deployable stent may be deployed to seal off the dissection. Failure to recognize a dissection may result in thrombosis of the access vessels with resulting ischemia of the involved lower extremity.

Retroperitoneal access techniques

Patients with small, calcified, tortuous artery or a combination of any of these factors may make femoral delivery of a transcatheter aortic valve device hazardous. The creation of a retroperitoneal conduit using a 10 mm graft allows such devices to be deployed safely without the risk of rupture or dissection of the ilio-femoral vessels. A retroperitoneal conduit is performed by making a 15 cm semi-lunar right flank incision four finger-breaths above the groin crease. Division of the external oblique, internal oblique, and transversus abdominus muscles is performed in the direction of their fibers. Extraperitoneal fascia and peritoneum are then retracted medially and dissection is carried out in the avascular plane of the retroperitoneum down to the level of the psoas muscle. All of the abdominal contents are then retracted medially with the help of a handheld retractor or an Omni retractor, providing excellent exposure of the lower infrarenal aorta, common iliac artery, and iliac bifurcation. The right common iliac artery along with the hypogastric and external iliac artery are identified and mobilized. Care is taken to spare the right urether, which crosses the common iliac artery before diving deep into the pelvis. A Rummel tourniquet is applied to control the proximal common iliac artery, external iliac artery, and origin of the hypogastric artery; alternatively vascular clamps can be applied for control. Heparin is usually given to the patient prior to clamping the vessels.

An arteriotomy is made on the common iliac artery with a no. 11 blade and extended with Pott's scissors close to the bifurcation of the hypogastric artery and the external iliac artery. A 10 mm conduit is then sewn in an end-to-side fashion using 5-0 prolene sutures (Fig. 13.5a). The 10 mm graft is subsequently tunneled through the retroperitoneal space beneath the inguinal ligament, and brought out through the groin incision used to expose the common femoral artery. The graft is subsequently flushed

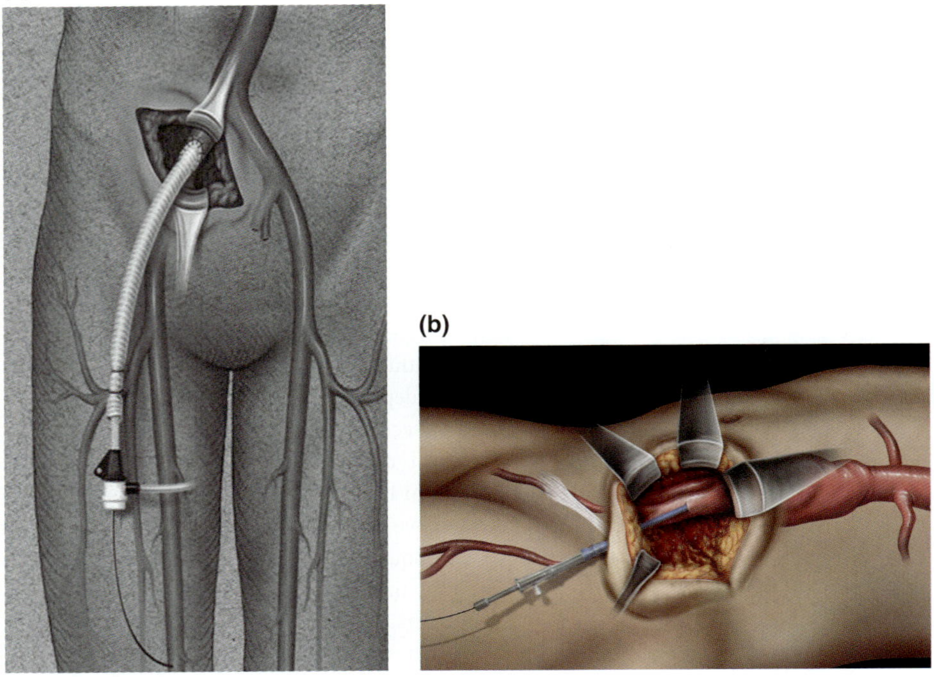

Fig. 13.5 (a) A 10 mm retroperitoneal iliac conduit sewn to the common iliac artery. (b) Direct iliac artery access with an introducer sheath through a retroperitoneal exposure.

and clamped at the groin incision, with the Rummel tourniquet released from the common iliac artery, external iliac artery, and hypogastric artery. The 10 mm conduit is subsequently looped with a Rummel tourniquet, ready to be punctured with an 18 gauge needle for access and the introduction of a guide wire and an introducer sheath. The introducer sheath is subsequently exchanged for a device sheath which is advanced into the distal aorta. The endoluminal graft is then introduced into the delivery sheath and deployed to the target area. Wires and sheaths are removed from the 10 mm conduit and the conduit is clamped.

The conduit can either be trimmed to the appropriate length and tied off as a stump or the distal end of the conduit can be sewn to the more distal iliac system in an end-to-end fashion as an interposition graft, or more commonly the conduit can be tunneled to the groin by tunneling the conduit under the inguinal ligament and performing either an end-to-end anastomosis or an ilio-femoral conduit. The ilio-femoral conduit is performed by making an arteriotomy on the adequately exposed common femoral artery after adequate proximal and distal control is achieved. An end-to-side anastomosis is constructed with a 5-0 prolene suture with adequate flushing maneuvers performed prior to completion of the anastomosis. The lilio-femoral conduit is the best for patients who may require further intervention for diffuse thoracic aneurysmal disease as the conduit may be reused through a simple infrainguinal incision. The groin incision is approximated in layers. The right flank incision is irrigated, a 10 Fr Jackson–Pratt drain is placed in the retroperitoneal space, and the incision is closed in layers. The same technique can be applied to the infrarenal aorta and thoracic aorta. Similarly, end-to-side grafting of a conduit to the axillary artery, as described elsewhere, to facilitate deep hypothermic circulatory arrest also provides excellent access to the thoracic aorta via the innominate [2].

Alternatively, a direct iliac artery access can be used via a retroperitoneal approach using a direct iliac artery puncture with an 18 gauge needle for the introduction of a guide wire and an introducer

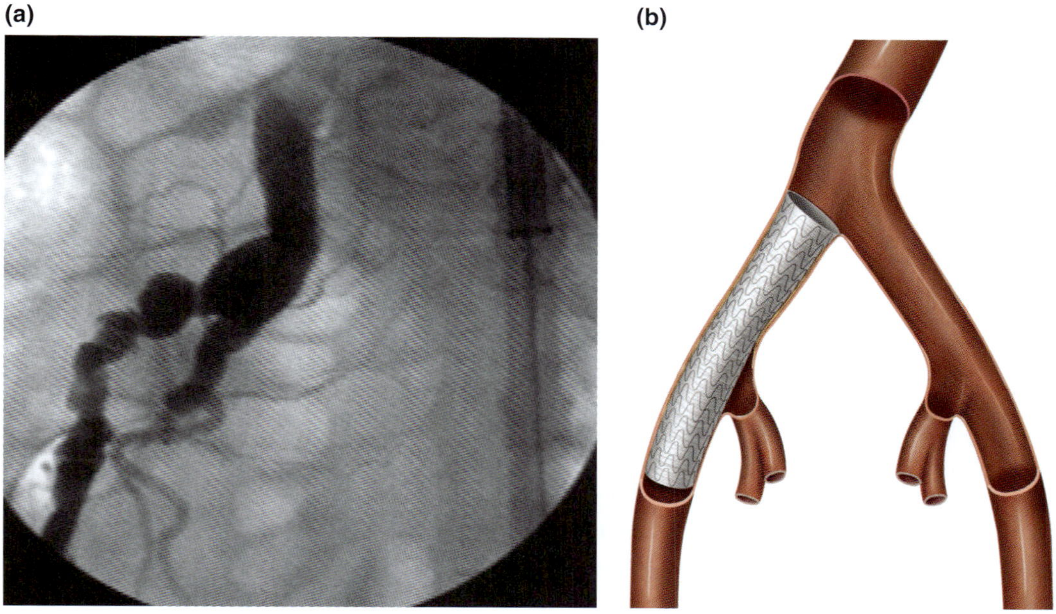

Fig. 13.6 (a) Angiogram demonstrating a small, tortuous left iliac artery. (b) The deployment of an endoconduit for the placement of a large access sheath.

sheath (Fig. 13.5b). The introducer sheath is subsequently exchanged for a device sheath which is advanced into the distal aorta. The transcatheter valve can then be introduced into the delivery sheath and deployed to the target area. Wires and sheaths are removed and the arteriotomy repaired in a standard fashion. The flank incision is irrigated, a 10 Fr Jackson–Pratt drain is placed in the retroperitoneal space, and the incision is closed in layers.

Deployment of an endoconduit in small calcified and tortuous iliac vessel

An endoconduit is an alternative percutaneous technique that can be used to deliver a transcatheter aortic valve in a patient with a small, calcified, or tortuous vessel instead of the conventional ilio-femoral conduit [8]. This technique can be applied in high-risk patients who have a relative contraindication to conventional open surgical techniques under general anesthesia. The endoluminal conduit technique allows aggressive balloon dilation of long segments of ilio-femoral stenosis without the risk of vessel rupture. The endoluminal graft conduit can be custom-assembled using grafts diameters of at least 8 mm and preferably 10 mm, and can be back-loaded into a delivery sheath and deployed via a femoral arteriotomy into the common iliac artery covering the origin of the internal iliac artery [1, 2]. Retrograde percutaneous access of the common femoral artery is performed with an 18 gauge needle in the usual fashion and a 0.035 inch glide wire is advanced under fluoroscopic guidance into the distal thoracic aorta after heparin is administered. A 9 Fr sheath is then exchanged for the needle. A retrograde angiographic picture of the iliac vessels is performed noting the size, tortuosity, and calcification. The presence of a small, severely calcific, or tortuous iliac vessel may preclude the introduction of a delivery sheath (Fig. 13.6a). An attempt may be made to pass the delivery sheath and if any resistance is noted the patient requires a retroperitoneal conduit or an endoconduit. Using the existing 9 Fr sheath balloon angioplasty can be performed to gently dilate the vessel. Subsequently, an endoluminal graft, most commonly an endoluminal graft (Viahbahn, W.L. Gore & Associates, Flagstaff, AZ) or an I-Cast stent-graft (Atrium Medical, Hudson, NH) (see Table 1.1) is deployed across the common iliac and external iliac artery covering the hypogastric vessels (Fig. 13.6b). Post-deployment balloon angioplasty is subsequently performed with a balloon to expand the endoluminal graft; this technique has been referred to as cracking and paving. The 9 Fr sheath is subsequently exchanged for a 20–24 Fr delivery sheath which is required to deliver the thoracic endoluminal graft.

Ventricular apical access techniques

The transapical route is an option for patients without transfemoral access and may have some advantages with respect to ease of device positioning and implantation, and in patients with ilio-occlusive peripheral vascular disease in which a conduit is not indicated or preferred. Advantages of the apical approach include that the size of the delivery system is not limited by the aorto-iliac occlusive disease. Passage through the transverse aortic arch, which is thought to be a cause of embolic stroke, is avoided and the working distance in the transapical approach is much shorter and improves the accuracy of valve deployment. Antegrade passage of wires, catheters, and sheaths through the stenotic aortic valve also simplifies the procedure.

Disadvantages of the transapical approach include pain from the thoracotomy site, contributing to postoperative respiratory compromise, and troublesome bleeding complications from the left ventricular apical site. Insertion of a femoral venous wire and an arterial 6 Fr sheath is strongly recommended to enable rapid cannulation for cardiopulmonary bypass using the Seldinger technique, if required [9].

A left anterolateral minithoracotomy is placed in the fifth or possibly sixth intercostal space (Fig. 13.7). The use of a soft tissue retractor can optimize exposure and minimize rib spreading. The apex of the left ventricle may occasionally be palpated prior to skin incision. Evaluation of a preoperative CT scan addressing the relationship of the apex to the chest wall can help with the positioning of the incision. Straight access to the apex should be achieved. If the apex is not visualized, then the next intercostal space should be opened through the same skin incision. In general, it is better for the incision to be a bit low rather than too high, since the apex can be distracted downward with pericardial traction sutures. The pericardium is opened longitudinally and stay sutures allow for good exposure of the apex. The position of the left anterior descending coronary artery should be confirmed and noted. An epicardial pacing wire is placed and tested for pacemaker capture. Two apical pursestring sutures (using 2-0prolene and a large needle with five interrupted Teflon pledgets (Ethicon Inc., Somerville, NJ)) are placed with sufficiently deep bites in the myocardium (approximately 3–5 mm, but not penetrating into the left ventricular cavity), close to the apex and lateral to the left anterior descending coronary artery. Care should be taken to be sure adequate bites are taken of the muscle and not just the epicardial fat. Placement of the sutures in the bare spot just above the apex on the anterior wall can achieve this more reliably. Fluoroscopy is used to visualize the aortic root and the aortic annulus in a perpendicular angle. All three aortic sinuses and aortic valve cusps should be in one plane. This is usually achieved using a left anterior oblique of approximately 10° and cranial approximately 10° position. The apex is punctured with a needle, and a soft guide wire is inserted antegrade across the stenotic aortic valve followed by a 14 Fr (30 cm long) soft-tip sheath that is placed across the aortic valve. The procedural steps of transcathere aortic valve replacement are then carried out.

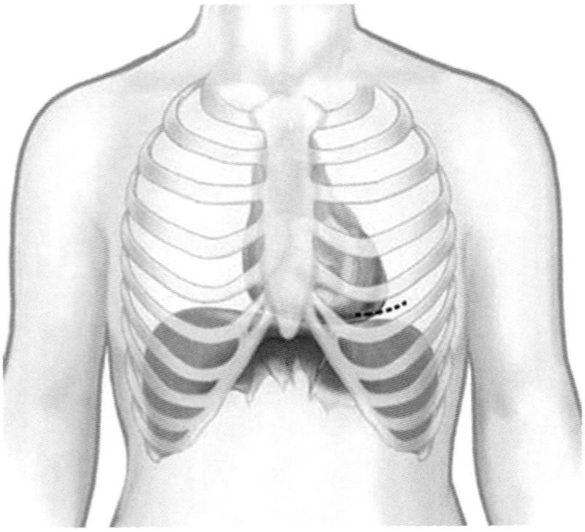

Fig. 13.7 Anterolateral thoracotomy through the fifth and sixth interspace.

After valve implantation, the apical sheath and guide wire are simultaneously retrieved. The apex is securely closed using the previously placed two pursestring sutures. Additional sutures may be required (usually with Teflon reinforcement) to achieve complete hemostasis. A final shot of contrast is given into the aortic root to confirm valve function once the guide wire has been removed. Protamine is then administered in a standard dose. The pericardium is slightly closed to additionally cover the apex. A pleural chest tube or soft drain is inserted. Once all bleeding is controlled and a long-acting local anesthetic is injected in the intercostal spaces, the chest wall and incision are closed in a routine fashion. Depending on local practice, the patient can be immediately extubated in the operating room or shortly thereafter upon transfer to the intensive care or postanesthetic care unit in the majority of cases.

Axillary artery access techniques

The axillary approach is simple and familiar to cardiac surgeons [10, 11]. The subclavian and proximal axillary arteries are usually good-sized vessels and are often free of atherosclerotic disease. This approach provides good stability of the sheath and valve delivery system, with what appears to be simpler device positioning and implantation relative to the transfemoral approach. A patent left internal thoracic artery graft is probably a contraindication to a left axillary approach. The potential to compromise innominate artery flow is also a relative contraindication to the right axillary approach.

The patient is placed in the standard supine position. For better exposure of the axillary artery, the arm is positioned near the body with the hand down to the side and the elbow slightly flexed, almost as if the hand were placed in an imaginary pants pocket. Arterial pressure is monitored via arterial lines placed routinely in both radial vessels. An infraclavicular skin incision 8–10 cm in length is made, running from a point just lateral to the sternal head of the clavicle to the upper deltopectoral groove. The pectoralis major fascia is incised and its fibers split, exposing the axillary vein. The pectoralis minor is retracted laterally. The axillary artery is easily exposed under the vein and gently mobilized for 2 cm, without touching the medial and lateral cords of the brachial plexus. An umbilical tape is looped around the artery, and gentle traction applied. After heparinization, the artery is cannulated either directly or indirectly through a longitudinal arteriotomy via a 10 mm woven Dacron graft anastomosed with a 5-0 polypropylene suture after a side-bite clamp has been applied across the artery. This graft can then be used as the access site for transcatheter valve deployment. Use of the left axillary artery is preferred as there is no occlusion of flow to the carotid arteries compared with using the right axillary artery.

Carotid artery access techniques

In rare instances when a patient is not a candidate for a ventricular apical approach and does not have femoral arteries for access due to ilio-femoral vascular occlusive disease or a subclavian/axillary artery available due to presence of a pacemaker or other device, a carotid artery approach can be performed.

In the carotid artery access technique, bilateral carotid arteries and the vertebrobasilar system is imaged to make sure there is no evidence of extracranial occlusive disease. The common carotid artery is exposed in a routine fashion, and heparin is given to the patient. The carotid artery is accessed with an 18 gauge needle and a soft glide wire threaded into the ascending aorta and a short 6 Fr sheath introduced. Using an angled Amplatzer catheter the aortic valve is crossed with a 0.035 inch straight guide wire. The wire is then exchanged for a 6 Fr pigtail catheter. A pigtail catheter is placed above the aortic valve through a retrograde femoral approach. Once gradients are obtained the pigtail catether in the ventricle is exchanged for a soft-tip curved 0.035 inch stiff Amplatz wire. The 6 Fr sheath is exchanged for the device sheath. The common carotid artery is clamped distally and the procedural steps for transcatheter aortic valve implantation are carried out. On completion of the procedure, the device is removed and the common carotid artery is repaired using traditional vascular closure techniques. The incision is closed in routine fashion.

Brachial artery access techniques

Access to the brachial or radial arteries carries not only a higher risk of complications, but the complications are generally more severe than those associated with femoral access. The arteries of the upper extremity have an enveloping fascial sheath. Therefore when a hematoma does occur, brachial plexopathies are more common. In addition, upper extremity vessels tend to spasm more frequently during manipulation, making access more challenging. Brachial access carries the added risk of distal ischemia and embolization over radial access. Although sheaths up to 6 or 7 Fr may be percutaneously placed in either vessel, radial access should be preferred over brachial because of a lower complication profile.

Open access should be used for larger sheaths or on smaller patients. The left brachial artery is preferred over the right so as to avoid the origin of the right common carotid artery. The arm is abducted on an arm board with the arm circumferentially prepped. The artery is palpated just proximal to the antecubital fossa where the biceps muscle thins out to its tendinous insertion. A 21 gauge micropuncture kit is preferred to the 18 gauge one due to the smaller size of the vessel. Catheter-over-wire exchange can then be performed to the desired sheath. Radial artery access is performed similarly to any arterial catheter placement. The artery is palpated at the lateral wrist and a 21 or 23 gauge needle is used to enter the vessel. A catheter-over-wire exchange is then performed. Sheaths of up to 6 Fr can be placed with relative safety. Long sheaths can help deal with the inherent vasospasm.

Conclusions

In conclusion, with the development of new endovascular technology for structural heart disease it is hoped that knowledge of the different approaches for deployment of transcatheter valves will lead to a larger number of patients considered high risk for traditional surgical aortic valves offered this new and exciting technology. The procedural learning curve is quite steep but as refinement in devices, imaging technology, and acquisition of transcatheter skills by surgeons continues to improve, transcatheter valve aortic valve replacement in the near future will become complimentary to open surgical aortic valve replacement [12].

References

1 Schwarz F, Baumann P, Manthey J, et al. The effect of aortic valve replacement on survival. Circulation 1982;66(5):1105–10.
2 Pai RG, Kapoor N, Bansal RC, et al. Malignant natural history of asymptomatic severe aortic stenosis: benefit of aortic valve replacement. Ann Thorac Surg 2006;82:2116–22.
3 Walther T, Dewey T, Borger MA, et al. Transapical aortic valve implantation: step by step. Ann Thorac Surg 2009;87(1):276–83.
4 Walther T, Falk V. Transcatheter aortic valve implantation – should we do it just because we can? EuroIntervention 2008;4(2):173–5.
5 Falk V, Schwammenthal EE, Kempfert J, et al. New anatomically oriented transapical aortic valve implantation. Ann Thorac Surg 2009;87(3):925–6.
6 Webb JG. Percutaneous aortic valve replacement will become a common treatment for aortic valve disease. J Am Coll Cardiol Interv 2008;1:122–6.
7 Diethrich EB, Ramaiah VG, Kpodonu J, et al. Endovascular and Hybrid Management of the Thoracic Aorta. A case-based approach, 1st edn. Oxford: Wiley Blackwell, 2008.
8 Kpodonu J, Rodriguez JA, Ramaiah VG, et al. Cracking and paving: a novel technique to deliver a thoracic endograft despite Ilio-femoral occlusive disease. J Card Surg 2009;24(2):188–90.
9 Walther T, Simon P, Dewey T, et al. Transapical minimally invasive aortic valve implantation: multicenter experience. Circulation 2007;116(Suppl 11):1240–5.
10 Asgar AW, Mullen MJ, Delahunty N, et al. Transcatheter aortic valve intervention through the axillary artery for the treatment of severe aortic stenosis. J Thorac Cardiovasc Surg 2009;137(3):773–5.
11 Kokotsakis J, Lazopoulo G, Milonakis M, et al. Right axillary artery cannulation for surgical management of the hostile ascending aorta. Tex Heart Inst J 2005;32(2):189–93.
12 Webb J. Impact of learning curve and next generation THV valves on procedural success. Presented at the annual EuroPCR meeting in Barcelona, Spain, 2008.

14

CHAPTER 14

Transfemoral transcatheter aortic valve replacement

Darren Mylotte[1]*, Giuseppe Martucci*[1]*, Ruediger Lange*[2] *& Nicolo Piazza*[1,2]

[1]Department of Interventional Cardiology at McGill University Health Center (MUHC), Royal Victoria Hospital, Montreal, Canada
[2]Department of Cardiac Surgery, German Heart Center Munich, Munich, Germany

Introduction

Somewhat surprisingly, transcatheter treatment of valvular heart disease was first conceived as far back as 1965. Davies devised a catheter-mounted cone-shaped valve as a potential therapy for aortic insufficiency [1], and paved the way for the development of a variety of transcatheter devices for the treatment of aortic insufficiency over the next 25–30 years [2–4]. Real progress in the field was not realized until 1986, when Professor Alain Cribier performed the first balloon aortic valvuloplasty (BAV) for the treatment of severe aortic stenosis [5]. Unfortunately, the impressive acute hemodynamic outcomes were diminished by valve restenosis, and symptoms typically recurred within 6–8 months of therapy [6–12]. Nevertheless, BAV demonstrated, for the first time, that transcatheter treatment of aortic stenosis was feasible, and with refinement could be an effective treatment for the 30–60% of patients who are refused surgery [13–16].

In 2002, some 15 years after performing the first BAV, Cribier implanted the first in-human balloon-expandable transcatheter heart valve. A first generation 23 mm bovine pericardial stent valve developed by Percutaneous Valve Technologies (Fort Lee, NJ), was implanted using a 24 Fr catheter delivery system [17]. The recipient was a 57-year-old man with refractory cardiogenic shock secondary to severe aortic stenosis, who was denied traditional aortic valve surgery (Fig. 14.1). Significant peripheral arterial disease necessitated antegrade implantation using a transvenous approach and transeptal puncture. After valve implantation, the transvalvular aortic gradient was <10 mmHg and the aortic valve area increased to 1.7 cm^2. Based on this initial success, the first series of 40 patients underwent implantation of a modified heart valve, the Cribier–Edwards valve, using an antegrade transeptal approach [18].

The challenging nature of antegrade transvenous transcatheter aortic valve implantation, and not infrequent hemodynamic instability encountered due to mitral valve tethering and injury, motivated the development of alternative implantation strategies. The retrograde approach via the femoral artery (transfemoral) and the antegrade approach via the apex of the left ventricle (transapical) were developed using the Edwards LifeSciences system (Irvine, CA) [19].

In July 2004, the CoreValve ReValving system (Paris, France) was first implanted (Fig. 14.2) [20]. Initially, these procedures were complex and

Endovascular and Hybrid Therapies for Structural Heart and Aortic Disease, First Edition.
Edited by Jacques Kpodonu and Raoul Bonan.

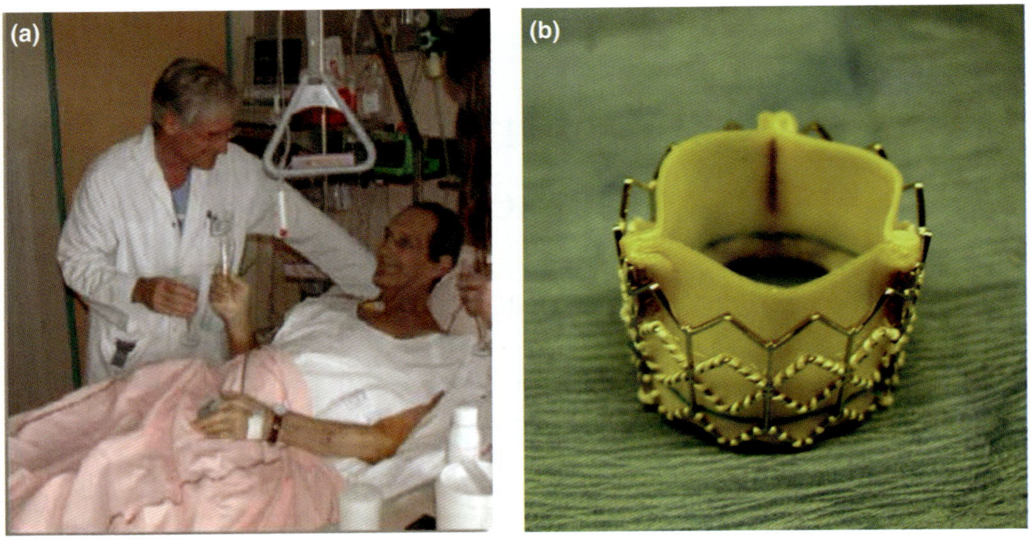

Fig. 14.1 (a) The first patient to undergo transcatheter aortic valve implantation (April 16, 2002) using the first generation balloon expandable valve (b) that housed trileaflet bovine pericardial leaflets. Image courtesy of the PCR-EAPCI Percutaneous Interventional Cardiovascular Medicine Textbook, 2012, Europa Publishing.

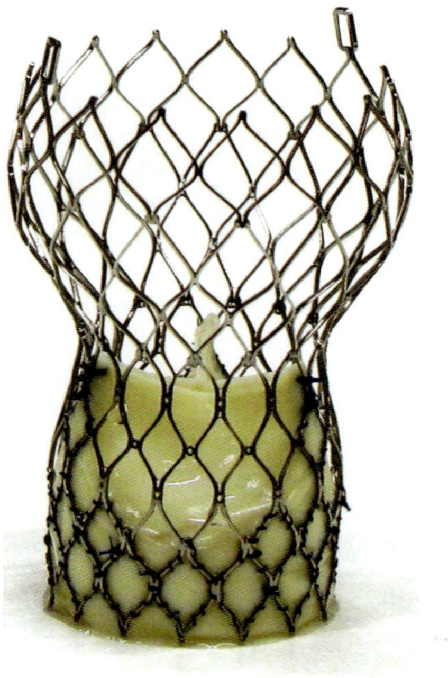

Fig. 14.2 The first generation CoreValve ReValving System bioprosthesis housing trileaflet bovine pericardial leaflets. The current third generation Medtronic CoreValve bioprosthesis houses leaflets made of porcine pericardium.

time consuming, requiring general anesthesia, cardiopulmonary bypass, and surgical cutdown of the femoral artery. However, downsizing of the delivery catheter and increasing operator experience soon saw the majority of procedures being performed percutaneously, under conscious sedation and local anesthesia, without cardiopulmonary support [21].

A wealth of knowledge has been acquired with respect to patient selection, procedural techniques, and post-procedure care over the last 10 years. These refinements have improved patient safety and procedural outcomes.

Patient selection

Transcatheter aortic valve replacement (TAVR) is currently indicated for high or prohibitive surgical risk patients with symptomatic calcific aortic stenosis (aortic valve area $<1.0\,cm^2$) requiring aortic valve replacement.

Clinical criteria

TAVR was developed to treat the high or prohibitive surgical risk patient. This risk is usually quantified using several cardiac surgical risk algorithms [22–34]. However, these risk models were developed using low to intermediate surgical risk patients and their reliability when applied to high or prohibitive surgical risk patients is unclear [35–38]. To date, the logistic EuroScore and the STS (Society of Thoracic Surgeons) Predicted Risk of Mortality score have directed enrolment of patients into

TAVR trials [22,33]. A logistic EuroScore ≥15% or STS score ≥10% define the high surgical risk patient for trial inclusion [39,40]. The logistic EuroScore tends to overestimate the observed mortality risk of high-risk patients by a factor of 2–3 [35,36], and therefore the STS score may be more reliable [58]. Evidently, clinical judgment should always supersede surgical risk algorithms [41].

Anatomical criteria

Pre-procedure screening of the peripheral arterial vasculature and aortic valvular complex (left ventricular outflow tract, aortic annulus, sinus of Valsalva, sinotubular junction, ascending aorta) is required. This is achieved using a combination of transthoracic and transesophageal echocardiography (TTE, TEE), multislice computed tomography (MSCT), and fluoroscopy/angiography [42]. These data determine the most appropriate access route (i.e. transfemoral, subclavian, apical, or direct aortic) and the transcatheter valve size [43].

Assessment of the arterial vasculature

Peripheral contrast angiography is the most practical, readily available, and cost effective modality for assessing the peripheral vasculature. In contrast, MSCT is associated with a higher contrast load, higher radiation exposure, and is more expensive. However, MSCT provides greater appreciation of vessel size, tortuosity, and calcific burden (Fig. 14.3) [44,45]. Using contrast angiography, a SFAR ratio (i.e. outer sheath diameter to femoral artery minimal luminal diameter ratio) of ≥1.05 was identified as a predictor of Valvular Academic Reseach Consortium (VARC) major vascular complications and 30-day mortality [46,47]. This ratio increased to 1.10 in non-calcified vessels and decreased to 1.00 in the presence of calcium. The utility of the SFAR criteria in MSCT is unclear.

Assessment of the aortic valve annulus

For the purposes of TAVR, the aortic valve annulus corresponds to a virtual ring formed by junction of the basal attachment points of the leaflets within the left ventricle (Fig. 14.4) [48]. This plane represents the transition from the left ventricular outflow tract into the aortic root. The non-circular shape of the aortic valve annulus has generated much debate about how best to measure its diameter for the purposes of transcatheter aortic valve size selection (Fig. 14.5) [49–51]. Currently, MSCT appears to be the most suitable method for assessment of aortic annulus dimensions. MSCT multiplanar reconstructions provide coronal, sagittal, and axial images of the aortic root [52,53]. On the axial view, the maximum and minimum diameter, perimeter, and area of the annulus can be measured. According to MSCT data, the mean difference between the maximum and minimum diameter of the non-circular aortic annulus is 6.5 mm (95% confidence interval, 5.7–7.2) [49,50]. Depending on the orientation, two-dimensional echocardiography appreciates only one view of the aortic annulus, and usually underestimates the annulus diameter with respect to MSCT. With this in mind, the use of two-dimensional measurements (TEE, TEE, contrast aortography) for transcatheter valve sizing is potentially problematic. Nevertheless, two-dimensional echocardiography remains the most commonly used method to assess the aortic valve annulus diameter, though a shift towards MSCT is emerging.

Approved device description

Current TAVR systems consist of three components: (i) the loading system; (ii) the delivery catheter; and (iii) the bioprosthetic aortic valve.

Edwards NovaFlex transfemoral system

The Edwards NovaFlex transfemoral system comprises the Edwards Sapien XT transcatheter heart valve (THV), the NovaFlex delivery system, the Edwards eSheath introducer sheath set, the Retroflex dilator kit, Retroflex balloon catheter, Crimper, and the Atrion inflation device (Fig. 14.6) [54,55].

The Edwards Sapien XT THV is a balloon-expandable valve consisting of a radiopaque cobalt-chromium frame, trileaflet bovine pericardial leaflets, and polyethylene terephthalate fabric skirt. The leaflets are manufactured according to *matching technology* and the Edwards Thermafix anticalcification process. The Edwards Sapien XT THV is currently available in four sizes (20, 23, 26, and 29 mm) and can be implanted in native annuli with diameters of 16–27 mm (Fig. 14.7). Novel features of the delivery system include: (i) the

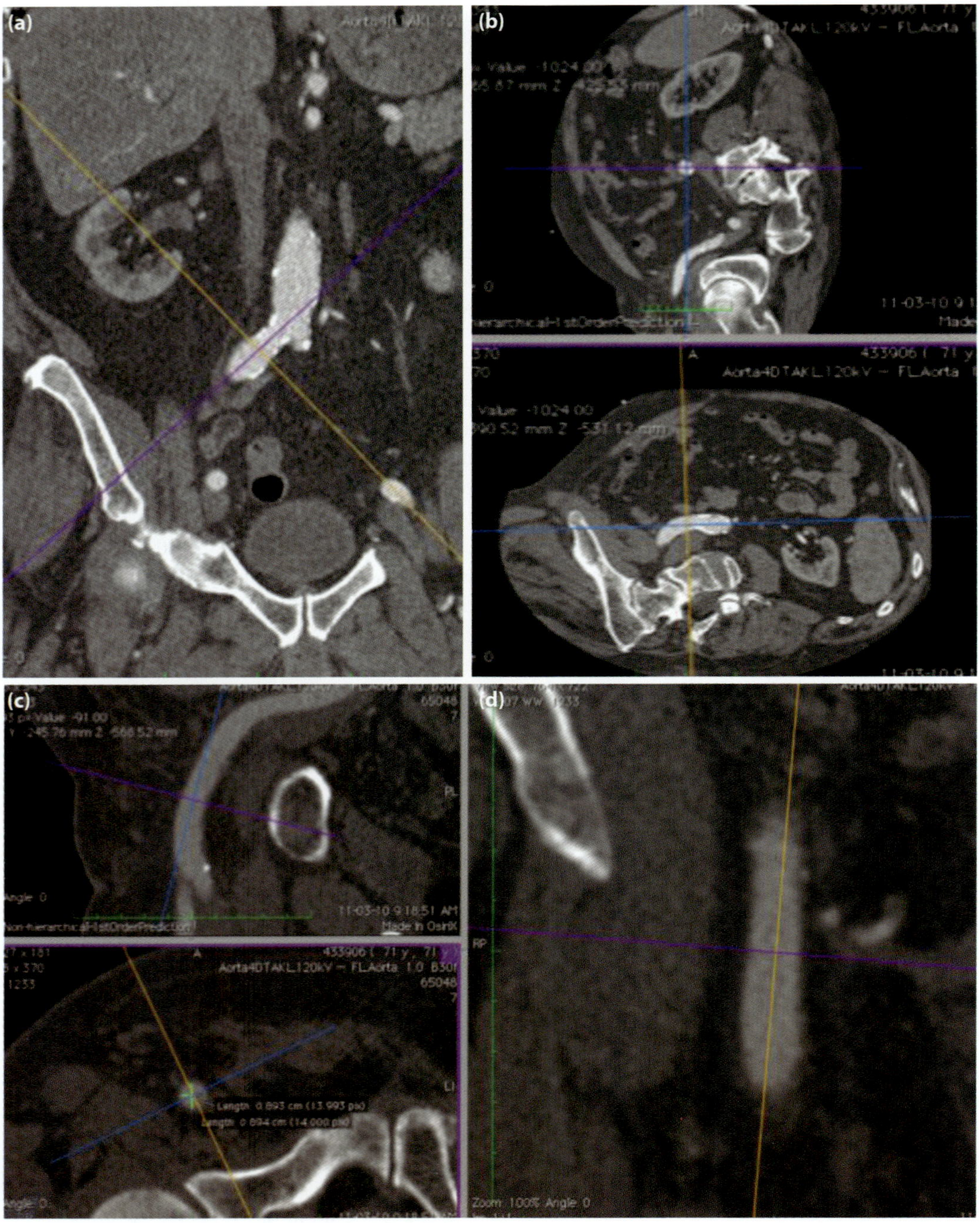

Fig. 14.3 MSCT scans provide the ability for 3D multiplanar reconstructions and therefore can provide superior information about minimum vessel diameter, tortuosity, and degree of calcification than a peripheral angiogram. (a, b) Cross-sectional measurements of the right common iliac artery. (c, d) Cross-sectional measurements of the right common femoral artery at the intended puncture site. Image courtesy of the PCR-EAPCI Percutaneous Interventional Cardiovascular Medicine Textbook, 2012, Europa Publishing.

deflectable NovaFlex delivery catheter, which has a tapered distal tip to facilitate crossing the native aortic valve; and (ii) the Edwards eSheath with dynamic expansion mechanism (DEM) that allows the sheath to transiently expand as the delivery system is advanced. The eSheath has an outer diameter of 6.6 mm (20 Fr) and 7.2 mm (21–22 Fr) for implantation of the 23 and 26 mm THVs, respectively.

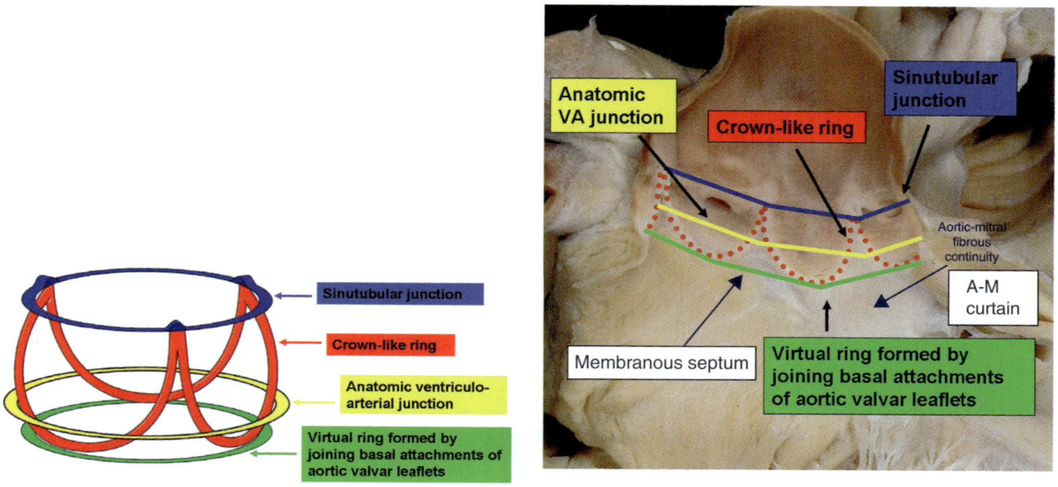

Fig. 14.4 The aortic root extends from the basal attachment points of the aortic valve leaflets (aortic annular plane) to their superior attachment points at the level of the sinutubular junction. There are three circular rings within the aortic root: (i) a virtual ring (i.e. without histologic demarcation) formed by joining the basal attachments of the aortic valvular leaflets; (ii) a ring at the anatomic ventriculo-arterial junction identified histologically as the transformation zone between aortic wall tissue and ventricular myocardium; and (iii) a ring at the sinutubular junction found at the apical attachment points of the aortic valvular leaflets. The "curtain-like" attachment line of the aortic valvular leaflets forms the crown-like ring. For purposes of transcatheter aortic valve sizing, it is the diameter of the virtual basal ring that is taken into consideration. Image courtesy of the PCR-EAPCI Percutaneous Interventional Cardiovascular Medicine Textbook, 2012, Europa Publishing.

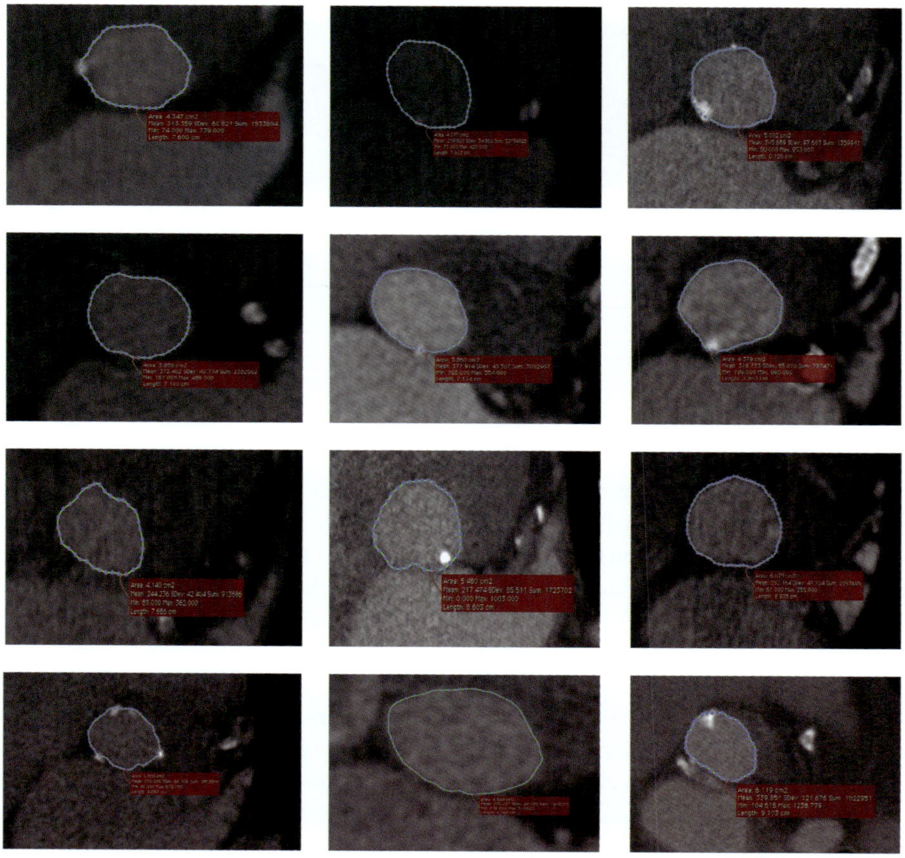

Fig. 14.5 MSCT axial cuts of the aortic annulus from 12 patients demonstrating that the aortic annulus is in fact non-circular. The difference between the maximum and minimum diameter measurements of the aortic annulus is on average 6.5 mm with a standard deviation of approximately 2 mm. The non-circularity of the aortic annulus limits applicability of two-dimensional imaging in estimating the annulus diameter for transcatheter valve sizing. Image courtesy of the PCR-EAPCI Percutaneous Interventional Cardiovascular Medicine Textbook, 2012, Europa Publishing.

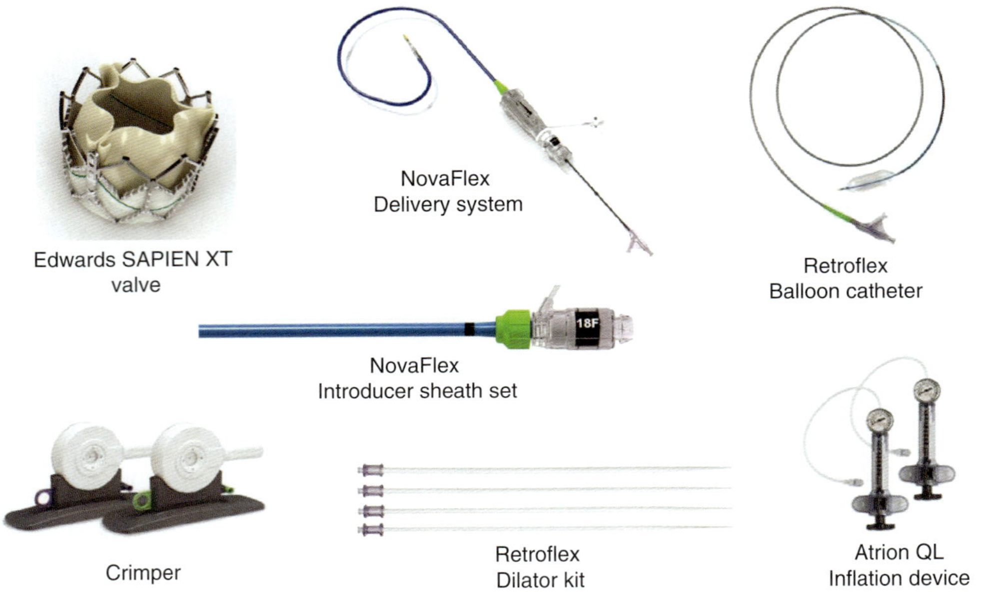

Fig. 14.6 Components of the transfemoral NovaFlex system.

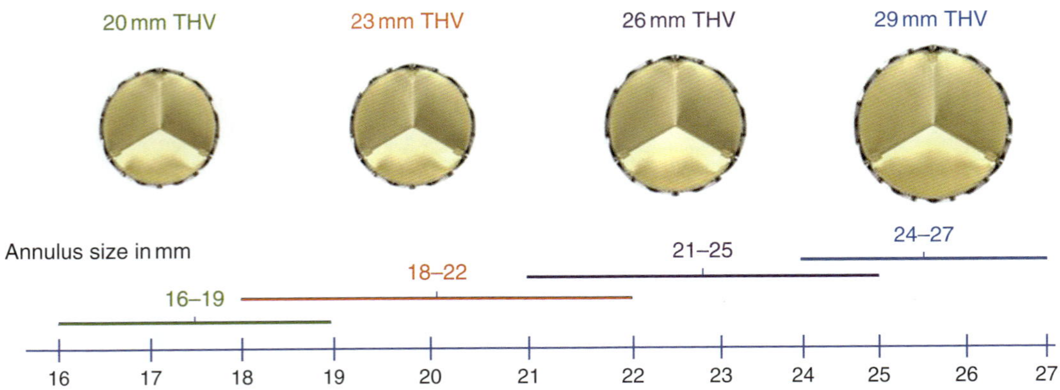

Fig. 14.7 The Edwards Sapien XT showing three of the available sizes.

Medtronic CoreValve system

The Medtronic CoreValve System comprises the CoreValve bioprosthesis, AccuTrak delivery catheter system, and a disposable loading system (Fig. 14.8).

The current (third generation) Medtronic CoreValve bioprosthesis is a self-expandable valve manufactured from a radiopaque nitinol support frame, trileaflet porcine pericardial leaflets, and porcine pericardium fabric skirt. From 2012, the valve leaflets will undergo tissue treatment with alpha-amino-oleic acid to reduce calcium deposition [56]. The nitinol support frame is a diamond cell pattern with various strut lengths and widths designed to expand to a non-uniform cylindrical "hour-glass" shape with three distinctive structure–function levels (Fig. 14.9). The inflow section has high radial force to anchor and seal against the native outflow tract and aortic valve to minimize paravalvular aortic regurgitation. The middle section houses the leaflets and has high hoop strength to minimize deformation and ensure optimal leaflet geometry. The outflow section sits in the ascending aorta, has low radial force, and functions to orient the prosthesis in the direction of blood flow.

The CoreValve is available in four sizes (23, 26, 29, and 31 mm) and can be implanted in native annuli with diameters ranging from 20 to 29 mm

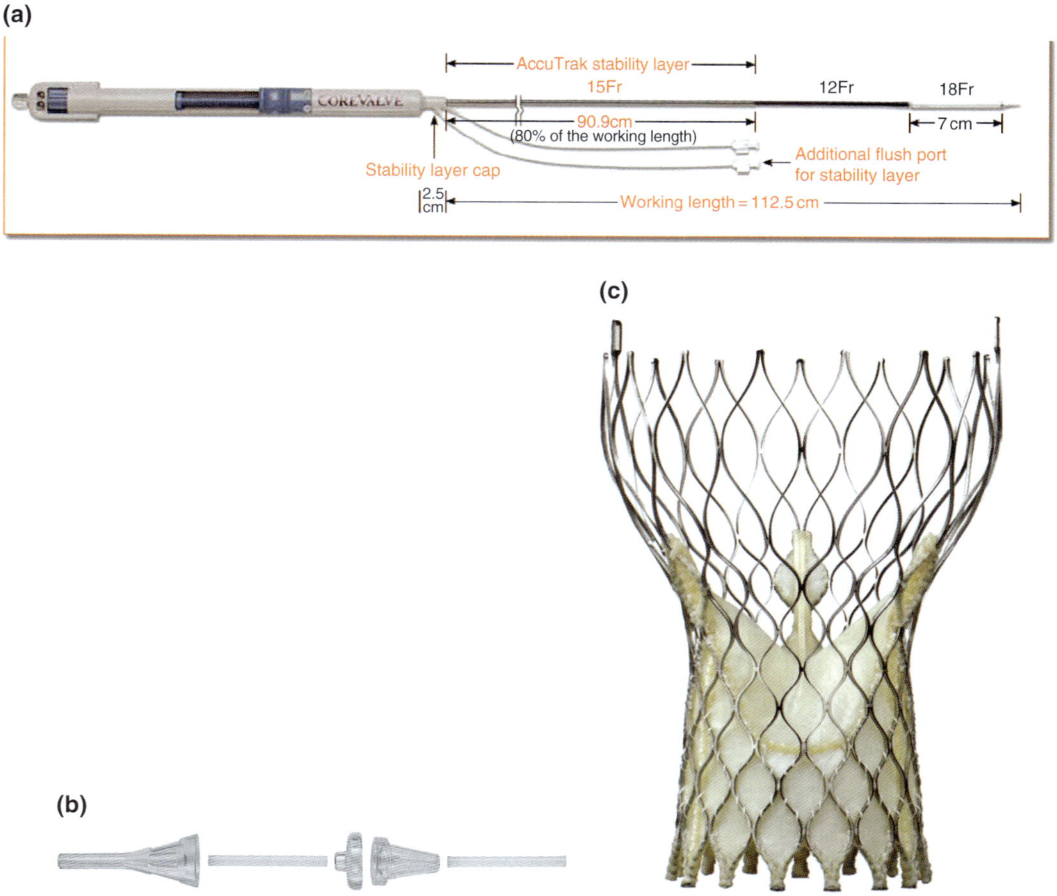

Fig. 14.8 The Medtronic CoreValve system comprises (a) the AccuTrak delivery catheter, (b) the five-piece disposable loading system, and (c) the bioprosthetic valve.

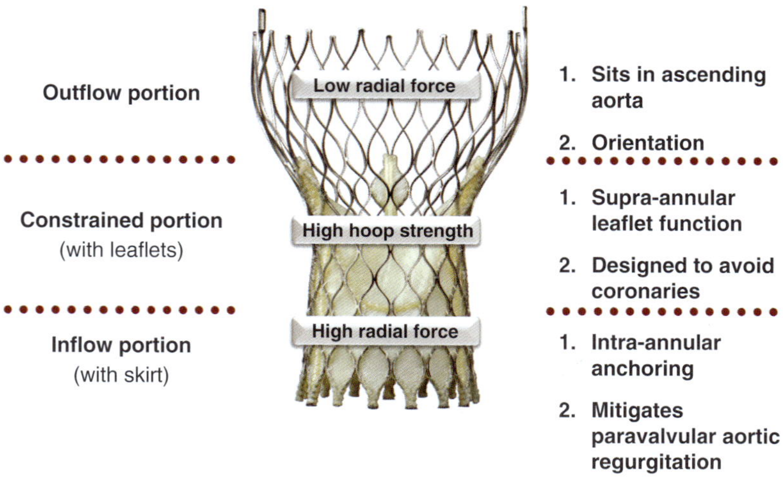

Fig. 14.9 The CoreValve bioprosthesis is characterized as a self-expanding multilevel frame with three distinct areas of form and function: (i) the inflow portion of the frame has high radial force and functions to anchor the prosthesis against the aortic annulus and aortic valve leaflets and together with the skirt creates a seal to mitigate paravalvular aortic regurgitation. (ii) The constrained portion of the frame houses the leaflets and has high hoop strength thereby resisting deformation and maintaining optimal leaflet geometry. Furthermore, this portion is constrained and was designed to avoid the coronary arteries. (iii) The outflow portion of the frame has low radial force and sits in the ascending aorta and was designed to orient the prosthesis in the direction of blood flow.

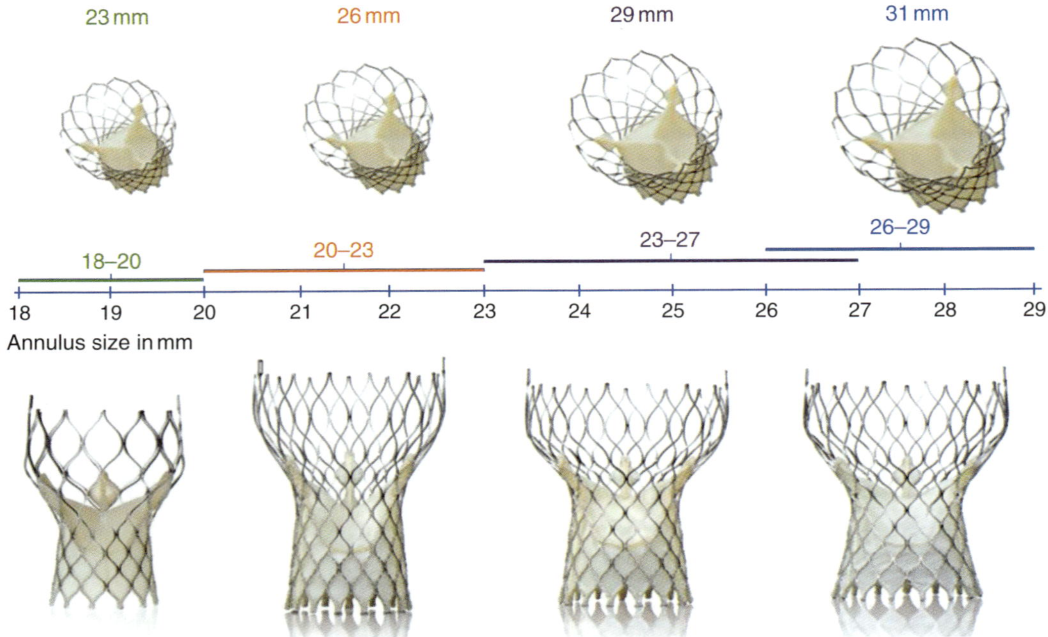

Fig. 14.10 The Medtronic CoreValve showing the four sizes currently available; in 2012.

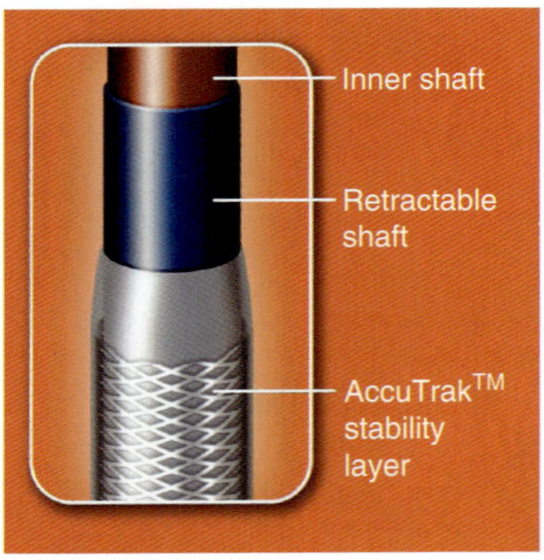

Fig. 14.11 The AccuTrak stability layer is an additional layer that isolates the retractable delivery sheath from the introducer and patient anatomy, thus providing a stable platform for deployment. The aim of the AccuTrak stability layer is to mitigate the forward motion (i.e. towards the ventricle) of the prosthesis during deployment which was characteristic of the predecessor generation of delivery catheter.

(Fig. 14.10). It can be implanted via the femoral artery, subclavian artery (57–59), and through a direct aortic access. The AccuTrak delivery catheter provides greater stability and precision during valve deployment than its predecessor and has an outer diameter of 18 Fr at its distal end (Fig. 14.11) [60].

Transfemoral TAVR: procedural steps

The generic steps involved in performing TAVR are outlined below [61,62].

1 **Anesthesia**: General or local anesthesia with mild sedation can be successfully used during TAVR [63–73].

2 **Anticoagulation**: Administer heparin to achieve and maintain an activated clotting time between 250 and 300 seconds. Typically, patients are loaded with 300 mg clopidogrel 24 hours prior to the procedure.

3 **Antibiotic prophylaxis**: Performed according to hospital protocol.

4 **Preparation of the prosthesis**: Both bioprostheses are gently agitated in sterile physiologic saline to remove the glutaraldehyde preservative. They are subsequently mounted and/or crimped onto the delivery system.

5 **Temporary pacemaker implantation**: A temporary pacemaker lead is placed into the right ventricle, and pacemaker function is assessed under rapid pacing, 160–180 beats/minute, such that systemic arterial pressure is reduced below 60 mmHg.

6 **Supra-aortic angiogram**: A pigtail catheter is placed in the non-coronary sinus to perform a supra-aortic angiogram. The C-arm is angulated to where the nadir of all three leaflets is in one plane,

perpendicular to the viewing angle. This is typically located in a left anterior oblique (approximately 10°) with some cranial or caudal (0–15°) angulation. Several ancillary devices can be used to facilitate the optimal viewing angle for implantation [74–77].

7 **Vascular access**: Vascular access may be performed using a surgical arterial cutdown or percutaneously with aid of pre-closure vascular devices [78]. Vascular pre-closure of the femoral arterial access site can be accomplished with one 10 Fr Prostar XL percutaneous vascular surgical system (Abbott, Park, IL) or two 6 Fr Perclose ProGlide suture-mediated closure system (Abbott, Park, IL). A single puncture of the anterior wall of the common femoral artery is recommended to avoid pre-closure vascular device failure. Contralateral contrast injections and ultrasound-guided puncture can assist vascular puncture.

8 **Vascular introducer sheath**: Introduction and advancement of the large bore vascular introducer sheath should be performed under fluoroscopic guidance over a stiff guide wire (Amplatz Extra-stiff or Super-stiff). Any resistance encountered while advancing the sheath should be carefully evaluated in order to avoid vascular complications.

9 **Crossing the native aortic valve**: A variety of catheters can be used to cross the native aortic valve. The Amplatz left 2 is usually selected in patients with an enlarged or a horizontal aortic root whereas the Amplatz left 1 is preferred in those with a small or vertical aortic root. Straight-tipped guide wires should be used to cross the valve. Once crossed, the straight guide wire is exchanged for a pre-shaped long Extra-stiff Amplatz guide wire (Cook Medical, Bloomington, IN; for Edwards Sapien) or Super-stiff Amplatz guide wire (Cook Medical; for Medtronic CoreValve). Pre-shaping of the distal tip is mandatory to reduce the risk of cardiac perforation.

10 **Pre-implant balloon aortic valvuloplasty**: The Edwards Sapien system is equipped with a custom retroflex 20 or 23 mm × 4 cm balloon dilation kit for the 23 and 26 mm valve sizes, respectively. For the 26 and 29 mm Medtronic CoreValve devices, 22 mm × 4 cm and 25 mm × 4 cm balloons are recommended for pre-implant dilation, respectively.

11 **Prosthesis positioning and deployment**:

- *Edwards Sapien XT*. The NovaFlex delivery system is advanced through the introducer sheath until the prosthesis exits the sheath. Valve alignment is then performed in the descending aorta and the delivery system is advanced, using the Flex Wheel to trasverse the aortic arch. The native aortic valve is crossed, the Flex Catheter retracted and the prosthesis positioned (50–60% ventricular). Under rapid pacing, to reduce the systolic aortic pressure <50 mmHg, the balloon is inflated, thus deploying the valve. After 4–5 seconds, the balloon is deflated and then the rapid pacing terminated. Finally, the delivery system is de-articulated and retracted across the aortic arch.
- *Medtronic CoreValve*. The CoreValve is advanced across the native aortic valve and is positioned such that its second horizontal radiopaque band lies at the level of the aortic annular plane. In this position, the valve lies approximately 4 mm below the annulus, the target implantation depth (Fig. 14.12). Once a baseline aortogram confirms the position of the prosthesis, the CoreValve is deployed in four steps (Fig. 14.13):

  (i) The micro knob is turned clockwise, until the radiopaque ring reaches the second radiopaque band of the prosthesis (Fig. 14.13b). An aortogram is then performed to confirm the prosthesis target depth of 4 mm. At this stage, the prosthesis can be repositioned either more cranial or caudal.

  (ii) The micro knob is turned until the inflow portion of the valve is 40–50% away from contacting the opposite annular surface (Fig. 14.13c). An aortogram is again performed to re-confirm target depth. Again, the prosthesis can be repositioned cranially or caudally.

  (iii) The micro knob is slowly rotated until the inflow portion of the prosthesis comes into contact with the opposite annular surface and an aortogram repeated. Further micro knob rotation is performed until the valve is three-fourths deployed and again an aortogram is performed. At this stage, slight cranial (but *not* caudal) repositioning of the CoreValve can be performed.

(iv) Further rotation of the micro knob is performed until complete deployment of the CoreValve is achieved.

- The stiff wire is withdrawn towards the tip of the nose cone and the delivery catheter is removed from the left ventricle. The macro knob is then used to recapture the nose cone in the descending aorta.

12 **Verify valve position and performance, and rule out potential complications**: After valve deployment and removal of the delivery catheters and guide wires, the cardiac rhythm and hemodynamic are carefully assessed. Severe bradycardia or

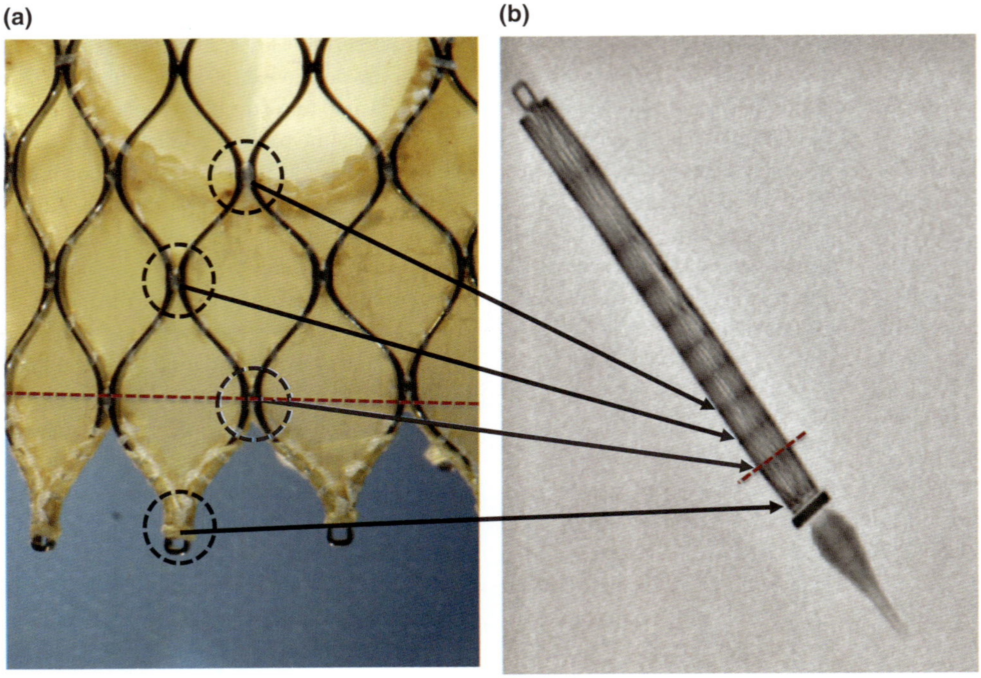

Fig. 14.12 The Medtronic CoreValve frame has a repeating diamond cell configuration. The junction between diamond cells, known as "nodes" (encircled in black in (a)); can be seen as horizontal radiopaque bands on the collapsed frame within the delivery catheter (b). The vertical distance between nodes at the inflow end is approximately 4 mm. The red dotted line represents an implantation depth of 4 mm (i.e. at the second horizontal radiopaque band). These horizontal radiopaque bands are used to guide positioning of the prosthesis during valve deployment.

high degrees of atrioventricular block will require immediate temporary pacing. A low aortic diastolic pressure (<35 mmHg), elevated left ventricular end-diastolic pressure, or near equalization of aortic diastolic and left ventricular end-diastolic pressures suggest significant prosthetic valve regurgitation. Valve performance should be assessed using contrast aortography and echocardiography. A supra-aortic angiogram in the right anterior oblique (RAO) position is recommended to evaluate valve position, estimate the degree of aortic regurgitation, and confirm patency of the coronary arteries. The severity and origin of aortic regurgitation is optimally assessed with TEE.

13 Vessel closure and hemostasis: Prior to securing the pre-closure sutures, it is strongly recommended that a safety wire be placed from the contralateral femoral artery down the ipsilateral femoral artery beyond the bifurcation [79]. This enables immediate intervention of the ipsilateral femoral artery in case of vascular injury. A final contrast angiography of the peripheral vessels should be performed to confirm hemostasis and rule-out vascular injury.

14 Post-procedural care: All patients should be monitored in an intensive care setting for 24–48 hours after valve implantation. Particular attention should be given to the neurologic status, cardiopulmonary function, renal function, and vascular/bleeding complications. Continuous telemetry monitoring is recommended for the duration of the hospital stay (4–10 days) [80,81].

TAVR-related complications

Complications associated with TAVR are classified as cardiac or non-cardiac in origin (Box 14.1).

Cardiac complications

Paravalvular aortic regurgitation

A degree of post-implant aortic regurgitation (paravalvular or transvalvular) is observed in 70–90% of TAVR recipients, though less than 5% of cases have moderate to severe aortic regurgitation [82–88].

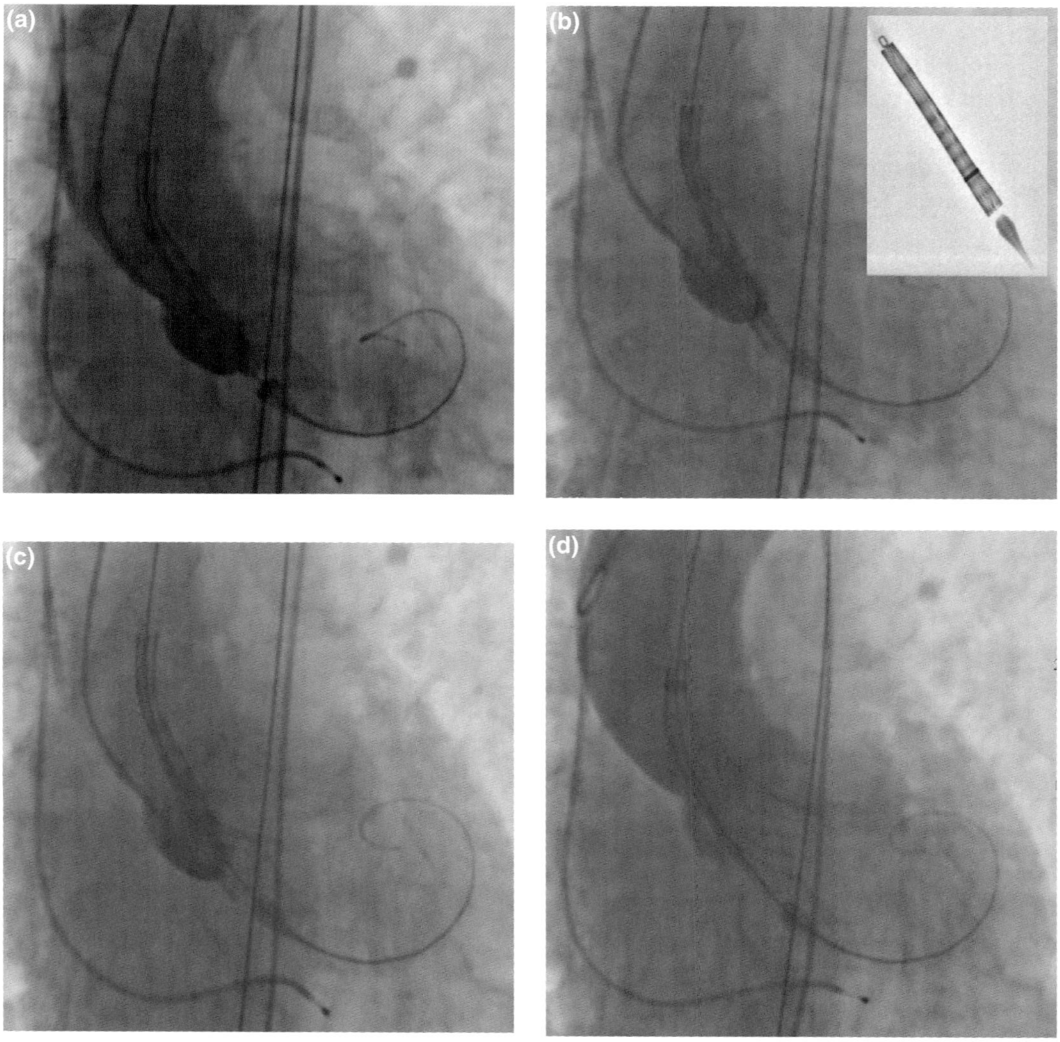

Fig. 14.13 Steps in deployment of the Medtronic CoreValve prosthesis. (a) The unsheathed prosthesis is positioned such that the second horizontal radiopaque band is at the level of the aortic annular plane. (b) Turn the micro knob until the radiopaque ring reaches the second radiopaque band of the prosthesis. (c) Slowly turn the micro knob until the inflow portion of the valve is 40–50% away from contacting the opposite annular surface. (d) Continue to slowly rotate the micro knob until the inflow portion of the prosthesis comes into contact with opposite annular surface. An aortogram may be repeated at this point; otherwise, continue to rotate the micro knob until the prosthesis is three-fourths deployed. Before retracting the delivery catheter verify that the loading hooks of the valve frame are detached from the delivery catheter; this is best appreciated in two orthogonal views. Image courtesy of the PCR-EAPCI Percutaneous Interventional Cardiovascular Medicine Textbook, 2012, Europa Publishing.

Mechanisms of aortic regurgitation include: (i) transcatheter valve undersizing [87,89]; (ii) malpositioning [90,91]; (iii) malapposition, under expansion or recoil of the transcatheter valve [92–94]; and (iv) malcoaptation or immobility of the valve leaflets [95–97]. Delayed severe aortic regurgitation has also been reported [98–100]. The mechanism of aortic regurgitation can usually be identified using TEE [85,101,102]. VARC recommends using an integrative echocardiographic approach when quantifying aortic regurgitation [101,102].

Management of significant aortic regurgitation depends on the underlying mechanism, though treatment may include post-implant dilation,

Box 14.1 Cardiac and non-cardiac complications of transcatheter aortic valve implantation

Cardiac
- Paravalvular aortic regurgitation
- Conduction abnormalities
- Atrial and ventricular arrhythmias
- Coronary obstruction
- Cardiac perforation
- Aortic root rupture
- Prosthetic valve dysfunction
- Embolization
- Transcatheter aortic valve thrombosis
- Transcatheter aortic valve endocarditis
- Mitral regurgitation and mitral valve injury

Non-cardiac
- Stroke
- Vascular injury
- Acute kidney injury

implantation of a second valve, or repositioning of the frame using a snare (Fig. 14.14). Conversion to surgical aortic valve replacement is required in less than 1% of cases.

Conduction disturbance

The anatomic proximity of the aortic valvular complex and the conduction system explains the potential for conduction disturbances following TAVR (Fig. 14.15) [48]. Indeed, the average distance between the nadir of the non-coronary aortic valve leaflet and the left bundle branch is only 6.3±2.4 mm (Fig. 14.15) [103]. New-onset left bundle branch block occurs in 30–65% of patients after Medtronic CoreValve implantation and in 7–18% [104–121] after Edwards Sapien implantation [122–124]. The long-term implications of new-onset left bundle branch block after TAVR are unclear however anecdotal evidence suggests that it has a negligible impact on 1-year survival. Approximately 15–47% [104–121] and 4–21% [122–124] of patients require a new permanent pacemaker after CoreValve and Edwards Sapien implantation, respectively. The most important predictors for new-onset conduction abnormalities after CoreValve implantation include a pre-existing right bundle branch block, baseline QRS duration (ms), and the depth of prosthesis implantation (mm) [104–111,113–115, 117–119,121,125,126]. A CoreValve implantation depth of <6 mm has been found to mitigate conduction disturbances [117]. Most patients needing a new permanent pacemaker are identified immediately after valve implantation; however, a small percentage of patients may present with delayed conduction block. Therefore, temporary pacing should be maintained for 48–72 hours, especially after CoreValve implantation. Indications for permanent pacemaker implantation after TAVR are based upon the European Society of Cardiology guidelines [127,128].

Cardiac arrhythmias

The reported rates of atrial fibrillation following TAVR vary considerably. A recent observational study found atrial fibrillation in 6% of patients following TAVR, as opposed to 33% in those undergoing surgical aortic valve replacement [129]. In contrast, another study found new-onset atrial fibrillation in 32% of patients undergoing TAVR. Importantly, new-onset atrial fibrillation is associated with higher rates of stroke/system embolism, though not with increased mortality [130].

Life-threatening ventricular arrhythmias (ventricular fibrillation/tachycardia) occur in up to 4% of TAVR patients [19,131]. Multiple ventricular ectopic beats can be induced by the left ventricular guide wire or delivery catheter, and can usually be terminated by repositioning. Defibrillator pads should be placed for the entirety of the procedure and maintained until the patient arrives in the intensive care unit.

Coronary obstruction

Occlusion of the left main coronary following TAVR occurs in less than 1% of cases [132–142]. Unsurprisingly, it frequently induces sudden hemodynamic compromise and death. The diagnosis is usually suspected on the basis of hemodynamics, electrocardiogram (ECG) pattern, and/or contrast aortography. Hemodynamic support and re-establishment of coronary perfusion is critical. The nature and severity of the coronary obstruction and hemodynamic status determines the mode of revascularization (percutaneous or surgical).

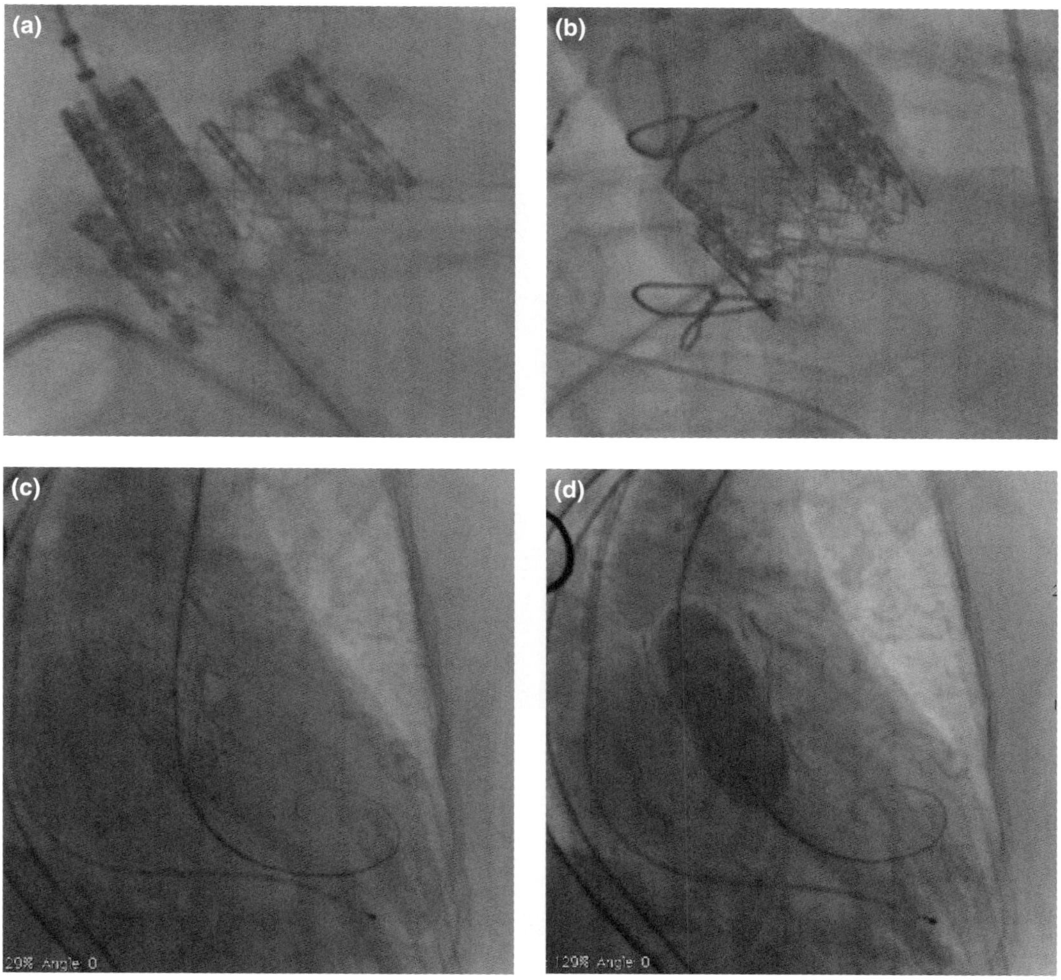

Fig. 14.14 (a) Severe paravalvular aortic regurgitation following low implantation of the Edwards Sapien prosthesis. (b) Transcatheter aortic valve-in-transcatheter aortic valve (TAV-in-TAV) implantation was successful in abolishing paravalvular aortic regurgitation. (c) Despite proper positioning, underexpansion of the CoreValve prosthesis due to severe bulky calcification led to severe paravalvular aortic regurgitation. (d) Post-implant dilation performed during rapid pacing was successful in abolishing the paravalvular aortic regurgitation. Image courtesy of the PCR-EAPCI Percutaneous Interventional Cardiovascular Medicine Textbook, 2012, Europa Publishing.

Possible mechanisms for coronary obstruction include: (i) impingement of the coronary ostia by the valve support structure; (ii) displacement of the native aortic valve leaflets towards the coronary ostia during valve deployment; and (iii) embolization from calcium, thrombus, air, and/or endocarditis. The width and height of the sinus of Valsalva, the height of the coronary ostia, and the bulkiness of the native leaflets play important roles in the pathogenesis of coronary occlusion following TAVR.

A contrast aortography during balloon aortic valvuloplasty may be performed to evaluate the potential for coronary obstruction. If the aortography suggests an increased risk for coronary obstruction, a safety coronary guide wire can be positioned into the coronary artery with the guiding catheter retracted into the ascending aorta during valve implantation.

Cardiac perforation

Cardiac perforation has been reported in 2–4% of patients undergoing TAVR [131,143,144]. Potential mechanisms include right or left ventricular injury due to the temporary pacemaker lead or stiff guide wire, respectively. Small hypertrophic

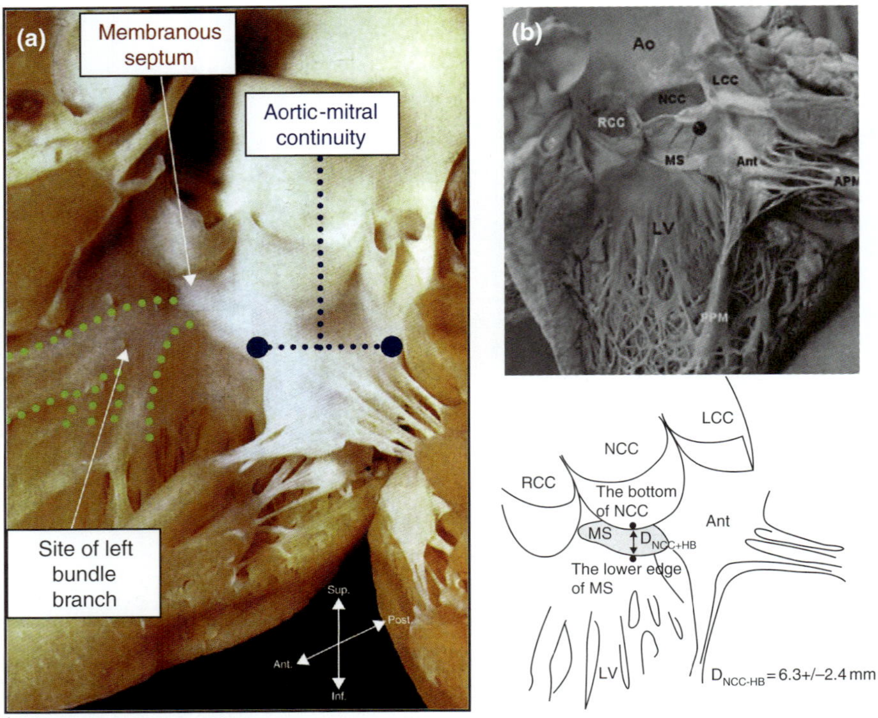

Fig. 14.15 (a) Human heart specimen of the left ventricular cavity, aortic valve, and ascending aorta. Note that the left bundle branch exits at the crest of the ventricular septum just beneath the membranous septum. (b) More specifically, the left bundle branch exits below the membranous septum approximately 6.3±2.4 mm from the bottom of the non-coronary cusp of the aortic valve. Coincidentally, several investigators have noted that conduction abnormalities following CoreValve implantation can be mitigated by implanting the prosthesis ≤6–8 mm from the aortic annular plane. Ant, anterior; Ao, aorta; LCC, left coronary cusp; LV, left ventricle; MS, membranous septum; NCC, non coronary cusp; PPM, posteromedial papillary muscle pacemaker; RCC, right coronary cusp. Green dotted line, site of left bundle branch block; blue dotted line, aortic mitral continuity. Image courtesy of the PCR-EAPCI Percutaneous Interventional Cardiovascular Medicine Textbook, 2012, Europa Publishing.

left ventricular cavities (commonly seen in elderly females), or inadequate pre-shaping or positioning of the left ventricular support wire may increase the risk for this complication. Positioning of the left ventricular stiff guide wire should be performed in the right anterior oblique projection and reassessed throughout the procedure. Cardiac perforation and cardiac tamponade are usually suspected on the basis of hypotension and/or a new pericardial effusion, and are diagnosed using TTE. Percutaneous pericardiocentesis and reversal of the anticoagulation are recommended.

Aortic annular rupture

Rupture of the annulus or aortic root is rare (<1%). This life-threatening complication is difficult to predict, but typically occurs during balloon inflation (pre-implant balloon aortic valvuloplasty or balloon-expandable valve implantation) (Fig. 14.16). A non-compliant aortic valvular complex, bulky calcification, and aggressive balloon/prosthesis oversizing are possible risk factors. Depending on its location, rupture may result in a ventricular septal defect, left ventricle-to-left atrial or left ventricle-to-right atrial shunt, or communication with the extracardiac space. Contrast aortography usually reveals contrast extravasation confirming the diagnosis. Emergent cardiopulmonary bypass support and surgical exploration is the management of choice.

Prosthetic valve dysfunction

Prosthetic valve dysfunction may manifest as symptoms and signs of valvular stenosis or regurgitation. Careful clinical history and examination coupled with echocardiography (TTE or TEE) are

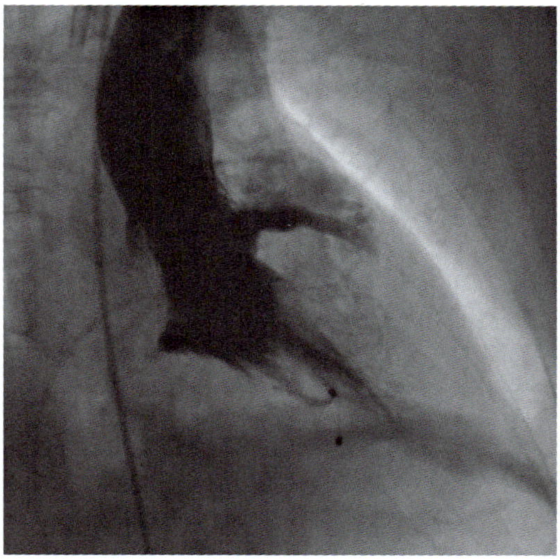

Fig. 14.16 Extravasation of contrast into the pericardial space due to aortic annular rupture. The injury likely occurred immediately after aggressive balloon aortic valvuloplasty. Image courtesy of the PCR-EAPCI Percutaneous Interventional Cardiovascular Medicine Textbook, 2012, Europa Publishing.

suggested to evaluate valve dysfunction [101,102]. Prosthetic valve dysfunction is graded as (i) normal, (ii) possible, or (iii) significant according to the VARC criteria [101,102]. To date, there are limited case reports describing degeneration of transcatheter valves [145,146].

Embolization

Transcatheter valve embolization usually occurs during valve implantation and appears to correlate with operator experience. Embolization may be caused by: (i) undersizing the prosthesis; (ii) malplacement of the prosthesis; (iii) improper rapid pacing during valve deployment or post-implant dilation; (iv) entanglement of a guide wire across the struts of the prosthesis during valve re-crossing; (v) entanglement of the nose cone with the inflow portion of the prosthesis upon retrieving the delivery catheter; and (vi) inadequate release of the loading hooks of the frame from the delivery catheter. Delayed embolization, presenting with unexpected hemodynamic compromise and severe aortic regurgitation, has also been described [98,99].

Thrombosis

Valve thrombosis is defined as any thrombus attached to or near an implanted valve that interrupts blood flow, interferes with valve function, or is sufficiently large to warrant treatment. Post-mortem studies of patients implanted with the Edwards Sapien and CoreValve prostheses have observed thrombotic material attached to the frame and/or leaflets [147]. To date, transcatheter aortic valve thrombosis has been reported in only three individual case reports [148–150].

Currently, dual antiplatelet therapy (aspirin and clopidogrel) is recommended for 6 months following TAVR, with aspirin continued indefinitely [131,151]. However, a single-center randomized study observed no differences in clinical outcomes between groups who received dual antiplatelet therapy for 3 months versus aspirin alone [152].

Endocarditis

The diagnosis of prosthetic valve endocarditis can be made using the Duke criteria for endocarditis, during reoperation, or on autopsy [101,102]. Several case reports of bacterial or fungal transcatheter aortic valve endocarditis have been reported involving both the Edwards Sapien and Medtronic CoreValve systems [153–159]. These cases underline the importance of adequate dental care prior to TAVR, the importance of pre-procedural antibiotics, and sterile techniques during the procedure.

Mitral valve injury

Mitral valve injury associated with retrograde TAVR is rare. Resistance during the passage of the delivery catheter into the left ventricle or observation of new mitral regurgitation on TEE should raise the suspicion of catheter entanglement within the mitral valve apparatus. Pre-procedural mitral regurgitation can be identified in up 75% of patients [160,161], and improves in approximately one-third of patients, and worsens in one-third following TAVR. Mitral annular calcification and deep implantation of the transcatheter valve into the left ventricular outflow tract have been associated with worsening mitral regurgitation [160–163].

Non-cardiac complications

Stroke

To date, observational series have reported 30-day stroke rates of 0–6% in patients undergoing TAVR [83,131,164–166]. In the randomized PARTNER Cohort A trial, the neurologic event rate (all strokes

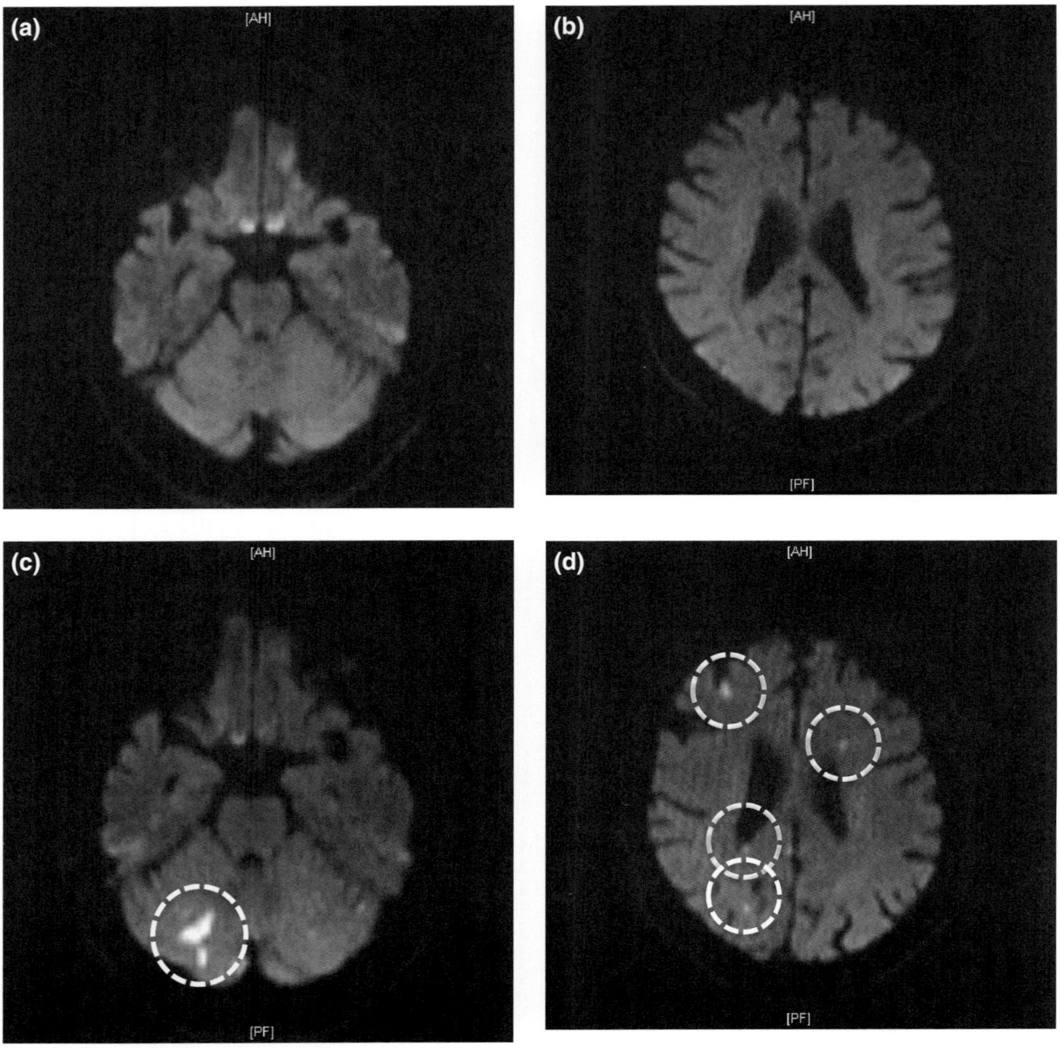

Fig. 14.17 (a, b) Diffusion-weighted MRI of the brain of a 79-year-old patient before undergoing TAVR. (c, d) corresponding diffusion-weighted MRI images of the same patient after a TAVR procedure showing multiple silent cerebral infarcts (encircled in white). Image courtesy of the PCR-EAPCI Percutaneous Interventional Cardiovascular Medicine Textbook, 2012, Europa Publishing.

or transient ischemic attack) was nearly two-fold higher in the TAVR than in the surgical group at 30 days and 1-year follow-up (5.5% versus 2.4% at 30 days, 8.3% versus 4.3% at 1 year) [151]. Similarly, in the randomized PARTNER Cohort B trial, the neurologic event rate was higher in the TAVR than in the medical therapy group at 30 days and 1 year (6.7% versus 1.7% at 30 days, 10.6% versus 4.5% at 1 year). Interestingly, one-third to one-half of strokes occurred between 2 and 30 days after the index procedure [131,151,167]. A history of cerebrovascular disease is an independent predictor of neurologic injury after TAVR [168].

Post-TAVR magnetic resonance imaging (MRI) studies have observed new and multiple silent cerebral infarcts in 68–83% of cases (Fig. 14.17) [169–174]. This suggests that most strokes after TAVR are embolic in nature, a hypothesis corroborated by a recent study using intra-procedural transcranial Doppler which found cerebral microemboli in all patients undergoing transapical TAVR [175]. Cerebral embolic protection devices such as the

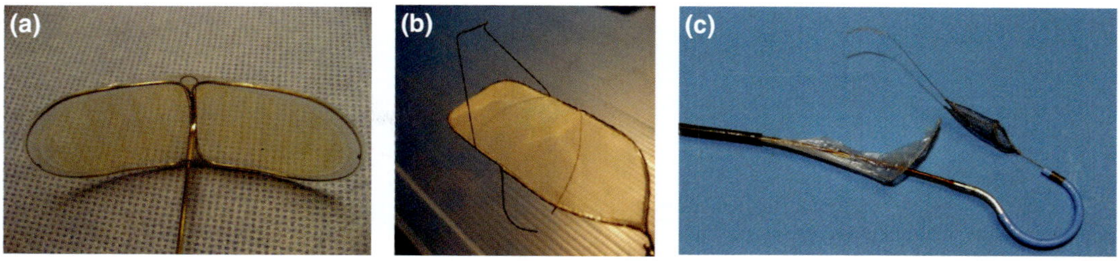

Fig. 14.18 (a) The Embrella device is implanted via a radial artery approach and sits across the aortic arch. (b) SMT embolic deflection device (SMT Research and Development, Herzliya Pituach, Israel) is implanted via a femoral arterial approach and sits across the aortic arch. (c) Montage System (Claret Medical, Santa Rosa, CA) is implanted via a radial approach and each basket sits within a carotid artery.

Embrella (Edwards LifeSciences, Irvine, CA) and Montage System (Claret Medical, Santa Rosa, CA) have been developed to prevent cerebral embolization and have received a European CE mark (Fig. 14.18) [176,177]. These devices have the potential to reduce the incidence of clinical stroke in TAVR recipients [178].

Vascular injury

Vascular complications have been reported in 2–30% of patients undergoing TAVR, and are associated with increased short-term mortality [46,179–182]. Vascular injuries may include dissection, rupture, thrombosis, stenosis, artery avulsion during sheath retraction, failure of vascular pre-closure, arterial-venous fistula, and/or pseudoaneurysms. Femoral and iliac artery complications occur with near equal frequency, though dissections occur more frequently in the femoral artery, and ruptures more common in the iliac artery [46]. Failure of vascular closure devices is an important source of minor vascular complications [180]. Treatment is again cause specific, and includes external femoral artery compression, prolonged balloon inflation, implantation of bare/covered stents, percutaneous endografts, or surgical repair. Guide wires are easily advanced from the contralateral femoral artery to delivery hemostatic occlusion balloons or stents when needed.

Serious vascular injuries can usually be avoided by: (i) careful vascular screening; (ii) low threshold for using non-femoral access; (iii) consideration for surgical cutdown; (iv) fluoroscopic guidance for advancing devices; and (v) never forcibly advancing materials. Ultrasound-guided femoral artery puncture may also reduce vascular injury [21].

Acute kidney injury

Chronic kidney failure is present in 10–25% of patients undergoing TAVR. Acute kidney injury (AKI) has been documented in 7–28% of patients following TAVR [80,183–187], and both baseline renal dysfunction and AKI have been associated with increased 30-day and 1-year mortality [183,185,186,188]. A variety of factors are predictive of AKI: history of hypertension, peripheral arterial disease, logistic EuroScore, pre-procedural creatinine level, and post-procedural aortic regurgitation >2+ [80,183–187]. Approximately 100–120 ml of contrast is used during a TAVR procedure, though the volume of contrast has not been linked to the development of AKI. The need for in-hospital renal replacement therapy has been reported in 1–10% of patients [183–187].

Clinical trial outcomes

Uniform definitions for clinical endpoints are of considerable importance when evaluating and summarizing current TAVR data.

Valvular Academic Research Consortium

The VARC was established to arrive at a consensus (i) on the most appropriate clinical endpoints reflecting device and patient effectiveness and safety, and (ii) to standardize the definition of endpoints for valve-related clinical trials [101,102,189].

Summary of TAVR clinical studies

Table 14.1 summarizes the clinical outcomes of selected TAVR studies [39,80,131,151,166,167,188,190–200].

Table 14.1 Summary of clinical outcomes with transcatheter aortic valve implantation.

Reference	Study sample size	Prosthesis type	Age (years)	Logistic EuroScore (%)	STS (%)	30-day mortality (%)	1-year mortality (%)	>1 year mortality (%) (as indicated)	Stroke (%)	MI and/or CO (%)	Vascular injury (%)	Bleeding (%)	Pacemaker implan- tation (%)	Acute renal injury/ dialysis* (%)	Tamponade (%)	New-onset atrial fibrilltion (%)	Conversion to surgery (%)
[193]	244	ES and MC	82.3 ± 7.3	25.6 ± 11.4	18.9 ± 12.8	12.7	–	–	3.6	1.2	7.3	–	11.8	–/1.6*	2.1	–	–
[200]	697	ES and MC	81.4 ± 6.3	20.5 ± 13.2	–	12.4	–	–	2.8	0.4	19.5	–	39.3	–	1.8	–	–
[60]	646	MDT CV	81.0 ± 6.6	23.1 ± 13.8	9.6 ± 3.5	8	–	–	1.9	0.6	1.9	–	9.3	–	1.4	–	0.5
[199]	200	ES and MC	82.0 ± 6.5	24.6 ± 15.3	6.4 ± 4.9	7.5	–	–	4.5	0.5	13.5	35.5	22.5	19/–	1.1	–	–
[196]	70	ES	84.7 ± 7.6	31.7 ± 16.0	9.6 ± 3.5	–	–	38.6 (3-year)	8.6 (3-year)	8.6 (3-year)	–	7.1 (3-year)	7.1 (3-year)	–	–	–	1.4 (3-year)
[80]	150	MC	81 ± 7	12.3 (9.1–18.4)	6.1 (3.7–12.5)	11	–	–	8	1.1	16	26	19	18.0/–	–	–	0
[188]	663	MC	81.0 ± 7.3	23.0 ± 13.7	–	5.9	15	–	1.2	0	2	–	17.4	–	1.2	–	0.8
[151]	348	ES	83.6 ± 6.8	29.3 ± 16.5	11.8 ± 3.3	3.4	24.2	–	4.7	0	17	9.3	3.8	1.2/2.9*	–	8.6	2.5
[81, 197]	1038	ES	81.2 ± 6.8	27.4 ± 15.1	–	8.5	23.9	–	2.5	0.6	12.8	–	7.1	–/4.3*	–	–	–
[192]	328	ES and MC	83.1 ± 6.1	28.0 ± 16.0	–	11	–	–	5	–	–	–	13	–/6*	–	–	–
[194]	136	MC	80.9	21.3	9.7	12.5	18.4	–	3.7	2.2	–	–	25	–	1.5	–	–
[190]	504	ES	81.2 ± 6.5	24 ± 16	11 ± 4	8.3	–	29 (2-year)	3.1	1.6	–	–	5.3	–	–	–	1.9
[195]	270	ES	83.3 ± 8.0	–	9.5	9.6	–	–	3.3	–	6.7	–	5.9	6.7/–	2.2	4.4	–
[167]	179	ES	83.1 ± 8.6	26.4 ± 17.2	11.2 ± 5.8	5	30.7	–	2.3	0	30.7	16.8	3.4	–/1.1*	–	0.6	0

CO, coronary occlusion; ES, Edwards Sapien system; MC, Medtronic CoreValue system; MI, myocardial infarction; STS, Society of Thoracic Surgeons.

PARTNER US Trial

The Placement of Aortic TraNscathetER Valve (PARTNER) US Trial was the first prospective, randomized-controlled trial for transcatheter heart valves. This trial consisted of two individually powered patient cohorts (Cohort A and B). In Cohort A, the Edwards Sapien prosthesis was compared with surgical aortic valve replacement in high-risk surgical patients with severe aortic stenosis [151]. In Cohort B, the Edwards Sapien THV was compared to best medical management in inoperable patients with severe aortic stenosis [167].

Cohort B results

In Cohort B, TAVR was superior to medical therapy and/or balloon aortic valvuloplasty for all-cause mortality at 1 year (31% versus 51%, P <0.001, number needed to treat (NNT)=5) and at 2 years (43% versus 68%, P <0.001, NNT=4) [167,201]. The observed rate of neurologic events (stroke and transient ischemic attack), were higher in the transcatheter group than in the medical group at 2-year follow-up (16% versus 6%, P=0.003), though the need for hospitalization was 38% lower in the TAVR group compared with the medical group (35% versus 73%, P <0.001). Quality of life, based on the Kansas City Cardiomyopathy Questionnaire (KCCQ) and SF-12 Health Survey, improved more in the transcatheter than standard therapy group at 30-days and 1-year follow-up [202]. At 12-month follow-up, total costs were significantly lower with TAVR compared with medical therapy: $29,352 versus $52,724 ($P$ <0.001) [203]. Incremental life expectancy of 1.9 years was noted with TAVR.

Cohort A results

In Cohort A, TAVR was non-inferior to surgical aortic valve replacement for all-cause mortality at 1 year (24% versus 27%, P=0.001 for non-inferiority) [151]. The rate of neurologic events was higher in the transcatheter group than in the surgical group at 30 days (5.5% versus 2.4%, P=0.04) and at 1 year (8.3% versus 4.3%, P=0.04). The rates of a composite of death from any cause or major stroke were comparable between the transcatheter group and surgical group at 30 days (6.9 versus 8.2%, P=0.52) and at 1 year (26.5 versus 28.0%, P=0.68). Both surgical aortic valve replacement and TAVR improved disease-specific and generic health-related quality of life over 1-year follow-up [204]. For patients eligible for the transfemoral approach, TAVR resulted in substantial quality of life benefit over surgery at 1 month with similar benefits at 6-month and 1-year follow-up.

Specific patient subgroups

Failing surgical bioprosthetic valves

Elective redo aortic valve surgery is associated with an operative mortality rate between 2% and 7%, though this increases to more than 30% in high-risk and non-elective patients [205–207]. In excess of 100 successful transcatheter aortic valve-in-surgical aortic valve (TAV-in-SAV) implantations have been reported with the Medtronic CoreValve and Edwards Sapien transcatheter heart valve for failing stented and stentless surgical bioprostheses [208].

Bicuspid valves

Congenital or acquired bicuspid aortic valve stenosis has been considered a contraindication to TAVR. However, several successful case reports have been documented [209–216]. Anecdotally, stenotic bicuspid aortic annuli are larger and more eccentric than stenotic tricuspid aortic valves, and thus MSCT is strongly recommended for transcatheter aortic valve sizing.

Lower surgical risk patients

Although TAVR was initially conceived for the treatment of high surgical risk or inoperable patients, a recent observational report observed a shift toward the selection of lower surgical risk patients for TAVR [217]. This paradigm shift was associated with significantly better clinical outcomes in the lower (mean STS score 4%) than higher (mean STS score 7%) surgical risk patients undergoing TAVR at 30-day and 6-month follow-up [218]. As further evidence of this move towards lower surgical risk patients, the SURTAVI (SURgical aortic valve replacement versus Transcatheter Aortic Valve Implantation) and PARTNER II trials are expected to randomize intermediate surgical risk patients with an STS score of 4–8% to TAVR or surgical aortic valve replacement.

Future transcatheter aortic valve platforms

Several novel transcatheter aortic valve designs are undergoing human trials. Table 14.2 summarizes these devices.

Table 14.2 A summary of various transcatheter aortic valves and their characteristics.

	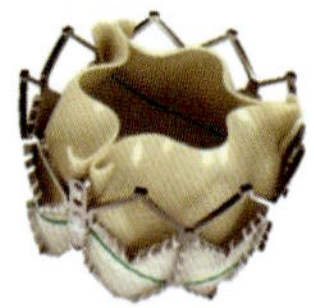	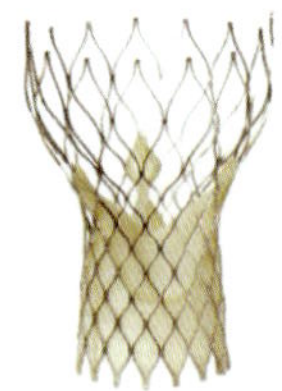	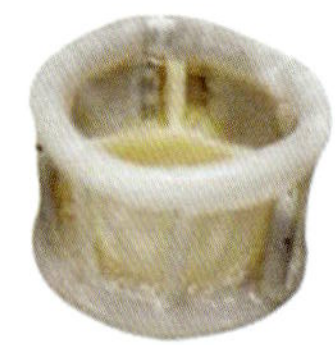	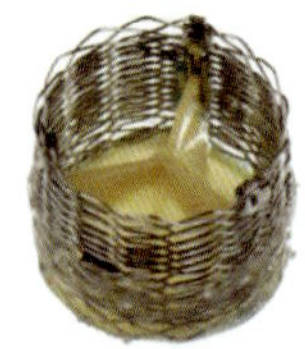	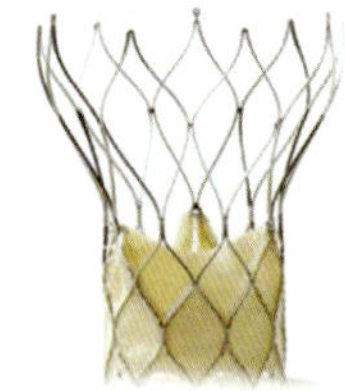
Manufacturer	Edwards SAPIEN XT	Medtronic CoreValve	Direct Flow Medical	Boston Scientific Sadra Medical	St. Jude Medical Portico
Access	TF, TA, DAo	TF, SC, DAo	TF	TF	TF
Deployment	Balloon-expandable	Self-expandable	Inflatable	Self-expandable	Self-expandable
Support structure	Cobalt chromium	Nitinol	Inflatable	Nitinol	Nitinol
Leaflets	Bovine pericardium	Porcine pericardium	Bovine pericardium	Bovine pericardium	Bovine pericardium
Skirt	Polyethylene terephalate	Porcine pericardium	Polyester	Polyurethane	Porcine pericardium
Delivery catheter	18F/19F	18F	18F	18F/20F	18F
R^3	No	Partially	Yes	Yes	Yes
	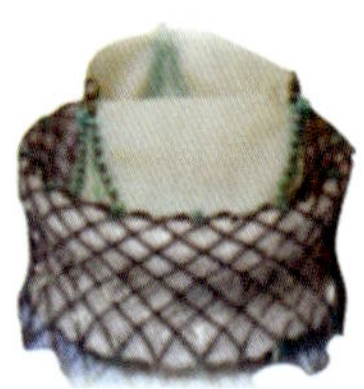	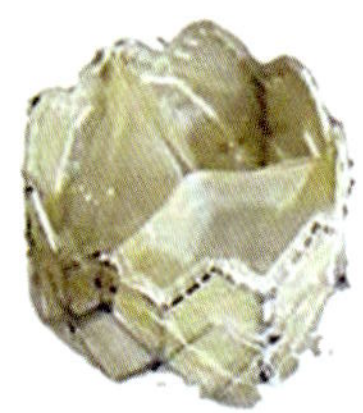	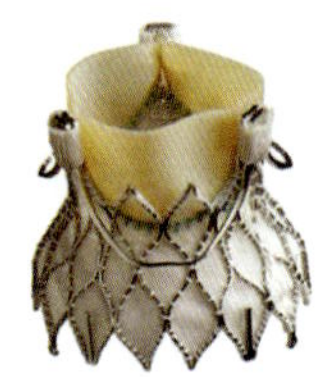	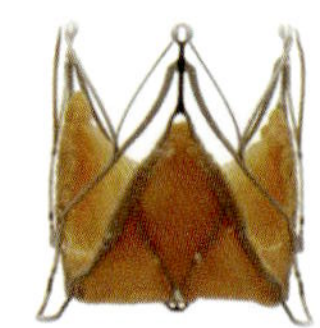	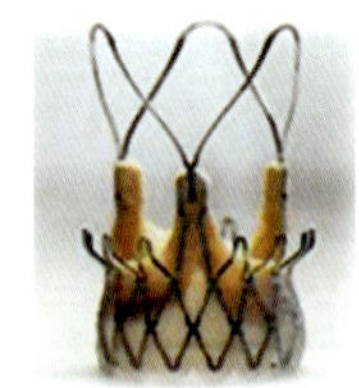
Manufacturer	Heart Leaflet Technology	Colibri Heart Valve	Medtronic Engager	Jena Valve Technology	Symetis Acurate System
Access	TF	TF	TA	TA	TA
Deployment	Self-expandable	Balloon-expandable	Self-expandable	Self-expandable	Self-expandable
Support structure	Nitinol	Stainless steel	Nitinol	Nitinol	Nitinol
Leaflets	Porcine pericardium	Porcine pericardium	Bovine pericardium	Porcine aortic root	?
Skirt	Braided polyester	Porcine pericardium	Polyester	Polyurethane	?
Delivery catheter	17F	14F/16F	26F	27F	?
R^3	Yes	No	No	Partially	Yes

Conclusions

Transcatheter aortic valve implantation has developed into a relatively mature, safe, and effective therapy for high or prohibitive surgical risk patients with severe aortic stenosis. Device evolution and increasing operator experience have led to improved clinical outcomes. An ever-growing array of clinical studies has improved our understanding of the etiology of cardiac and non-cardiac complications. Meticulous patient selection, procedural techniques, and post-procedure care will further reduce these serious events. Compared with surgical aortic valve replacement, paravalvular aortic regurgitation, stroke, and conduction abnormalities are more common. A variety of novel transcatheter aortic valves are in development.

Conflict of interest statement

Nicolo Piazza is a consultant and proctor for Medtronic CoreValve.

References

1 Davies H. Catheter mounted valve for temporary relief of aortic insufficiency. Lancet 1965;1:250.
2 Moulopoulos SD, Anthopoulos L, Stamatelopoulos S, et al. Catheter-mounted aortic valves. Ann Thorac Surg 1971;11:423–30.
3 Phillips SJ, Ciborski M, Freed PS, et al. A temporary catheter-tip aortic valve: hemodynamic effects on experimental acute aortic insufficiency. Ann Thorac Surg 1976;21:134–7.
4 Matsubara T, Yamazoe M, Tamura Y, et al. Balloon catheter with check valves for experimental relief of acute aortic regurgitation. Am Heart J 1992;124:1002–8.
5 Cribier A, Savin T, Saoudi N, et al. Percutaneous transluminal valvuloplasty of acquired aortic stenosis in elderly patients: an alternative to valve replacement? Lancet 1986;1:63–7.
6 Drobinski G, Lechat P, Metzger JP, et al. Results of percutaneous catheter valvuloplasty for calcified aortic stenosis in the elderly. Eur Heart J 1987;8:322–8.
7 Serruys PW, Luijten HE, Beatt KJ, et al. Percutaneous balloon valvuloplasty for calcific aortic stenosis. A treatment 'sine cure'? Eur Heart J 1988;9:782–94.
8 Safian RD, Berman AD, Diver DJ, et al. Balloon aortic valvuloplasty in 170 consecutive patients. N Engl J Med 1988;319:125–30.
9 Block PC, Palacios IF. Clinical and hemodynamic follow-up after percutaneous aortic valvuloplasty in the elderly. Am J Cardiol 1988;62:760–3.
10 Berland J, Cribier A, Savin T, et al. Percutaneous balloon valvuloplasty in patients with severe aortic stenosis and low ejection fraction. Immediate results and 1-year follow-up. Circulation 1989;79:1189–96.
11 Letac B, Cribier A, Eltchaninoff H, et al. Evaluation of restenosis after balloon dilatation in adult aortic stenosis by repeat catheterization. Am Heart J 1991;122:55–60.
12 Otto CM, Mickel MC, Kennedy JW, et al. Three-year outcome after balloon aortic valvuloplasty. Insights into prognosis of valvular aortic stenosis. Circulation 1994;89:642–50.
13 Charlson E, Legedza AT, Hamel MB. Decision-making and outcomes in severe symptomatic aortic stenosis. J Heart Valve Dis 2006;15:312–21.
14 Pellikka PA, Sarano ME, Nishimura RA, et al. Outcome of 622 adults with asymptomatic, hemodynamically significant aortic stenosis during prolonged follow-up. Circulation 2005;111:3290–5.
15 Lung B, Cachier A, Baron G, et al. Decision-making in elderly patients with severe aortic stenosis: why are so many denied surgery? Eur Heart J 2005;26:2714–20.
16 Bouma BJ, van Den Brink RB, van Der Meulen JH, et al. To operate or not on elderly patients with aortic stenosis: the decision and its consequences. Heart 1999;82:143–8.
17 Cribier A, Eltchaninoff H, Bash A, et al. Percutaneous transcatheter implantation of aortic valve prosthesis for calcific aortic stenosis: first human case description. Circulation 2002;106:3006–8.
18 Cribier A, Eltchaninoff H, Tron C, et al. Treatment of calcific aortic stenosis with the percutaneous heart valve: mid-term follow-up from the initial feasibility studies: the French experience. J Am Coll Cardiol 2006;47:1214–23.
19 Webb JG, Chandavimol M, Thompson CR, et al. Percutaneous aortic valve implantation retrograde from the femoral artery. Circulation 2006;113:842–50.
20 Hijazi Z, Ruiz C, Bonhoeffer P, et al. Transcatheter Valve Repair, 1st edn. New York: Informa Healthcare, 2006.
21 de Jaegere P, van Dijk L, Laborde JC, et al. True percutaneous implantation of the CoreValve aortic valve prosthesis by the combined use of ultrasound guided vascular access, Prostar XL and the TandemHeart. Eurointervention 2007;2:500–5.
22 O'Brien SM, Shahian DM, Filardo G, et al. The Society of Thoracic Surgeons 2008 cardiac surgery risk models: part 2 – isolated valve surgery. Ann Thorac Surg 2009;88:S23–42.
23 Kuduvalli M, Grayson AD, Au J, et al. A multi-centre additive and logistic risk model for in-hospital mortality following aortic valve replacement. Eur J Cardiothorac Surg 2007;31:607–13.
24 Hannan EL, Wu C, Bennett EV, et al. Risk index for predicting in-hospital mortality for cardiac valve surgery. Ann Thorac Surg 2007;83:921–9.

25 Rankin JS, Hammill BG, Ferguson TB, Jr, et al. Determinants of operative mortality in valvular heart surgery. J Thorac Cardiovasc Surg 2006;131:547–57.
26 Nilsson J, Algotsson L, Hoglund P, et al. Comparison of 19 pre-operative risk stratification models in open-heart surgery. Eur Heart J 2006;27:867–74.
27 Jin R, Grunkemeier GL, Starr A. Validation and refinement of mortality risk models for heart valve surgery. Ann Thorac Surg 2005;80:471–9.
28 Ambler G, Omar RZ, Royston P, et al. Generic, simple risk stratification model for heart valve surgery. Circulation 2005;112:224–31.
29 Nowicki ER, Birkmeyer NJ, Weintraub RW, et al. Multivariable prediction of in-hospital mortality associated with aortic and mitral valve surgery in northern New England. Ann Thorac Surg 2004;77:1966–77.
30 Gardner SC, Grunwald GK, Rumsfeld JS, et al. Comparison of short-term mortality risk factors for valve replacement versus coronary artery bypass graft surgery. Ann Thorac Surg 2004;77:549–56.
31 Florath I, Rosendahl UP, Mortasawi A, et al. Current determinants of operative mortality in 1400 patients requiring aortic valve replacement. Ann Thorac Surg 2003;76:75–83.
32 Edwards FH, Peterson ED, Coombs LP, et al. Prediction of operative mortality after valve replacement surgery. J Am Coll Cardiol 2001;37:885–92.
33 Nashef SA, Roques F, Michel P, et al. European system for cardiac operative risk evaluation (EuroSCORE). Eur J Cardiothorac Surg 1999;16:9–13.
34 Parsonnet V, Dean D, Bernstein AD. A method of uniform stratification of risk for evaluating the results of surgery in acquired adult heart disease. Circulation 1989;79:I3–12.
35 Osswald BR, Gegouskov V, Badowski-Zyla D, et al. Overestimation of aortic valve replacement risk by EuroSCORE: implications for percutaneous valve replacement. Eur Heart J 2009;30:74–80.
36 Leontyev S, Walther T, Borger MA, et al. Aortic valve replacement in octogenarians: utility of risk stratification with EuroSCORE. Ann Thorac Surg 2009;87:1440–5.
37 Dewey TM, Brown D, Ryan WH, et al. Reliability of risk algorithms in predicting early and late operative outcomes in high-risk patients undergoing aortic valve replacement. J Thorac Cardiovasc Surg 2008;135:180–7.
38 Brown ML, Schaff HV, Sarano ME, et al. Is the European System for Cardiac Operative Risk Evaluation model valid for estimating the operative risk of patients considered for percutaneous aortic valve replacement? J Thorac Cardiovasc Surg 2008;136:566–71.
39 Lefevre T, Kappetein AP, Wolner E, et al. One year follow-up of the multi-centre European PARTNER transcatheter heart valve study. Eur Heart J 2011;32:148–57.
40 Buellesfeld L, Gerckens U, Schuler G, et al. 2-year follow-up of patients undergoing transcatheter aortic valve implantation using a self-expanding valve prosthesis. J Am Coll Cardiol 2011;57:1650–7.
41 Piazza N, Wenaweser P, van Gameren M, et al. Relationship between the logistic EuroSCORE and the Society of Thoracic Surgeons Predicted Risk of Mortality score in patients implanted with the CoreValve ReValving system – a Bern-Rotterdam Study. Am Heart J 2010;159:323–9.
42 Delgado V, Ewe SH, Ng AC, et al. Multimodality imaging in transcatheter aortic valve implantation: key steps to assess procedural feasibility. Eurointervention 2010;6: 643–52.
43 Piazza N, de Jaegere P, Manoharan G, et al. Patient selection for the CoreValve ReValving System. In: Serruys P, Piazza N, Cribier A, Webb J, Laborde JC, de Jaegere P (eds) Transcatheter Aortic Valve Implantation: tips and tricks to avoid failure. New York: Informa Healthcare, 2011, p. 82.
44 Nietlispach F, Leipsic J, Al-Bugami S, et al. CT of the iliofemoral arteries using direct aortic contrast injection: proof of feasibility in patients screened towards percutaneous aortic valve replacement. Swiss Med Wkly 2009;139:458–62.
45 Eltchaninoff H, Kerkeni M, Zajarias A, et al. Aorto-iliac angiography as a screening tool in selecting patients for transfemoral aortic valve implantation with the Edwards SAPIEN bioprosthesis. Eurointervention 2009;5:438–42.
46 Hayashida K, Lefevre T, Chevalier B, et al. Transfemoral aortic valve implantation new criteria to predict vascular complications. JACC Cardiovasc Interv 2011;4:851–8.
47 Piazza N, Serruys PW, Lange R. Getting safely in and out of a transcatheter aortic valve implantation procedure vascular complications according to the valvular academic research consortium criteria. JACC Cardiovasc Interv 2011;4:859–60.
48 Piazza N, de Jaegere P, Schultz C, et al. Anatomy of the aortic valvar complex and its implications for transcatheter implantation of the aortic valve. Circ Cardiovasc Intervent 2008;1:74–81.
49 Schultz CJ, Moelker A, Piazza N, et al. Three dimensional evaluation of the aortic annulus using multislice computer tomography: are manufacturer's guidelines for sizing for percutaneous aortic valve replacement helpful? Eur Heart J 2010;31:849–56.
50 Tops LF, Wood DA, Delgado V, et al. Noninvasive evaluation of the aortic root with multislice computed tomography implications for transcatheter aortic valve replacement. JACC Cardiovasc Imaging 2008;1:321–30.
51 Ng AC, Yiu KH, Ewe SH, et al. Influence of left ventricular geometry and function on aortic annular dimensions as assessed with multi-detector row computed

tomography: implications for transcatheter aortic valve implantation. Eur Heart J 2011;32:2806–13.
52 Schultz C, Moelker A, Tzikas A, et al. The use of MSCT for the evaluation of the aortic root before transcutaneous aortic valve implantation: the Rotterdam approach. Eurointervention 2010;6:505–11.
53 Schultz CJ, Moelker AD, Tzikas A, et al. Cardiac CT: necessary for precise sizing for transcatheter aortic implantation. Eurointervention 2010;6(Suppl G):G6–13.
54 Nietlispach F, Wijesinghe N, Wood D, et al. Current balloon-expandable transcatheter heart valve and delivery systems. Catheter Cardiovasc Interv 2010;75:295–300.
55 Rodes-Cabau J, Delarochelliere R, Dumont E. First-in-man transcatheter aortic valve implantation of a 20-mm edwards SAPIEN XT valve: one step forward for the treatment of patients with severe aortic stenosis and small aortic annulus. Catheter Cardiovasc Interv 2012;79:789–93.
56 Chen W, Schoen FJ, Levy RJ. Mechanism of efficacy of 2-amino oleic acid for inhibition of calcification of glutaraldehyde-pretreated porcine bioprosthetic heart valves. Circulation 1994;90:323–9.
57 Vavuranakis M, Vrachatis DA, Toutouzas K, et al. Successful percutaneous aortic valve implantation via a stenotic left subclavian artery access. Heart Vessels 2010;25:359–62.
58 Munoz-Garcia AJ, Alonso-Briales JH, Such-Martinez M, et al. Left subclavian artery approach to CoreValve aortic prosthesis implantation. Rev Esp Cardiol 2010;63:121–2.
59 Ruge H, Lange R, Bleiziffer S, et al. First successful aortic valve implantation with the CoreValve ReValving System via right subclavian artery access: a case report. Heart Surg Forum 2008;11:E323–4.
60 Sarkar K, Ussia GP, Tamburino C. Transcatheter aortic valve implantation for severe aortic regurgitation in a stentless bioprosthetic valve with the core valve revalving system – technical tips and role of the Accutrak system. Catheter Cardiovasc Interv 2011;78:485–90.
61 de Jaegere P, Piazza N, Tzikas A, et al. Implantation of the CoreValve ReValving System. In: Serruys P, Piazza N, Cribier A, Webb J, Laborde J, de Jaegere P (eds) Transcatheter Aortic Valve : tips and tricks to avoid failure, 1st edn. New York: Informa Healthcare, 2011, pp. 183–97.
62 Nietlispach F, Webb J. Implantation of the Edwards SAPIEN valve. In: Serruys P, Piazza N, Cribier A, Webb J, Laborde J, de Jaegere P (eds) Transcatheter Aortic Valve Implantation, 1st edn. New York: Informa Healthcare, 2011, pp. 198–206.
63 Hutchinson N. Sedation vs general anaesthesia for the 'high-risk' patient – what can TAVI teach us? Anaesthesia 2011;66:965–8.
64 Motloch LJ, Rottlaender D, Reda S, et al. Local versus general anesthesia for transfemoral aortic valve implantation. Clin Res Cardiol 2012;101:45–53.
65 Dehedin B, Guinot PG, Ibrahim H, et al. Anesthesia and perioperative management of patients who undergo transfemoral transcatheter aortic valve implantation: an observational study of general versus local/regional anesthesia in 125 consecutive patients. J Cardiothorac Vasc Anesth 2011;25:1036–43.
66 Covello RD, Landoni G, Zangrillo A. Anesthetic management of transcatheter aortic valve implantation. Curr Opin Anaesthesiol 2011;24:417–25.
67 Guinot PG, Depoix JP, Tini L, et al. [Transcutaneous aortic valve implantation: anesthetic and perioperative management]. Ann Fr Anesth Reanim 2011;30:734–42.
68 Vavuranakis M, Voudris V, Vrachatis DA, et al. Transcatheter aortic valve implantation, patient selection process and procedure: two centres' experience of the intervention without general anaesthesia. Hellenic J Cardiol 2010;51:492–500.
69 Guinot PG, Depoix JP, Etchegoyen L, et al. Anesthesia and perioperative management of patients undergoing transcatheter aortic valve implantation: analysis of 90 consecutive patients with focus on perioperative complications. J Cardiothorac Vasc Anesth 2010;24:752–61.
70 Covello RD, Ruggeri L, Landoni G, et al. Transcatheter implantation of an aortic valve: anesthesiological management. Minerva Anestesiol 2010;76:100–8.
71 Behan M, Haworth P, Hutchinson N, et al. Percutaneous aortic valve implants under sedation: our initial experience. Catheter Cardiovasc Interv 2008;72:1012–15.
72 Bergmann L, Kahlert P, Eggebrecht H, et al. Transfemoral aortic valve implantation under sedation and monitored anaesthetic care – a feasibility study. Anaesthesia 2011;66:977–82.
73 Fassl J, Walther T, Groesdonk HV, et al. Anesthesia management for transapical transcatheter aortic valve implantation: a case series. J Cardiothorac Vasc Anesth 2009;23:286–91.
74 Wood DA, Tops LF, Mayo JR, et al. Role of multislice computed tomography in transcatheter aortic valve replacement. Am J Cardiol 2009;103:1295–301.
75 Tzikas A, Schultz C, Van Mieghem NM, et al. Optimal projection estimation for transcatheter aortic valve implantation based on contrast-aortography: validation of a Prototype Software. Catheter Cardiovasc Interv 2010;76:602–7.
76 Dvir D, Kornowski R. Percutaneous aortic valve implantation using novel imaging guidance. Catheter Cardiovasc Interv 2010;76:450–4.
77 Kurra V, Kapadia SR, Tuzcu EM, et al. Pre-procedural imaging of aortic root orientation and dimensions: comparison between X-ray angiographic planar

imaging and 3-dimensional multidetector row computed tomography. JACC Cardiovasc Interv 2010;3:105–13.
78 Cockburn J, de Belder A, Brooks M, et al. Large calibre arterial access device closure for percutaneous aortic valve interventions: use of the prostar system in 118 cases. Catheter Cardiovasc Interv 2012;79:143–9.
79 Sharp AS, Michev I, Maisano F, et al. A new technique for vascular access management in transcatheter aortic valve implantation. Catheter Cardiovasc Interv 2010; 75:784–93.
80 Nuis RJ, Piazza N, Van Mieghem NM, et al. In-hospital complications after transcatheter aortic valve implantation revisited according to the valve academic research consortium definitions. Catheter Cardiovasc Interv 2011;78:457–67.
81 Conradi L, Seiffert M, Treede H, et al. Transcatheter aortic valve implantation versus surgical aortic valve replacement: a propensity score analysis in patients at high surgical risk. J Thorac Cardiovasc Surg 2012;143:64–71.
82 Clavel MA, Webb JG, Pibarot P, et al. Comparison of the hemodynamic performance of percutaneous and surgical bioprostheses for the treatment of severe aortic stenosis. J Am Coll Cardiol 2009;53:1883–91.
83 Himbert D, Descoutures F, Al-Attar N, et al. Results of transfemoral or transapical aortic valve implantation following a uniform assessment in high-risk patients with aortic stenosis. J Am Coll Cardiol 2009;54:303–11.
84 Jilaihawi H, Chin D, Spyt T, et al. Prosthesis-patient mismatch after transcatheter aortic valve implantation with the Medtronic-Corevalve bioprosthesis. Eur Heart J 2010;31:857–64.
85 Moss RR, Ivens E, Pasupati S, et al. Role of echocardiography in percutaneous aortic valve implantation. JACC Cardiovasc Imaging 2008;1:15–24.
86 Jabbour A, Ismail TF, Moat N, et al. Multimodality imaging in transcatheter aortic valve implantation and post-procedural aortic regurgitation: comparison among cardiovascular magnetic resonance, cardiac computed tomography, and echocardiography. J Am Coll Cardiol 2011;58:2165–73.
87 Detaint D, Lepage L, Himbert D, et al. Determinants of significant paravalvular regurgitation after transcatheter aortic valve: implantation impact of device and annulus discongruence. JACC Cardiovasc Interv 2009;2:821–7.
88 Moat NE, Ludman P, de Belder MA, et al. Long-term outcomes after transcatheter aortic valve implantation in high-risk patients with severe aortic stenosis: the U.K. TAVI (United Kingdom Transcatheter Aortic Valve Implantation) Registry. J Am Coll Cardiol 2011;58:2130–8.
89 Schultz C, Rossi A, van Mieghem N, et al. Aortic annulus dimensions and leaflet calcification from contrast MSCT predict the need for balloon post-dilatation after TAVI with the Medtronic CoreValve prosthesis. Eurointervention 2011;7:564–72.
90 Ong SH, Mueller R, Gerckens U. Sequential CoreValve implantation for a mal-positioned prosthesis during transcatheter aortic valve implantation. Catheter Cardiovasc Interv 2011;77:1071–5.
91 Zahn R, Schiele R, Kilkowski C, et al. Correction of aortic regurgitation after transcatheter aortic valve implantation of the Medtronic CoreValveTM prosthesis due to a too-low implantation, using transcatheter repositioning. J Heart Valve Dis 2011;20:64–9.
92 Litzler PY, Cribier A, Zajarias A, et al. Surgical aortic valve replacement after percutaneous aortic valve implantation: what have we learned? J Thorac Cardiovasc Surg 2008;136:697–701.
93 Al-Attar N, Ghodbane W, Himbert D, et al. Unexpected complications of transapical aortic valve implantation. Ann Thorac Surg 2009;88:90–4.
94 Takagi K, Latib A, Al-Lamee R, et al. Predictors of moderate-to-severe paravalvular aortic regurgitation immediately after CoreValve implantation and the impact of postdilatation. Catheter Cardiovasc Interv 2011;78:432–43.
95 Al-Attar N, Himbert D, Vahanian A, et al. Severe intraprosthetic regurgitation by immobile leaflet after transcatheter aortic valve implantation. Eur J Cardiothorac Surg 2011;39:591–2.
96 Zahn R, Schiele R, Kilkowski C, et al. Severe aortic regurgitation after percutaneous transcatheter aortic valve implantation: on the importance to clarify the underlying pathophysiology. Clin Res Cardiol 2010; 99:193–7.
97 Miranda-Balbuena N, Araji OA, Gutierrez-Martin MA, et al. Management of aortic valve dysfunction after transapical approach using the technique "valve after valve". Ann Thorac Surg 2011;92:1102–4.
98 Clavel MA, Dumont E, Pibarot P, et al. Severe valvular regurgitation and late prosthesis embolization after percutaneous aortic valve implantation. Ann Thorac Surg 2009;87:618–21.
99 Baumbach H, Hill S, Hansen M, et al. Severe aortic insufficiency after transapical aortic valve implantation. Ann Thorac Surg 2011;92:728–9.
100 Pagnotta P, Ferrante G, Presbitero P. Rescue "valve in valve" implantation after late onset corevalve cusp rupture leading to acute massive aortic insufficiency. Catheter Cardiovasc Interv 2012;in press.
101 Leon MB, Piazza N, Nikolsky E, et al. Standardized endpoint definitions for transcatheter aortic valve implantation clinical trials: a consensus report from the Valve Academic Research Consortium. Eur Heart J 2011;32:205–17.
102 Leon MB, Piazza N, Nikolsky E, et al. Standardized endpoint definitions for Transcatheter Aortic Valve

Implantation clinical trials: a consensus report from the Valve Academic Research Consortium. J Am Coll Cardiol 2011;57:253–69.

103 Igawa O, Adachi M, Yano A, et al. Anatomical information for catheter ablation concerning the relationship between the aortic non-coronary cusp and the His-bundle. Circ J 2009;257:73.

104 Aktug O, Dohmen G, Brehmer K, et al. Incidence and predictors of left bundle branch block after transcatheter aortic valve implantation. Int J Cardiol 2011;160:26–30.

105 Baan J, Jr, Yong ZY, Koch KT, et al. Factors associated with cardiac conduction disorders and permanent pacemaker implantation after percutaneous aortic valve implantation with the CoreValve prosthesis. Am Heart J 2010;159:497–503.

106 Bleiziffer S, Ruge H, Horer J, et al. Predictors for new-onset complete heart block after transcatheter aortic valve implantation. JACC Cardiovasc Interv 2010;3:524–30.

107 Calvi V, Puzzangara E, Pruiti GP, et al. Early conduction disorders following percutaneous aortic valve replacement. Pacing Clin Electrophysiol 2009;32(Suppl 1):S126–30.

108 Erkapic D, Kim WK, Weber M, et al. Electrocardiographic and further predictors for permanent pacemaker requirement after transcatheter aortic valve implantation. Europace 2010;12:1188–90.

109 Ferreira ND, Caeiro D, Adao L, et al. Incidence and predictors of permanent pacemaker requirement after transcatheter aortic valve implantation with a self-expanding bioprosthesis. Pacing Clin Electrophysiol 2010;33:1364–72.

110 Fraccaro C, Buja G, Tarantini G, et al. Incidence, predictors, and outcome of conduction disorders after transcatheter self-expandable aortic valve implantation. Am J Cardiol 2011;107:747–54.

111 Guetta V, Goldenberg G, Segev A, et al. Predictors and course of high-degree atrioventricular block after transcatheter aortic valve implantation using the CoreValve Revalving system. Am J Cardiol 2011;108:1600–5.

112 Haworth P, Behan M, Khawaja M, et al. Predictors for permanent pacing after transcatheter aortic valve implantation. Catheter Cardiovasc Interv 2010;76:751–6.

113 Khawaja MZ, Rajani R, Cook A, et al. Permanent pacemaker insertion after CoreValve transcatheter aortic valve implantation: incidence and contributing factors (the UK CoreValve Collaborative). Circulation 2011;123:951–60.

114 Koos R, Mahnken AH, Aktug O, et al. Electrocardiographic and imaging predictors for permanent pacemaker requirement after transcatheter aortic valve implantation. J Heart Valve Dis 2011;20:83–90.

115 Latsios G, Gerckens U, Buellesfeld L, et al. "Device landing zone" calcification, assessed by MSCT, as a predictive factor for pacemaker implantation after TAVI. Catheter Cardiovasc Interv 2010;76:431–9.

116 Nuis RJ, Van Mieghem NM, Schultz CJ, et al. Timing and potential mechanisms of new conduction abnormalities during the implantation of the Medtronic CoreValve System in patients with aortic stenosis. Eur Heart J 2011;32:2067–74.

117 Piazza N, Nuis RJ, Tzikas A, et al. Persistent conduction abnormalities and requirements for pacemaking six months after transcatheter aortic valve implantation. Eurointervention 2010;6:475–84.

118 Piazza N, Onuma Y, Jesserun E, et al. Early and persistent intraventricular conduction abnormalities and requirements for pacemaking after after percutaneous replacement of the aortic valve. J Am Coll Cardiol Interv 2008;1:310–16.

119 Roten L, Wenaweser P, Delacretaz E, et al. Incidence and predictors of atrioventricular conduction impairment after transcatheter aortic valve implantation. Am J Cardiol 2010;106:1473–80.

120 Rubin JM, Avanzas P, del Valle R, et al. Atrioventricular conduction disturbance characterization in transcatheter aortic valve implantation with the CoreValve prosthesis. Circ Cardiovasc Interv 2011;4:280–6.

121 Jilaihawi H, Chin D, Vasa-Nicotera M, et al. Predictors for permanent pacemaker requirement after transcatheter aortic valve implantation with the CoreValve bioprosthesis. Am Heart J 2009;157:860–6.

122 Godin M, Eltchaninoff H, Furuta A, et al. Frequency of conduction disturbances after transcatheter implantation of an Edwards Sapien aortic valve prosthesis. Am J Cardiol 2010;106:707–12.

123 Gutierrez M, Rodes-Cabau J, Bagur R, et al. Electrocardiographic changes and clinical outcomes after transapical aortic valve implantation. Am Heart J 2009;158:302–8.

124 Sinhal A, Altwegg A, Pasupati S, et al. Atrioventricular block after transcatheter balloon expandable aortic valve implantation J Am Coll Cardiol Interv 2008;1: 305–309.

125 Koektuerk B, Schaefer U, Bergmann M, et al. Acquired conduction disturbances after percutaneous aortic valve replacement. Circulation 2009;120:S307.

126 Saia F, Lemos PA, Bordoni B, et al. Transcatheter aortic valve implantation with a self-expanding nitinol bioprosthesis: prediction of the need for permanent pacemaker using simple baseline and procedural characteristics. Catheter Cardiovasc Interv 2011;79:712–19.

127 Epstein AE, DiMarco JP, Ellenbogen KA, et al. ACC/AHA/HRS 2008 guidelines for device-based therapy of cardiac rhythm abnormalities: a report of the American

College of Cardiology/American Heart Association Task Force on Practice Guidelines (Writing Committee to Revise the ACC/AHA/NASPE 2002 Guideline Update for Implantation of Cardiac Pacemakers and Antiarrhythmia Devices) developed in collaboration with the American Association for Thoracic Surgery and Society of Thoracic Surgeons. J Am Coll Cardiol 2008;51:e1–62.

128 Vardas PE, Auricchio A, Blanc JJ, et al. Guidelines for cardiac pacing and cardiac resynchronization therapy. The Task Force for Cardiac Pacing and Cardiac Resynchronization Therapy of the European Society of Cardiology. Developed in collaboration with the European Heart Rhythm Association. Europace 2007;9:959–98.

129 Motloch LJ, Reda S, Rottlaender D, et al. Postprocedural atrial fibrillation after transcatheter aortic valve implantation versus surgical aortic valve replacement. Ann Thorac Surg 2012;93(1):124–31.

130 Amat-Santos IJ, Rodes-Cabau J, Urena M, et al. Incidence, predictive factors, and prognostic value of new-onset atrial fibrillation following transcatheter aortic valve implantation. J Am Coll Cardiol 2012;59(2):178–88.

131 Piazza N, Grube E, Gerckens U, et al. Procedural and 30-day outcomes following transcatheter aortic valve implantation using the third generation (18 F) CoreValve ReValving System – results from the Multicenter, Expanded Evaluation Registry 1-year following CE mark approval. Eurointervention 2008;4:242–9.

132 Fiorina C, Curello S, Maffeo D, et al. Management of acute left main obstruction after transcatheter aortic valve replacement: the "tunnel technique." Cardiovasc Revasc Med 2012;13(2):142 e5–9.

133 Gurvitch R, Cheung A, Bedogni F, et al. Coronary obstruction following transcatheter aortic valve-in-valve implantation for failed surgical bioprostheses. Catheter Cardiovasc Interv 2011;77:439–44.

134 Kapadia SR, Svensson L, Tuzcu EM. Successful percutaneous management of left main trunk occlusion during percutaneous aortic valve replacement. Catheter Cardiovasc Interv 2009;73:966–72.

135 Kukucka M, Pasic M, Dreysse S, et al. Delayed subtotal coronary obstruction after transapical aortic valve implantation. Interact Cardiovasc Thorac Surg 2011;12:57–60.

136 Webb JG. Coronary obstruction due to transcatheter valve implantation. Catheter Cardiovasc Interv 2009; 73:973.

137 Gogas BD, Zacharoulis AA, Antoniadis AG. Acute coronary occlusion following TAVI. Catheter Cardiovasc Interv 2011;77:435–8.

138 Saia F, Marrozzini C, Marzocchi A. Displacement of calcium nodules of the native valve as a possible cause of left main occlusion following transcatheter aortic valve implantation. J Invasive Cardiol 2011;23:E106–9.

139 Gerckens U, Latsios G, Mueller R, et al. Left main PCI after trans-subclavian CoreValve implantation. Successful outcome of a combined procedure for management of a rare complication. Clin Res Cardiol 2009;98:687–90.

140 Bagur R, Dumont E, Doyle D, et al. Coronary ostia stenosis after transcatheter aortic valve implantation. JACC Cardiovasc Interv 2010;3:253–5.

141 Bartorelli AL, Andreini D, Sisillo E, et al. Left main coronary artery occlusion after percutaneous aortic valve implantation. Ann Thorac Surg 2010;89:953–5.

142 Stabile E, Sorropago G, Cioppa A, et al. Acute left main obstructions following TAVI. Eurointervention 2010;6:100–5.

143 Lange R, Bleiziffer S, Piazza N, et al. Incidence and treatment of procedural cardiovascular complications associated with trans-arterial and trans-apical interventional aortic valve implantation in 412 consecutive patients. Eur J Cardiothorac Surg 2011;40:1105–13.

144 Webb JG, Pasupati S, Humphries K, et al. Percutaneous transarterial aortic valve replacement in selected high-risk patients with aortic stenosis. Circulation 2007; 116:755–63.

145 Ong SH, Mueller R, Iversen S. Early calcific degeneration of a CoreValve transcatheter aortic bioprosthesis. Eur Heart J 2012;33(5):586.

146 Hammerstingl C, Nickenig G, Grube E. Treatment of a degenerative stenosed CoreValve(®) aortic bioprosthesis by transcatheter valve-in-valve insertion. Catheter Cardiovasc Interv 2012;79(5):748–55.

147 Virmani R, Bonan R, Nakazawa G, et al. Accumulation of worldwide experience with postmortem studies of transcatheter aortic valve implantation – what should we be avoiding? In: Serruys P, Piazza N, Cribier A, Webb J, Laborde J (eds) Transcatheter Aortic Valve Implantation: tips and tricks to avoid failure. New York: Informa Healthcare, 2011, pp. 18–39.

148 Tay EL, Gurvitch R, Wijeysinghe N, et al. Valve thrombosis after transcatheter heart valve implantation. Eurointervention 2011;7:170–1.

149 Kefer J, Astarci P, Renkin J, et al. Images and case reports in interventional cardiology. Thrombotic aortic restenosis after transapical Sapien valve implantation. Circ Cardiovasc Interv 2010;3:289–92.

150 Trepels T, Martens S, Doss M, et al. Images in cardiovascular medicine. Thrombotic restenosis after minimally invasive implantation of aortic valve stent. Circulation 2009;120:e23–4.

151 Smith CR, Leon MB, Mack MJ, et al. Transcatheter versus surgical aortic-valve replacement in high-risk patients. N Engl J Med 2011;364:2187–98.

152 Ussia GP, Scarabelli M, Mule M, et al. Dual antiplatelet therapy versus aspirin alone in patients undergoing transcatheter aortic valve implantation. Am J Cardiol 2011;108:1772–6.
153 Head SJ, Dewey TM, Mack MJ. Fungal endocarditis after transfemoral aortic valve implantation. Catheter Cardiovasc Interv 2011;78:1017–19.
154 Carnero-Alcazar M, Maroto Castellanos LC, Carnicer JC, et al. Transapical aortic valve prosthetic endocarditis. Interact Cardiovasc Thorac Surg 2010;11:252–3.
155 Gotzmann M, Mugge A. Fatal prosthetic valve endocarditis of the CoreValve ReValving System. Clin Res Cardiol 2011;100:715–17.
156 Santos M, Thiene G, Sievers HH, et al. Candida endocarditis complicating transapical aortic valve implantation. Eur Heart J 2011;32:2265.
157 Comoglio C, Boffini M, El Qarra S, et al. Aortic valve replacement and mitral valve repair as treatment of complications after percutaneous core valve implantation. J Thorac Cardiovasc Surg 2009;138:1025–7.
158 Wong DR, Boone RH, Thompson CR, et al. Mitral valve injury late after transcatheter aortic valve implantation. J Thorac Cardiovasc Surg 2009;137:1547–9.
159 Rafiq I, Parthasarathy H, Tremlett C, et al. Infective endocarditis caused by Moraxella nonliquefaciens in a percutaneous aortic valve replacement. Cardiovasc Revasc Med 2011;12:184–6.
160 Tzikas A, Piazza N, van Dalen BM, et al. Changes in mitral regurgitation after transcatheter aortic valve implantation. Catheter Cardiovasc Interv 2010; 75:43–9.
161 De Chiara B, Moreo A, De Marco F, et al. Influence of CoreValve ReValving System implantation on mitral valve function: an echocardiographic study in selected patients. Catheter Cardiovasc Interv 2011;78:638–44.
162 Durst R, Avelar E, McCarty D, et al. Outcome and improvement predictors of mitral regurgitation after transcatheter aortic valve implantation. J Heart Valve Dis 2011;20:272–81.
163 Hekimian G, Detaint D, Messika-Zeitoun D, et al. Mitral regurgitation in patients referred for transcatheter aortic valve implantation using the Edwards Sapien prosthesis: mechanisms and early postprocedural changes. J Am Soc Echocardiogr 2012;25(2):160–5.
164 Webb JG, Altwegg L, Boone RH, et al. Transcatheter aortic valve implantation: impact on clinical and valve-related outcomes. Circulation 2009;119:3009–16.
165 Rodes-Cabau J, Webb JG, Cheung A, et al. Transcatheter aortic valve implantation for the treatment of severe symptomatic aortic stenosis in patients at very high or prohibitive surgical risk: acute and late outcomes of the multicenter Canadian experience. J Am Coll Cardiol 2010;55:1080–90.
166 Thomas M, Schymik G, Walther T, et al. One-year outcomes of cohort 1 in the Edwards SAPIEN Aortic Bioprosthesis European Outcome (SOURCE) registry: the European registry of transcatheter aortic valve implantation using the Edwards SAPIEN valve. Circulation 2011;124:425–33.
167 Leon MB, Smith CR, Mack M, et al. Transcatheter aortic-valve implantation for aortic stenosis in patients who cannot undergo surgery. N Engl J Med 2010;363:1597–607.
168 Tay EL, Gurvitch R, Wijesinghe N, et al. A high-risk period for cerebrovascular events exists after transcatheter aortic valve implantation. JACC Cardiovasc Interv 2011;4:1290–7.
169 Astarci P, Glineur D, Kefer J, et al. Magnetic resonance imaging evaluation of cerebral embolization during percutaneous aortic valve implantation: comparison of transfemoral and trans-apical approaches using Edwards Sapiens valve. Eur J Cardiothorac Surg 2011;40:475–9.
170 Kahlert P, Knipp SC, Schlamann M, et al. Silent and apparent cerebral ischemia after percutaneous transfemoral aortic valve implantation: a diffusion-weighted magnetic resonance imaging study. Circulation 2010; 121:870–8.
171 Ghanem A, Muller A, Nahle CP, et al. Risk and fate of cerebral embolism after transfemoral aortic valve implantation: a prospective pilot study with diffusion-weighted magnetic resonance imaging. J Am Coll Cardiol 2010;55:1427–32.
172 Rodes-Cabau J, Dumont E, Boone RH, et al. Cerebral embolism following transcatheter aortic valve implantation: comparison of transfemoral and transapical approaches. J Am Coll Cardiol 2011;57:18–28.
173 Arnold M, Schulz-Heise S, Achenbach S, et al. Embolic cerebral insults after transapical aortic valve implantation detected by magnetic resonance imaging. JACC Cardiovasc Interv 2010;3:1126–32.
174 Fairbairn TA, Mather AN, Bijsterveld P, et al. Diffusion-weighted MRI determined cerebral embolic infarction following transcatheter aortic valve implantation: assessment of predictive risk factors and the relationship to subsequent health status. Heart 2012; 98(1):18–23.
175 Drewș T, Pasic M, Buz S, et al. Transcranial Doppler sound detection of cerebral microembolism during transapical aortic valve implantation. Thorac Cardiovasc Surg 2011;59:237–42.
176 Etienne PY, Papadatos S, Pieters D, et al. Embol-x intraaortic filter and transaortic approach for improved cerebral protection in transcatheter aortic valve implantation. Ann Thorac Surg 2011;92:e95–6.
177 Nietlispach F, Wijesinghe N, Gurvitch R, et al. An embolic deflection device for aortic valve interventions. JACC Cardiovasc Interv 2010;3:1133–8.

178 Macdonald S. New embolic protection devices: a review. J Cardiovasc Surg (Torino) 2011;52:821–7.

179 Tchetche D, Dumonteil N, Sauguet A, et al. Thirty-day outcome and vascular complications after transarterial aortic valve implantation using both Edwards Sapien and Medtronic CoreValve bioprostheses in a mixed population. Eurointervention 2010;5:659–65.

180 Van Mieghem NM, Nuis RJ, Piazza N, et al. Vascular complications with transcatheter aortic valve implantation using the 18 Fr Medtronic CoreValve System: the Rotterdam experience. Eurointervention 2010;5:673–9.

181 Ducrocq G, Francis F, Serfaty JM, et al. Vascular complications of transfemoral aortic valve implantation with the Edwards SAPIEN prosthesis: incidence and impact on outcome. Eurointervention 2010;5:666–72.

182 Kahlert P, Al-Rashid F, Weber M, et al. Vascular access site complications after percutaneous transfemoral aortic valve implantation. Herz 2009;34:398–408.

183 Elhmidi Y, Bleiziffer S, Piazza N, et al. Incidence and predictors of acute kidney injury in patients undergoing transcatheter aortic valve implantation. Am Heart J 2011;161:735–9.

184 Bagur R, Webb JG, Nietlispach F, et al. Acute kidney injury following transcatheter aortic valve implantation: predictive factors, prognostic value, and comparison with surgical aortic valve replacement. Eur Heart J 2010;31:865–74.

185 Nuis RJ, Van Mieghem NM, Tzikas A, et al. Frequency, determinants, and prognostic effects of acute kidney injury and red blood cell transfusion in patients undergoing transcatheter aortic valve implantation. Catheter Cardiovasc Interv 2011;77:881–9.

186 Sinning JM, Ghanem A, Steinhauser H, et al. Renal function as predictor of mortality in patients after percutaneous transcatheter aortic valve implantation. JACC Cardiovasc Interv 2010;3:1141–9.

187 Aregger F, Wenaweser P, Hellige GJ, et al. Risk of acute kidney injury in patients with severe aortic valve stenosis undergoing transcatheter valve replacement. Nephrol Dial Transplant 2009;24:2175–9.

188 Tamburino C, Capodanno D, Ramondo A, et al. Incidence and predictors of early and late mortality after transcatheter aortic valve implantation in 663 patients with severe aortic stenosis. Circulation 2011;123:299–308.

189 Piazza N, Cutlip DE, Onuma Y, et al. Clinical endpoints in transcatheter aortic valve implantation: a call to ARC for standardised definitions. Eurointervention 2009;5:29–31.

190 Kempfert J, Rastan A, Holzhey D, et al. Transapical aortic valve implantation: analysis of risk factors and learning experience in 299 patients. Circulation 2011; 124:S124–9.

191 D'Onofrio A, Rubino P, Fusari M, et al. Clinical and hemodynamic outcomes of "all-comers" undergoing transapical aortic valve implantation: results from the Italian Registry of Trans-Apical Aortic Valve Implantation (I-TA). J Thorac Cardiovasc Surg 2011;142:768–75.

192 Bosmans JM, Kefer J, De Bruyne B, et al. Procedural, 30-day and one year outcome following CoreValve or Edwards transcatheter aortic valve implantation: results of the Belgian national registry. Interact Cardiovasc Thorac Surg 2011;12:762–7.

193 Eltchaninoff H, Prat A, Gilard M, et al. Transcatheter aortic valve implantation: early results of the FRANCE (FRench Aortic National CoreValve and Edwards) registry. Eur Heart J 2011;32:191–7.

194 Grube E, Buellesfeld L, Mueller R, et al. Progress and current status of percutaneous aortic valve replacement: results of three device generations of the CoreValve Revalving System. Circ Cardiovasc Interv 2008; 1:167–75.

195 Gurvitch R, Tay EL, Wijesinghe N, et al. Transcatheter aortic valve implantation: lessons from the learning curve of the first 270 high-risk patients. Catheter Cardiovasc Interv 2011;78:977–84.

196 Gurvitch R, Wood DA, Tay EL, et al. Transcatheter aortic valve implantation: durability of clinical and hemodynamic outcomes beyond 3 years in a large patient cohort. Circulation 2010;122:1319–27.

197 Thomas M, Schymik G, Walther T, et al. Thirty-day results of the SAPIEN aortic Bioprosthesis European Outcome (SOURCE) Registry: a European registry of transcatheter aortic valve implantation using the Edwards SAPIEN valve. Circulation 2010;122:62–9.

198 Walther T, Kempfert J, Rastan A, et al. Transapical aortic valve implantation at 3 years. J Thorac Cardiovasc Surg 2012;143(2):326–31.

199 Wenaweser P, Pilgrim T, Roth N, et al. Clinical outcome and predictors for adverse events after transcatheter aortic valve implantation with the use of different devices and access routes. Am Heart J 2011;161:1114–24.

200 Zahn R, Gerckens U, Grube E, et al. Transcatheter aortic valve implantation: first results from a multi-centre real-world registry. Eur Heart J 2011;32:198–204.

201 Makkar RR. Two-Year Outcomes of Transcatheter Aortic Valve Replacement (TAVR) in "Inoperable" Patients With Severe Aortic Stenosis: The PARTNER Trial. San Francisco: Transcatheter Cardiovascular Therapeutics (TCT), 2011.

202 Reynolds MR, Magnuson EA, Lei Y, et al. Health-related quality of life after transcatheter aortic valve replacement in inoperable patients with severe aortic stenosis. Circulation 2011;124:1964–72.

203 Reynolds M. Lifetime Cost Effectiveness of Implantatiob Compared with Standard Care in Inoperable Patients: Results from the PARTNER Trial (Cohort B). New Orleans: American Heart Association, 2011.

204 Cohen D. Health-Related Quality of Life After Transcatheter vs. Surgical Aortic Valve Replacement in High-Risk Patients with Severe Aortic Stenosis – Results from the PARTNER Trial (Cohort A). San Francisco: Transcatheter Cardiovascular Therapeutics (TCT), 2011.

205 Jamieson WR, Burr LH, Miyagishima RT, et al. Re-operation for bioprosthetic aortic structural failure – risk assessment. Eur J Cardiothorac Surg 2003;24:873–8.

206 Vogt PR, Brunner-LaRocca H, Sidler P, et al. Reoperative surgery for degenerated aortic bioprostheses: predictors for emergency surgery and reoperative mortality. Eur J Cardiothorac Surg 2000;17:134–9.

207 Christiansen S, Schmid M, Autschbach R. Perioperative risk of redo aortic valve replacement. Ann Thorac Cardiovasc Surg 2009;15:105–10.

208 Piazza N, Bleiziffer S, Brockmann G, et al. Transcatheter aortic valve implantation for failing surgical aortic bioprosthetic valve: from concept to clinical application and evaluation (part 2). JACC Cardiovasc Interv 2011;4:733–42.

209 Kochman J, Huczek Z, Koltowski L, et al. Transcatheter implantation of an aortic valve prosthesis in a female patient with severe bicuspid aortic stenosis. Eur Heart J 2012;33(1):112.

210 Wijesinghe N, Ye J, Rodes-Cabau J, et al. Transcatheter aortic valve implantation in patients with bicuspid aortic valve stenosis. JACC Cardiovasc Interv 2010;3: 1122–5.

211 Ferrari E, Locca D, Sulzer C, et al. Successful transapical aortic valve implantation in a congenital bicuspid aortic valve. Ann Thorac Surg 2010;90:630–2.

212 Chiam PT, Chao VT, Tan SY, et al. Percutaneous transcatheter heart valve implantation in a bicuspid aortic valve. JACC Cardiovasc Interv 2010;3:559–61.

213 Unsworth B, Malik I, Mikhail GW. Recognising bicuspid aortic stenosis in patients referred for transcatheter aortic valve implantation: routine screening with three-dimensional transoesophageal echocardiography. Heart 2010;96:645.

214 Delgado V, Tops LF, Schuijf JD, et al. Successful deployment of a transcatheter aortic valve in bicuspid aortic stenosis: role of imaging with multislice computed tomography. Circ Cardiovasc Imaging 2009;2:e12–3.

215 Jilaihawi H, Asgar A, Bonan R. Good outcome and valve function despite Medtronic-corevalve underexpansion. Catheter Cardiovasc Interv 2010;76:1022–5.

216 Raja Y, Holloway B, Doshi SN. Symmetrical expansion of an Edwards Sapien valve in a congenitally bicuspid aortic valve. Heart 2011;97:1113.

217 Lange R, Bleiziffer S, Mazzitelli D, et al. Improvements in transcatheter aortic valve implantation outcomes in lower surgical risk patients: a glimpse into the future. J Am Coll Cardiol 2012;59:280–7.

218 Lange R, Bleiziffer S, Mazzitelli D, et al. Improvements in transcatheter aortic valve implantation outcomes in lower surgical risk patients a glimpse into the future. J Am Coll Cardiol 2011;157(5):860–6.

15

CHAPTER 15

Transapical valve technology for aortic stenosis

Jurg Grunenfelder[1], *Theodoros Kofidis*[2], *Andre Plass*[1] *& Volkmar Falk*[1]

[1] Clinic for Cardiovascular Surgery, University Hospital Zurich, Zurich, Switzerland
[2] Department of Cardiac, Thoracic and Vascular Surgery, National University Heart Center, Singapore

Introduction

The development of new technology in valve and stent manufacture has recently led to the introduction of a novel treatment for severe aortic valve stenosis without the need for sternotomy and cardiopulmonary bypass (CPB) [1,2]. Transcatheter aortic valve replacement (TAVR) may potentially offer advantages to patients and healthcare providers, since a much faster discharge from the hospital and return to functional status is being advocated. However, the procedure is quite complex and long-term outcomes are not yet known. In addition, the conditions and environment in which TAVR is carried out are substantially different from surgical aortic valve replacement (AVR). Therefore, a team approach between cardiologist, cardiac surgeon, and cardiac anesthesiologist is essential to implement this new technology safely and successfully into clinical routine. After early experience in animal models, the first human percutaneous transcatheter aortic valve implantation was performed in 2002 by Cribier [3]. Since then, equipment and techniques have evolved rapidly, and to date more than 10,000 transfemoral (TF) implants of the CoreValve prosthesis (Medtronic, Minneapolis, MN) and approximately a similar number of TF and transapical (TA) implants of the Edwards Sapien prosthesis (Edwards Lifesciences, Irvine, CA) have been reported worldwide.

Aortic stenosis

Calcific aortic stenosis is the most common indication for surgical valve replacement in the United States [4]. With the decline of acute rheumatic fever, calcific aortic stenosis has become the most common reason for valvular disease in the Western world. Several epidemiologic studies identified risk factors for aortic valve disease which are similar to those of vascular atherosclerosis, such as hypertension, smoking, elevated cholesterol levels, male gender, as well as renal failure [5,6]. Aortic valve calcification is a complex pathologic process that starts at the base of the aortic cusp, primarily in response to endothelial damage caused by blood flow shear stress, and is followed by inflammatory cell infiltration, lipid and calcium deposition, and activation of osteoblast-like cells [7–9]. Disease progression might be potentially modifiable by anti-inflammatory and lipid-lowering therapy [10,11]. However, if the disease is progressive, calcification usually spreads to the leaflet tips causing thickening, stiffening, and restricted movement of the leaflets. The cardinal symptoms consist of the classic triad including chest pain, shortness of

Endovascular and Hybrid Therapies for Structural Heart and Aortic Disease, First Edition.
Edited by Jacques Kpodonu and Raoul Bonan.

breath, and lightheadedness. Survival of patients with symptomatic aortic stenosis is dismal [12,13] and the treatment of choice is aortic valve replacement [14]. Current indication for AVR is largely based on the development of angina, dyspnea, or syncope [15] and successful AVR results in good long-term prognosis [16,17]. However, management of severe aortic stenosis in the absence of symptoms is challenging. Whereas lack of symptom recognition might potentially carry a high risk of death [18], unselected and premature AVR is associated with the risk of surgery and valve prosthesis complications. The fact that almost every third patient with severe aortic stenosis is asymptomatic [19,20] makes a reliable risk estimation and appropriate AVR indication and timing a common and important clinical challenge.

In the future pre-emptive AVR might emerge as the treatment of choice; however, this will be dependent on the (yet unproven) superiority of the watchful waiting strategy and the advances in prosthetic aortic valve design and percutaneous valve replacement.

Devices available for TAVR

The plurality in manufacture of devices for transapical aortic valve implantation derives from the need to improve upon the limitations of existing concepts. It is also an indication of a rapidly expanding field of interest and practice, as involved physicians ponder expanding the application of TAVR to younger and healthier patients. However, the market is still dominated by the prototype TAVR device and its derivates, the Edwards (formerly Cribier) Sapien valve [21]. The valve is designed for delivery both through the retrograde, transfemoral, as well as antegrade transapical approach [22,23].

Edwards Sapien and Sapien XT transcatheter heart valve system

The pioneering idea that led to the development of the Sapien transcatheter heart valve (THV) was first conceived by French Cardiologist Dr. Alain Cribier of Rouen, France. He employed a team of engineers led by Stanton Rowe and Stanley Rabinovitch to manufacture a balloon-expandable valve and implant it in a patient who would have been too fragile for open heart surgery. Despite good function of the implanted valve, the patient died of vascular complications [3]. The manufacturer PVI (Percutaneous Valve Products) was acquired by Edwards in 2005. A range of evolutionary developments in the valve and introduction systems occurred following systematic clinical implants by Dr. John Webb, who focused on the retrograde, transfemoral approach, and produced the world's biggest series [23–25], and by Dr. Lichtenstein et al. who carried out transapical implantations [26]. Dr. Walther of Leipzig, Germany has reported on a large series of transapically treated high-risk patients with results comparable to those of the percutaneous approach [27,28].

The Edwards Sapien THV (Video 15.1) comprises three pericardial leaflets of bovine origin which are hand-sewn onto a stainless steel frame using polytetrafluoroethylene (PTFE) sutures (Fig. 15.1) [22]. The organic parts of the valve are selected

(a)

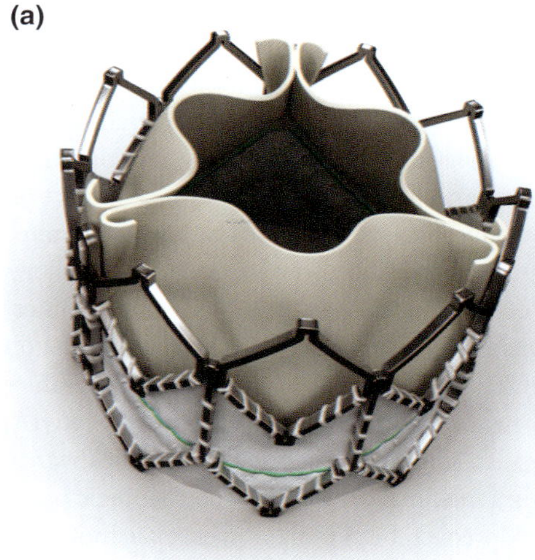

(b)

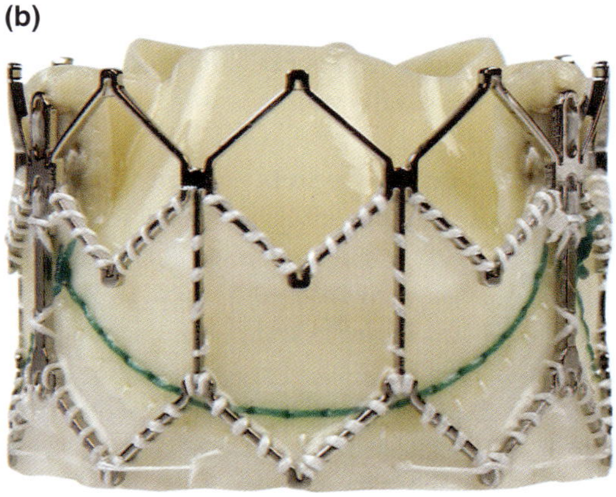

Fig. 15.1 (a, b) Edwards Sapien XT prosthesis.

from special, durable areas of the bovine pericardial sack, fixed with glutaraldehyde and treated with the proprietary Edwards ThermaFix process, which eliminates more than 98% of calcium-binding sites on the tissue surface. The metallic frame undergoes durability testing in compliance with international ISO standards. The waving pattern is designed to retain the expanded state and interlink with the calcification processes of the aortic valve annulus, which are presupposed for positioning stability. The valve exists in two sizes, 23 and 26 mm in diameter [22,29]. Further improvement has generated the Edwards Sapien XT THV, which features a wider waving pattern of a cobalt-chromium compound that mounts leaflets, also made of bovine pericardium. The Edwards XT resulted from extensive engineering and testing steps to enhance the valve design, ease of use, positioning, and patients' demands. Edwards is currently developing a 29 mm valve for use in patients with wider annuli. The CE mark for the Edwards Sapien XT THV was received in March 2010, and the product is now ubiquitously distributed on the market. The cobalt-chromium frame is superior in radial strength and long-term durability, and is supposed to minimize impact on the surrounding aortic tissues. The low profile aims at reducing the risk of coronary obstruction, allowing access for future percutaneous coronary interventions and avoiding disturbance of the conduction system. The 23 and 26 mm Sapien XT THVs feature frame heights of 14.3 and 17.2 mm, respectively. The leaflet shape is also proprietary to Edwards, offering a maximal orifice area and rheologic properties. Moreover, high radial forces are achieved by 3D computer modeling which determines the optimal cobalt-chrome frame shape and pattern to maximize leaflet endurance and resistance to superficial tears and asymmetric workload [30].

Ascendra 2 delivery system

The introduction system has involved in parallel to the THV itself. The new Ascendra 2 delivery sheath size has been reduced by 30%, from 26 to 22 Fr [30]. The Ascendra and Ascendra 2 delivery systems are designed to enhance procedural control through the apex. First, the reduced diameter allows for easier introduction and closure of the apical incision. The antegrade, metered, and short-distance delivery sheath allows for a direct and streamlined access. The Ascendra 2 delivery system employs a new push-button loader for easy de-airing and improved hemostatic control. The prominent novelty though is a new handle design for single-handed valve delivery, as the second hand of the surgeon is released to hold the sheath at the entry through the apex. The components necessary for the introduction of the Sapien XT valve are: the Ascendra 2 delivery system (Fig. 15.2a), the Ascendra 2 introducer sheath set (Fig. 15.2b), the Ascendra balloon aortic valvuloplasty catheter, the Edwards crimper, and the Atrion QL2530 inflation device (Video 15.2).

The Medtronic Engager TAVR System

The Medtronic Engager (formerly Ventor) TAVR system was designed for transapical use. Animal studies have been accomplished, and the device has gone through first-in-man implantation successfully by Falk et al. in Leipzig, Germany [31]. It is currently undergoing clinical trials [32]. The system is manufactured by Medtronic Ventor Technologies Ltd in Netanya, Israel, while the delivery system is manufactured by Medtronic Ireland. It comprises of an aortic valve bioprosthesis and a delivery system (Fig. 15.3) [32]. The valve leaflets are harvested from bovine pericardium sewn on polyester and expanded PTFE. The frame consists of nitinol, which is compressed and

(a)

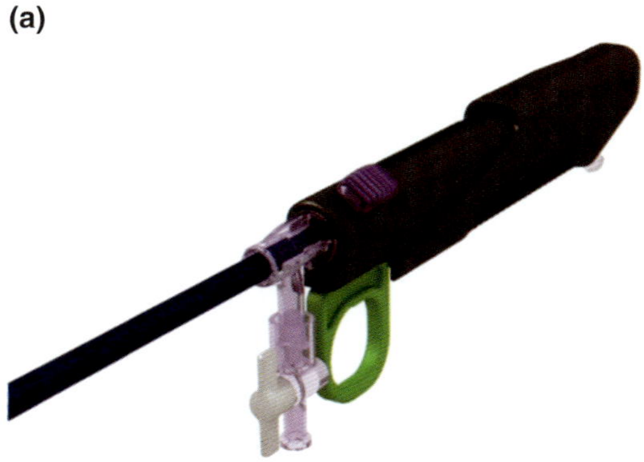

(b)

Fig. 15.2 **(a)** Edwards Ascendra 2 delivery system. **(b)** Edwards Ascendra 2 introducer sheath.

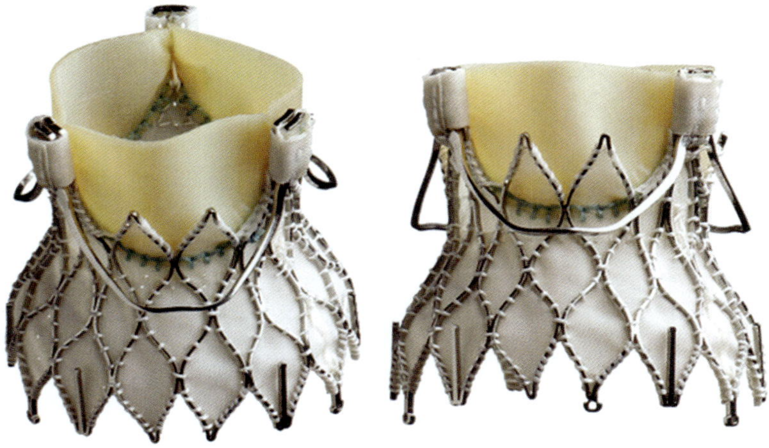

Fig. 15.3 Medtronic Engager valve.

expands thermosensitively. The same frame involves two parts, a main frame and a support frame, which are coupled to form the commissural posts of the prosthesis. The main frame further comprises of three components, a "throat" that comes to lie within the aortic valve annulus, the diverging commissural extensions, and an adaptable inlet which seals the left ventricular outflow tract off against regurgitation. The prosthesis has a maximal inlet diameter of 28 mm, a waist diameter of 18 mm, and a diameter at the outlet of 23 mm. The shape is dynamic and aims at minimizing pressure loss at the inlet and recovering pressure at the outlet. The valve design facilitates periannular implantation with minimal risk of coronary obstruction. When the prosthesis assumes final position, the total length is 24 mm with approximately one-third sitting subannularly. Thereby, the support arms form an arch that fits into the sinuses, while the commissural posts towering opposite to the native valve's commissures. The Engager valve is produced in three sizes, which cover the range of annulus diameters between 19 and 29 mm [31, 32].

The Medtronic Engager transcatheter delivery system comprises a pointed tip, a cup, and an introducer carrying a flushing port at its base, which are all mounted around a straight delivery shaft (Fig. 15.4). Its bottom end, the actual handle, comprises a distal knob and a proximal knob, which are turned by the surgeon to facilitate controlled release, and, finally, another flushing port at the very end (Fig. 15.5).

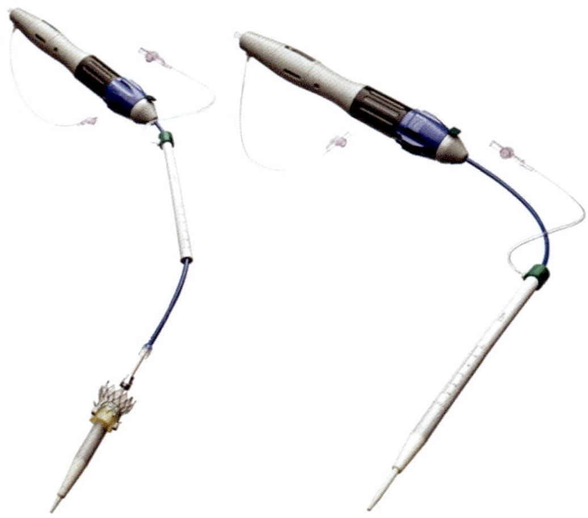

Fig. 15.4 Medtronic Engager delivery system.

The in vitro studies so far have shown comparable durability and hemodynamic findings to a Hancock II 23 mm controller valve. The Medtronic Engager prosthesis has demonstrated lower transvalvular gradients and higher effective orifice area (EOA) compared with the controls. A single-arm study to evaluate feasibility and safety in the notoriously selected high-risk target population was performed. The study involved three investigational sites, 30 patients with a minimal EuroScore of >9 points, hence a logistic EuroScore of at least 11% mortality. The results of the first-in-man (FIM) trial show feasibility (97% device success) and outcomes comparable to the leading transcatheter

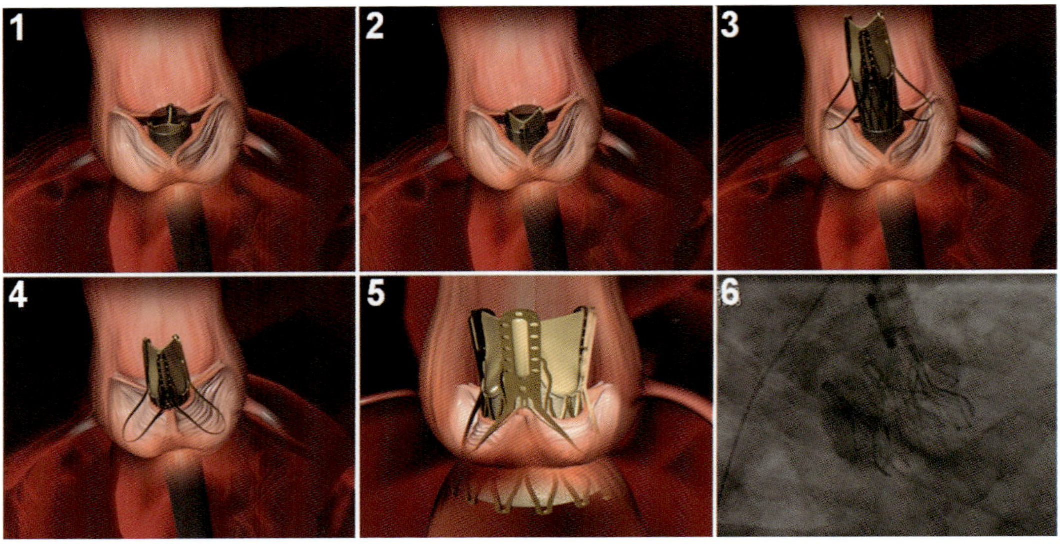

Fig. 15.5 Medtronic Engager stepwise implantation. 1 and 2, the commissural posts of the crimped prosthesis are rotated until aligned with the native commissures; 3, when prosthetic and native commissures are aligned, the support arms are released directly above the sinuses; 4, the system is pulled back until the support arms engage against the sinuses; 5, unsheathing of the mainframe results in self-expanding release of the device and deployment is completed; 6, deployed device *in situ* (aortography).

devices on the market. Aortic dissections occurred in four cases, spurring improvements in the design of the delivery system to avoid this complication [32] (Video 15.3).

JenaValve

The company JenaValve Technology (Munich, Germany) has designed two TAVR concepts, one for transapical and one for transfemoral implantation. The system components are a catheter delivery system, a self-expanding nitinol stent, and a valve (Fig. 15.6). The TA system includes a porcine root valve. Dr. Hendrik Treede at the University Heart Centre in Hamburg has performed the first two implantations. In September 2010 approval was received and the consecutive CE trial was designed to test feasibility and safety of the TAVR system, with 70 patients involved [33].

The JenaValve features feelers, which can be advanced, rotated, repositioned, or retracted into the sheath. In this mode the physician can "feel" and locate the optimal position in the presumed "landing zone," allowing for more accurate placement of the prosthesis. The additional JenaClip mechanism provides twofold advantages: first, it enhances anchoring to prevent migration, and second, it prevents excessive radial force at the annulus. It is also claimed to reduce mitral valve distortion and heart block. Furthermore, the clip mechanism as designed can contain annular calcifications and reduces the risk of coronary flow impairments. The commissure posts are flexible

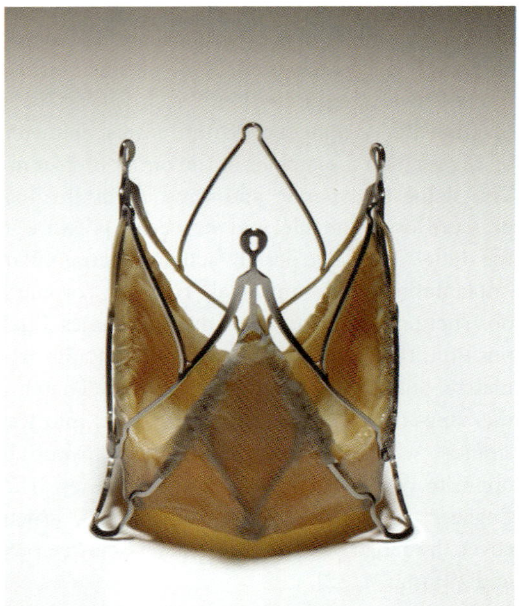

Fig. 15.6 JenaValve.

and support the valve leaflets. The company envisions achieving reduced tissue stresses during valve closure, and therefore better valve durability. A series of sizes up to a diameter of 27 mm is in production to cover a wide range of patients [34].

JenaValve delivery system

The prominent feature is that rapid pacing is not required for the deployment procedure. The shorter transapical system carries a flexible tip for the apical path and to prevent aortic wall trauma.

(a)

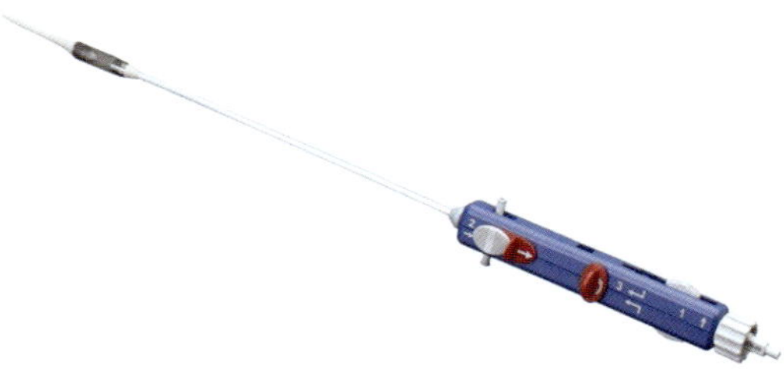

(b)

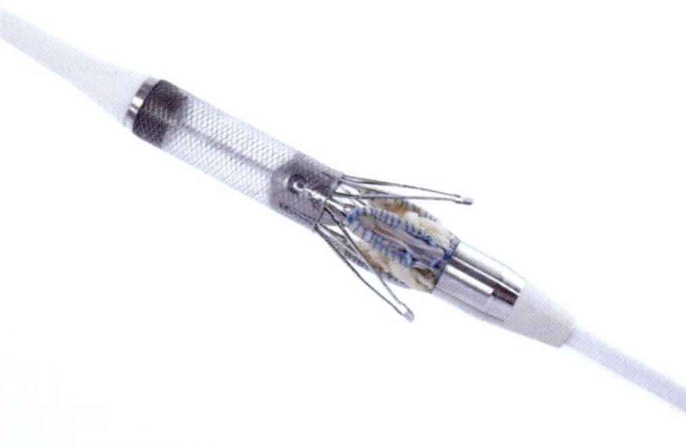

(c)

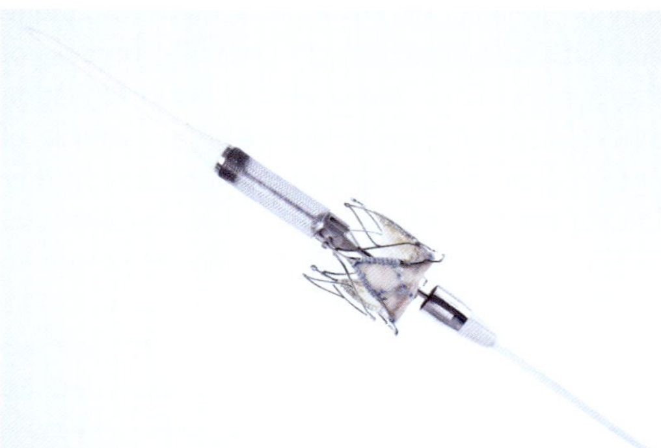

Fig. 15.7 **(a)** JenaValve delivery system. **(b, c)** JenaValve partially and fully unsheathed.

The valve can still be retrieved following expansion of the feelers (Fig. 15.7) [34].

Symetis Acurate valve

The Symetis Acurate valve is a porcine trileaflet valve mounted on a self-expanding nitinol stent (Fig. 15.8). The stent comprises the body of the stent at the inflow portion and an upper anchoring crown with stabilization arches that self-align the valve in the ascending aorta. The delivery sequence releases first the stabilization arms, then the superior crown, and lastly the body of the stent (Fig. 15.9). Until now, clinical results are limited and a multicenter pivotal study trial is being planned.

Patient selection

Pre-procedural evaluation of patients for TAVR is crucial to select the patients that will benefit the most and to ensure they are being exposed to the least risk possible during the procedure. Transcatheter aortic valve implantation (TAVI) is intended to be used in symptomatic patients with severe aortic stenosis who are at high risk for conventional surgery due to comorbid conditions or who are considered inoperable. However, defining high-risk surgical patients is not easy and therefore

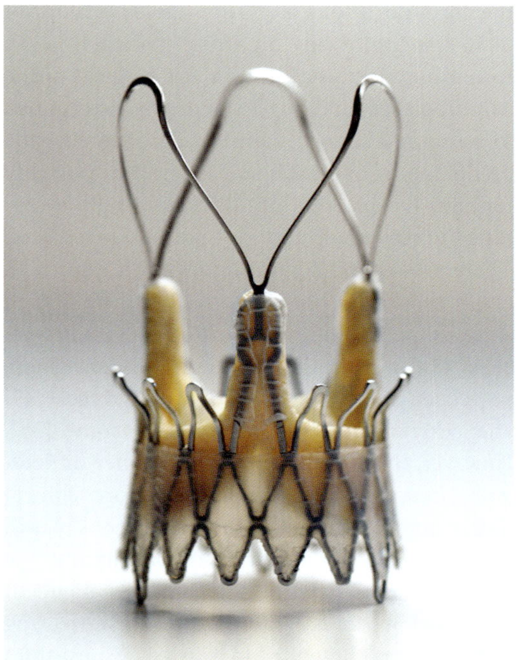

Fig. 15.8 Symetis Acurate valve.

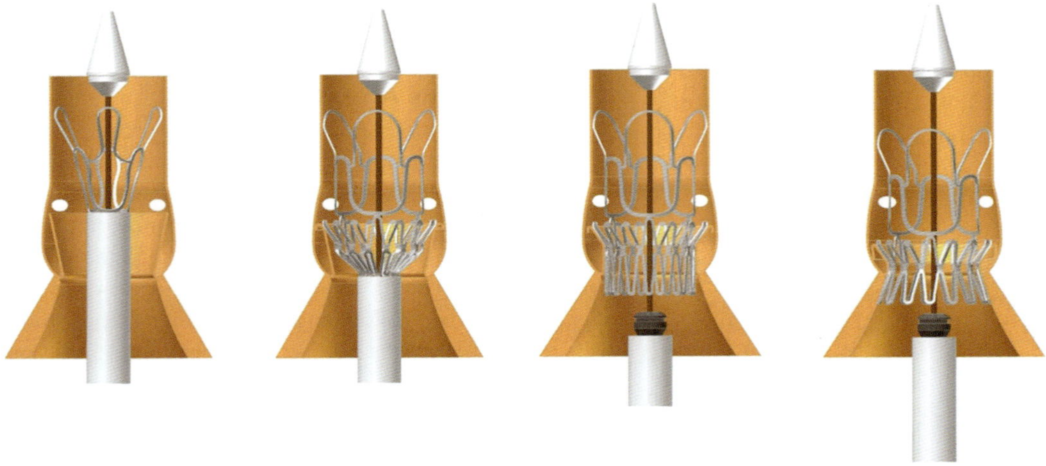

Fig. 15.9 Stepwise implantation of the self-expanding Symetis Acurate valve.

TAVR has led to a renewed interest in cardiac surgical risk modeling. In general most centers use the Society of Thoracic Surgery (STS) risk score >10 and/or a logistic EuroScore >20 to select their patients, since there are no validated risk models for the purposes of TAVI. Osswald et al. have shown that although the logistic EuroScore can adequately stratify patients into low, intermediate, or high risk, it overestimates the absolute 30-day mortality rate by a factor of 2–3 (especially in high-risk patients) [35]. Regarding risk stratification for surgical aortic valve replacement, the STS score was determined to be more accurate than the EuroScore in the prediction of operative and long-term mortality for high-risk patients [36]. Patients can be at very high operative mortality risk yet have low scores. There are several comorbidities not captured in either the EuroScore or the STS scoring system such as porcelaine aorta, chest wall radiation, chest wall deformities, frailty, and others. There have been attempts to quantify frailty index [37] and correlate frailty index with outcome [38]. However, the analysis of frailty is rather difficult and often not quantifiable. Therefore clinical judgment of experienced cardiac surgeons plays a key role in assessing operative mortality in these cases as well as to define "inoperable" patients. It is important to emphasize that these scoring systems are not intended to be used as substitutes for clinical decision making.

Recent National Institute for Health and Clinical Excellence (NICE) guidelines and licensing regulations have restricted the use of TAVR to selected patients, who are either deemed to be at greatly increased risk of death or severe complications from conventional open surgery, or who are not suitable for surgical AVR [39]. However, the fact that a patient is deemed inoperable conventionally does not necessarily imply that he or she is a candidate for TAVI.

The following patients are ideal for TAVR: patients >80 years with previous sternotomy for coronary artery bypass surgery and patent grafts which might get damaged during re-sternotomy and dissection of retrosternal adhesions. There are also a number of patients not even referred for surgery or turned down after surgical assessment due to their poor medical condition. These patients may be suitable for TAVR, with the transfemoral approach being particularly favorable, because of the avoidance of postoperative hypoventilation owing to pain. Careful anesthetic assessment of potential candidates in conjunction with further investigation may lead to successful management of patients who previously had no alternative to medical therapy.

There are a number of relative contraindications to TAVR, which may change as technology evolves. These include: bicuspid aortic valve (because the altered anatomy makes secure placement of the transcatheter valve potentially unstable), endocarditis, severe mitral or tricuspid valve regurgitation, left ventricular or atrial thrombus, aortic annular dimensions outside the manufacturers' range (device-specific), and an ascending aorta of >45 mm.

The evaluation results of patients are reviewed by a multidisciplinary team who then decide on the most appropriate and unbiased treatment option and approach (transfemoral/transapical/conventional surgery/medical therapy) to achieve maximum patient outcome [40].

Adequate vascular access is one of the most important determinants of procedural success. Aorto-ilio-femoral angiography and computed tomographic angiography provide the most useful information to predict feasibility of the TF approach. Precise vessel measurements are performed in multiple sites starting from the common femoral artery. A minimal diameter of 8 mm for a 24 Fr sheath, 7 mm for a 22 Fr sheath, and of 6 mm for a 18 Fr sheath is required. Excessive vessel tortuosity can prevent the large sheaths from advancing into the abdominal or thoracic aorta. Also, tortuosity with marked long calcifications does not allow the advancement of large sheaths. However, tortuosity without calcifications, which can be straightened by a wire, does not preclude the procedure.

If the minimal diameter, the tortuosity, and the vessel calcifications do not prohibit the advancement of the necessary large sheaths, the patients are assigned to the TF approach. On the other hand, if the likelihood of an unsuccessful insertion of sheaths and the retrograde advancement of the large catheter into the aortic valve is low, the TA approach is preferred. In general, there are no real contraindications for the TA approach except for severe skin lesions on the left chest, thrombus in the apex of the left ventricle, and a left ventricular aneurysm.

Procedure details

General considerations

Since catheter-based procedures target patients and conditions of high risk, particular attention and special preparatory steps are required [41]. The preparatory "checklist" starts with discussion of the indication in an interdisciplinary team of a cardiologist, cardiac surgeon, and anesthesiologist [42]. Next, imaging modalities are employed and findings discussed in a similar setting. Of paramount importance are the imaging counts for annulus size, coronary height, configuration of the aorta and calcific changes, the left ventricle (LV) to aorta angle, eventual LV thrombus formation, size of the LV, and position of the left ventricular apex. Once the patient is deemed eligible for the procedure and scheduled for it, a hybrid operation theater or a hybrid-similar functionality with anesthesiology and cardiopulmonary presence is warranted [43]. The anesthesiologist must have professional echocardiography skills to provide on-line transesophageal echocardiography (TEE) imaging at all times, to carry out measurements, and to contribute to differential diagnosis and trouble shooting in case of complications [42,44]. The perfusionist should be on standby in the room with the CPB device ready to connect in case of conversion [41].

The patient is placed in a slightly rotated, lateral decubitus position (c. 15°) with the left submammary region most prominent to line up with the direction of the incoming sheath. The leading cardiac surgeon and eventually his assistant stand to the patient's right, while the assisting cardiologist (or any colleague with adequate catheter and angiography table skills) places him/herself on the opposite side. Before surface disinfection, a TEE is performed to locate the exact projection of the LV apex on the body surface, and a marking is made to delineate the site of the incision. The size of the annulus is confirmed in two planes for the appropriate choice of valve and the patient is disinfected. The incision is carried out as marked (usually 5–6 cm), most frequently in the fifth or sixth left parasternal, submammary intercostal space. Some surgeons will prefer to use a soft tissue retractor, others do not. In most cases, selective unilateral lung ventilation is not required. Next, the pericardial fat tissue is resected, a pericardiotomy performed, and the pericardial stay sutures placed. As the surgeon focuses on the left anterolateral thoracotomy, a minimum of 150 U/heparin/kg body weight is administered and the cardiologist enters the femoral artery and places a femoral arterial sheath, aortic root pigtail, and femoral venous wire as a safety net. Next, the apical entry site is defined. Here, a distinction has to be made between the anatomic apex as the utmost tip of the cardiac muscle helix, and the actual entry point into the left ventricle. The latter is usually a muscular region of 2 × 3 cm, slightly to the left of the anatomic apex, which projects in direct line with the TEE position of the aortic annulus, and lies safely lateral to the septum to avoid its penetration. Often, a gauze is placed deep into the pericardium, lateral to the LV, or an additional deep pericardial stay stitch is carried out to lift and centralize the apex safely into the vision field, and to avoid later derangements of the optimal position. An epicardial pacemaker electrode is placed laterally towards the right ventricle, if accessible, otherwise anywhere outside the field of action. The apical closure suture is then placed. Two modes are recommended. One involves two large felt-reinforced U-sutures at 90° to each other, resulting in a rectangular distribution of traction, leaving enough space for penetration in the middle. The other one – most frequently used – involves two continuous circular pursestring stitches starting from antidiametric points on the apex. These pursestrings are loaded with one new pledget every time the needle exits the myocardium, on every bite. Hence, the closure traction is more circular in this manner. Both techniques have in common two things. First, that the "bites" must be deep and vertical into the myocardium, and not superficial, as they could otherwise fail and tear through the LV, especially in the frail tissue of an 80+ year old. Second, they are usually performed with a 2.0 or 3.0 polypropylene suture. A tear of these sutures through the LV occurs in less than 5% of cases, and may result in conversion with median sternotomy. For this reason, fatty epicardium should be avoided, because it masks the underlying myocardium and may mislead the surgeon to take too shallow bites through the actual muscle, resulting in a high risk of LV rupture.

Once the apex is secured, and the hemodynamics are stable, the order is given to prepare the application catheter and start crimping the valve. This process is kept in parallel steps with the surgical part, and optimal synchronization is usually achieved. Next, the LV apex is punctured, and a soft, then stiff, wire (0.035 inches) is propagated into the LV and passes through the aortic valve down to the descending aorta. The next step is the balloon valvuloplasty under a short period of rapid pacing (this applies for the Edwards Sapien and Medtronic Engager valves). The rapid pacing frequency usually lies between 160 and 200 beats/min. Often enough, the selected frequency is not optimal for that particular patient and may result in persistently high blood pressure (blood pressure does not drop below mean 50 mmHg), that prohibits expansion of the balloon. Next, the introduction sheath is placed and optimally comes to lie in the LV down to the 4–5 cm marking. The valve carrier shaft enters next and positions the prosthesis across the aortic valve annulus. The general principle is for the valve to be in an axial position at one-third above and two-thirds below the annulus. A severely calcified, fluoroscopically visible native valve will offer more checkpoints to facilitate correct positioning. Note that every annulus is different, the LA/aortic angulation varies, and the calcifications are not symmetric. Also, there are fluoroscopy scanner projection differences that have to be considered. A meticulous study of the unreleased prosthesis′ position in multiple planes is recommended. TEE can provide some help, in spite of poor resolution and ultrasound effects, which obscure the picture. Also, the dynamics of valve release need to be considered, as ballooning of the prosthesis will redirect its position, may push it higher or lower, and alter its axial orientation. Complications may arise from misplacement, such as aortic valve regurgitation (valve too low), coronary ostial obstruction (valve too high), or valve migration (valve distorted in its axial orientation). Presumably, growing experience will offset these limitations.

Next, the balloon is fully inflated during another short period of rapid pacing. It is recommended to let the heart and hemodynamics recover after every session of rapid pacing to allow for sufficient myocardial perfusion, before the next procedural step is undertaken. The stiff wire should be retained in place until the final valve position is reached or for the eventual need to re-balloon and dilate the valve, in case of non-optimal anchorage in the surrounding calcified tissue, with persisting significant aortic valve regurgitation (2+). Besides, it prevents malrotation of the valve. At this point, the final position of the prosthesis is assessed by TEE, with particular attention to existing aortic valve regurgitation (two planes), the freedom of movement of the anterior mitral valve leaflet (120°, longitudinal section), and the final shape of the valve (cross-section), which should be approximately circular, without indentations and asymmetries. Finally, one or more shots of contrast medium (15–20 ml) are administered to confirm patency of the coronary ostiae, and the degree of residual aortic valve regurgitation. The ultimate result can only be concluded following removal of the guide wire, which may cause a significant regurgitant jet. Next, the sheath is removed, and the pursestring tied. A curved chest tube is placed in the pleura. The ribs are reapproximated with a single or two strong vicryl stitches (lung prolapse has been reported), followed by wound closure in three layers. Some surgeons may prefer to administer intercostal lidocaine for pain control. Early extubation is desired [32,41,45].

Specific considerations

The sequence above largely applies for the Edwards Sapien and Sapien XT valves (Video 15.2). The Medtronic Engager delivery system comprises an introducer sheath, which contains the dilator, around a guide wire [31,32,41]. The Engager valve is inserted into the "overtube" via a wedge-shaped entrance. Fluoroscopically guided retraction and positioning occurs while the valve is still in the overtube, until the commissural posts assume the correct position. Once the delivery system leaves the overtube, the Engager support arms are exposed in the aortic root, and expand laterally into the coronary sinuses. The position is verified fluoroscopically in various planes. If necessary, rotation and repositioning of the commissural posts against the commissures can be applied. A short period of rapid pacing follows, during which constant pull is applied until the valve is released.

In a single-armed FIM study to test feasibility and safety, 30 patients who complied with the European Society of Cardiology guidelines participated. Valve positioning was achieved in 29 of these patients with reasonable procedure and fluoroscopy times. The peak-to-peak gradients compared to existing biological heart valve prostheses on the market, and paravalvular leackage was mild in the majority of cases (80%). The overall 6-month survival was 56.7%. One drawback was the event of an aortic dissection in four patients, of which three had to undergo urgent surgery. The valve was subsequently redesigned to counteract this risk, whereby the straight and rigid delivery system was abandoned in favur of a delivery system with a flexible shaft for over-the-wire tracking, and facilitation of coaxial alignment with the aorta. A protective cover over the commissural posts secured the posts until the valve's final position could be confirmed, before the main frame is released. Several more structural modifications have been implemented to increase space between the support arms and main frame, increase radial strength at the waist, and to improve conformance with the native root anatomy [32].

The JenaValve has special structural features, such as a double layer system of three clips in two rows, one for valve fixation onto the frame, and the other for anchoring purposes. During placement, the catheter sheath is pushed forward (for the TA implantation of the JenaValve), whereby three feelers are released and manipulated by the surgeon by tactile feedback behind the calcified valve and into the sinuses (Video 15.4). Once achieved, the sheath is pushed further; the anchoring system assumes its annular position, and the valve is fully released. The JenaClip stent then expands to provide retention force, at which point the prosthesis is fully functional. The JenaValve does not require rapid ventricular pacing. Retrieval is possible until final release of the prosthesis. Feelers and the JenaClip stent provide anchoring, and prevent migration of the valve either way. The FIM trial was performed in Hamburg in 2010 while approval for more extensive patient studies was obtained mid-2010 [33,34].

In summary, the transapical procedure is gaining weight in the transcatheter valve field, with outcomes and complication rates comparable to the transfemoral procedure. This is achieved through an optimized orchestration of surgeon, cardiologist, anesthetist, and perfusionist teams and fast response and backup algorithms in case of failure. The future trends clearly point towards a plethoric armamentarium of devices and delivery systems with access decreasing to a fully endoscopic route, and the portfolio expanding to include repeat and mitral valve procedures. Ultimately, as we are already entering the post-pioneering and experimental phase, optimal results can only be reached in a structured and integrated training system.

Imaging requirements

Preoperative imaging

Potential candidates for TAVR undergo a systematic work-up protocol which includes:

- Transthoracic (TTE) or transesophageal echocardiography (TEE) to determine aortic valve morphology (bicuspid/tricuspid), extent and location of calcifications, annulus size, size of the left ventricular outflow tract (LVOT), size of the sinus of Valsalva, and to assess mitral/tricuspid valve and left ventricular function.
- Coronary angiography including angioplasty if necessary to treat proximal flow-limiting lesions.
- Aorto-ilio-femoral angiography to assess tortuosity and diameter of the aorta, iliac and femoral arteries.
- Multislice computed tomography (MSCT) for evaluating the degree of calcification of the ilio-femoral arteries, the abdominal and thoracic aorta, as well as the extent and the location of calcifications of the aortic valve, to measure the dimensions of the LVOT, the aortic annulus, and the ascending aorta.

Pre- and intraoperative imaging is of utmost importance for procedural planning and execution. Preoperative information on vascular access sites, quality and tortuosity of the femoral artery, as well as the aorta, are important. Furthermore, the relation of the apex to the chest wall, angulation of the left ventricle, and the LVOT in relation to the aortic root have to be determined in order to plan for the ideal access site (intercostal space). Angulation of the left ventricle and LVOT in relation to the aortic root can be easily visualized by MSCT (Fig. 15.10) and the distance of the coronary ostia from the aortic annulus can be adequately measured (Fig. 15.11). The ventriculo-aortic angle can only be appreciated in the right anterior oblique (RAO) view, but not in the left anterior oblique (LAO) view, since the latter looks at this angulation en face (Fig. 15.12). In addition the anatomy of the aortic valve leaflets, the leaflet calcification, and the distribution and geometry of the calcification are assessed and give more information on predicting the ease of implantation (Fig. 15.13).

As for all cardiac procedures, the extent of concomitant coronary artery disease and concomitant valvular pathology, as well as left ventricular function, have to be known. To what extent percutaneous coronary intervention has to be performed prior to valve implantation is based on the risk to the myocardium during the valve procedure, which is, however, currently under debate.

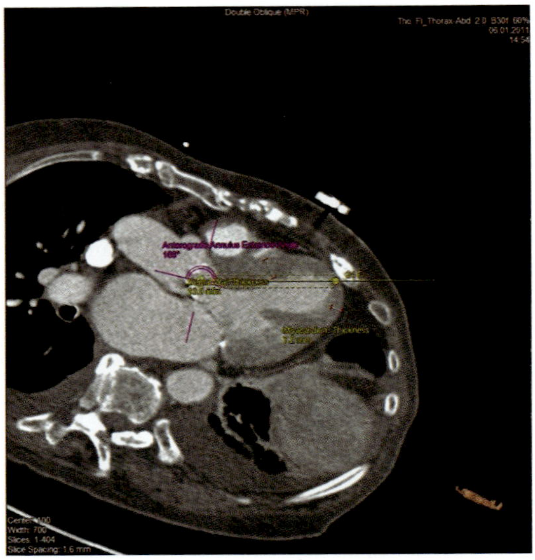

Fig. 15.10 MSCT scan showing the ventriculo-aortic angle from the transapical access in a double oblique multiplanar rendered view.

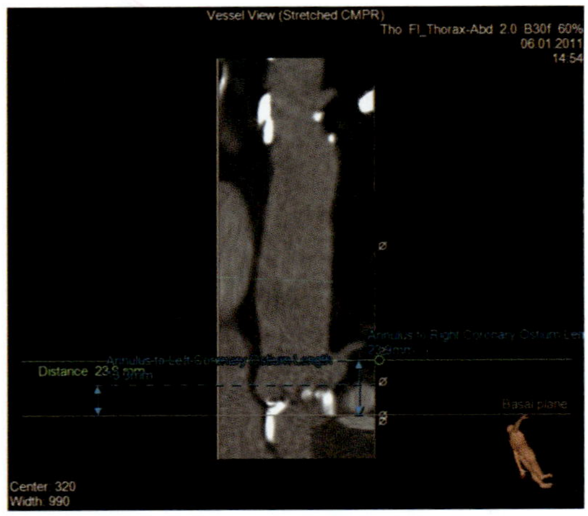

Fig. 15.11 MSCT scan showing the aortic root and indicating distances from the aortic annulus to the right and left coronary ostia.

One of the key imaging requirements for a successful transcatheter aortic valve implantation is an accurate measurement of the aortic annulus. The aortic valve annulus is often elliptical and the differences in the minimum and maximum diameter can

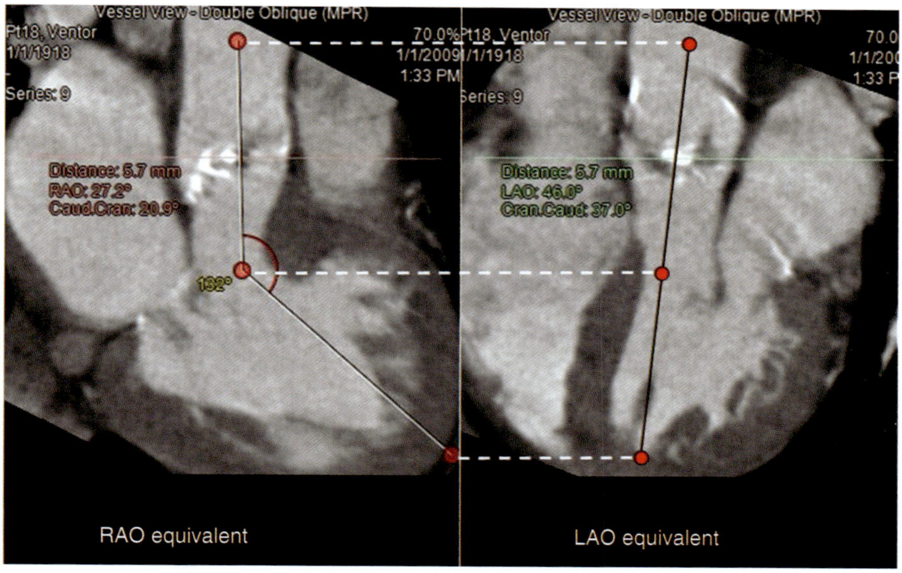

Fig. 15.12 MSCT scan showing the ventriculo-aortic angle from RAO/LAO projections.

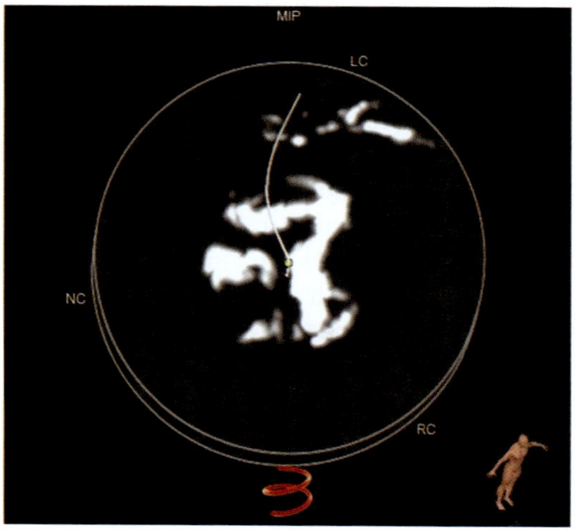

Fig. 15.13 MSCT scan showing an asymmetric annulus calcification pattern.

lead to substantial differences in the selection of prosthesis size and subsequent undersizing or oversizing. Annulus measurements are usually performed during TTE or TEE [46,47]. Recently, it has been suggested that MSCT also could provide detailed information on the shape and diameter of the aortic annulus [48]. In the literature different definitions of the diameter of the aortic valve are used: the minimal diameter D_{min}, the maximal diameter D_{max}, the mean diameter D_{mean} $(D_{max}+D_{min}/2)$ and diameter cross-sectional area $(D_{csa}=2 \times (CSA/\Pi)^{0.5}$. If MSCT measurements are used D_{mean} and D_{csa} produce the best approximation of a one-dimensional radius for valve selection [49]. Which modality is superior and should be used for choosing the appropriate prosthesis size remains to be determined, but the use of TEE as a reference is associated with good clinical results [50].

Intraoperative imaging

Fluoroscopy is used to monitor guide wire placement for TAVI. To confirm correct wire placement within the left ventricle (especially to rule out interference with the subvalvular apparatus of the mitral valve), TEE can be supportive. Accurate valve positioning is the most crucial step of the implantation to achieve an optimal sealing of the annulus with the stented valve. Furthermore, the occlusion to the coronary ostia as well as the impairment of the mitral valve has to be avoided. To ensure this, online imaging is required that allows for identification of the coronary ostia and the aortic annulus. The gold standard for imaging during valve placement is fluoroscopy. C-arm angulation is an important factor for obtaining reliable and conclusive images. The optimal projection is perpendicular to the annulus plane and orthogonal to the line through both commissures (see Fig. 15.6) which can already be determined prior to the procedure through dedicated planning workflow software for TAVR (3mensio Medical Imaging BV, Bilthofen, the Netherlands).

Throughout the implantation process, TEE is used to monitor left ventricular function, which may deteriorate after valvuloplasty due to acute onset of aortic valve regurgitation, and to detect cardiac tamponade. Post-implant valve position is confirmed with TEE and angiography. To assess valve competence and potential paravalvular regurgitation TEE is best used, whereas obstruction or occlusion of the coronary arteries is best seen in angiography of the aortic root.

Complications

Heart block

The most common complication after TAVI is third-degree atrioventricular block with an incidence reported of up to 36% [51–53], presumably as a consequence of the pressure applied on the conducting tissues located subendocardially in the left ventricular outflow tract and interventricular septum. Early experience suggests that prostheses extending further in the ventricle are associated with a higher incidence of conduction abnormalities, most likely new-onset left bundle branch block [54].

Paravalvular leaks

Mild and moderate degrees of paravalvular leaks seem to be well tolerated and clinically significant hemolysis has not been observed so far [55]. On the other hand, moderate to severe or severe paravalvular leaks, although infrequent, are likely to be hemodynamically significant. The initial sign is typically low aortic diastolic pressure. Rising ventricular filling pressure might lead to myocardial ischemia and ventricular dysfunction due to a significantly higher workload on the left ventricle, which seems to be more pronounced in TAVI paravalvular leakages compared with equivalently sized surgically implanted bioprosthesis [56].

Valve embolization

Valve embolization immediately after deployment is generally the result of a major error in valve positioning or inadequate rapid ventricular pacing and subsequent ejection of the valve by an effective ventricular contraction during deployment. Embolization to the aorta is usually well tolerated as long as the guide wire is in the descending aorta, preventing the valve from flipping over to obstruct antegrade flow. In this situation the valve can be repositioned with a partially inflated valvuloplasty balloon into a stable position somewhere in the aorta (ideally in the descending aorta). Embolization into the left ventricle is very rare, but in such cases surgical removal is the only option [57].

Apical access issues

Direct access to the left ventricle is typically obtained through an intercostal minithoracotomy. The most common concern related to the incision is chest wall discomfort and associated respiratory compromise with prolonged ventilation [58]. On completion of the procedure, the apical access site is closed with preinserted pledgeted sutures. Short bursts of rapid ventricular pacing might be helpful during tying the pursestring sutures. Management of large tears at the apex or the left ventricular free wall might require institution of cardiopulmonary support. In rare cases pseudoaneurysm formation at the apex has been observed weeks to months after the procedure. Although pseudoaneurysms are initially asymptomatic, they typically progress and might require intervention later [59].

Stroke

The most frequent etiology of stroke is atheroembolism from the ascending aorta or the aortic arch from catheters or wires. Other potential causes include embolism from the aortic valve during valvuloplasty. Repeated or overly aggressive valvuloplasty might be associated with an increased risk of embolization of calcific material from the aortic valve and should be avoided [60,61]. The incidence of stroke varies as a consequence of the learning curve and the evolution in technique but also the sophistication of the neurologic assessment. With current devices stroke rate ranges from 0% to 10%, suggesting that stroke rate is lower with the transapical access due to less manipulation of the aorta and the aortic arch [62–64].

Coronary obstruction

Coronary obstruction might occur if the valve frame or the sealing cuff is placed directly over a coronary ostium, which is, however, exceedingly rare. Of more concern is the possibility of displacing a bulky, calcified native leaflet over a coronary ostium. Although this is potentially fatal, some cases have been successfully managed by immediate percutaneous angioplasty on emergently placed cardiopulmonary bypass [43]. The risk of coronary occlusion is usually low although difficult to predict. It most likely depends on the bulkiness of the native leaflets, height of the coronary ostium from the annulus, and the dimension of the sinus of Valsalva which can be assessed by MSCT [65].

Annular and root rupture

Rupture of the aortic annulus is a rare complication of TAVI with subsequent hemodynamic collapse. Excessive balloon dilation and aggressive valve oversizing in combination with the presence of extensive annular (especially subcommissural) calcification might increase the likelihood of annular rupture. A tear created at the level of the valve inflow can result in a ventricular septal defect or left ventricular-to-left atrial shunt, whereas a root rupture will likely cause cardiac tamponade requiring emergent cardiopulmonary bypass and surgical repair [58].

Future evolution of TAVR and new devices

Since the results of the first randomized trials (PARTNER trial) are published comparing a cohort of patients with severe aortic stenosis treated with TAVI and standard medical therapy, and with the expectation that technology is definitely to improve within the next few years, the indication for TAVI is likely to shift to a younger population [66,67]. However, controlled randomized clinical trials will be required beforehand. The interdisciplinary nature of TAVR, combining aspects of both surgical and interventional therapies, presents special challenges and requires an enlightened and collaborative approach to the development of clinical research recommendations and endpoint definitions. The VARC (Valve Academic Research Consortium) initiative has been founded in an attempt to achieve the necessary consensus among the various subspecialties, such that this innovative treatment modality may be evaluated objectively and according to practical endpoint definitions [68].

Another interesting population are patients with degenerated xenografts. While this problem is less frequent with the current generation of biologic valves, the trend for implantation in younger patient groups will generate an increasing patient cohort requiring a second operation. Redo AVR can be performed with excellent results, but alternative techniques may further decrease the risks associated with redo aortic valve surgery. Especially after root replacement, redo AVR can be challenging. A few studies demonstrated that for both mitral and aortic valve xenografts TAVR can be performed successfully. The so-called valve-in-valve concept makes use of the stent of the implanted xenograft that serves as a marker during implantation of the transcatheter valve [69–71]. This concept has also already been applied in an experimental setting as valve-in-a-ring for late mitral valve replacement after late failure of mitral valve repair [71]. Another promising approach is the transcatheter placement of autologous tissue engineered valved stents. A proof of concept has recently been demonstrated. This approach may have important implications for the correction of congenital cardiac malformations [72].

In the absence of randomized trials and the few data on matched comparisons showing similar results for TAVR as for patients undergoing conventional surgery [28], TAVR can currently be considered an alternative approach for selected high-risk patients with severe aortic stenosis.

References

1 Vahanian A, Alfieri OR, Al-Attar N, et al. Transcatheter valve implantation for patients with aortic stenosis: a position statement from the European Association of Cardiothoracic Surgery (EACTS) and the European Society of Cardiology (ESC), in collaboration with the European Association of Percutaneous Cardiovascular Interventions (EAPCI). Eur J Cardiothorac Surg 2008;34:1–8.

2 Walther T, Chu MW, Mohr FW. Transcatheter aortic valve implantation: time to expand? Curr Opin Cardiol 2008;23:111–16.

3 Cribier A, Eltchaninoff H, Bash A, et al. Percutaneous transcatheter implantation of an aortic valve prosthesis for calcific aortic stenosis: first human case description. Circulation 2002;106:3006–8.
4 Lindroos M, Kupari M, Heikkilä J, et al. Prevalence of aortic valve abnormalities in the elderly: an echocardiographic study of a random population sample. J Am Coll Cardiol 1993;21:1220–5.
5 Otto CM, Lind BK, Kitzman DW, et al. Association of aortic-valve sclerosis with cardiovascular mortality and morbidity in the elderly. N Engl J Med 1999;341:142–7.
6 Aronow WS, Ahn C, Kronzon I. Association of valvular aortic stenosis with symptomatic peripheral arterial disease in older persons. Am J Cardiol 2001;88:1046–7.
7 Agmon Y, Khandheria BK, Jamil Tajik A, et al. Inflammation, infection, and aortic valve sclerosis: Insights from the Olmsted County (Minnesota) population. Atherosclerosis 2004;174:337–42.
8 Olsson M, Dalsgaard CJ, Haegerstrand A, et al. Accumulation of T lymphocytes and expression of interleukin-2-receptors in nonrheumatic stenotic aortic valves. J Am Coll Cardiol 1994;23:1162–70.
9 Rajamannan NM, Subramaniam M, Rickard D, et al. Human aortic valve calcification is associated with an osteoblast phenotype. Circulation 2003;107:2181–4.
10 Cowell SJ, Newby DE, Prescott RJ, et al. Scottish Aortic Stenosis and Lipid Lowering Trial, Impact on Regression (SALTIRE) Investigators. A randomized trial of intensive lipid-lowering therapy in calcific aortic stenosis. N Engl J Med 2005;352:2389–97.
11 Moura LM, Ramos SF, Zamorano JL, et al. Rosuvastatin affecting aortic valve endothelium to slow the progression of aortic stenosis. J Am Coll Cardiol 2007; 49:554–61.
12 Turina J, Hess O, Sepulcri F, et al. Spontaneous course of aortic valve disease. Eur Heart J 1987:8:471–83.
13 Kelly TA, Rothbart RM, Cooper CM, et al. Comparison of outcome of asymptomatic to symptomatic patients older than 20 years of age with valvular aortic stenosis. Am J Cardiol 1988;61:123–30 .
14 Lindblom D, Lindblom U, Qvist J, et al. Long-term relative survival rates after heart valve replacement. J Am Coll Cardiol 1990;15:566–73.
15 Bonow RO, Carabello BA, Kanu C, et al. ACC/AHA 2006 guidelines for the management of patients with valvular heart disease: a report of the American College of Cardiology/American Heart Association Task Force on Practice Guidelines (writing committee to revise the 1998 Guidelines for the Management of Patients With Valvular Heart Disease): developed in collaboration with the Society of Cardiovascular Anesthesiologists: endorsed by the Society for Cardiovascular Angiography and Interventions and the Society of Thoracic Surgeons. Circulation 2006;114:e84–231.
16 Rosenhek R, Binder T, Porenta G, et al. Predictors of outcome in severe asymptomatic aortic stenosis. N Engl J Med 2000;343:611–17.
17 Pai RG, Kapoor N, Bansal RC, et al. Malignant natural history of asymptomatic severe aortic stenosis: benefit of aortic valve replacement. Ann Thorac Surg 2006;82:2116–22.
18 Chizner MA, Pearle DL, deLeon AC, Jr. The natural history of aortic stenosis in adults. Am Heart J 1980;99:419–24.
19 Pellikka PA, Sarano ME, Nishimura RA, et al. Outcome of 622 adults with asymptomatic, hemodynamically significant aortic stenosis during prolonged follow-up. Circulation 2005;111:3290–5
20 Baumgartner H. What influences the outcome of valve replacement in critical aortic stenosis? Heart 2005;91:1254–6.
21 Chiam PT, Ruiz CE. Percutaneous transcatheter aortic valve implantation: evolution of the technology. Am Heart J 2009;157:229–42.
22 Walther T, Simon P, Dewey T, et al. Transapical minimally invasive aortic valve implantation: multicenter experience. Circulation 2007;116(11 Suppl):I240–5.
23 Webb JG, Chandavimol M, Thompson CR, et al. Percutaneous aortic valve implantation retrograde from the femoral artery. Circulation 2006;113:842–50.
24 Leon MB, Smith CR, Mack M, et al. Transcatheter aortic-valve implantation for aortic stenosis in patients who cannot undergo surgery. N Engl J Med 2010; 363:1597–607.
25 Webb JG, Altwegg L, Boone RH, et al. Transcatheter aortic valve implantation: impact on clinical and valve-related outcomes. Circulation 2009;119:3009–16.
26 Wong DR, Ye J, Cheung A, et al. Technical considerations to avoid pitfalls during transapical aortic valve implantation. J Thorac Cardiovasc Surg 2010;140:196–202.
27 Wendler O, Walther T, Nataf P, et al. Trans-apical aortic valve implantation: univariate and multivariate analyses of the early results from the SOURCE registry. Eur J Cardiothorac Surg 2010;38:119–27.
28 Walther T, Schuler G, Borger MA, et al. Transapical aortic valve implantation in 100 consecutive patients: comparison to propensity-matched conventional aortic valve replacement. Eur Heart J 2010;31:1398–403.
29 Walther T, Dewey T, Wimmer-Greinecker G, et al. Transapical approach for sutureless stent-fixed aortic valve implantation: experimental results. Eur J Cardiothorac Surg 2006;29:703–8.
30 Webb JG, Altwegg L, Masson JB, et al. A new transcatheter aortic valve and percutaneous valve delivery system. J Am Coll Cardiol 2009;53:1855–8.
31 Falk V, Schwammenthal EE, Kempfert J, et al. New anatomically oriented transapical aortic valve implantation. Ann Thorac Surg 2009;87:925–6.

32 Falk V, Walther T, Schwammenthal E, et al. Transapical aortic valve implantation with a self-expanding anatomically oriented valve. Eur Heart J 2011;32(7):878–87.
33 Trahan R. JenaValve Technology initiates multicenter CE-mark study for its transapical TAVI system. San Francisco: Business Wire, 2010 (updated November 2, 2010, cited January 17, 2011). Available from http://www.businesswire.com/news/home/20101102006317/en/JenaValve-Technology-Initiates-Multicenter-CE-Mark-Study-Transapical.
34 JenaValve™ Technology. Technology – unique features. Munich: © JenaValve™ Technology GmbH, 2010, 2011 (cited January 17, 2011). Available from http://www.jenavalve.de/index.php?id=Technology&subid=Unique%20Features&PHPSESSID=97a6c9ab9658d714aa332720cd58deb7.
35 Osswald BR, Gegouskov V, Badowski-Zyla D, et al. Overestimation of aortic valve replacement risk by EuroSCORE: implications for percutaneous valve replacement. Eur Heart J 2009;30:74–80.
36 Dewey TM, Brown D, Ryan WH, et al. Reliability of risk algorithms in predicting early and late operative outcomes in high-risk patients undergoing aortic valve replacement. J Thorac Cardiovasc Surg 2008; 135:180–187.
37 Purser JL, Kuchibhatla MN, Fillenbaum GG, et al. Identifying frailty in hospitalized older adults with significant coronary artery disease. J Am Geriatr Soc 2006;54:1674–81.
38 Jones DM, Song X, Rockwood K. Operationalizing a frailty index from a standardized comprehensive geriatric assessment. J Am Geriatr Soc 2004;52:1929–33.
39 National Institute of Health and Clinical Excellence. Transcatheter aortic valve implantation for aortic stenosis: guidance. London: NICE, June 2008, abstract no. IPG 266.
40 Dewey TM, Brown DL, Das TS, et al. High-risk patients referred for transcatheter aortic valve implantation: management and outcomes. Ann Thorac Surg 2008;86: 1450–6.
41 Walther T, Dewey T, Borger MA, et al. Transapical aortic valve implantation: step by step. Ann Thorac Surg 2009;87:276–83.
42 Ruel M, Dickie S, Chow BJ, Labinaz M. Interventional valve surgery: building a team and working together. Semin Thorac Cardiovasc Surg 2010;22:145–9.
43 Walther T, Falk V, Kempfert J, et al. Transapical minimally invasive aortic valve implantation; the initial 50 patients. Eur J Cardiothorac Surg 2008;33:983–8.
44 Heinze H, Sier H, Schafer U, et al. Percutaneous aortic valve replacement: overview and suggestions for anesthestic management. J Clin Anesth 2010;22:373–8.
45 Ferrari E, von Segesser LK. Transcatheter aortic valve implantation (TAVI): state of the art techniques and future perspectives. Swiss Med Wkly 2010;140:w13127.
46 Fan CM, Liu X, Panidis JP, et al. Prediction of homograft aortic valve size by transthoracic and transesophageal two-dimensional echocardiography. Echocardiography 1997;14:345–8.
47 Moss RR, Ivens E, Pasupati S, et al. Role of echocardiography in percutaneous aortic valve implantation. JACC Cardiovasc Imaging 2008;1:15–24.
48 Tops LF, Wood DA, Delgado V, et al. Noninvasive evaluation of the aortic root with multislice computed tomography implications for transcatheter aortic valve replacement. JACC Cardiovasc Imaging 2008;1:321–30.
49 Schultz CJ, Moelker A, Piazza N, et al. Three dimensional evaluation of the aortic annulus using multislice computer tomography: are manufacturer's guidelines for sizing for percutaneous aortic valve replacement helpful? Eur Heart J 2010;31:849–56.
50 Messika-Zeitoun D, Serfaty JM, Brochet E, et al. Multimodal assessment of the aortic annulus diameter. J Am Coll Cardiol 2010;55:186–94.
51 Thomas M, Schymik G, Walther T, et al. Thirty-day results of the SAPIEN aortic Bioprosthesis European Outcome (SOURCE) Registry: a European registry of transcatheter aortic valve implantation using the Edwards SAPIEN valve. Circulation 2010;122:62–9.
52 Eltchaninoff H, Prat A, Gilard M, et al.; on behalf of the FRANCE Registry Investigators. Eur Heart J 2011;32:191–7.
53 Sinhal A, Altwegg L, Pasupati S, et al. Atrioventricular block after transcatheter balloon expandable aortic valve implantation. JACC Cardiovasc Interv 2008;1:305–9.
54 Piazza N, Onuma Y, Jesserun E, et al. Early and persistent intraventricular conduction abnormalities and requirements for pacemaking after percutaneous replacement of the aortic valve. JACC Cardiovasc Interv 2008;1:310–16.
55 Murphy CJ, Pasupati S, Webb JG. Hemolysis after transcatheter balloon-expandable aortic valve insertion. Can J Cardiol 2007;23:260.
56 Azadani AN, Jaussaud N, Matthews PB, et al. Energy loss due to paravalvular leak with transcatheter aortic valve implantation. Ann Thorac Surg 2009;88:1857–63.
57 Tuzcu ME. Transcatheter aortic valve replacement malposition and embolization: innovation brings solutions also new challenges. Catheter Cardiovasc Interv 2008;71:579–80.
58 Walther T, Falk V, Borger MA, et al. Minimally invasive transapical beating heart aortic valve implantation – proof of concept. Eur J Cardiothorac Surg 2007;31:9–15.
59 Masson JB, Kovac J, Schuler G, et al. Transcatheter aortic valve implantation. JACC Cardiovasc Interv 2009;2:811–20.
60 Berry C, Cartier R, Bonan R. Fatal ischemic stroke related to non permissive peripheral artery access for

percutaneous aortic valve replacement. Catheter Cardiovasc Interv 2007;69:56–63.
61 Isner J. Acute catastrophic complications of balloon aortic valvuloplasty: the Mansfield scientific aortic valvuloplasty registry investigators. J Am Coll Cardiol 1991;17:1436–44.
62 Svensson LG, Dewey T, Kapadia S, et al. United States feasibility study of transcatheter insertion of a stented aortic valve by the left ventricular apex. Ann Thorac Surg 2008;86:46–54.
63 Cribier A, Eltchaninoff H, Tron C, et al. Treatment of calcific aortic stenosis with the percutaneous heart valve: mid-term follow-up from the initial feasibility studies: the French experience. J Am Coll Cardiol 2006; 47:1214–23.
64 Grube E, Schuler G, Buellesfeld L, et al. Percutaneous aortic valve replacement for severe aortic stenosis in high-risk patients using the second- and current third-generation self-expanding CoreValve prosthesis: device success and 30-day clinical outcome. J Am Coll Cardiol 2007;50:69–76.
65 Lu TL, Huber CH, Rizzo E, et al. Ascending aorta measurements as assessed by ECG-gated multi-detector computed tomography: a pilot study to establish normative values for transcatheter therapies. Eur Radiol 2009;19:664–9.
66 Leon MB, Smith CR, Mack M, et al.; PARTNER Trial Investigators. Transcatheter aortic-valve implantation for aortic stenosis in patients who cannot undergo surgery. N Engl J Med 2010;363:1597–607.
67 Lefèvre T, Kappetein AP, Wolner E, et al.; on behalf of the PARTNER EU Investigator Group. One year follow-up of the multi-centre European PARTNER transcatheter heart valve study. Eur Heart J 2011;32:148–57.
68 Leon MB, Piazza N, Nikolsky E, et al. Standardized endpoint definitions for transcatheter aortic valve implantation clinical trials: a consensus report from the Valve Academic Research Consortium. Eur Heart J 2011;32:205–17.
69 Seiffert M, Franzen O, Conradi L, et al. Series of transcatheter valve-in-valve implantations in high-risk patients with degenerated bioprostheses in aortic and mitral position. Catheter Cardiovasc Interv 2010;76:608–15.
70 Webb JG, Wood DA, Ye J, et al. Transcatheter valve-in-valve implantation for failed bioprosthetic heart valves. Circulation 2010;121:1848–57.
71 Kempfert J, Blumenstein J, Chu MW, et al. Minimally invasive off-pump valve-in-a-ring implantation: the atrial transcatheter approach for re-operative mitral valve replacement after failed repair. Eur J Cardiothorac Surg 2009;35:965–9.
72 Schmidt D, Dijkman PE, Driessen-Mol A, et al. Minimally invasive implantation of living tissue engineered heart valves. J Am Coll Cardiol 2010;56:510–20.

Videoclips

This chapter contains the following videoclips:

Video 15.1 Animation Edwards Ascendra 2 system.

Video 15.2 Case presentations: Edwards Ascendra 2 transapical heart valve (Sapien XT 23 mm).

Video 15.3 Case presentations: Medtronic Engager transapical heart valve (Engager 26 mm).

Video 15.4 Animation of the transapical deployment of the JenaValve.

They can be accessed at www.wiley.com/go/valverepair.

16

CHAPTER 16

Axillary/subclavian access for transcather aortic valve replacement

Gilles Lemesle[1], Arnaud Sudre[1] & Thomas Modine[2]

[1] Service de Cardiologie B et Centre Hémodynamique, Pôle de Cardiologie, Hôpital Cardiologique, CHRU de Lille, France

[2] Service de Chirurgie Cardio-vasculaire, Pôle de Chirurgie Cardio-vasculaire, Hôpital Cardiologique, CHRU de Lille, France

Introduction

Patient selection plays a crucial role in the success of transcather aortic valve replacement (TAVR) [1–5]. Vascular access is of major interest and patient selection requires a complete study of the different arterial access points. Today, the trans-femoral route is recommended to be the first vascular access of choice in all TAVR procedures. In some patients, the ilio-femoral artery and/or abdominal aorta anatomy does not allow TAVR through the femoral approach. Small peripheral arteries (diameter less than 6 mm), severe peripheral artery disease, and severe ilio-femoral and/or aorta tortuosities may render the ilio-femoral approach difficult or even impossible (Fig. 16.1). Indeed, these parameters greatly increase the risk of implantation failure or vascular injury that contributes significantly to mortality and morbidity associated with transfemoral TAVR [1–5].

Although there has been a reduction in the sheath size for the different available percutaneous aortic valve implantation (PAVI) devices, they are still relatively big. The Edwards Sapien Retroflex system is a 18 French or 24 Fr delivery catheter system [1–3]. As shown in Fig. 16.2, the Medtronic CoreValve revalving system (Minneapolis, MN) is a smaller 18 Fr delivery catheter system [4,5] that subsequently permits the use of the axillary/subclavian access as a second option when the ilio-femoral access is either impossible or too risky [6–11]. Up to date, little is known about the safety of this approach for PAVI procedures compared with the ilio-femoral access The chapter reviews the technical issues related to this specific access route.

General considerations

Since the first case of TAVR through the axillary/subclavian access with the Medtronic CoreValve revalving system was published in 2008 [11], the technique has continued to evolve with a rapid degree of adoption [6–10]. Assessing the safety and the feasibility of the axillary/subclavian route requires, however, a complete analysis from the skin to the aortic valve. In contrast to the ilio-femoral arteries, axillary and subclavian arteries are usually relatively free of disease even in elderly people and are frequently good-sized vessels. Axillary and subclavian arteries fulfill anatomic criteria in most patients eligible for

Endovascular and Hybrid Therapies for Structural Heart and Aortic Disease, First Edition.
Edited by Jacques Kpodonu and Raoul Bonan.

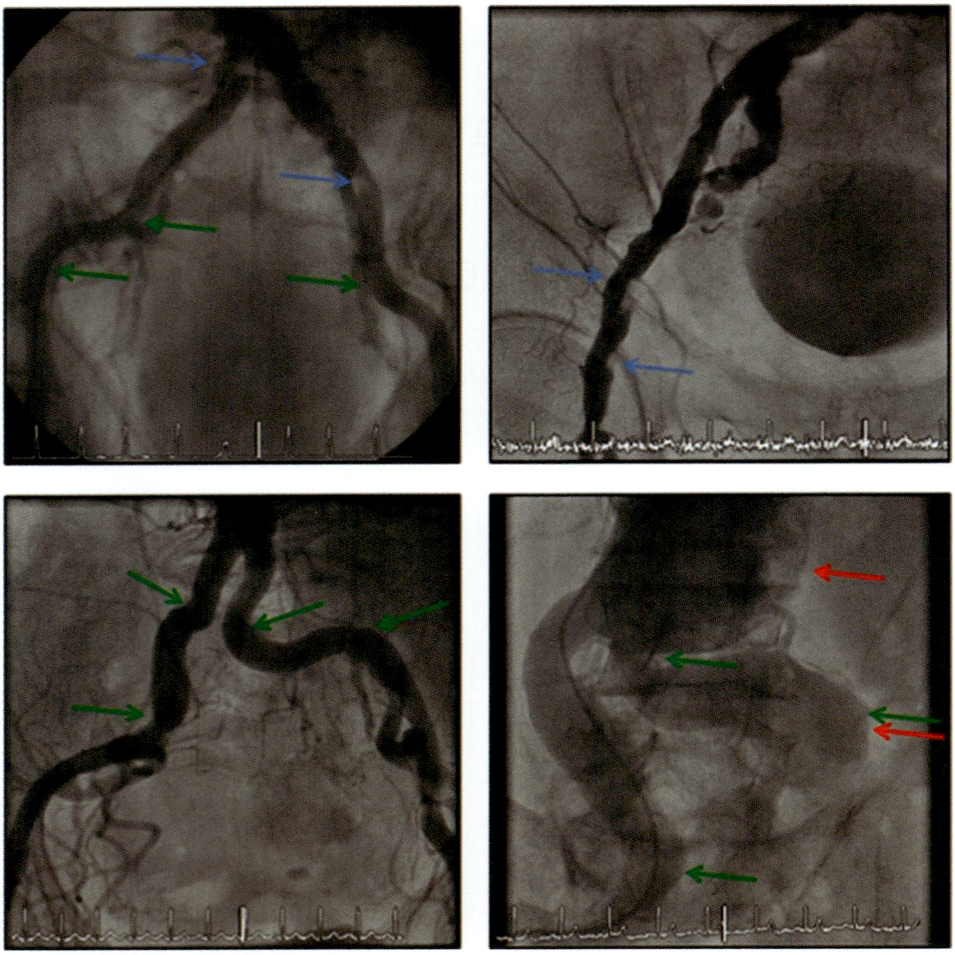

Fig. 16.1 Examples of ilio-femoral artery and/or abdominal aorta anatomies that do not allow percutaneous aortic valve implantation. Blue arrows indicate significant atherosclerotic disease reducing the lumen to less than 6 mm in diameter. Green arrows indicate severe tortuosities. Red arrows indicate severe artery aneurysm.

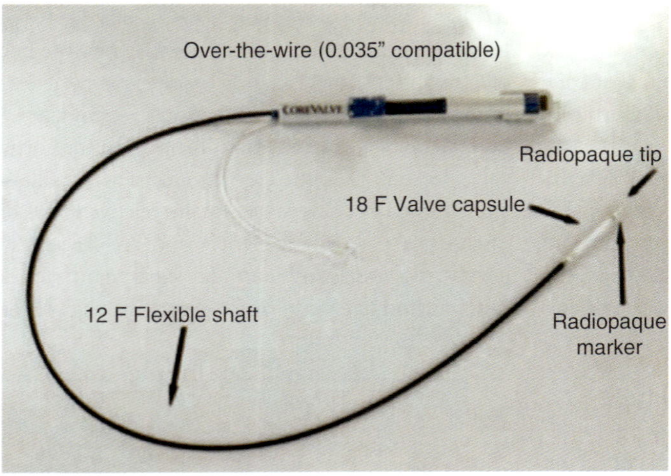

Fig. 16.2 Medtronic CoreValve revalving system, an 18 Fr delivery catheter system.

TAVR. Just as a reminder, there are some anatomic criteria that exclude the axillary/subclavian route with regard to the risk of vessel injury.

Contraindications, as for the ilio-femoral route, include:

- Vessel diameter <6 mm.
- Severe tortuosity.
- Severe disease and/or circumferential calcifications.

Patient selection and imaging

Parameters to be assessed for TAVR (such as patient comorbidities, aortic valve anatomy, aortic root and ascending aorta anatomy, coronary artery disease, left ventricular function and volume, etc.), have to be analyzed prior to any PAVI procedure through the axillary/subclavian route.

Skin assessment

A simple physical examination is required in order to establish local skin integrity and to eliminate any local infection process and/or skin injury. In addition, operators have to make sure that no obstacle, such as pacemakers, will make it impossible for surgical access, hence a careful assessment of the clavicular is needed.

(a)

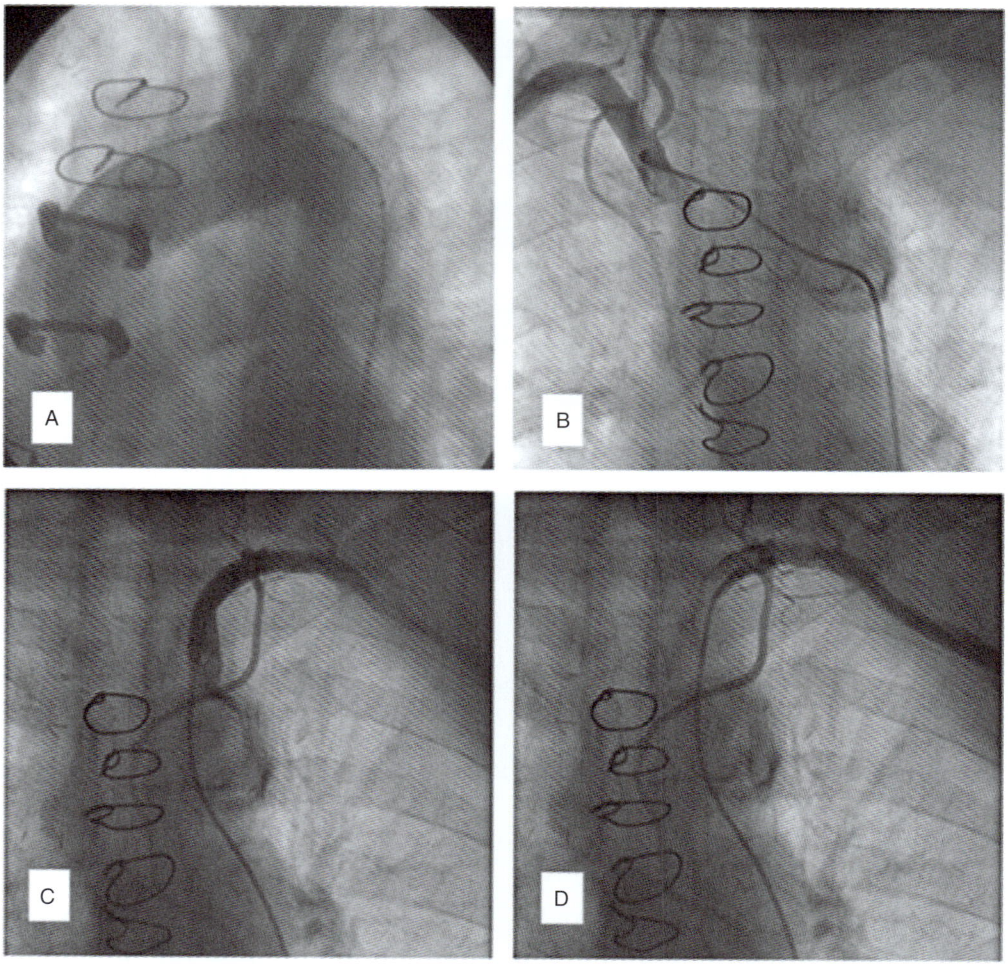

Fig. 16.3 (a) Examples of assessment of the subclavian arteries by angiogram: A, aortic arch angiogram allowing a perfect analysis of the origin of the left subclavian artery; B, angiogram of the right subclavian artery; C and D, angiogram of the left subclavian artery. (b) Examples of assessment of the subclavian arteries by a CT scanner. (c) Examples of assessment of the subclavian arteries by MRI.

(b)

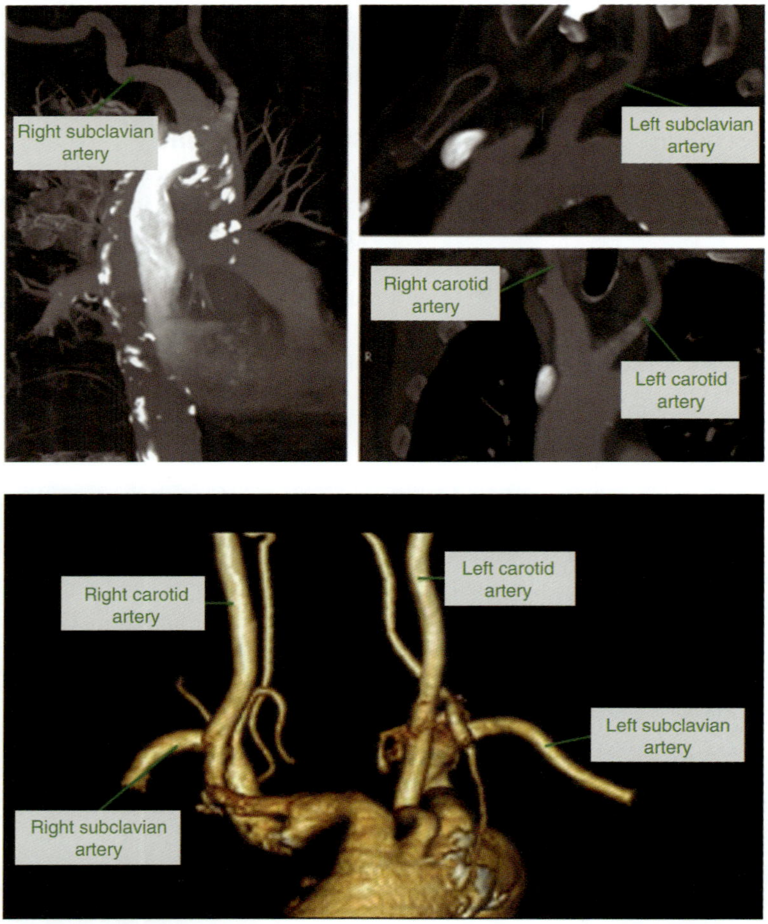

(c)

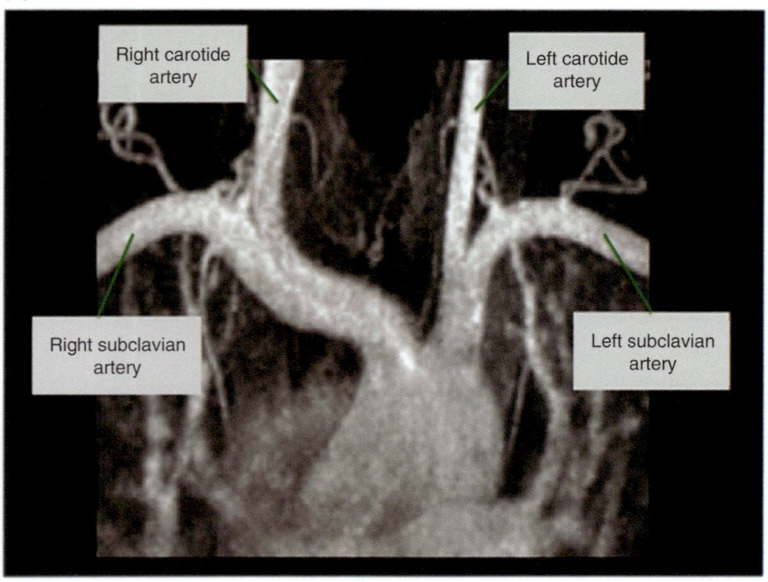

Fig. 16.3 *(Continued).*

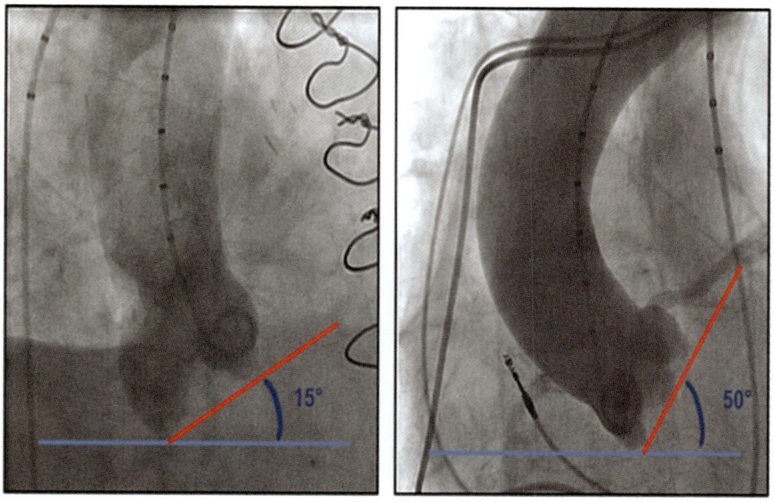

Fig. 16.4 Examples of angle between the aortic valve annulus (red line) and the horizontal line (blue line).

Vessel assessment

Vessel assessment is one of the major points required prior to considering a patient for TAVR. Similar to assessment of the ilio-femoral arteries, angiograms (Fig. 16.3a), computed tomography (CT) scans (Fig. 16.3b), and/or magnitude resonance imaging (MRI) (Fig. 16.3c) provide accurate data on the diameter, tortuosities, and degree of disease and calcifications of the axillary and subclavian arteries. Special care should be taken to look at the origin of the subclavian artery and to any bifurcations, where significant disease and/or calcifications are more frequently found. In addition, the relationship to the vertebral, carotid, and mammary arteries has to be clearly individualized, especially in patients with patent graft.

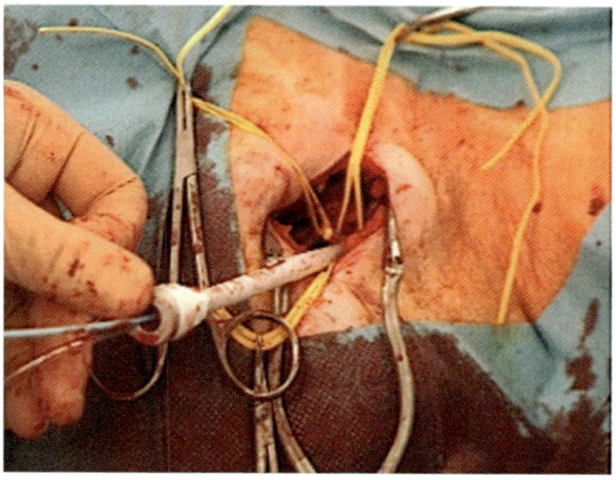

Fig. 16.5 Left subclavian surgical access (infraclavicular incision), with an 18 Fr sheath insertion.

Although the left axillary/subclavian artery is the preferred route, the right axillary/subclavian artery is also feasible and safe. The right axillary/subclavian artery access, however, needs additional anatomic criteria to be checked. Due to the wire and valve catheter stiffness, the valve catheter tends to be at a vertical angle to the native aortic valve annulus, especially when the right axillary/subclavian artery is used as access. Other authors have reported that TAVR through the right axillary/subclavian artery is almost impossible when the aortic root becomes more horizontal (i.e. the aortic valve annulus becomes more vertical). An angle greater than 25° between the aortic valve annulus plan and the horizontal line disqualifies the use of the right axillary/subclavian approach (Fig. 16.4) [7,9].

Surgical access

As direct manual compression is ineffective for axillary/subclavian arteries in case of closure failure, percutaneous access is not recommended and a surgical access is mandatory.

The axillary/subclavian access is very familiar to cardiovascular surgeons. The vessels are usually approached through an infraclavicular incision

(Fig. 16.5). In patients with an implanted pacemaker in that area, supraclavicular incision could be used, taking into consideration the proximity to the nervous brachial plexus origin. The infraclavicular incision is well tolerated and causes little discomfort, thus allowing very early mobilization. Most of the time, the axillary/subclavian access is done under general anesthesia. Such a vascular access could, however, be done under local anesthesia in an experienced team.

Advantages of the use of the axillary/subclavian access

Most axillary and subclavian arteries are good-sized vessels and are often free of significant disease and calcifications, even in sicker and older people. They subsequently fulfill the implantation criteria in most of the patients.

Secondly, the shorter distance between the arterial access point and the aortic valve compared to the ilio-femoral access usually provides better stability of the delivery catheter. This improves the accuracy of positioning the valve and reduces procedure time (Fig. 16.6). An optimal position of the prosthetic valve is of major interest to reduce the risk of valve embolization, para-valvular insufficiency, and coronary artery obstruction.

Thirdly, axillary and/or subclavian artery access and repair are familiar to all cardiovascular surgeons, with a limited risk of vascular complications and local bleeding.

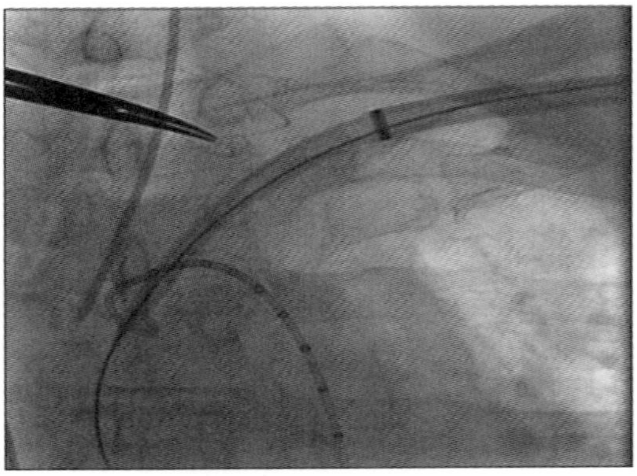

Fig. 16.6 An 18 Fr sheath in place in the left subclavian artery, with a short distance between the end of the sheath and the aortic valve annulus allowing a perfect positioning of the valve.

Limitations of the axillary/subclavian access

Similar to the ilio-femoral route, vessel diameter <6 mm, severe tortuosity, severe disease, and circumferential calcifications are contraindications. In addition, the presence of a pacemaker may increase the risk of pacemaker damage and/or infection, hence it is recommend that the other subclavian artery be used instead. Finally, the presence of a patent and functional internal mammary artery graft is also reported as a potential contraindication to the use of the axillary/subclavian route because of the risk of graft occlusion or injury.

In the presence of a patent graft, some criteria have to be strictly respected with regard to the risk of axillary and/or subclavian artery dissection or ostial graft occlusion. Should the axillary/subclavian access be used an artery diameter of >6.5 mm (rather than 6 mm) is needed, there should be an absence of circumferential calcifications or extensive atherosclerotic disease close to the graft origin, and an absence of atherosclerotic lesions requiring peripheral balloon angioplasty.

Conclusions

Among patients eligible for PAVI, some do not meet the criteria for the transfemoral approach. The Medtronic CoreValve revalving system is an 18 Fr delivery catheter system that allows axillary/subclavian access as a second option when ilio-femoral access is either impossible or too risky. The axillary/subclavian approach is indeed feasible and safe for TAVR using the Medtronic CoreValve revalving system allowing especially perfect stability of the device and an easier valve positioning compared to the transfemoral route. It requires, however, an experienced team and a complete check-up from the skin to the aortic valve in order to eliminate all limitations and/or contraindications of the technique.

References

1 Cribier A, Eltchaninoff H, Bash A, et al. Percutaneous transcatheter implantation of an aortic valve prosthesis for calcific aortic stenosis: first human case description. Circulation 2002;106:3006–8.

2 Cribier A, Eltchaninoff H, Tron C, et al. Treatment of calcific aortic stenosis with the percutaneous heart

valve: mid-term follow-up from the initial feasibility studies: the French experience. J Am Coll Cardiol 2006;47:1214–23.

3 Cribier A, Eltchaninoff H, Tron C, et al. Early experience with percutaneous transcatheter implantation of heart valve prosthesis for the treatment of end-stage inoperable patients with calcific aortic stenosis. J Am Coll Cardiol 2004;43:698–703.

4 Grube E, Schuler G, Buellesfeld L, et al. Percutaneous aortic valve replacement for severe aortic stenosis in high-risk patients using the second- and current third-generation self-expanding CoreValve prosthesis: device success and 30-day clinical outcome. J Am Coll Cardiol 2007;50:69–76.

5 Piazza N, Grube E, Gerckens U, et al. Procedural and 30-day outcomes following transcatheter aortic valve implantation using the third generation (18 Fr) corevalve revalving system: results from the multicentre, expanded evaluation registry 1-year following CE mark approval. EuroIntervention 2008;4:242–9.

6 Asgar AW, Mullen MJ, Delahunty N, et al. Transcatheter aortic valve intervention through the axillary artery for the treatment of severe aortic stenosis. J Thorac Cardiovasc Surg 2009;137:773–5.

7 De Robertis F, Asgar A, Davies S, et al. The left axillary artery – a new approach for transcatheter aortic valve implantation. Eur J Cardiothorac Surg 2009;36:807–12.

8 Fraccaro C, Napodano M, Tarantini G, et al. Expanding the eligibility for transcatheter aortic valve implantation the trans-subclavian retrograde approach using: the III generation CoreValve revalving system. JACC Cardiovasc Interv 2009;2:828–33.

9 Modine T, Obadia JF, Choukroun E, et al. Transcutaneous aortic valve implantation using the axillary/subclavian access: feasibility and early clinical outcomes. J Thorac Cardiovasc Surg 2011;141(2):487–9.

10 Petronio AS, De Carlo M, Bedogni F, et al. Safety and efficacy of the subclavian approach for transcatheter aortic valve implantation with the CoreValve Revalving System. Circ Cardiovasc Interv 2010;3(4):359–66.

11 Ruge H, Lange R, Bleiziffer S, et al. First successful aortic valve implantation with the CoreValve ReValving System via right subclavian artery access: a case report. Heart Surg Forum 2008;11:E323–4.

17

CHAPTER 17

Aortic valve replacement and transvalvular aortic valve replacement

Thierry Folliguet[1] & François Laborde[2]

[1] Pôle Territorial Lorrain Chirurgie Cardiaque Vasculaire et Transplantation Institut, Lorrain du Coeur et des Vaisseaux Louis Mathieu Centre Hospitalier U, Vandoeuvre, Les Nancy Cedex 54511, France

[2] Department of Cardiovascular Surgery, Institut Mutualiste Montsouris, Paris, France

Introduction

Aortic valve replacement with biological heart valves is the treatment of choice for aortic valve stenosis when it is symptomatic or with severe aortic stenosis ($\leq 0.6\,cm^2/m^2$), or with left ventricular dysfunction for older patients [1,2]. However, percutaneous valve replacement with a sutureless valve has been performed since 2002 [3], and is proposed for high-risk patients. By introducing a less invasive technique it is hypothesized that mortality and survival would be lower than when treated by conventional aortic valve replacement. Recently, sutureless aortic valve replacements have been performed through sternotomy with excellent results. In this article we will discuss the different options available and the current results of all the available techniques.

Porcine bioprostheses were originally used and progressively abandoned due to their poor long-term resistance with high levels of valvular obstruction [4,5]. Pericardial bioprostheses were therefore developed and the first generation of these had a high rate of structural deterioration, leading to the discontinuance of their use [6], and modifications were made in the design and manufacturing methods [7–9].

Many clinical reports have shown excellent reports with pericardial valves with very low gradient and improved long-term durability compared with porcine bioprostheses, with results up to 20 years [10–18]. However, all these valves are mounted on a stent with a Dacron cuff which allows the prosthesis to be sutured to the aortic annulus. In order to improve hemodynamics, especially in a small annulus (19–21 mm), stentless bioprostheses have been developed [19–22]. After removing the entire calcified aortic leaflet, the prosthesis is inserted with a single or double line of sutures placed in the annulus and on the aortic wall [20]. These valves provide a greater effective orifice area and a lower gradient for the same annular diameter [21,23–27], without any changes in survival at long-term follow-up [28].

Development of prostheses

Therefore, in order to simplify surgical implantation sutureless prostheses were designed. Two different prostheses have been implanted surgically either through a sternotomy or a mini-incision. These are the 3f Enable (ATS, Minneapolis, MN) and the Perceval S (Sorin, Saluggia, Italy).

The 3f Enable consists of a tubular structure assembled from three equal sections of equine

Endovascular and Hybrid Therapies for Structural Heart and Aortic Disease, First Edition.
Edited by Jacques Kpodonu and Raoul Bonan.

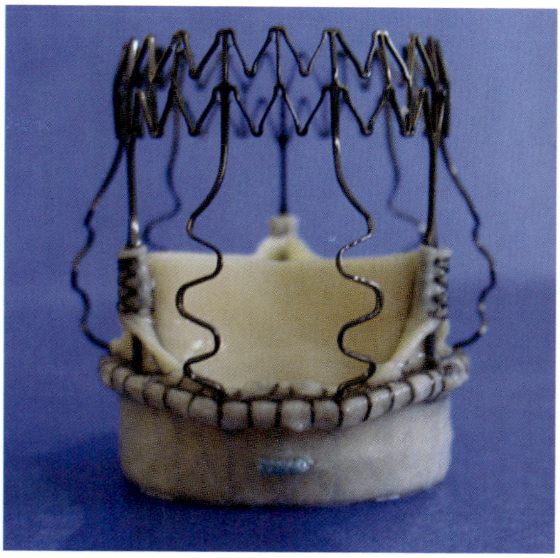

Fig. 17.1 Perceval S prosthesis.

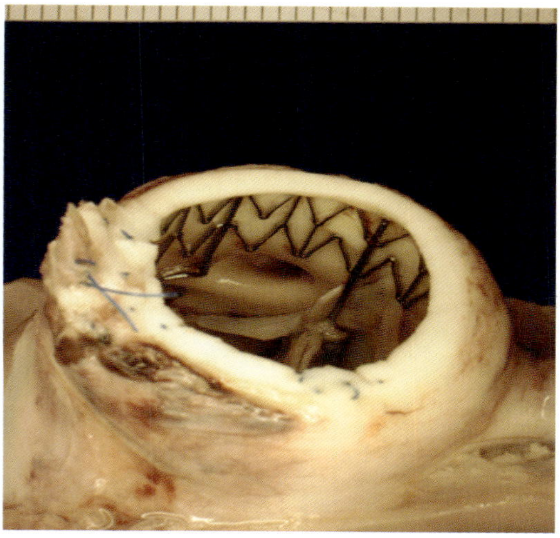

Fig. 17.2 Coronary orifice after implantation of the Perceval S prosthesis.

pericardial tissue mounted on a self-expanding nitinol frame [29]. The nitinol frame contributes to the fixation of the device in the deployed location by virtue of outward radial forces inherent in the nitinol material. A polyester flange has been incorporated at the inflow aspect to minimize the potential of paravalvular leaks and migration. There are currently four sizes available: 21, 23, 25, and 27 mm.

The Perceval S valve (Fig. 17.1) is a prosthetic valve comprising a functional component in bovine pericardium fixed in a metal cage made of a superelastic alloy. The cage design is characterized by two ring segments, on the proximal and distal end, and a number of connecting elements designed to support the valve and to allow prosthesis anchoring to the aortic root, in the sinuses of Valsalva (Fig. 17.2) [30]. The material used for the cage is an equiatomic alloy of nitinol. This material is able to accept strong deformation and return to its original shape after the force is removed. Therefore the cage can be compressed for the implantation and is then released to reach its final diameter. The functional valve component is a bovine pericardium valve, fixed into the cage by sutures (Fig. 17.3).

For the initial study two valve sizes (21 and 23 mm) were available for annulus sizes 19–23 mm. Both these valves were implanted with cardiopulmonary bypass through a surgical incision under general anesthesia. The diseased native aortic valve was removed and the aortic annulus completely decalcified.

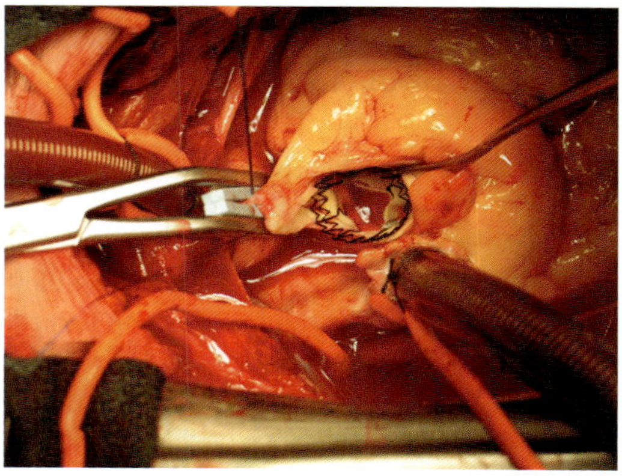

Fig. 17.3 Perceval S during implantation, after deployment.

Transcatheter aortic valve replacement (TAVR) is an expanding therapeutic option for high-risk patients who are not considered to be suitable candidates for surgery [3]. There are currently two devices that can be implanted: the Edwards Sapien valve (Edwards Lifesciences, Irvine, CA) and the CoreValve revalving system (Medtronic, Minneapolis, MN).

The CoreValve aortic bioprosthesis (Fig. 17.4) is the third generation of a trileaflet, porcine pericardial tissue valve, mounted and sutured in a self-expanding nitinol frame, which is 53 or 55 mm long, depending on the valve size. There are currently two valve sizes for annuli, from 20 to 27 mm. The frame is

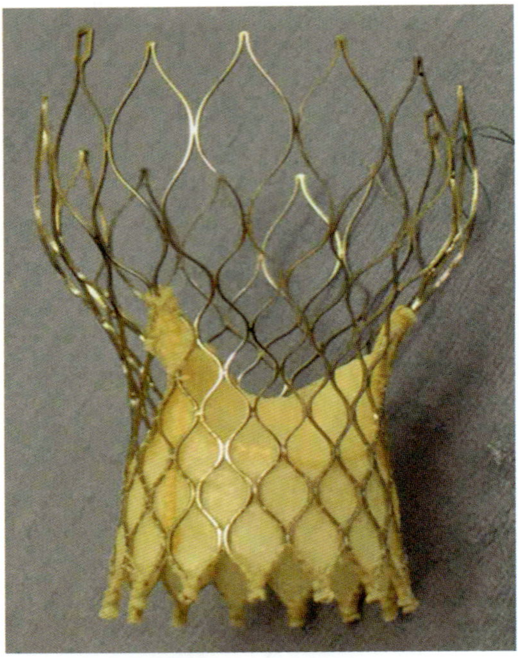

Fig. 17.4 CoreValve aortic bioprosthesis.

divided into three distinct zones of radial force. The lower portion has a high radial force to expand and exclude the calcified leaflets and to avoid recoil. This portion extends into the left ventricular outflow tract. The middle portion features high loop strength and is the area of valvular attachment. The frame is constrained in order to avoid the coronary arteries. The upper portion of the frame has low radial force and is flared outward to make contact with the ascending aorta, which serves to align the valve to blood flow. The porcine pericardial tissue is hand sutured to the nitinol stent and chemically processed using standard tissue fixation.

The CoreValve is implanted in the annulus with a valve portion supra-annular. The implantation is performed transfemorally (or trans-subclavian) via an 18 Fr (6 mm) delivery catheter. The technique is performed in the cath lab or hybrid room under echocardiographic and radiologic guidance without cardiopulmonary bypass, with or without general anesthesia. The aortic valve is first dilated with an aortic balloon under rapid pacing followed by the deployment of the prosthesis.

The other device is the Edwards Sapien valve (Fig. 17.5) which consists of three pericardial leaflets, initially equine and currently bovine,

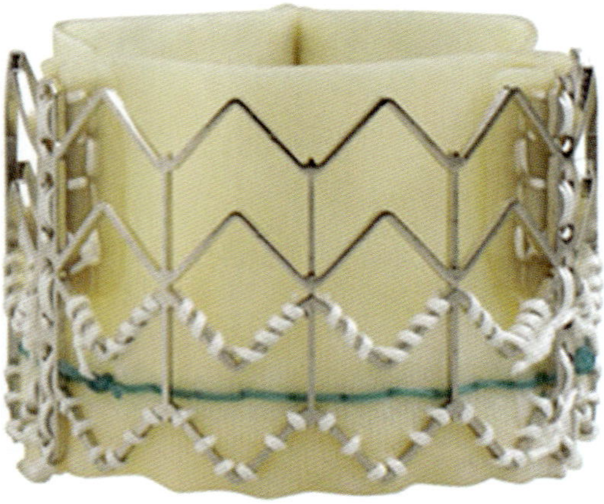

Fig. 17.5 Edwards Sapien valve.

mounted within a tubular, slotted, stainless steel, balloon-expandable stent. It is currently available in 23 and 26 mm sizes, necessitating, for the transfemoral approach, respectively, 22 and 24 Fr introducer sheaths; for the transapical approach this measurement was 33 Fr and is now 26 Fr. The Edwards transcatheter valve is a balloon-expandable stented valve, which can be placed either transfemorally or transapically. The valve is placed intra-annular and currently two sizes are available: 23 and 26 mm.

Results

Transcatheter valve replacement

Since the first in-man surgery, performed by Alain Cribier in 2002, over 5000 high-risks patients with severe symptomatic aortic stenosis have been treated using TAVR [31–35]. Patients treated with this technique are usually older with high comorbidities (Logistic EuroScore ≥20%) or with contra-indications for surgery. The procedural success varies between 78% and 100%, but varies with experience [33,35–38]. The mortality at 30 days ranges from 5% to 20%, with various complications such as myocardial infarction in 2–11%, strokes in 3–9%, vascular complications in 10–15%, and atrioventricular block in 4–30% [34,35]. Mild to moderate aortic regurgitation, usually paravalvular, is seen in 50% of cases. Long-term survival rates up to 1 year are reported in a limited number of patients, with mortality from 10% to 20% in the transfemoral approach, and 26–42% in the transapical approach, reflecting the higher comorbidity in the latter group [33,34,36–38]. The majority of deaths are due to comorbidities.

Analysis of the devices in patients who died during the first year post implant, shows fibrin deposition and inflammatory response early after valve implantation followed by late neointimal coverage with progressive regression of the inflammatory response over time. The results of the transapical approach are somewhat different [37, 38]. Although less patients are being treated with this approach it is usually offered when the transfemoral approach is contraindicated, such as in severe peripheral vascular disease. The implantation success rate is around 90%, with a rate of perioperative conversion of 9–12% depending on the experience of the team. The mortality is higher, at 13–18%, reflecting higher risk patients, but the stroke rate is less (0–6%) than with the transfemoral approach, probably due to less manipulation in the aortic arch.

Sutureless surgical valves

The 3f Enable aortic valve has been successfully implanted in 32 patients [39] after being tested in animals [40]. This included patients with isolated aortic stenosis or with concomitant cardiac pathologies. The mean age was 78 ± 3 years with a mean Logistic EuroScore of 13.7; the Society of Thoracic Surgeons (STS) score revealed a mean risk for mortality of 16.4 ± 6.4%. Thirty patients had a successful implantation of the device, with one patient showing mild paravalvular leak. The transvalvular gradients at discharge were 9 mmHg and remained low at 6 months. It is of interest that the gradients did not correlate to the size of the valve prosthesis, even months after surgery.

Between April 2007 and February 2008, the Perceval S valve was implanted in 30 high-risk patients. All patients had significant aortic valve disease and 14 had concomitant coronary artery disease (Table 17.1). Patients had to be older than 75 years old and had a EuroScore >5 (Table 17.2). Exclusion criteria included reoperation. The institutional Review Boards of the University Hospitals gave approval for this study. All the patients gave informed consent. There were no intra-procedural deaths (Table 17.3). The valves were firmly positioned under visual control in all the patients. Fourteen patients received concomitant coronary revascularization.

Table 17.1 Indications and contraindications for the sutureless Perceval S.

Indications	*Contraindications*
Age ≥75 years Aortic valve stenosis at high surgical risk and candidate for a standard surgical intervention of aortic valve replacement with biological prosthesis NYHA functional class III and IV Small and calcific aortic root/anulus	Aneurysmal dilation or dissection of the ascending aorta requiring correction Aortic annulus size after decalcification, not suitable for a 21 or 23 mm valve implantation (by direct intraoperative measurement)

NYHA, New York Heart Association.

Table 17.2 Patients' characteristics for the Perceval S initial study.

Patients characteristics	
Age (years)	81 (76–88)
Sex	22 female, 8 male
NYHA status	Class III, 28 patients (93.3%); class IV, 2 patients (26.7%)
Aortic valve pathology:	
Aortic stenosis	23 (76.7%)
Combined pathology	7 (23.3%)
Coronary artery disease	14
EuroScore (Logistic) (%)	12.01 ± 8.29 (5.7–49.94)
Ejection fraction (%)	61 ± 11 (45–79)
Height (cm)	160 ± 7.5 (147–178)
Weight (kg)	71 ± 15(47–110)
Body mass index	1.7 ± 0.2 (1.31–2.17)

NYHA, New York Heart Association.

One patient died during hospital stay. Autopsy, however, revealed no valve-related pathologies; the valve was seated appropriately inside the aortic annulus with patent coronary ostia. Two patients died within the 3-month follow-up, one due to an accident, the other due to multiorgan failure. Complications within 1 month of follow-up were: cardiac tamponade due to mediastinal bleeding (n = 1), an atrioventricular conduction block (n = 1), wound infection (n = 1), and gastrointestinal bleeding (n = 1). There was one case of peripheral thromboembolism. All patients received an echocardiography control before discharge. All

Table 17.3 Intraoperative characteristics for the Perceval S study.

Intra/postoperative data	*With concomitant CABG (n = 14)*	*Isolated AVR (n = 16)*
CPB time (min)	73 (41–130)	46 (34–60)
X clamp time (min)	42 (21–79)	29 (23–55)
Valve size (mm)		21 mm: 11 patients; 23 mm: 19 patients

AVR, aortic valve replacement; CABG, coronary artery bypass graft; CPB, cardiopulmonary bypass.

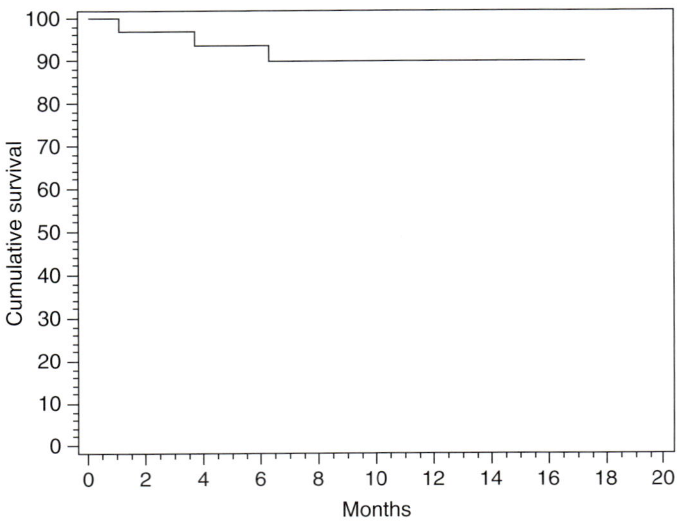

Fig. 17.6 Survival of patients in the Perceval S study.

surviving patients showed a good functioning aortic valve prosthesis, with two cases of mild paravalvular leakage intravalvular and two cases of mild paravalvular insufficiency (Fig. 17.6). No migration or dislodgement of the prostheses have occurred during further follow-up. Transvalvular gradients were low up to 1-year follow-up (Fig. 17.7) and effective orifice area increased from 0.9 to 1.6 cm^2 (Fig. 17.8). All patients improved after surgery as assessed by New York Heart Association (NYHA) class up to 12 months follow-up (Table 17.4).

Discussion

In view of these published results it is unclear if TAVR is a safe procedure compared with surgical aortic valve replacement. In the recent series the 1-month mortality rates range from 6% to 7% in transfemoral and 11% to 19% in transapical approaches. It is unclear what the operative mortality of these patients would have been if operated on conventionally, since many reports have shown that EuroScore overpredicts mortality. It is generally admitted that EuroScore overestimates the risk by a factor of 2–3, with the STS score being more predictive of the risk [41]. On the other hand, recent reports on surgical outcome in such high-risk populations of elderly patients has shown that aortic valve replacement can safely be performed, applying recent advances in cardio-surgical techniques. These include minimal access to valve replacement as well as optimization of myocardial preservation. Recent published series have shown that an operative mortality of 2% can be attained in octogenarians [42–44].

Several issues are still of concern, including how crimping of the valves affects long-term durability. How does bovine pericardium behave in the long term? How does para-aortic insufficiency affect the ventricle, especially in small hypertrophic ventricle? These interesting questions have been addressed by Azadani et al. [45] recently. They showed that substantial energy loss during diastole occurs due to transcatheter aortic valve (TAV)

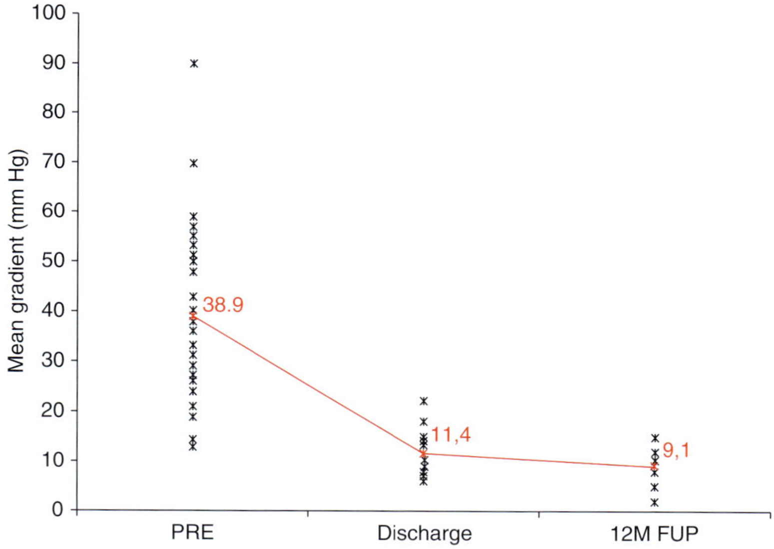

Fig. 17.7 Perceval S study: gradients pre- and postoperative at discharge and at 12-month follow-up (FUP).

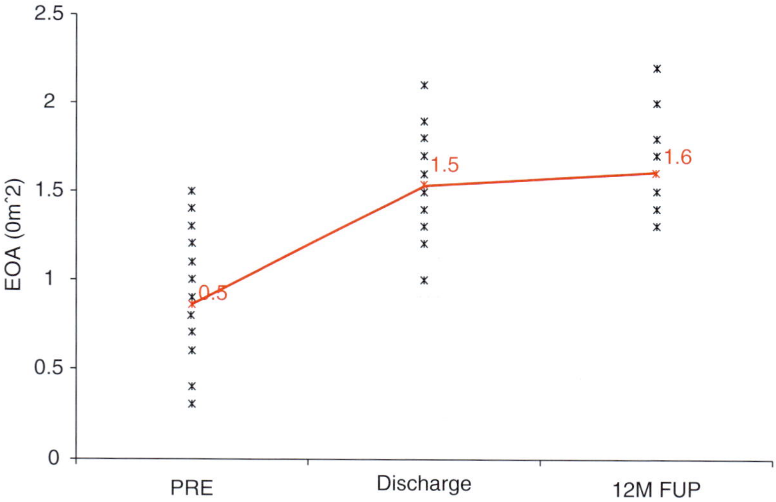

Fig. 17.8 Perceval S. Effective orifice area (EOA) at discharge and at 12-month follow-up (FUP).

Table 17.4 NYHA class during follow-up in patients in the Perceval S study.

NYHA class	*Preoperative*	*6-month follow-up*	*12-month follow-up*
Class I	–	60%	60%
Class II	–	34%	40%
Class III	93.3%	4%	–
Class IV	6.7%	–	–

NYHA, New York Heart Association.

paravalvular leakage [45]. This imposes a significantly higher workload on the left ventricle than on the surgical aortic valve replacement of equivalent bioprosthetic size. To reduce the incidence and severity of paravalvular leak, the oversizing technique (i.e. the choice of a prosthesis size of at least 2 mm more than that of the aortic annulus diameter) has been proposed and proved to be effective [32]. However, oversizing can still lead to paravalvular leakage [32] and can also be associated with prosthetic mismatch leading to high postoperative gradients [46].

Also, in vitro studies have shown that stenosis leads to significant forces of TAV during systole with increased shear stress [47].

Why is there such a high incidence of heart block and how is that altering cardiac physiology compared to a normal sinus rhythm heart with a conventional bioprosthesis? Most of the devices are not optimally deployed and not in a circular fashion. How does that affect long-term durability, since we know flow turbulence causes calcification and early pericardial tear? Finally, what significance has mismatch on the medium and long-term effect? Several in vitro studies have shown that a small TAV (19 and 21 mm) can generate a high pressure gradient creating hemodynamic complications [46], and that shear stresses on the TAV were greatest during peak systolic flow with stress concentrations on the tips of the leaflets [47].

Based on the data available to date, this percutaneous approach has to be reserved for high-risk patients [48–50]. In all studies sutureless aortic valves were implanted following thorough surgical removal of the diseased valve, as done with conventional valve replacement. The approach therefore allows for a sutureless valve implantation under direct visual control. Using these techniques, the first experience in 30 patients at three different locations in Europe, would suggest an extremely secure valve positioning with no problems of diminished blood flow to the coronary ostia. Also, these valves are associated with minimal incidence of paravalvular leakage as seen in both series. In 14 of the patients described, a simultaneous coronary bypass grafting could be done without adding any risk to the patient.

With these significant advances compared with conventional valve implantation, including suture anchoring of the valve, the rate of stroke as well as the rate of dialysis was extremely low. These are two main risk factors for postoperative morbidity and mortality that obviously can be reduced by applying this new technique.

The data acquired in this small series of patients admitted for aortic valve replacement clearly indicate sutureless aortic valve implantation to be a future asset of valve implantation [30]. With an operative mortality of 3.3% in this clearly at-risk population it does favorably compare to interventional techniques including both the transfemoral and the transapical approach. It also allows for simultaneous coronary bypass grafting, thereby adding to a broader spectrum of indications when compared with interventional techniques. The data also suggest that proper explantation of a diseased valve followed by sutureless implantation may result in a better outcome when compared with balloon dilation of a diseased severely calcified aortic valve. Removing the annulus and suturing the prosthesis can be performed in most patients with excellent results, a low incidence of strokes (1–3%) and of atrioventricular block, and minimal paravalvular insufficiency [42].

Safety concerns

There are a number of theoretical concerns with the sutureless bioprosthesis. Since all of these devices require crimping the bioprosthesis, questions remains concerning long-term failure of these valves compared to other bioprostheses mounted on a rigid stent and not crimped. Secondary endpoints should include valve area and transvalvular gradient measurement, paravalvular leaks, device migration, emergency valve-in-valve implantation, conversion to conventional surgery, and vascular complications.

A few cases have shown fibrin deposition and an inflammatory response early after valve implantation, followed by neointimal coverage with progressive regression of the inflammatory response over time.

Surgical aortic valve replacement represents the gold standard of treatment in patients with aortic valve stenosis. Often, symptomatic patients have significant comorbidities. In such subsets of candidates, conventional surgical replacement may pose a high perioperative risk. Nevertheless, modern techniques of aortic valve implantation need to be measured against the background of most recently published series of conventional surgery in the subgroups of patients [51].

Conclusions

Further experience is needed to find out the potential of these devices for either an open or a minimal invasive approach. Furthermore the sutureless devices appear to be ideal for patients with severe calcification of the aortic root and/or patients requiring concomitant procedures in whom a reduced bypass time is mandatory.

At this point, however, careful patient selection and echocardiographic assessment is crucial in choosing a device. Correct sizing of the valve is critical to minimize paravalvular leakage and this should be performed with transesophageal echocardiography.

Also long-term studies are needed to evaluate echocardiographic results of this new prosthesis. Surgery should be offered to patients with no contraindications since it offers better results and long-term survival, while TAVR should be performed in high-risk patients after careful assessment in order to choose the best approach (transfemoral, transapical or transaxillary).

Sutureless bioprostheses represent an extremely promising field. When implanted surgically (Video 17.1) they allow a marked decrease in circulatory assistance time as well as cardiac arrest, which is extremely important in elderly and high-risk patients. The transcatheter approach of implanting these devices can be offered to very high-risk patients or to those with contraindications for surgery.

References

1 Bonow RO, Carabello BA, Kanu C, et al. ACC/AHA 2006 guidelines for the management of patients with valvular heart disease: a report of the American College of Cardiology/American Heart Association Task Force on Practice Guidelines (writing committee to revise the 1998 Guidelines for the Management of Patients With Valvular Heart Disease): developed in collaboration with the Society of Cardiovascular Anesthesiologists: endorsed by the Society for Cardiovascular Angiography and Interventions and the Society of Thoracic Surgeons. Circulation 2006;114:e84–231.

2 Vahanian A, Baumgartner H, Bax J, et al. Guidelines on the management of valvular heart disease: the Task Force on the Management of Valvular Heart Disease of the European Society of Cardiology. Eur Heart J 2007;28:230–68.

3 Cribier A, Eltchaninoff H, Bash A, et al. Percutaneous transcatheter implantation of aortic valve prosthesis for calcific aortic stenosis: first human case description. Circulation 2002;106:3006–8.

4 Jamieson WR, Burr LH, Munro AI, et al. Carpentier-Edwards standard porcine bioprosthesis: a 21-year experience. Ann Thorac Surg 1998;66:S40–3.

5 Eric Jamieson WR, Marchand MA, Pelletier CL, et al. Structural valve deterioration in mitral replacement surgery: comparison of Carpentier-Edwards supra-annular porcine and perimount pericardial bioprostheses. J Thorac Cardiovasc Surg 1999;118:297–304.

6 Grabenwoger M, Grimm M, Leukauf C, et al. Failure mode of a new pericardial valve prosthesis (Sorin Pericarbon). A morphological study. Eur J Cardiothorac Surg 1994;8:470–6.

7 Pelletier LC, Carrier M, Leclerc Y, et al. Porcine versus pericardial bioprostheses: a comparison of late results in 1,593 patients [see comments]. Ann Thorac Surg 1989;47:352–61.

8 Gonzalez-Lavin L, Gonzalez-Lavin J, Chi S, et al. The pericardial valve in the aortic position ten years later. J Thorac Cardiovasc Surg 1991;101:75–80.

9 Valente M, Ius P, Bortolotti U, et al. Pathology of the pericarbon bovine pericardial xenograft implanted in humans. J Heart Valve Dis 1998;7:180–9.

10 Boeken U, Litmathe J, Kurt M, et al. Hemodynamic performance and clinical consequences of aortic valve replacement with 21-mm sized pericardial bioprostheses. Thorac Cardiovasc Surg 2005;53:281–4.

11 Yankah CA, Pasic M, Musci M, et al. Aortic valve replacement with the Mitroflow pericardial bioprosthesis: durability results up to 21 years. J Thorac Cardiovasc Surg 2008;136:688–96.

12 Dunning J, Graham RJ, Thambyrajah J, et al. Stentless vs. stented aortic valve bioprostheses: a prospective randomized controlled trial. Eur Heart J 2007;28:2369–74.

13 Sjogren J, Gudbjartsson T, Thulin LI. Long-term outcome of the MitroFlow pericardial bioprosthesis in the elderly after aortic valve replacement. J Heart Valve Dis 2006;15:197–202.

14 Pomar JL, Jamieson WR, Pelletier LC, et al. Mitroflow pericardial bioprosthesis experience in aortic valve replacement> or =60 years of age. Ann Thorac Surg 1998;66:S53–6.

15 Dellgren G, David TE, Raanani E, et al. Late hemodynamic and clinical outcomes of aortic valve replacement with the Carpentier-Edwards Perimount pericardial bioprosthesis. J Thorac Cardiovasc Surg 2002;124:146–54.

16 Puvimanasinghe JP, Takkenberg JJ, Eijkemans MJ, et al. Prognosis after aortic valve replacement with the Carpentier-Edwards pericardial valve: use of microsimulation. Ann Thorac Surg 2005;80:825–31.

17 Pavoni D, Badano LP, Musumeci SF, et al. Results of aortic valve replacement with a new supra-annular pericardial stented bioprosthesis. Ann Thorac Surg 2006;82:2133–8.

18 Puvimanasinghe JP, Takkenberg JJ, Eijkemans MJ, et al. Comparison of Carpentier-Edwards pericardial and supraannular bioprostheses in aortic valve replacement. Eur J Cardiothorac Surg 2006;29:374–9.

19 David TE, Puschmann R, Ivanov J, et al. Aortic valve replacement with stentless and stented porcine valves: a case-match study. J Thorac Cardiovasc Surg 1998;116:236–41.

20 Repossini A, Kotelnikov I, Bouchikhi R, et al. Single-suture line placement of a pericardial stentless valve. J Thorac Cardiovasc Surg 2005;130:1265–9.

21 Beholz S, Dushe S, Konertz W. The Freedom SOLO valve: superior hemodynamic results with a new stentless pericardial valve for aortic valve replacement. J Heart Valve Dis 2007;16:49–55; discussion 55.

22 Casabona R, De Paulis R, Zattera GF, et al. Stentless porcine and pericardial valve in aortic position. Ann Thorac Surg 1992;54:681–684; discussion 685.

23 Grubitzsch H, Linneweber J, Kossagk C, et al. Aortic valve replacement with new-generation stentless pericardial valves: short-term clinical and hemodynamic results. J Heart Valve Dis 2005;14:623–9.

24 de Kerchove L, Glineur D, El Khoury G, et al. Stentless valves for aortic valve replacement: where do we stand? Curr Opin Cardiol 2007;22:96–103.

25 Kunadian B, Vijayalakshmi K, Thornley AR, et al. Meta-analysis of valve hemodynamics and left ventricular mass regression for stentless versus stented aortic valves. Ann Thorac Surg 2007;84:73–8.

26 Bove T, Van Belleghem Y, Francois K, et al. Stentless and stented aortic valve replacement in elderly patients: factors affecting midterm clinical and hemodynamical outcome. Eur J Cardiothorac Surg 2006;30:706–13.

27 Miraldi F, Spagnesi L, Tallarico D, et al. Sorin stentless pericardial valve versus Carpentier-Edwards Perimount pericardial bioprosthesis: is it worthwhile to struggle? Int J Cardiol 2007;118:253–5.

28 Kallikourdis A, Jacob S. Is a stentless aortic valve superior to conventional bioprosthetic valves for aortic valve replacement? Interact Cardiovasc Thorac Surg 2007;6:665–72.

29 Cox JL, Ad N, Myers K, et al. Tubular heart valves: a new tissue prosthesis design – preclinical evaluation of the 3F aortic bioprosthesis. J Thorac Cardiovasc Surg 2005;130:520–7.

30 Shrestha M, Khaladj N, Bara C, et al. A staged approach towards interventional aortic valve implantation with a sutureless valve: initial human implants. Thorac Cardiovasc Surg 2008;56:398–400.

31 Cribier A, Eltchaninoff H, Tron C, et al. Early experience with percutaneous transcatheter implantation of heart valve prosthesis for the treatment of end-stage inoperable patients with calcific aortic stenosis. J Am Coll Cardiol 2004;43:698–703.

32 Cribier A, Eltchaninoff H, Tron C, et al. Treatment of calcific aortic stenosis with the percutaneous heart valve: mid-term follow-up from the initial feasibility studies: the French experience. J Am Coll Cardiol 2006;47: 1214–23.

33 Webb JG, Pasupati S, Humphries K, et al. Percutaneous transarterial aortic valve replacement in selected high-risk patients with aortic stenosis. Circulation 2007;116:755–63.

34 Webb JG, Chandavimol M, Thompson CR, et al. Percutaneous aortic valve implantation retrograde from the femoral artery. Circulation 2006;113:842–50.

35 Grube E, Schuler G, Buellesfeld L, et al. Percutaneous aortic valve replacement for severe aortic stenosis in high-risk patients using the second- and current third-generation self-expanding CoreValve prosthesis: device success and 30-day clinical outcome. J Am Coll Cardiol 2007;50:69–76.

36 Lichtenstein SV, Cheung A, Ye J, et al. Transapical transcatheter aortic valve implantation in humans: initial clinical experience. Circulation 2006;114:591–6.

37 Ye J, Cheung A, Lichtenstein SV, et al. Six-month outcome of transapical transcatheter aortic valve implantation in the initial seven patients. Eur J Cardiothorac Surg 2007;31:16–21.

38 Walther T, Falk V, Kempfert J, et al. Transapical minimally invasive aortic valve implantation; the initial 50 patients. Eur J Cardiothorac Surg 2008;33:983–8.

39 Martens S, Ploss A, Sirat S, et al. Sutureless aortic valve replacement with the 3f Enable aortic bioprosthesis. Ann Thorac Surg 2009;87:1914–17.

40 Mueller XM, von Segesser LK. A new equine pericardial stentless valve. J Thorac Cardiovasc Surg 2003;125: 1405–11.

41 Dewey TM, Brown D, Ryan WH, et al. Reliability of risk algorithms in predicting early and late operative outcomes in high-risk patients undergoing aortic valve replacement. J Thorac Cardiovasc Surg 2008;135:180–7.

42 Ionescu A, Fraser AG, Butchart EG. Prevalence and clinical significance of incidental paraprosthetic valvar regurgitation: a prospective study using transoesophageal echocardiography. Heart 2003;89:1316–21.

43 Svensson LG, Dewey T, Kapadia S, et al. United States feasibility study of transcatheter insertion of a stented aortic valve by the left ventricular apex. Ann Thorac Surg 2008;86:46–54; discussion 54–45.

44 Walther T, Simon P, Dewey T, et al. Transapical minimally invasive aortic valve implantation: multicenter experience. Circulation 2007;116:I240–5.

45 Azadani AN, Jaussaud N, Matthews PB, et al. Valve-in-valve implantation using a novel supravalvular transcatheter aortic valve: proof of concept. Ann Thorac Surg 2009;88:1864–9.

46 Azadani AN, Jaussaud N, Matthews PB, et al. Aortic valve-in-valve implantation: impact of transcatheter- bioprosthesis size mismatch. J Heart Valve Dis 2009;18:367–73.

47 Dwyer HA, Matthews PB, Azadani A, et al. Computational fluid dynamics simulation of transcatheter aortic valve degeneration. Interact Cardiovasc Thorac Surg 2009;9:301–8.

48 Rosengart TK, Feldman T, Borger MA, et al. Percutaneous and minimally invasive valve procedures: a scientific statement from the American Heart Association Council on Cardiovascular Surgery and Anesthesia, Council on Clinical Cardiology, Functional Genomics and Translational Biology Interdisciplinary Working Group, and Quality of Care and Outcomes Research Interdisciplinary Working Group. Circulation 2008;117:1750–67.

49 Dewey TM, Brown DL, Das TS, et al. High-risk patients referred for transcatheter aortic valve implantation: management and outcomes. Ann Thorac Surg 2008;86:1450–1456; discussion 1456–7.

50 Vahanian A, Alfieri O, Al-Attar N, et al. Transcatheter valve implantation for patients with aortic stenosis: a position statement from the European association of cardio-thoracic surgery (EACTS) and the European Society of Cardiology (ESC), in collaboration with the European Association of Percutaneous Cardiovascular Interventions (EAPCI). EuroIntervention 2008;4:193–9.

51 Mehta RH, Grab JD, O'Brien SM, et al. Bedside tool for predicting the risk of postoperative dialysis in patients undergoing cardiac surgery. Circulation 2006;114:2208–16; quiz 2208.

Videoclip

This chapter contains the following videoclip:

Video 17.1 Surgical implantation of the Perceval S sutureless aortic valve prosthesis.

It can be accessed at www.wiley.com/go/Valverepair.

18

CHAPTER 18

Transcatheter mitral leaflet repair

Francesco Maisano[1], *Joerg Seeburger*[2], *Paolo Denti*[3], *Friedrich W. Mohr*[2] *& Ottavio Alfieri*[3]

[1]Cardiothoracic and Vascular Institute, San Raffaele Hospital, Milan, Italy
[2]Heart Center, Leipzig University, Leipzig, Germany
[3]Department of Cardiac Surgery, San Raffaele Hospital, Milan, Italy

Introduction

Surgical mitral repair is based on the concept of the combination of leaflet repair and annuloplasty. Initial experience with leaflet repair is based on two concepts: edge-to-edge repair and neochordae implantation. This chapter will focus on the initial preclinical and clinical experience with these procedures.

Edge-to-edge procedure

The edge-to-edge technique was introduced about two decades ago by Ottavio Alfieri as an alternative option for treating mitral regurgitation (MR) due to complex lesions [1,2]. The technique simply consists of the suture of the opposing leaflet edges at the site of the regurgitation (Fig. 18.1). If the suture is positioned centrally, a double orifice valve is created. The technique is versatile and effective for both degenerative and functional MR [3,4].

The intrinsic simplification of mitral valve repair introduced by the edge-to-edge technique suggested a possible application in the endovascular field some years ago [2]. Two technologies have been developed to reproduce the surgical edge-to-edge with a catheter-based approach: the Mobius system and the MitraClip system.

Mobius program: from direct access to fully percutaneous suture-based transcatheter edge-to-edge

The Mobius project was initiated by Edwards Lifesciences (Irvine, CA), and developed a suture-based device designed to closely replicate the surgical procedure. The initial device was a surgical tool designed to be used on the beating heart. The device was only tested in preclinical trials, and was never used in humans. The device was placed through an access cannula port into the left atrium and then through the mitral valve. A pistol-grip firing mechanism was incorporated to trigger suction and suture. The tip of the device contained lumens for two sutures and their needles, as well as for two suction channels used to grasp the mitral valve leaflets (Fig. 18.2). The system was connected to a wall-mounted suction (Fig. 18.3). The procedure was performed under general anesthesia, through a left thoracotomy approach to expose the left atrium. A pursestring suture was done on the dome of the left atrium and the access cannula (with hemostasis valve) was inserted. The device was then introduced in the left atrium and advanced across the mitral valve. Under echo guidance the tip of the device was positioned in the middle of the valve. Using pressure monitoring, the tip was positioned in the "transition" area, where the pressure waveform was intermediate between the ventricular and the atrial pattern,

Endovascular and Hybrid Therapies for Structural Heart and Aortic Disease, First Edition.
Edited by Jacques Kpodonu and Raoul Bonan.

identifying the level of the coaptation of the leaflets. The device was then oriented under echo guidance until the suction ports would be facing the leaflet edges (Fig. 18.4). When orientation and longitudinal position were optimized, suction was activated and leaflet grasped. Grasping was confirmed by both echocardiography and by evidence of no blood flow through the suction port and its tubing. When optimal grasping was confirmed, needles perforated the leaflets and carried the sutures. The sutures were exteriorized and subsequently tied using a knot-pusher.

The system never entered into clinical trial because of the development of a catheter designed with the same functionalities of the surgical tool, but miniaturized to allow a fully percutaneous approach (Fig. 18.5). The system was extensively tested in animals [5]. The procedure was conducted under general anesthesia, using intracardiac echocardiography (ICE) guidance (Fig. 18.6) [6]. The experimental set-up included a bilateral femoral vein percutaneous approach, with a 22 Fr sheath in the right groin (to insert the therapy catheter) and a 10 Fr sheath in the left groin (for the introduction of the ICE catheter. The procedure was performed

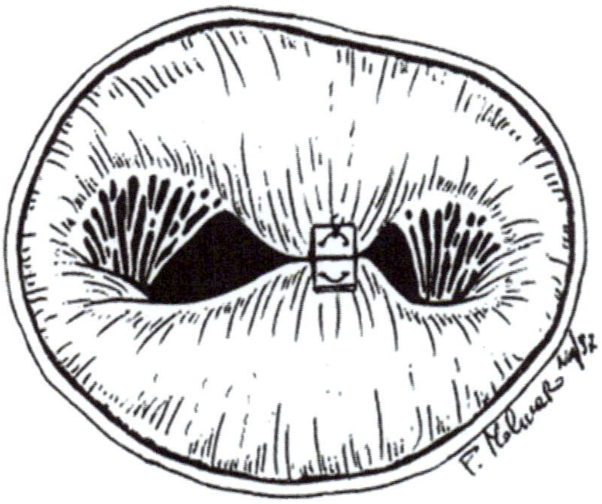

Fig. 18.1 The edge-to-edge technique used as a double orifice repair.

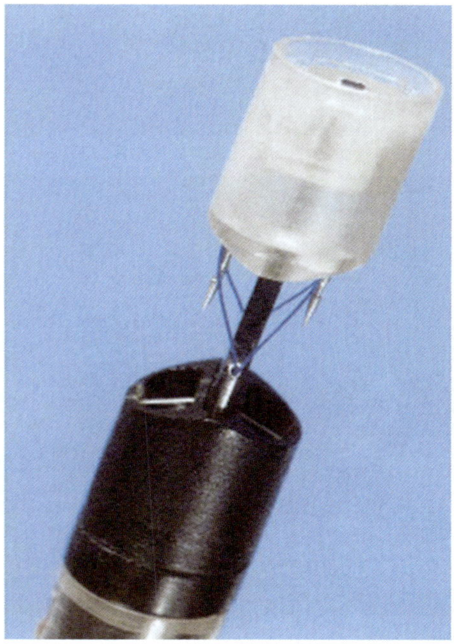

Fig. 18.2 The tip of the edge-to-edge device contains lumens for two sutures and their needles

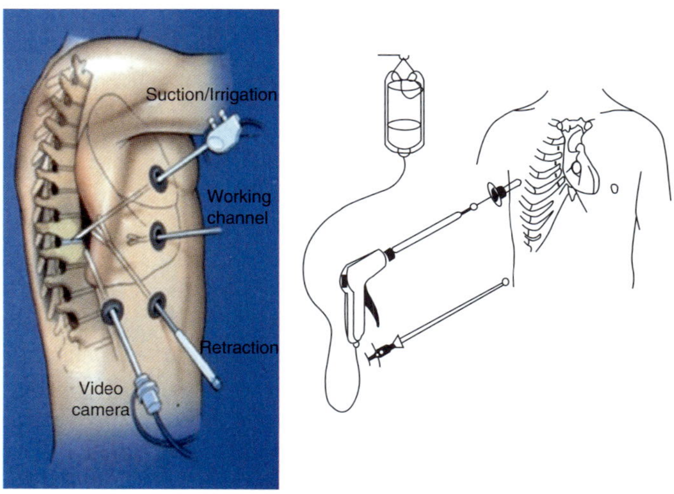

Fig. 18.3 The edge-to-edge system connected to wall-mounted suction.

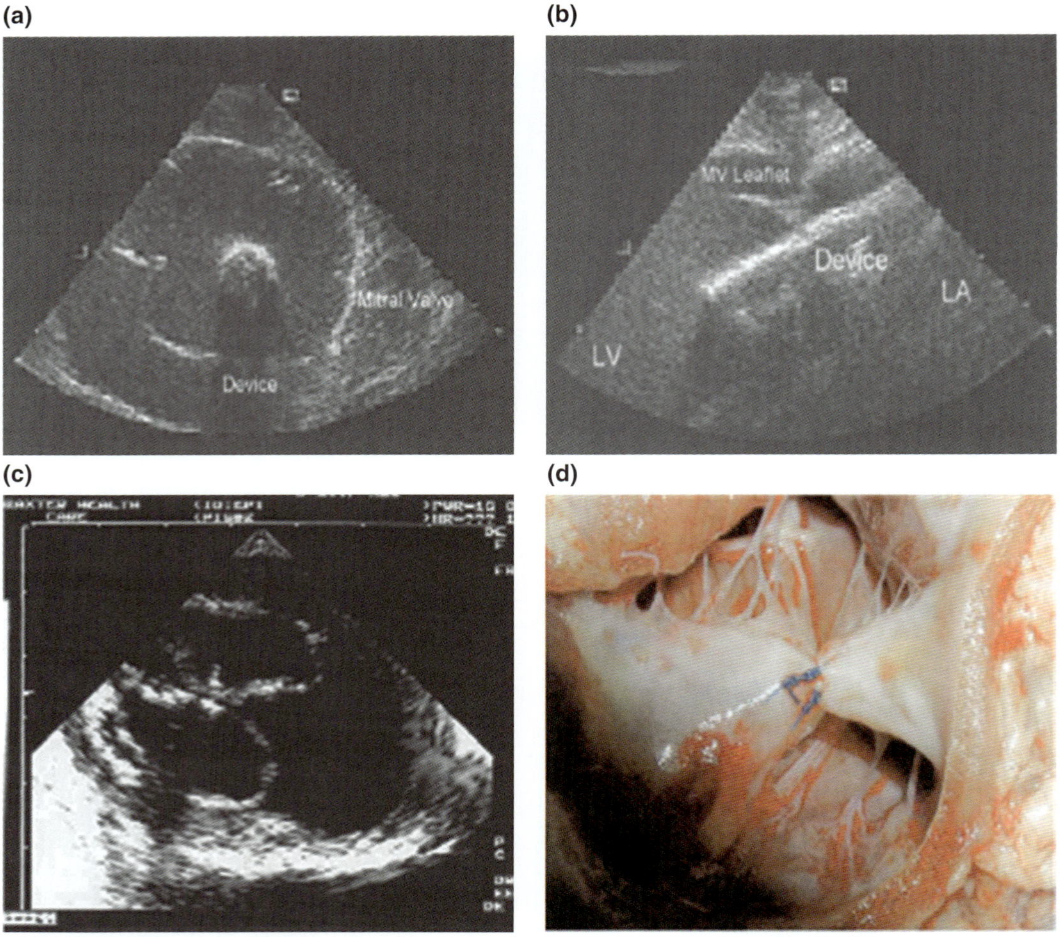

Fig. 18.4 (**a, b**) Echocardiographic images of the edge-to-edge device in the left atrium (LA). The device is oriented under echo guidance until the suction ports are facing the leaflet edges. When orientation and longitudinal position is optimized, suction is activated and the leaflet grasped. Needles then perforate the leaflets and carry the sutures. The sutures are exteriorized and subsequently tied using a knot-pusher. (c, d) The final result: (c) echo, and (d) anatomic. LV, left ventricle.

similarly to the surgical direct approach, with few differences. The first step included a precise echo-guided transeptal puncture aiming at the posterior/superior aspect of the fossa ovalis to allow better manipulation of the device inside of the small left atrium of the pigs. Septal crossing through a naturally patent foramen ovale was avoided since the tissue tunnel would prevent the device being effectively manipulated to orient the therapy catheter towards the leaflets. A 17 or 21 Fr steerable guide-catheter was inserted in the left atrium and a 0.0018 inch guide wire positioned in the descending aorta using a floating balloon technique. The therapy catheter was then inserted over the wire into the left atrium and facing the mitral leaflets. The leaflet capture was obtained in a sequential manner, since the catheter had a single suction and suture port. The edges of the opposing leaflets were captured sequentially, rotating the device 180°, and trying to keep the system aligned to the first capture. Once bilateral capture was achieved, the therapy catheter was retrieved and sutures were exteriorized. Then leaflet approximation was obtained by a nitinol clip delivered with a fastener catheter, designed to fasten the sutures, deploy the clip, and cut the suture at the tip of the clip to get the final result of

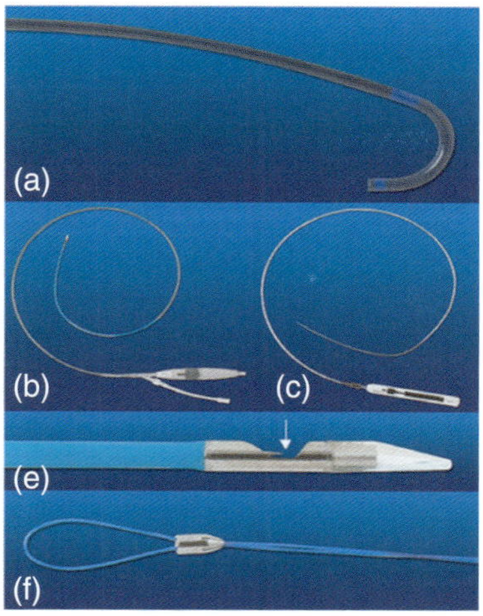

Fig. 18.5 The Mobius leaflet repair suture delivery system comprising a 17 Fr guide catheter (a), a 10 Fr therapy catheter (b), and a 7 Fr fastener catheter designed to deploy the suture clip and cut the suture (c). (d) The zoomed view of the end of the therapy catheter showing an orifice (white arrow) which is used to suction the mitral leaflet and deliver the suture. (e) The nitinol suture clip that is delivered over the suture before the suture is cut above the suture clip.

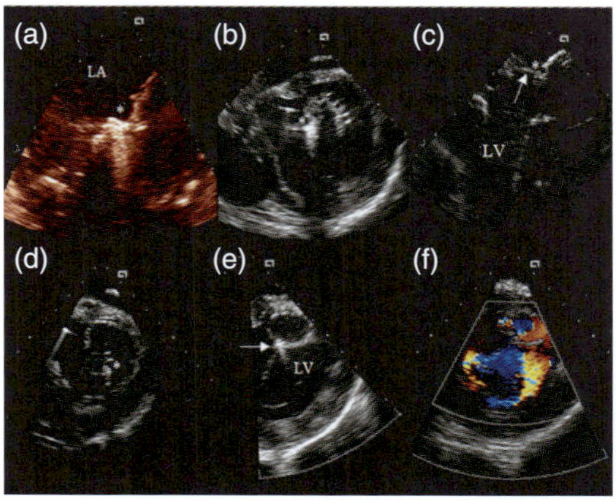

Figure 18.6 Echocardiographic images obtained from an intracardiac imaging catheter in the right atrium showing short axis views of the mitral valve (b, d–f), and in the left atrium (LA) showing long axis views of the mitral valve (a, c). The orifice of the therapy catheter is shown by a white asterisk in panels (a–d). Panels (a–d) show the therapy catheter orifice directed towards the anterior mitral leaflet and (d) shows it directed against the posterior mitral leaflet. The white arrow in (c) points at the anterior mitral leaflet caught in the therapy catheter orifice by vacuum. The figure-of-8 appearance of the mitral valve along with a central suture clip (white arrow) is shown in panel (e). Panel (f) show color flow Doppler across two separate orifices of the mitral valve. LV, left ventricle.

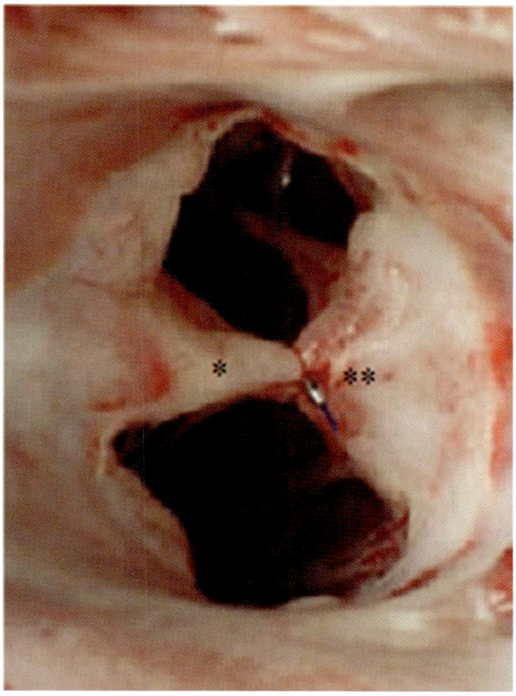

Fig. 18.7 View of the mitral valve from the left atrial aspect after heart explantation. The single black asterisk represents the anterior mitral valve leaflet and double black asterisks represent the posterior mitral valve leaflet.

a suture-based double orifice mitral valve (Fig. 18.7). The main complexity of the procedure was the challenge of proper echocardiographic visualization of the therapy catheter, since orientation of the suction port towards the target segment of the mitral leaflet was critical for a successful capture. In addition, the sequential approach resulted in asymmetric captures in some animals, particularly in the early stages of the development.

The device has been tested in a small cohort of patients in a multicenter pivotal trial [7]. Endovascular suture-based double orifice mitral repair was feasible with an acute reduction in the severity of MR by at least one grade in nine of 15 patients. At 30 days improvement in MR appeared durable in six patients, while the others experienced delayed failure due to suture detachment. Short durability was probably driven by the inadequacy of leaflet capture due to the small profile of the suction port, and to the potential for asymmetric sequential capture leading to excessive tension on the sutures. Both issues were also related to the inadequacy of imaging. At the time of the trial, live 3D echocardiography was still unavailable. The small profile and the design of the catheter were not ideal for echo visualization. Also, quantification of leaflet capture as well as topographic assessment of suture positioning was insufficient to ensure durable leaflet approximation. For these reasons and due to the ongoing initial promising results of the MitraClip, the program was discontinued. Subsequently, the same technology has been used to perform transapical neochordae implantation in the animal model [8], with no further development into clinical practice.

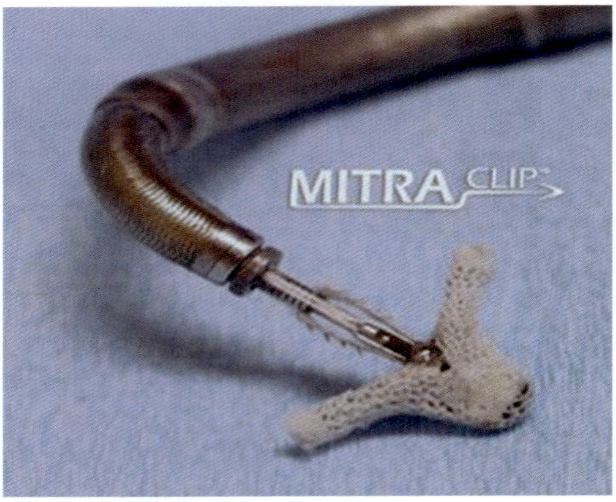

Fig. 18.8 The MitraClip device.

MitraClip: the first successful percutaneous leaflet repair system

MitraClip has been developed by Evalve, Inc., a company based in California, and recently acquired by Abbott Laboratories (Abbott Park, IL). The clip is a soft tissue fixation device (Figs 18.8 and 18.9), covered by polyester and designed to be modified into three configurations: closed, grasping, and inverted (Fig. 18.10). The outside dimension is 4 mm when closed, while it is 20 mm in the grasping position. The clip arm is designed to engage 8 mm of the free edge of the leaflets (to create an 8 mm coaptation surface) on each side. In the open position, it is echo-reflecting with minimal artifacts, and, therefore, is used to grasp and immobilize the central mitral leaflet scallops by retraction of the delivery catheter. Each arm has an opposing "gripper" that aids in securing the leaflets in the clip by means of small multipronged friction elements. After the leaflet is captured between an arm on the ventricular side and a gripper on the atrial side, the clip is closed in a locked position. Once a functioning double-orifice mitral valve is confirmed with echocardiography, the clip is detached. The handle at the user end of the delivery catheter actuates the arms and grippers, the locking mechanism, and the detachment of the clip device (Video 18.1).

The initial animal studies were conducted in isolated pig hearts, followed by chronic animal experiments to evaluate the long-term effect of the

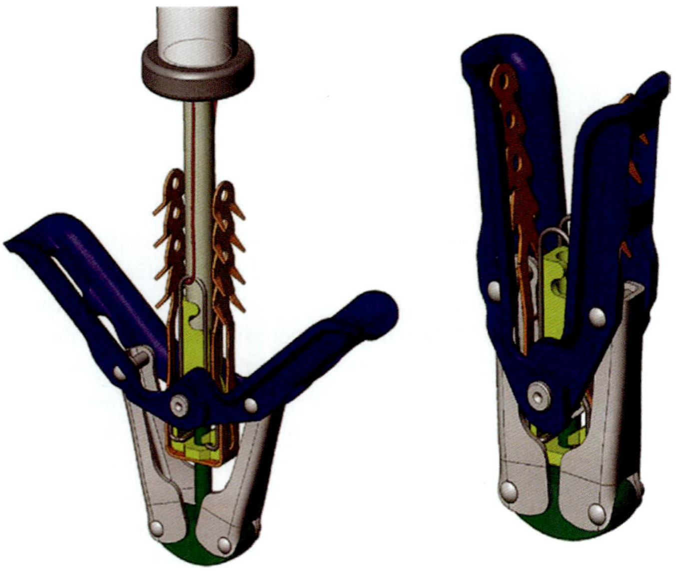

Fig. 18.9 Components of the MitraClip. On the inner portion of the clip is a U-shaped gripper that matches up to each arm and helps to stabilize the leaflets from the atrial aspect as they are captured during closure of the clip arms. Leaflet tissue is secured between the closed arms and each side of the gripper, and the clip is then closed and locked to effect and maintain coaptation of the two leaflets.

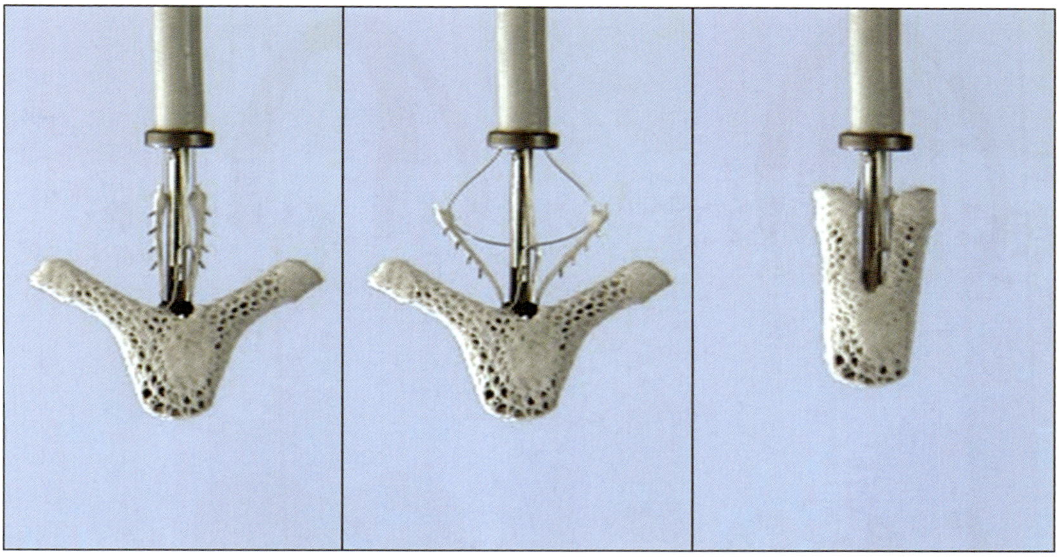

Fig. 18.10 Possible configuration of the clip: open (leaflet), grasping, and closed (from right to left). The inverted position is not shown.

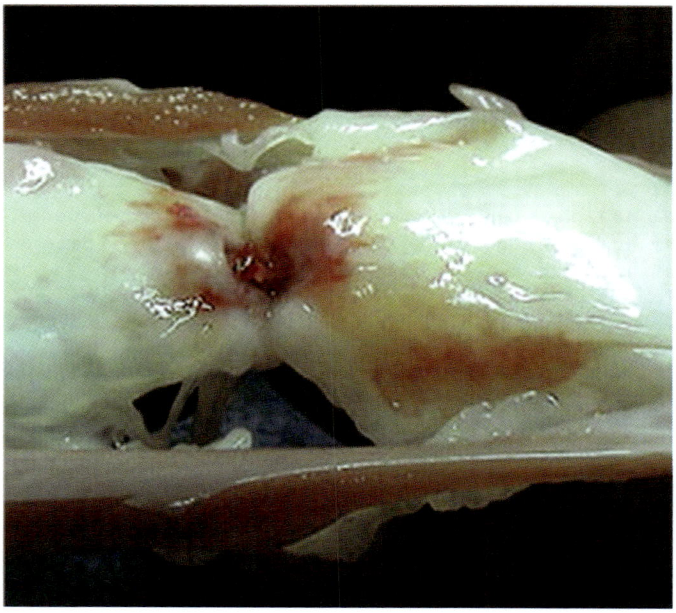

Fig. 18.11 Growth of a tissue bar onto the septolateral axis of the valve.

clip on the leaflet tissue. In 2004, Fann et al. reported the initial healing effects of the MitraClip in the chronic animal model [9], suggesting that the clip implant was inducing a fibrous bar (Fig. 18.11) on the septolateral axis of the anterior and posterior leaflets, perpendicular to the plane of the coaptation. This bar has been suggested to support the annular dimension and avoid ongoing dilation of the annulus following clip implant. More recently, Luk et al. [10] reported the long-term histopathology findings of the healing process of the clip in an animal model. Twenty-one clips with surrounding leaflet tissue were examined at up to 52 weeks. Both the atrial and ventricular surfaces showed tissue growth, proportional to time of implant. Endothelialization and fibrous encapsulation of the clip into the surrounding tissue

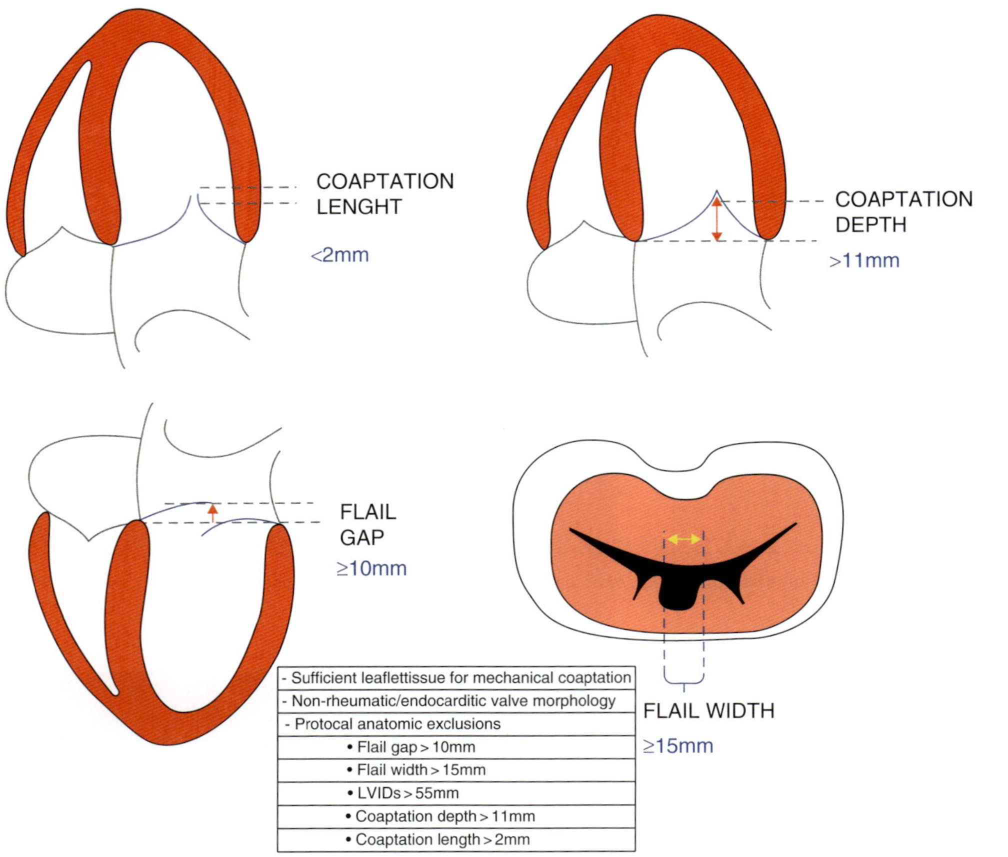

Fig. 18.12 Key anatomic inclusion criteria include a regurgitant jet origin associated with the A2 to P2 segments of the mitral valve and, for patients with functional MR, the coaptation length must be at least 2 mm. The coaptation depth must be <11 mm. If a flail leaflet exists, the flail gap must be ≤10 mm, and the flail width must be ≤15 mm. These anatomic characteristics are necessary for sufficient leaflet tissue for mechanical coaptation when the MitraClip device is used. LVID, Left Ventricular Internal Diameter.

was seen as early as 12 weeks after the implant. These findings suggest that the clip is incorporated early into the native tissue and that endothelialization occurs within weeks from the implant, reducing the risk of embolization and of thromboembolism.

To date, more than 1500 patients have been treated worldwide with this technology, which is CE marked in Europe and therefore available for clinical practice. Selection is fundamental, and it includes clinical as well as anatomic factors (Fig. 18.12). Firstly, to be eligible, patients should demonstrate central MR, originating from the A2 and P2 segments. Single-leaflet as well as bileaflet lesions are treatable, and the device is designed to treat both degenerative and functional MR. Since the creation of a double orifice configuration reduces mitral valve area approximately by half, a baseline valve area less than 4 cm^2 is considered a relative contraindication. However, the most critical factor related to post-procedural increased transvalvular gradients is the presence of thickened leaflets, as in rheumatic disease. In the other cases, mitral stenosis is rarely observed after the procedure, regardless of the etiology or the number of clips implanted [11]. In patients with functional MR, the coaptation length at echo should be at least 2 mm, and the coaptation depth should be less than 10 mm. In patients with degenerative MR, the width of the flail or prolapsing segment should be less than 15 mm and the distance between the opposing leaflet free edges (flail gap) should be less than 10 mm to allow proper leaflet capture and amount of leaflet insertion in the clip. Such anatomic inclusion criteria have to be considered as relative;

as experience increases, when the procedure is performed beyond the above-mentioned boundaries, higher incidence of early and late failure should be expected with the currently available clip design. In the future, new designs will probably expand the current indications. Anatomic assessment should be performed by a trained echocardiographist, and it is usually based on both two-dimensional and 3D transesophageal examination. When the diagnostic procedure is performed under sedation, the degree of the regurgitant jet as well as its geometry could be different from that observed when the patient is awake, therefore only mild sedation is usually performed in this case.

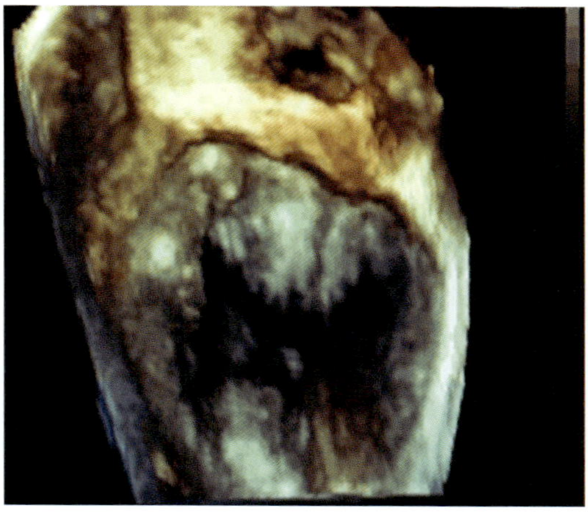

Fig. 18.13 3D echo image of the ideal position for puncture of the atrial septum.

The procedure is performed under general anesthesia, since it is completely transesophageal echo-guided. In the future, however, less invasive echo guidance is expected to become available and this introduces the possibility of performing the procedure under local anesthesia with sedation. Prior to the implant, the patient is prepared in a similar fashion as for an open surgical mitral valve procedure. The patient is anesthetized and a transesophageal echocardiography (TEE) probe is placed. Prior to sterile draping, an indwelling urinary catheter is placed and preparations are made to maintain normothermia. Also prior to sterile draping, a Plexiglas plate and a lift are placed under and over the right lower extremity, respectively. The right femoral vein and left femoral artery and vein or the right internal jugular veins are cannulated for hemodynamic assessment and monitoring.

From the right femoral venous puncture, a TEE-guided transeptal cannulation of the left atrium via puncture of the interatrial septum is performed. Transeptal puncture is performed usually in the superior and posterior corner of the fossa ovalis (Fig. 18.13). The distance between the tenting and the mitral valve is assessed prior to puncture, to confirm that the device will have enough trajectory to reach the valve and to travel above and under the annular level in order to safely and effectively grasp the leaflets (Fig. 18.14). Once the optimal location of the transeptal puncture is confirmed, the septum is punctured and the patient is heparinized to

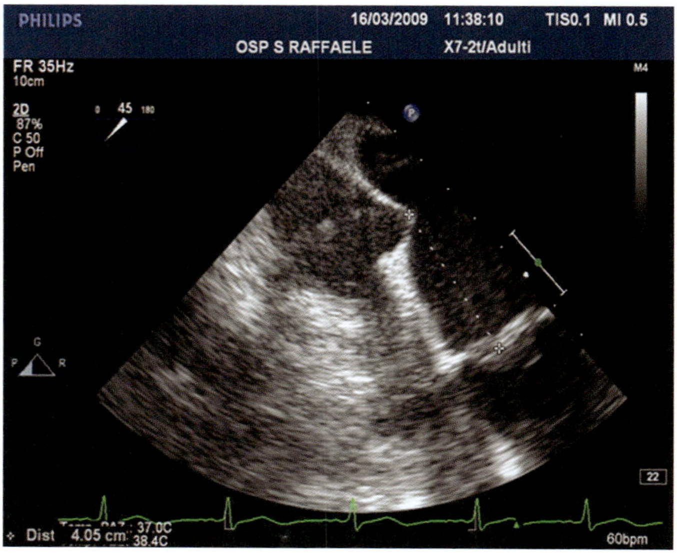

Fig.18.14 Final check by a four-chamber view incorporating the septum and the free edge of the mitral valve at the site of regurgitation. Ideally, the distance between the tenting and the mitral valve should be between 3 and 4 cm to allow enough space for the delivery system to move above the mitral valve leaflets in a perpendicular fashion.

achieve an activated clotting time (ACT) of at least 250 seconds. A 260 cm exchange length J-tipped (0.0035 inch Amplatz Super-stiff) guide wire is placed through the transeptal catheter into the left atrium and the left atrial transeptal catheter is then removed. The percutaneous femoral vein entry site is dilated with a 16 Fr dilator and the steerable guide catheter–dilator assembly is inserted over the guide wire under TEE guidance (Figs 18.15 and 18.16). During this step, continuous echo guidance is ensured to avoid inadvertent lesions of either the roof of the atrium or left atrial appendage. Once the guide catheter is in position, the handle is secured in the sterile stabilizer placed on top of the previously placed lift. The dilator and guide wire are removed together and the guide is de-aired. The clip delivery system (CDS) (Fig. 18.17) is inserted through the steerable guide catheter under fluoroscopic and TEE guidance, again checking for eventual collisions of the system with left atrial

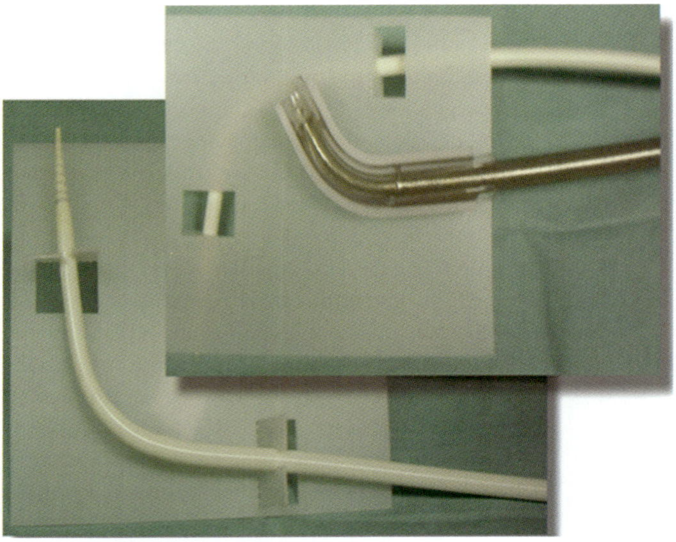

Fig. 18.15 Tip of the steerable guide catheter and dilator.

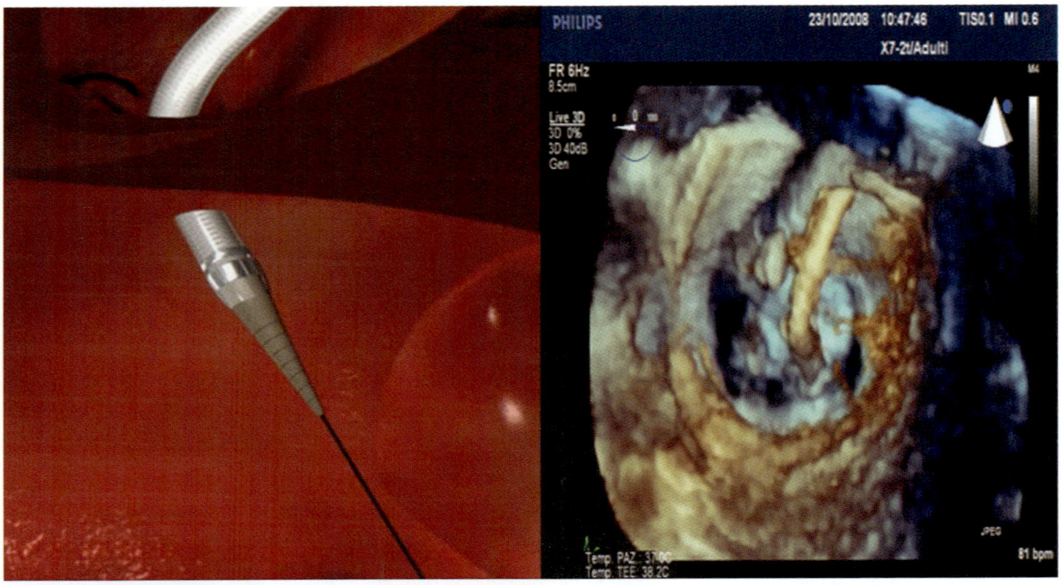

Fig. 18.16 Animation and 3D real view of the insertion of a guide catheter through the atrial septum.

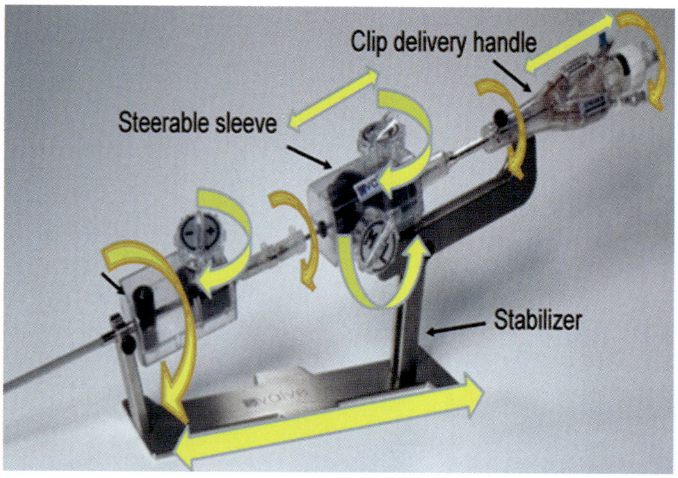

Fig. 18.17 Possible 3D movements of the clip delivery system and guide catheter.

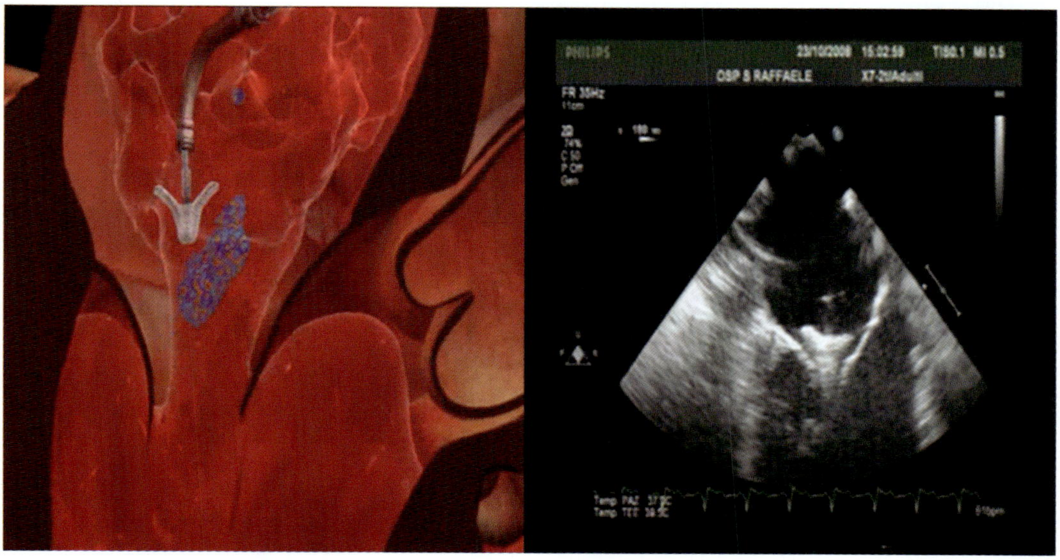

Fig. 18.18 Device opening and alignment (two-chamber view).

structures. The steerable guide catheter and CDS are positioned in the left atrium for clip deployment using echocardiographic and fluoroscopic guidance. The CDS is then steered towards the mitral valve, pointing at the tip of the left ventricle. The maneuver is performed under both echo and fluoroscopic guidance. Once the CDS is coaxial with the long axis of the heart, the clip is advanced above the annular level and opened. The clip arms of the MitraClip are then oriented perpendicularly relative to the line of coaptation. Clip orientation is checked in two 2D views (two-chamber view and long axis left ventricular outflow tract view; Fig. 18.18) and eventually in live 3D anatomic view to confirm proper alignment (Fig. 18.19). Once alignment is confirmed, the relative position of the clip to the regurgitant orifice is determined, and the clip is positioned at the level of the origin of the regurgitant jet. The clip is then advanced below the annular level, usually during an apnea to minimize the movement artifact due to artificial ventilation (Fig. 18.20). Clip arms are partially closed to enhance grasping and the mitral valve leaflets are grasped. Then the MitraClip is partially closed to induce leaflet coaptation of the leaflets and to reduce MR (Fig. 18.21). Quality of the grasp, valve

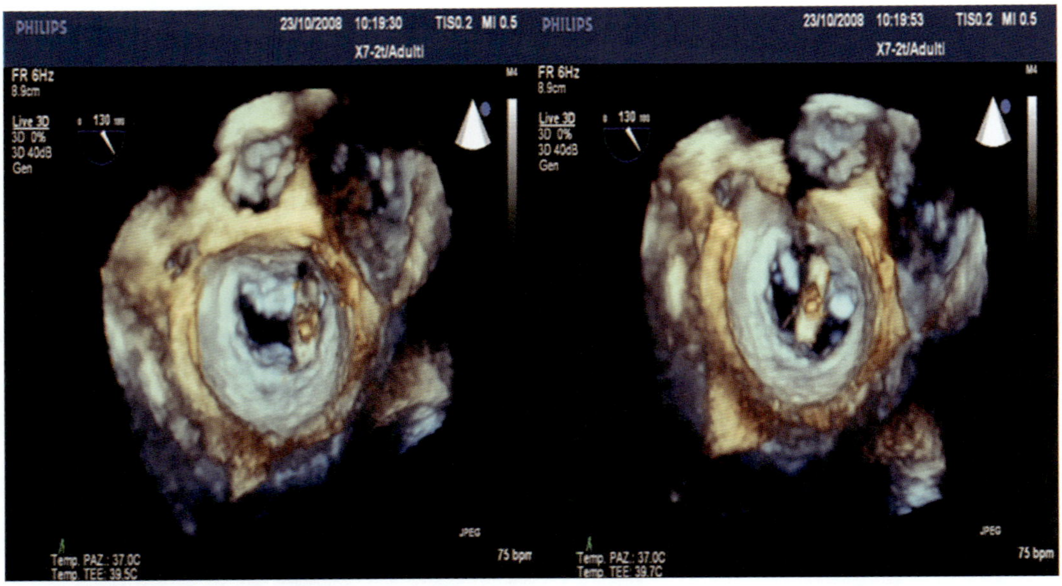

Fig. 18.19 Real 3D echo surgical view of the clip (right position is on the right).

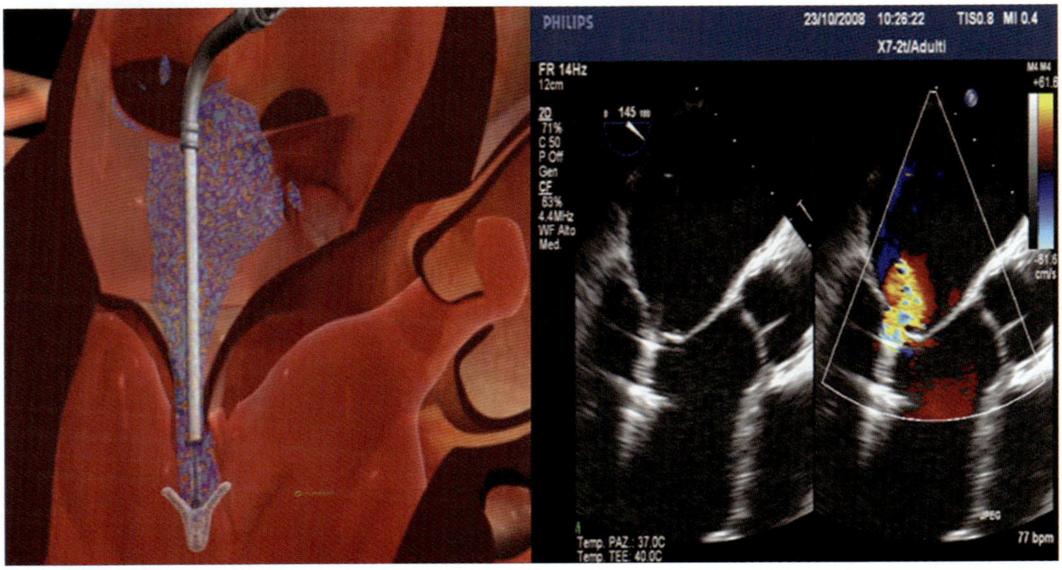

Fig. 18.20 Device advancement onto the ventricle and determination of the best position.

function, and adequacy of repair (reduction of MR) are assessed using echocardiography and fluoroscopy if desired (Fig. 18.22). The clip is closed further as needed under real-time MR assessment (Fig. 18.23). If necessary, the clip is repositioned to reduce MR further. When the physician determines that an optimal result has been achieved, the clip is deployed and the delivery catheters are removed. A second clip may be placed as needed to further reduce MR. Usually a two-clip strategy is decided in advance, based on the anatomic and functional aspect of the valve. In this case, the first clip is positioned relatively off-set from the middle of the origin of the jet to allow the second clip to complete leaflet approximation and reduction of MR. The patient is recovered from

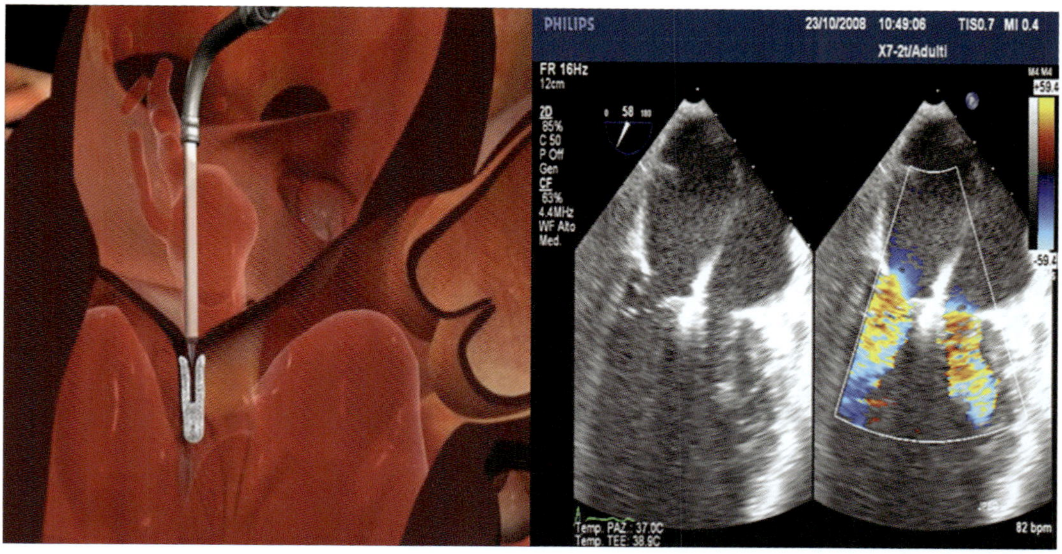

Fig. 18.21 Clip closure and double orifice assesment for evaluation of adequacy of repair.

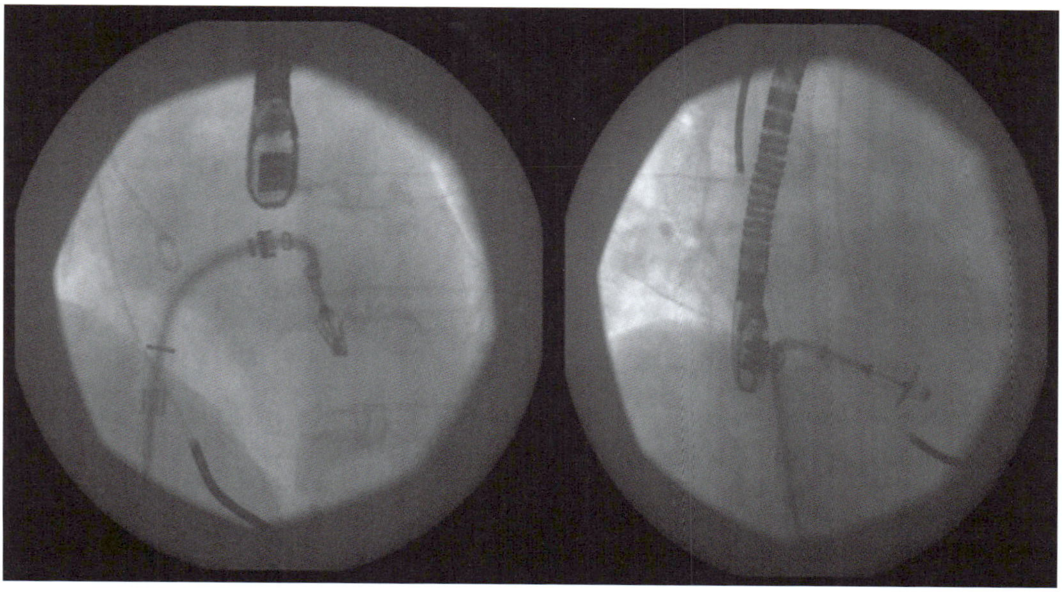

Fig.18.22 Fluoroscopic control of advancement and placement of the clip.

general anesthesia in the appropriate environment. Usually high-risk patients require a short stay in the intensive care unit. Short-term antiplatelet therapy is required after clip placement (Plavix for 30 days and aspirin for 6 months).

The initial experience of the use of the MitraClip in humans has been reported by Feldmann et al. [12]. The data from 107 patients enrolled into either the EVEREST (Endovascular Valve Edge-to-edge REpair STudy) I feasibility trial or the EVEREST II trial (roll-in patients, non-randomized) were prospectively collected. Most patients (79%) had degenerative MR or mixed disease as compared with 23 patients with pure functional MR (21%). All patients were surgical candidates by the definition of the study. Primary endpoints were analyzed for the per protocol population, defined as patients receiving a clip implant with a reduction

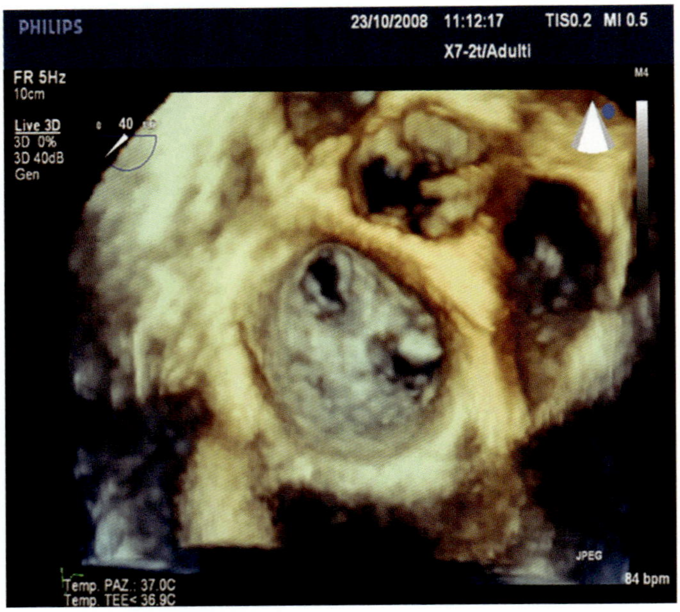

Fig. 18.23 Real 3D echo of the final result.

of MR to ≤2+ in a scale of 0 to 4+. This was also defined as acute procedural success (APS). The composite primary safety endpoint was major adverse events at 30 days, defined as freedom from the following: death, myocardial infarction, non-elective cardiac surgery for adverse events, renal failure, transfusion of more than 2 U of blood, reoperation for failed surgery, stroke, gastrointestinal complications requiring surgery, ventilation for 48 hours, deep wound infection, septicemia, and new onset of permanent atrial fibrillation. The composite primary efficacy endpoint was freedom from MR ≥2+, freedom from cardiac surgery for valve dysfunction, and freedom from death at 12 months. The median age was 71 years. One clip was placed in 65 patients (61%), two clips in 31 patients (29%) while 11 patients received no clip due to either inability to reduce MR (11 patients) or due to transeptal puncture complications (three patients). There was no intra-procedural mortality, while 10 patients had a major adverse event at 30 days including one hospital death. Mitral valve area by planimetry decreased from $5.7 \pm 1.5\,cm^2$ at baseline to $3.2 \pm 1.2\,cm^2$ at discharge and $3.5 \pm 1.1\,cm^2$ at 12 months. No patient had clip embolization, but partial clip detachment (defined as the detachment of one leaflet from the clip) occurred in 10 patients: in three cases during the procedure, in nine cases within 30 days. Only in one case was partial clip detachment noted at 6 months follow-up. Acute procedural success was achieved in 79 patients (74%). Patients with functional MR achieved 83% APS. The flow of patients from the point of clip procedure to the hospital discharge is presented in Fig. 18.24. Of those patients achieving APS, 66% had stable MR reduction at 12 months. Overall, 32 patients had surgery after the clip attempt. The flowchart depicting the outcomes of the patients who had surgery after a clip attempt is shown in Fig. 18.25. Successful mitral repair following clip removal was performed in 21 patients, as long as 18 months following the percutaneous procedure. The composite primary efficacy endpoint was 66%. Clinical symptoms were improved in 74% of the patients, 21% had no change, and 6% had worsened symptoms. In the APS cohort, the freedom from death was 95.9%, 94.0%, and 90.1% at 1, 2, and 3 years, and Kaplan–Meier freedom from surgery was 88.5%, 83.2%, and 76.3% at 1, 2, and 3 years, respectively (Fig. 18.26).

The EVEREST II controlled randomized trial has been recently completed and the clinical data reported at the American College of Cardiology by Ted Feldman. The study design involved 279

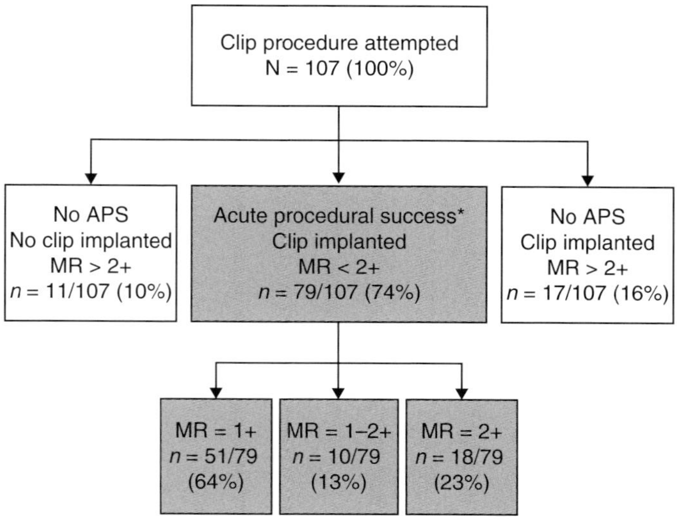

Fig. 18.24 Efficacy results through discharge. This chart shows the flow of patients from the point of clip procedure attempt through to hospital discharge. Acute procedural success (APS) is defined as the placement of one or more clips resulting in a discharge mitral regurgitation (MR) severity of ≤2+, as determined by the Core Laboratory.

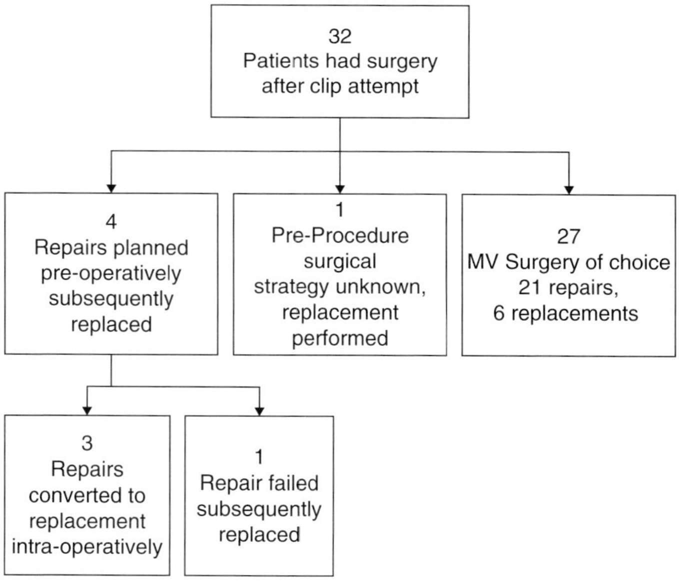

Fig. 18.25 Surgical patient flowchart depicting the outcomes of patients who had surgery after a clip attempt. MV, mitral valve.

patients enrolled at 37 sites. Patients had to be surgical candidates, with significant MR and to be anatomically eligible for the MitraClip procedure. Exclusion criteria included acute myocardial infarction within 12 weeks before the procedure, need for other cardiac surgery, renal insufficiency (serum creatinine level above 2.5 mg/ml), endocarditis, and rheumatic disease. When fulfilling the criteria (Table 18.1) the patients were randomized in a 2 : 1 fashion to surgery. This resulted in 184 and 95 patients enrolled in the device and surgical arms, respectively. Patients were followed up with routine echocardiography at discharge, 30 days, 6 months, 1 year, 18 months, and annually through 5 years. Echocardiographic assessment was performed through a core lab. The mean age was 68 years in the overall population. There were no significant differences in the clinical characteristics of the two groups (Tables 18.2 and 18.3). Etiology was degenerative in about 75% of the patients. Mean ejection fraction was 60%, and 50% of patients

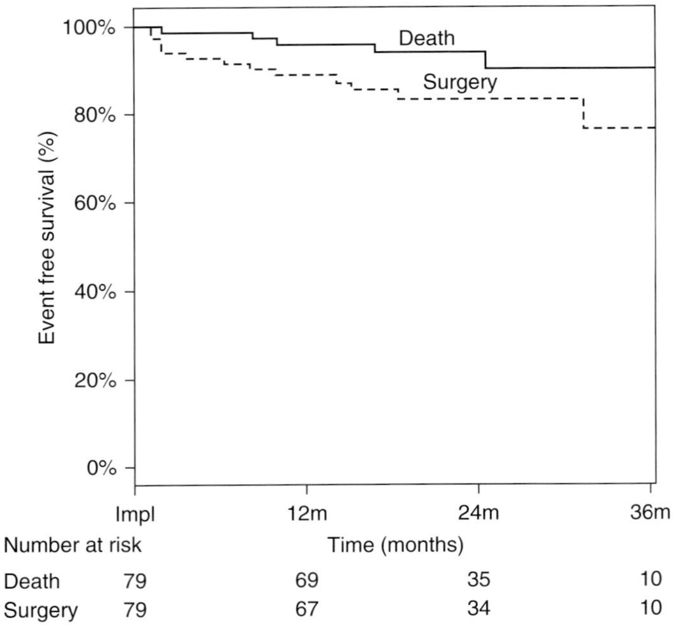

Fig. 18.26 Kaplan–Meier curves for patients with acute procedure success; freedom from death and freedom from surgery are depicted.

Table 18.1 Inclusion and exclusion criteria for the EVEREST II randomized clinical trial.

EVEREST II Randomized clinical trial	
Key inclusion/exclusion criteria	
Inclusion	*Exclusion*
• Candidate for MV surgery	• AMI within 12 weeks
• Moderate to severe (3+) or severe (4+) MR	• Need for other cardiac surgery
– Symptomatic	• Renal insufficiency
○ >25% EF & LVSD ≤55 mm	– Creatinine >2.5 mg/dl
– Asymptomatic with one or more of the following	• Endocarditis
○ LVEF 25–60%	• Rheumatic heart disease
○ LVSD ≥40 mm	• MV anatomic exclusions
○ New onset atrial fibrillation	– Mitral valve area <4.0 cm^2
○ Pulmonary hypertension	– Leaflet flail width (≥15 mm) and gap (≥10 mm)
	– Leaflet tethering/coaptation depth (>11 mm) and length (<2 mm)

AMI, acute myocardial infarction; EF, ejection fraction; LVEF, left ventricular ejection fraction; LVSD, left ventricular systolic diameter; MR, mitral regurgitation; MV, mitral valve.

were in New York Heart Association (NYHA) class III or IV. The primary endpoints were safety, defined as rate of major adverse events at 30 days, and effectiveness, defined as freedom from the combined outcome of death, mitral valve surgery, or reoperation for mitral valve dysfunction and MR >2+ at 12 months. The analysis was conducted on the per protocol cohort and a superiority hypothesis for safety (prespecified margin 6%) and a non-inferiority hypothesis (prespecified margin 31%) were made. In the device group 178 patients were treated and APS was achieved in 137 patients, while in the control group out of 95 randomized, 80 patients were

Table 18.2 Baseline characteristics of patients in the EVEREST II randomized clinical trial.

	EVEREST II Randomized clinical trial		
	Baseline demographics & co-morbidities		
	Device (%)	*Control (%)*	
	n=184	*n*=95	*P*
Age (mean)	67.3 years	65.7 years	0.32
Male	62.5	66.3	0.60
Congestive heart failure	90.8	77.9	<0.01
Coronary artery disease	47.0	46.3	>0.99
Myocardial infarction	21.9	21.3	>0.99
Angina	31.9	22.2	0.12
Atrial fibrillation	33.7	39.3	0.42
Cerebrovascular disease	7.6	5.3	0.62
Peripheral vascular disease	6.5	11.6	0.17
Cardiomyopathy	17.9	14.7	0.61
Hypercholesterolemia	61.0	62.8	0.80
Hypertension	72.3	78.9	0.25
Moderate to severe renal disease	3.3	2.1	0.72
Diabetes	7.6	10.5	0.50
Previous cardiovascular surgery	22.3	18.9	0.54
MR severity: 3+ to 4+	95.7	92.6	0.48
MR etiology: degenerative / functional	73 / 27	73 / 27	0.81

MR, mitral regurgitation.

Table 18.3 Demographic comparison of EVEREST II population and patients underwent mitral surgical repair or replacement according to the Society of Thoracic Surgeon (STS) database.

	EVEREST II Randomized clinical trial			
	Demographic comparison			
	EVEREST II	*2008 STS database*		*Isolated 1st elective*
	RCT			*Operation for MR**
	n=279	*Repair*	*Replace*	*High volume hospitals (>140/Years)*
Age years (mean)	68	60	61	59
≥65 years	58%	37%	45%	n/a
≥75 years	32%	n/a	n/a	0%
NYHA class III or IV	50%	26%	45%	n/a
CHF	86%	41%	58%	n/a
Hypertension	75%	60%	67%	43%
Diabetes mellitus	9%	13%	23%	6.5%
COPD / Chronic lung disease	15%	17%	29%	n/a
EF (mean)	60%	53%	55%	56%

COPD, chronic obstructive pulmonary disease; EF, ejection fraction; MR, mitral regurgitation; NYHA, New York Heart Association; RCT, randomized controlled trial.

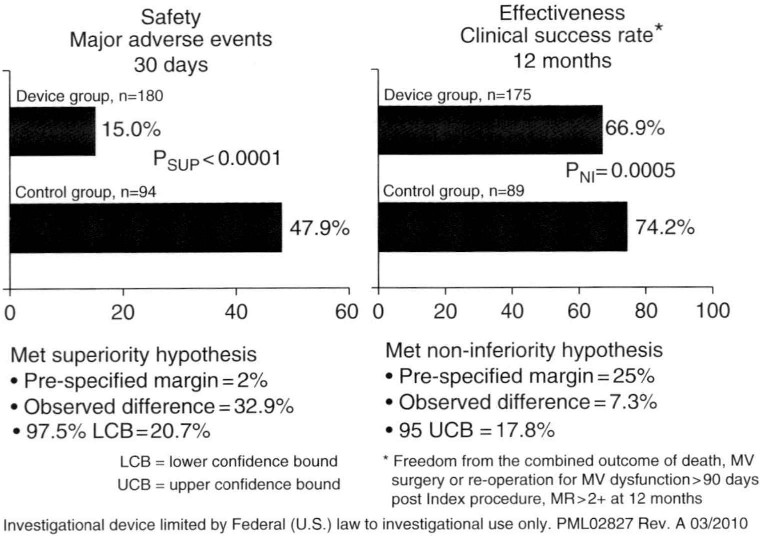

Fig. 18.27 Meeting of non-inferiority and superiority criteria in per protocol and intention to treat cohort. MR, mitral regurgitation; MV, mitral valve.

treated. The MitraClip treatment met the superiority hypothesis with an observed margin of 47.4%: major adverse events were 9.6% in the device group and 57% in the control group (*P* <0.0001). Also, the non-inferiority hypothesis was met, with an observed difference of 15.4% due to the evidence of the composite outcome of clinical success in 72.4% and 87.8% in the device and the control groups, respectively (Fig. 18.27). In the device group, major events were a gastrointestinal complication requiring surgery in one patient, and 12 patients requiring more than 2 units of blood elements. In the surgical control group, there were two deaths, two strokes, one reoperation for re-entry for bleeding, four patients requiring prolonged mechanical ventilation, and 42 (53%) patients requiring transfusions with more than 2 units of blood elements (Table 18.4). The study also demonstrated that patients undergoing MitraClip experienced reverse remodeling at 12 months with reduction of ventricular volumes, as well as improvement of symptoms and of quality of life assessed by the SF-36 survey (Fig. 18.28) [13].

Although the results of the EVEREST trial are interesting, the real world scenario is developing in a different way. Since the acquisition of the CE mark, MitraClip use in Europe is expanding. However, unlike the early experience in the EVEREST I and II trials, MitraClip is mostly used in Europe to treat functional mitral regurgitation. Unlike degenerative MR, surgical treatment of functional MR is suboptimal, with high risk and a high recurrence rate at 1 year. As a consequence, MitraClip offers an alternative with a lower risk for this specific population of patients. Most patients treated have comorbidities, previous open heart surgery, and other conditions increasing the risk of conventional surgery. Initial results appear to be promising [14,15] even though the procedure has been performed in patients with anatomic and clinical characteristics beyond the limits of the EVEREST inclusion criteria. However, no conclusion should be made until longer follow-up is available and controlled trials and registries are available.

Transapical beating heart chordal replacement

Chordal replacement with implantation of polytetrafluoroethylene (PTFE) sutures is an established repair technique in open heart surgery with excellent short- and long-term results [16–19]. Aiming at a complete percutaneous procedure, the NeoChord DS1000 device has

Table 18.4 30-day major adverse events (MAE) in the EVEREST II randomized clinical trial.

EVEREST II RCT: Primary safety endpoint		
Per protocol cohort		
	# Patients experiencing event	
	Device group	*Control group*
30 Days MAE, non-hierarchical	*(n = 136)*	*(n = 79)*
Death	0	2 (2.5%)
Major stroke	0	2 (2.5%)
Reoperation of mitral valve	0	1 (1.3%)
Urgent / emergent CV surgery	0	4 (5.1%)
Myocardial infarction	0	0
Renal failure	0	0
Deep wound infection	0	0
Ventilation >48 hours	0	4 (5.1%)
New onset permanent atrial fibrillation	0	0
Septicemia	0	0
GI complication requiring surgery	1 (0.7%)	0
All transfusions ≥2 units*	12 (8.8%)	42 (53.2%)
TOTAL % of patients with MAE	**9.6%**	**57.0%**
**P*<0.0001 if include Major Bleeding only	*P*<0.0001* (95% CI 34.4%, 60.4%)	

CI, confidence interval; CV, cardiovascular; GI, gastrointestinal.

been developed to realize transapical implantation of neochordae and thus enable beating heart mitral valve (MV) repair.

Procedure and technical details

The concept of beating heart transapical implantation of neochordae to the MV has been introduced and proven in acute and chronic animal studies by a group from the Mayo Clinic [20] and confirmed by Maisano et al. [8]. This group, in cooperation with the start-up company NeoChord Inc. (Minnetonka, MN), developed the DS1000 device (Fig. 18.29). Regarding clinical application, a transapical access to the MV is used to introduce the device into the left ventricle and left atrium (Figs 18.30 and 18.31). Then the device enables grasping of a mitral leaflet and deployment of a PTFE suture to the edge of the respective mitral valve leaflet. This is achieved by an adjustable gripper-like tip of the device with two jaws (Figs 18.30 and 18.31). After grasping the leaflet, the quality of tissue between the two jaws can be assessed using the device monitor. When confirming a good grasp with enough tissue (or a poor grasp with no tissue) betwseen the jaws, the four lights on the monitor reflect the white color of the leaflet tissue (red color of the blood). A needle to puncture the leaflet and retract the suture as well as an exchangeable cartridge for loading of the PTFE suture is installed within the device. After application of the PTFE neochordae to the leaflet, the device is retracted, both ends of the suture are pulled exteriorly of the apex, and a slip knot is tied and pulled tight to enable secure fixation of the suture onto the leaflet margin (Fig. 18.32). A free needle is then used to anchor the two ends of the suture individually over an additional felt pledget to the apex of the heart after adjusting the ideal length of the neochordae (Videos 18.2–18.6).

Pre-clinical experience comprises acute and chronic animal studies. During the animal trials, the NeoChord DS1000 has proven to be applicable for transapical replacement of chordae tendinae to the MV on the arrested as well as on the beating heart. The device monitor to confirm leaflet grasp, in particular, has been shown to be extremely valuable. Regarding the handling and procedural

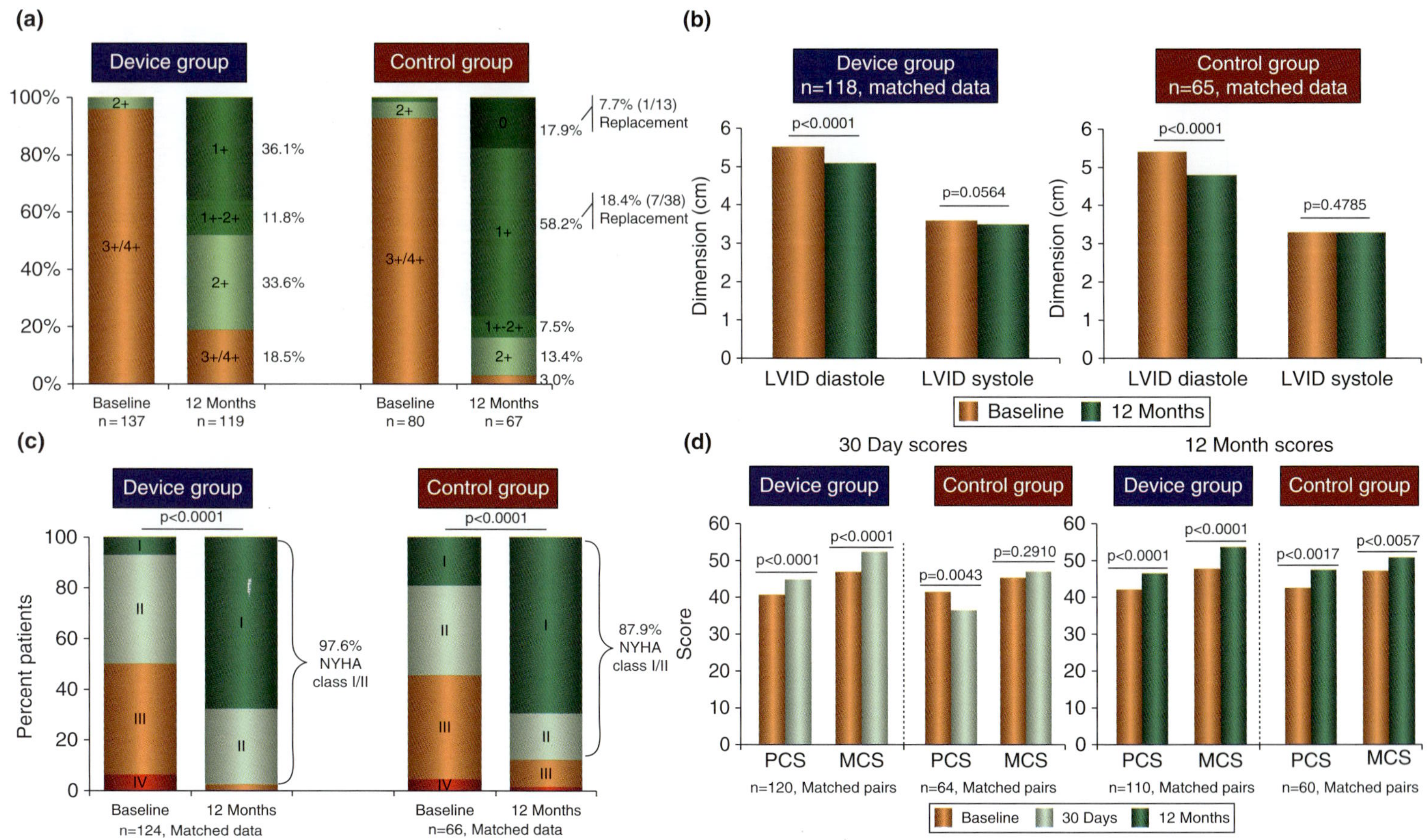

Fig. 18.28 Everest II 1-year results: difference between device and control groups in the per protocol cohort showing (a) mitral regurgitation, (b) left ventricular dimension, (c) functional status and (d) quality of life. LVID, Left Ventricular Internal Diameter; MCS, Mental Component Summary score; NYHA, New York Heart Association; PCS, Physical Component Summary score.

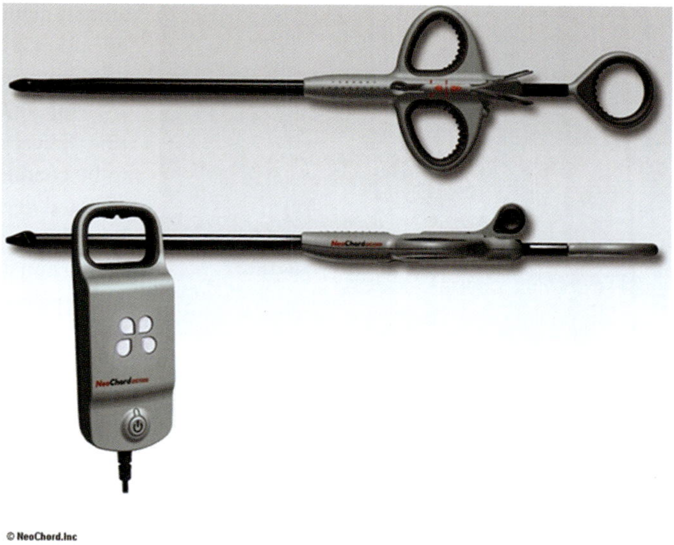

Fig. 18.29 The NeoChord DS1000 device for the application of neochordae to the mitral valve. The device is shown in two dimensions with the monitor that is used to confirm sufficient grasp.

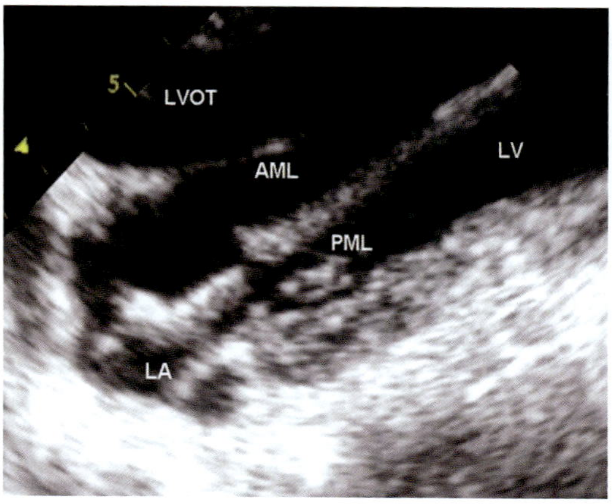

Fig. 18.30 The NeoChord DS1000 delivery system within the left atrium in an echocardiographic long axis view of an acute animal model. The device has been introduced through the apex of the heart and the jaws of the device are open towards the anterior mitral leaflet. When aiming for the posterior leaflet the device needs to be twisted for 180°. AML, anterior mitral leaflet; LA, left atrium; LV, left ventricle; LVOT, left ventricular outflow tract; PML, posterior mitral leaflet.

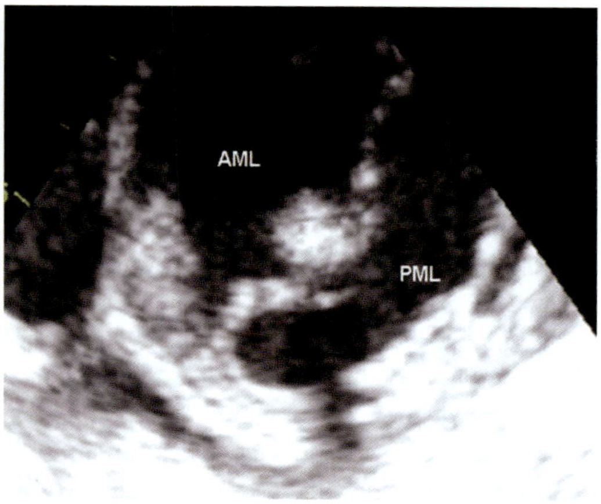

Fig. 18.31 The device is seen at the level of coaptation of the mitral valve (MV) leaflets at the level of the A2/P2 segment. The short axis view allows for easy orientation regarding the segments of the MV. AML, anterior mitral leaflet; PML, posterior mitral leaflet.

success of the device, surgical workflow analysis was performed during acute animal studies. The implantation procedure was divided into three different phases – phase I: introduction of the device from the apex into the left atrium; phase II: grasping of the mitral leaflet; phase III: fixation of the neochordae to the leaflet and retraction of the device. Successful grasping of the leaflet was achieved roughly every second attempt and showed overall a high procedural success. Regarding longevity and security of leaflet fixation of the neochordae, the chronic model showed no chordae rupture or any significant leaflet injury on cadaver examination at 60-day follow-up. Thus overall pre-clinical experience shows promising results for further application in man.

This newly developed technique is currently under investigation for human use in the Transapical Artificial Chordae Tendinae (TACT) trial. Primary endpoints of the study are the safety of the device and procedure, deployment and fixation of

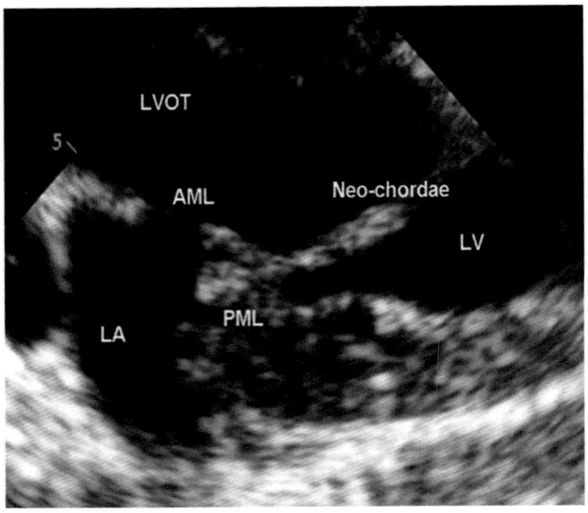

Fig. 18.32 After deploying the neochordae to the posterior leaflet, the device is retracted through the apical access. The neochordae is then suspended between the posterior mitral leaflet (PML) and apex of the heart at the desired length. AML, anterior mitral leaflet; LA, left atrium; LV, left ventricle; LVOT, left ventricular outflow tract.

neochordae to the mitral leaflet, and reduction of mitral regurgitation. Furthermore, relevant clinical parameters such as bleeding, recovery time, and level of pain are evaluated.

The main inclusion criterion for this study is an isolated P2 prolapse of the posterior leaflet resulting in grade 3+ or 4+ MR with clinical symptoms. Patients with additional MV pathologies such as massive dilation of the MV annulus, complex leaflet anatomy with indentations, perforation of leaflets, commissural prolapse, etc. are supposedly not eligible for inclusion. Furthermore patients with concomitant heart diseases such as atrial fibrillation, tricuspid valve regurgitation, or coronary artery disease are excluded. Thus an ideal patient would be a "healthy" young person with an isolated narrow P2 prolapse and severe MR but dyspnoea only on exertion, no comorbidities, and referred for surgery. This, however, is a rather small patient group in everyday cardiac surgical clinical practice. Nevertheless, the potential benefits of this repair technique are considered to be vast especially since current guidelines for patients with significant MR due to degenerative disease suggest performing MV repair at a reference center at the onset of symptoms and before structural cardiac changes such as an increase in ventricular size occurs. Correction of an anterior or even bileaflet prolapse is conceivable but so far only pursued in animal models. However, in an ideal candidate, the operation is hoped to completely restore native valve anatomy and physiologic valve function.

Before the introduction of this technique into routine clinical practice, proof of concept in humans has to be conducted. Despite the simplicity of the concept and device, numerous drawbacks and potential hazards exist: (i) procedural failure with the need for conversion to open heart surgery; (ii) incomplete MV repair without reduction of MR to at least grade 1+ or less; and (iii) injury of the mitral valve leaflets or chordae tendinae, the aortic valve, left atrium, ventricle, or other structures. Next to these potential major complications several obstacles may emerge during the implantation procedure: (i) exact positioning of the neochordae to the prolapsing segment; (ii) incomplete re-suspension of the leaflet without reduction of the MR; (iii) length adjustment of the neochord to eliminate prolapse but at the same time prevent additional restriction of the leaflet; and (iv) overall incomplete repair.

As a conclusion, transapical beating heart implantation of neochordae represents a promising new MV repair technique. Clinical evaluation is currently ongoing and initial steps towards fully percutaneous neochordae implantation are reported in early pre-clinical studies.

References

1 Alfieri O, Maisano F, De Bonis M, et al. The double-orifice technique in mitral valve repair: a simple solution for complex problems. J Thorac Cardiovasc Surg 2001;122(4):674–81.

2 Maisano F, Torracca L, Oppizzi M, et al. The edge-to-edge technique: a simplified method to correct mitral insufficiency. Eur J Cardiothorac Surg 1998;13(3):240–5; discussion 5–6.

3 De Bonis M, Lapenna E, La Canna G, et al. Mitral valve repair for functional mitral regurgitation in end-stage dilated cardiomyopathy: role of the "edge-to-edge" technique. Circulation 2005;112(9 Suppl):I402–8.

4 De Bonis M, Lorusso R, Lapenna E, et al. Similar long-term results of mitral valve repair for anterior compared with posterior leaflet prolapse. J Thorac Cardiovasc Surg 2006;131(2):364–70.

5 Naqvi TZ, Buchbinder M, Zarbatany D, et al. Beating-heart percutaneous mitral valve repair using a transcatheter endovascular suturing device in an animal model. Catheter Cardiovasc Interv 2007;69(4):525–31.

6 Naqvi TZ, Zarbatany D, Molloy MD, et al. Intracardiac echocardiography for percutaneous mitral valve repair in a swine model. J Am Soc Echocardiogr 2006;19(2):147–53.

7 Webb JG, Maisano F, Vahanian A, et al. Percutaneous suture edge-to-edge repair of the mitral valve. EuroIntervention 2009;5(1):86–9.

8 Maisano F, Michev I, Rowe S, et al. Transapical endovascular implantation of neochordae using a suction and suture device. Eur J Cardiothorac Surg 2009;36(1):118–22; discussion 22–3.

9 Fann JI, St Goar FG, Komtebedde J, et al. Beating heart catheter-based edge-to-edge mitral valve procedure in a porcine model: efficacy and healing response. Circulation 2004;110(8):988–93.

10 Luk A, Butany J, Ahn E, et al. Mitral repair with the Evalve MitraClip device: histopathologic findings in the porcine model. Cardiovasc Pathol 2009;18(5):279–85.

11 Herrmann HC, Kar S, Siegel R, et al. Effect of percutaneous mitral repair with the MitraClip device on mitral valve area and gradient. EuroIntervention 2009;4(4):437–42.

12 Feldman T, Kar S, Rinaldi M, et al. Percutaneous mitral repair with the MitraClip system: safety and midterm durability in the initial EVEREST (Endovascular Valve Edge-to-Edge REpair Study) cohort. J Am Coll Cardiol 2009; 54(8):686–94.

13 Sedrakyan A, Vaccarino V, Elefteriades JA, et al. Health related quality of life after mitral valve repairs and replacements. Qual Life Res 2006;15(7):1153–60.

14 Tamburino C, Ussia GP, Maisano F, et al. Percutaneous mitral valve repair with the MitraClip system: acute results from a real world setting. Eur Heart J 2010;31(11):1382–9.

15 Ranzen O, Baldus S, Rudolph V, et al. Acute outcomes of MitraClip therapy for mitral regurgitation in high-surgical-risk patients: emphasis on adverse valve morphology and severe left ventricular dysfunction. Eur Heart J 2010; 31(11):1373–81.

16 Seeburger J, Falk V, Borger MA, et al. Chordae replacement versus resection for repair of isolated posterior mitral leaflet prolapse. Ann Thorac Surg 2009;87(6):1715–20.

17 Zussa C, Frater RW, Polesel E, et al. Artificial mitral valve chordae: experimental and clinical experience. Ann Thorac Surg 1990;50(3):367–73.

18 Frater RW, Vetter HO, Zussa C, et al. Chordal replacement in mitral valve repair. Circulation 1990;82 (5 Suppl):IV125–30.

19 David TE, Bos J, Rakowski H. Mitral valve repair by replacement of chordae tendineae with polytetrafluoroethylene sutures. J Thorac Cardiovasc Surg 1991;101(3): 495–501.

20 Bajona P, Katz WE, Daly RC, et al. Beating-heart, off-pump mitral valve repair by implantation of artificial chordae tendineae: an acute in vivo animal study. J Thorac Cardiovasc Surg 2009;137(1):188–93.

Videoclips

This chapter contains the following videoclips:

Video 18.1 MitraClip procedure.
Videos 18.2–18.6 Transapical neochord procedure.

They can be accessed at www.wiley.com/go/Valverepair.

19

CHAPTER 19

Mitral valve: valvuloplasty for mitral stenosis/mitral regurgitation and available devices

Hasan Jilaihawi & Saibal Kar
Cedars-Sinai Heart Institute, Los Angeles, CA, USA

Anatomic aspects of the mitral valve

The mitral valve apparatus is a complex structure consisting of three components: the leaflets, chordae tendiniae, and the left ventricular papillary muscles (Fig. 19.1). Its normal functioning is attributable to the complex yet efficient interaction of these individual components throughout the cardiac cycle [1]. The normal mitral valve opens with the rise in left atrial pressure during left ventricular diastole allowing blood from the left atrium to fill the decompressed left ventricle. In early systole the rapid rise in left ventricular pressure closes the mitral valve with an upward force, while its competency is facilitated by the subvalvular apparatus transmitting a downward force on the leaflets so that they remain closed in late systole. This cohesive coordination of mitral valve function is disrupted in pathologic states. An understanding of the anatomic relations of the mitral valve to its neighboring structures is central to the success of all mitral interventions (Fig. 19.2).

Leaflets and annulus

The mitral annulus is the anatomic junction of the left atrium and the left ventricle and acts as a point of insertion for the anterior and posterior leaflets. The anterior mitral leaflet has a semi-lunar shape and occupies around 40% of the mitral annular circumference. It has a medial location and its neighboring structures are the left and right fibrous trigones (Fig. 19.1), part of the fibrous skeleton of the heart, which connect it to the left and non-coronary cusps of the aortic valve respectively; this continuity is often referred to as the aortic–mitral curtain. The posterior leaflet of the mitral valve is U-shaped and occupies approximately 60% of the annular circumference. It has a lateral location and is encircled by the coronary sinus and left circumflex coronary artery. In contrast to the anterior annulus, the posterior annulus does not have adjacent fibrous structures and the fibrous skeleton here is less developed.

The posterior leaflet is divided into three scallops. These are often referred to as P1 (anterolateral), P2 (middle), and P3 (posteromedial) scallops. The corresponding portions of the anterior leaflet are referred to as theh A1, A2, and A3 segments. The anterolateral and posteromedial commissures are the points where the anterior and posterior leaflets come together at their lateral and medial aspects, respectively (Fig. 19.1).

Subvalvular apparatus

The subvalvular apparatus consists of the chordae tendiniae, which connect the mitral valve to

Endovascular and Hybrid Therapies for Structural Heart and Aortic Disease, First Edition.
Edited by Jacques Kpodonu and Raoul Bonan.

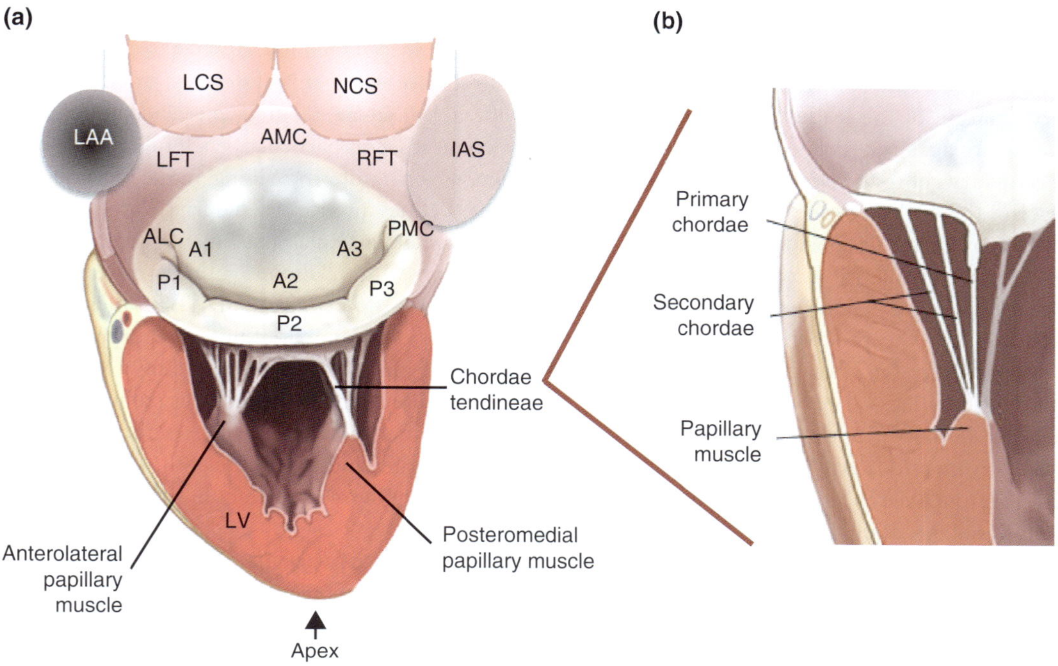

Fig. 19.1 Schematic of the mitral valve. (a) A longitudinal cross-section of the left ventricle, demonstrating the anatomic relationships of the mitral valve. The anterior leaflet is subdivided into three segments (A1, A2, A3), that correspond to the three scallops of the posterior leaflet (P1, P2, P3). ALC, anterolateral commissure; AMC, aortic–mitral curtain; IAS, inter-atrial septum; LAA, left atrial appendage; LCS, left coronary sinus; LFT, left fibrous trigone; NCS, non-coronary sinus (of aortic root); PMC, posteromedial commisure; RFT, right fibrous trigone. (b) The chordae tendiniae and their papillary muscle attachment. Adapted from Castillo et al. [81] with permission from Elsevier.

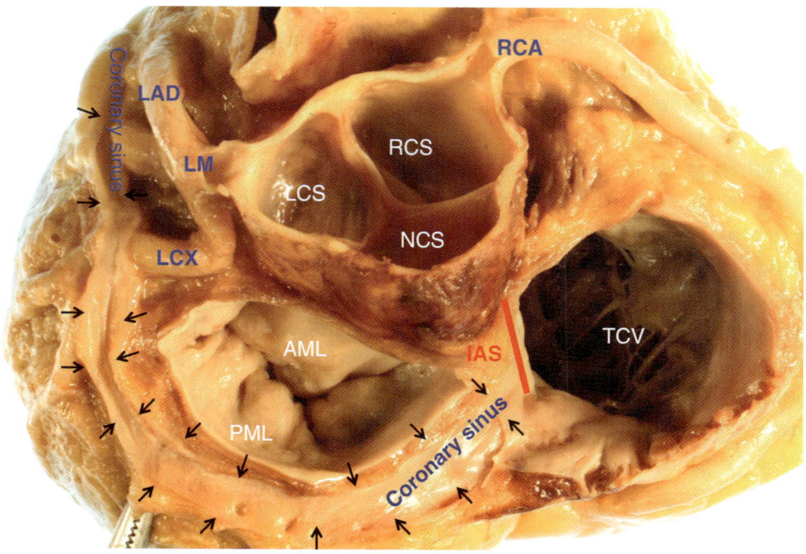

Fig. 19.2 Anatomic relations of the mitral valve. Arrows delineate the coronary sinus, which passes posteriorly to the posterior mitral leaflet (PML), and has a course that often crosses that of the left circumflex coronary artery (LCX). The anterior mitral leaflet (AML) is in close proximity to the left (LCS) and non-coronary (NCS) sinuses of the aortic valve. IAS, inter-atrial septum; LAD, left anterior descending artery; LM, left main stem; RCA, right coronary artery; RCS, right coronary sinus; TCV, tricuspid valve. Photograph of the pathologic specimen provided by Dr. Renu Virmani, CV Path Institute, Gaithersberg, MD.

the left ventricle via the papillary muscles, thereby inextricably linking their function (Fig. 19.1). Primary chordae are inserted to the free margin of the leaflets and function to prevent prolapse of the edges of each leaflet. Secondary chordae insert on the ventricular surface of the leaflets and relieve any excess tension they may carry. In considering patients for percutaneous mitral valve repair, the presence of intact primary and secondary chordae are required for the procedure to be feasible. The posterior leaflet has additional stabilizing tertiary chordae.

The chordae of both leaflets are linked to two papillary muscles, anterolateral and posteromedial, arising from the mid left ventricular walls. Ischemia and resultant dysfunction of the posteromedial papillary muscle in particular can result in ischemic mitral regurgitation and is classically seen in circumflex disease. Calcification of the subvalvular apparatus may be seen in rheumatic mitral valve disease and may contribute to leaflet restriction and is also a predictive factor for a poor response to surgical and transcatheter mitral valvotomy in predominant stenosis.

Imaging of the mitral valve

Echocardiography

The mitral valve was the first to have its disease diagnosed with echocardiography (mitral stenosis in 1968) and this remains the principal imaging modality for both diagnostic and interventional purposes [2]. There are two principal approaches to echocardiography – transthoracic (TTE) and transesophageal (TEE) – which are useful as simple non-invasive screening and diagnostic tools for the evaluation and quantification of the severity of mitral valve disease. The precise details pertaining to evaluation of the two principal disease processes, mitral stenosis and regurgitation, will be discussed later in the relevant sections.

TTE is used primarily as a gold standard for severity quantification (Fig. 19.3). TEE provides additional severity information where imaging windows are poor by TTE. It also offers clarity for the understanding of anatomic morphology and for intra-procedural guidance.

The relatively novel modality of 3D TEE deserves special mention. Applied to estimation of mitral valve area in mitral stenosis, it does not provide a real advantage for experienced operators, whereas it seems particularly helpful for less experienced operators, providing more reproducible data. It does improve a description of valvular anatomy, in particular assessment of commissural splitting with balloon mitral valvuloplasty (Fig. 19.4) [3]. In contrast, 3D TEE is increasingly used in the assessment of mitral regurgitation [4] and is of immense value in guiding novel transcatheter procedures targeting this pathology, with the potential to make complex structural interventions safer and more efficient [5]. This will be discussed in more detail later in the chapter.

Computed tomography

Multidetector computed tomography (MDCT) presently has the highest image quality of all non-invasive imaging modalities to visualize cardiac morphology due to its spatial resolution, clarity, and completeness of data [6]. However, for the mitral valve it lacks the temporal resolution (around 200 ms) relative to echocardiography (10 ms or less). A direct quantitative comparison between echocardiography and MDCT in mitral stenosis revealed a slight overestimation ($0.20 \pm 0.17\,cm^2$) of echocardiographic planimetry data for the mitral orifice area [7]. A recent study applying MDCT to mitral regurgitation demonstrated superior image quality relative to echocardiography [8], clearly showing morphological changes in valve leaflets such as tenting, but adding little on a practical level to information obtainable by TEE. It did, however, provide greater spatial resolution and hence superior imaging of the subvalvular apparatus, in particular the papillary muscles, although this additional information has at present an unclear utility in a clinical setting. Cardiac CT is of value in guiding suitability for transcatheter mitral valve repair by the coronary sinus approach and assesses with clarity the relation of the coronary sinus to the mitral annulus and the circumflex coronary artery (see Fig. 19.2) [9–11]. However, mitral annular dimension as measured by CT correlates poorly with traditional anatomic measures by echocardiography [12], which remains the preferred modality for this purpose.

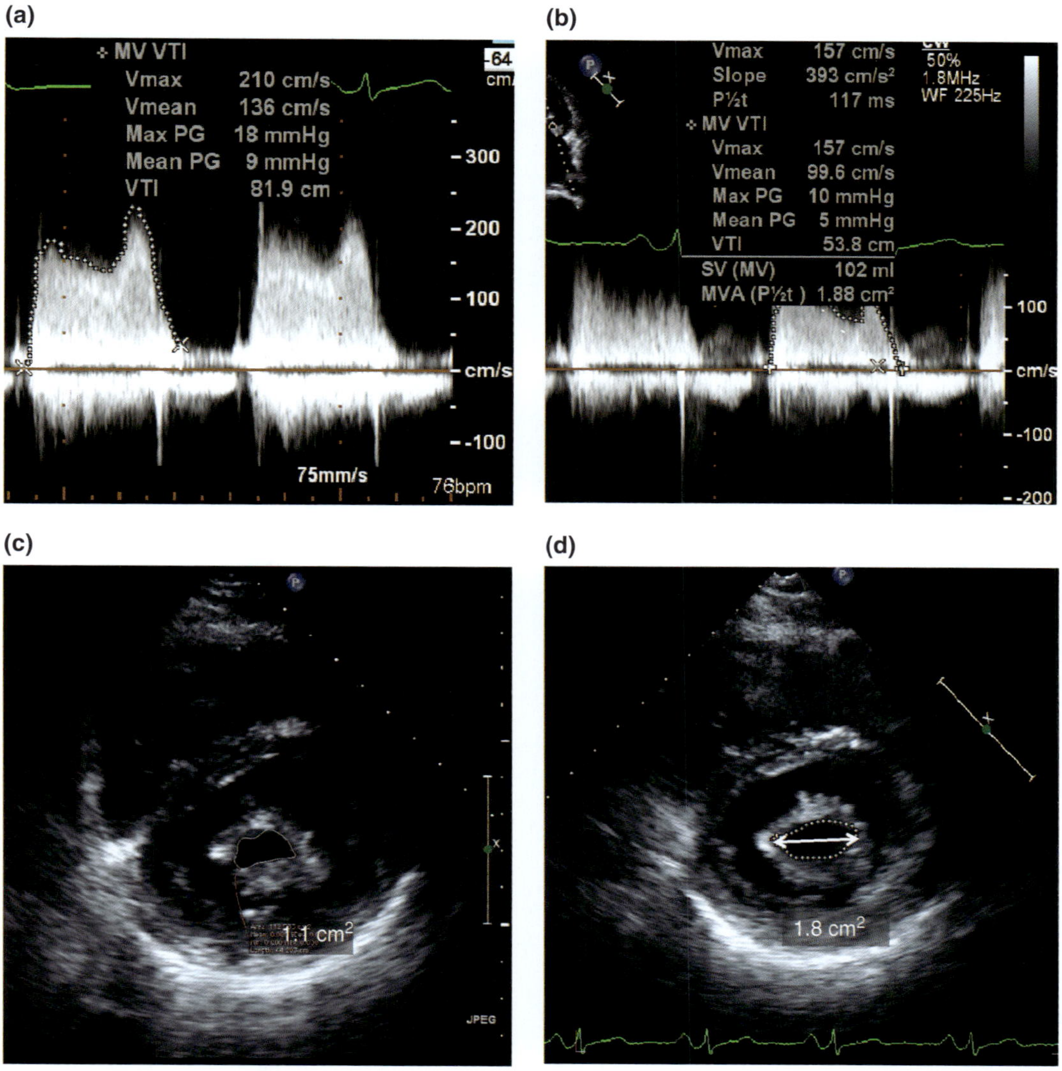

Fig. 19.3 TEE and severity assessment of mitral stenosis. Continuous wave Doppler demonstrating moderate–severe (a, c) and mild mitral stenosis (b, d), before and after percutaneous transvenous mitral valvuloplasty (PTMV), respectively (see Table 19.1). The mechanism of action of PTMV can be seen to be commissural splitting, with a longitudinal expansion of the mitral orifice observed (arrow).

Magnetic resonance imaging

Like CT, cardiac magnetic resonance imaging (MRI) has been applied effectively to the assessment of the anatomic relations used for the transcatheter coronary sinus approach to mitral annuloplasty [13]. It has additional strengths in the evaluation of the severity of mitral regurgitation [14,15] and left ventricular function and volume [16], thus offering the potential for comprehensive information in a single examination. It has more recently been used for the assessment of specific subsets of mitral valve disease such as mitral valve prolapse, where it may provide additional prognostic data with regard to arrhythmogenic potential, and has been used to measure other variables that may be of relevance to mitral regurgitation such as annular dimension [17].

(a)

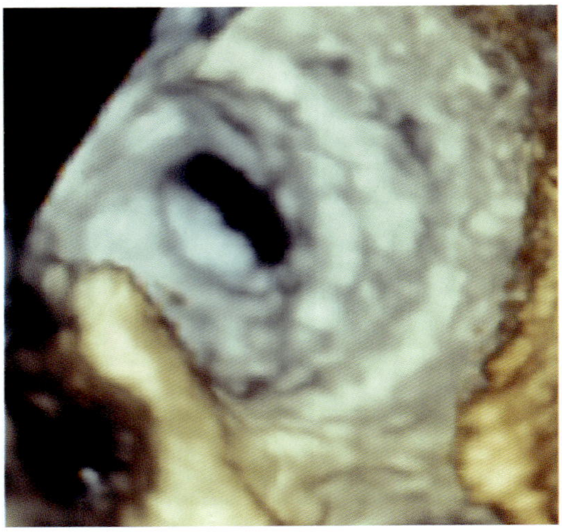

(b)

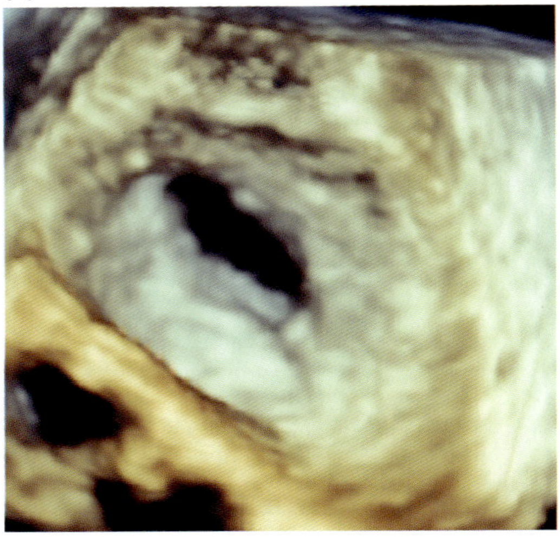

Fig. 19.4 3D TEE demonstration of commissural splitting by PTMV. The post-dilation 3D en face image shows the mitral orifice to have expanded longitudinally (b) in relation to the pre-dilation image (a).

Valvuloplasty for mitral stenosis

Mitral stenosis, a disease with principally a rheumatic etiology, was first described over 300 years ago by French anatomist Vieussens in 1705. It was the first valve lesion to be successfully treated by surgery by Harvard surgeon Elliot Cutler in 1923, using a knife through the wall of the left ventricle (LV) [2]. This was later superseded by the open valvotomy transauricular approach and later by the closed valvotomy approach through the left ventricular apex.

In 1982, mitral stenosis was the first valve lesion to be treated with percutaneous mitral balloon valvuloplasty (PMBV), by Japanese surgeon Kanji Inoue (see Fig. 19.4) [18], and this approach has now become the mainstay of treatment for the vast majority of patients with significant mitral stenosis. In anatomically suitable patients, it has consistently been shown to be equivalent in efficacy to surgical valvotomy approaches and has reduced associated morbidity considerably. Closed valvotomy is performed in some Asian countries when PMBV is considered an expensive option. Open valvotomy allows controlled reconstruction of the valves, and simultaneous tricuspid valve repair or mitral valve repair to be done if necessary, and is still recommended if there is concomitant severe tricuspid regurgitation, or in the absence of anatomic suitability for PMBV (see below).

Table 19.1 Severity grading of mitral stenosis.

	Mild	*Moderate*	*Severe*
Mean gradient (mmHg)	<5	5–10	>10
Pulmonary artery systolic pressure (mmHg)	<30	30–50	>50
Valve area (cm^2)	>1.5	1.0–1.5	<1.0

Modified from Bonow et al. [19] with permission from Lippincott Williams & Wilkins.

Although rheumatic fever and its associated rheumatic mitral valve disease have declined dramatically in developed countries, mitral stenosis still remains a common pathology in the developing world, which accounts for two-thirds of the world's population. In developed countries the disease is seen in older patients with greater comorbidities and as a result there is a higher likelihood of complicated outcomes following PMBV. PMBV is also known as percutaneous transvenous mitral commissurotomy (PTMC) and percutaneous transvenous mitral valvuloplasty (PTMV).

Patient evaluation

The evaluation of the severity of mitral stenosis involves an assessment of gradient, area, and pulmonary pressure (Table 19.1) [19]. The normal mitral valve area (MVA) is 4–6 cm^2 and a gradient

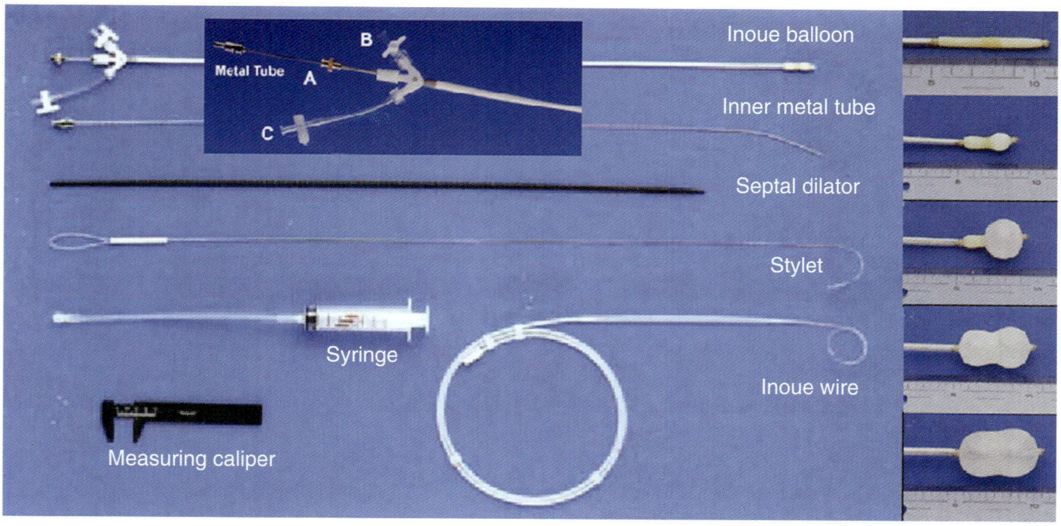

Fig. 19.5 The Inoue balloon system (Toray Industries, Inc., Tokyo, Japan). The measuring caliper is used to verify the dimensions of the syringe-inflated Inoue balloon prior to introduction into the body. The inner metal tube slenderizes the Inoue balloon (top right). When the inner tube is removed, the Inoue balloon expands distally first, then proximally, when inflated (right panel, lower four images). The inner lumen of the Inoue catheter (A) permits pressure measurements, blood sampling, or insertion of the inner metal tube, guide wire or stylet. The outer lumen connects proximally with a two-way stopcock (B) (used to connect the catheter to the syringe), and a vent (C). Adapted from www.ptmv.org.

is rare unless the valve is less than 2 cm^2. Severe (MVA <1 cm^2, mean gradient >10 mmHg) or moderate (MVA 1.0–1.5 cm^2, mean gradient 5–10 mmHg) symptomatic mitral stenosis indicate clinical suitability. Symptoms usually start when the MVA reduces to 1.5 cm^2, and most patients have obvious symptoms when the area is less than 1 cm^2. In asymptomatic patients, high-risk features that support PBV are severe pulmonary arterial hypertension at rest or with exercise, clinically significant increase in pulmonary artery wedge pressure with exercise, history of thromboemboli, a very large left atrium, new-onset atrial fibrillation, or evidence for right heart dysfunction.

Anatomic scores for predicting the likelihood of immediate success of PMBV include the 16-point Wilkins score [20] and the simpler 3-point Cormier score [21]. These include echocardiographic assessments of leaflet mobility, valvular and subvalvular thickening, and echocardiographic and fluoroscopic evaluations of calcification. A Wilkins score of more than 8 is predictive of a low rate of success following PMBV, whereas a Cormier echocardiographic score of less than 2 predicts success. As PMBV relies on the concept of commissural splitting, a valve with a bilateral commissural fusion benefits more than a valve without any commissural fusion, in which rigid or calcified leaflets or diseased subvalvular apparatus may fracture following PMBV. Although operators vary in their use of intra-procedural echocardiography, pre-procedural TEE is a prerequisite, both for the aforementioned anatomic assessment of suitability and to identify patients with left atrial and left atrial appendage thrombus in whom PMBV is prohibitive. Our own practice involves a peri-procedural TEE.

Clinical variables predicting immediate success include no prior commissurotomy, low New York Heart Association (NYHA) functional class, sinus rhythm, absence of mitral regurgitation, and lower effective balloon dilating area [21]. Contraindications to PMBV include persistent left atrial or left atrial appendage thrombus, more than moderate mitral regurgitation, massive or bicommissural calcification, severe tricuspid valve disease, and severe concomitant coronary artery disease requiring bypass surgery [22].

Available devices

Inoue's balloon (Fig. 19.5) was the first to be applied to PMBV and remains the most widely used device for this purpose worldwide. Other

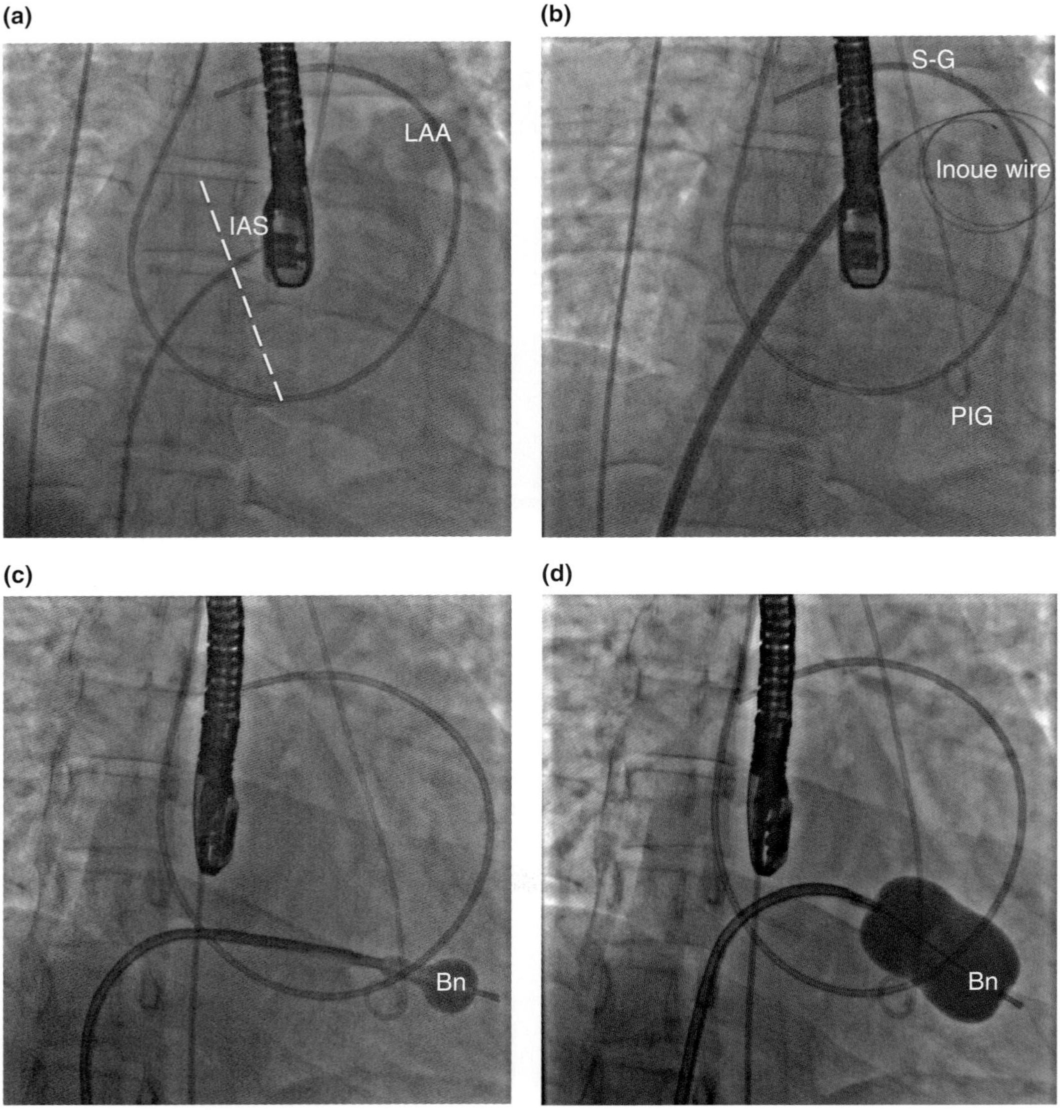

Fig. 19.6 Fluoroscopic imaging of the stepwise technique of PTMV. After performing transeptal puncture (a), the Inoue wire is advanced to the left atrium (b), over which the dilator is advanced to stretch the inter-atrial septum (IAS). The Inoue balloon (Bn) is then advanced over the Inoue wire into the left atrium (LA), and the Inoue wire is removed and replaced by the stylet, which is used to direct the balloon into the left ventricle (c). The distal end of the balloon is then inflated and pulled back, ensuring the tip is free and not trapped in the chordae. The balloon is then fully inflated (d), deflated and pulled back into the LA, where the pressures can be compared to those of the left ventricle (LV), determining a LA : LV gradient. LAA, left atrial appendage.

devices used include cylindrical balloons, first used in India [23], the double balloon, first used in Saudi Arabia [24], and Cribier's metallic commissurotome [25,26]. The metallic commissurotome has the benefit of resterilization with an associated cost saving.

Procedure

The Inoue balloon procedure is a cath lab procedure performed with fluoroscopic and echocardiographic guidance (Fig. 19.6). In some centers it is performed under general anesthesia with fluoroscopy/TEE guidance or under local anesthesia with pre-procedural TEE to verify the absence of left atrial thrombus and intra-procedural fluoroscopy guidance with or without intra-procedural TTE. In the present era, transeptal puncture is usually performed under TEE guidance, precisely localizing it to the fossa. TEE accurately guides this, minimizes complications, and detects complications such as tamponade early. When performed under fluoroscopy guidance, a pigtail is positioned in the aortic root. Right anterior oblique (RAO), anteroposterior (AP) and lateral views are most useful. In the RAO view, the needle should lie just anterior to the spine, in the AP view just below the pigtail catheter, and in the lateral view midway between the pigtail and posterior margin of the cardiac silhouette.

Extremely large atria may mandate different shapes and sizes of transeptal needle. The needle is advanced using the pressure waveform to verify passing into the left atrium. The whole system is then advanced by 1 cm, the dilator advanced a further 1 cm and then the transeptal catheter advanced well into the left atrium. The needle is then withdrawn. The arterial pigtail is advanced into the LV, calculating a baseline gradient.

The Inoue wire, with its special loop design, is then positioned in the left atrium. This is used to advance the Inoue dilator, dilating groin, and septum. The slenderized Inoue balloon is advanced, the silver inner metal tube retracted 2–3 cm, allowing the system to be advanced to the zenith of the wire's curve. The gold tube is then retracted, making the balloon floppy and allowing it to be advanced further. In the RAO projection, the customized stylet has a shepherd's crook shape and is then advanced and torqued anticlockwise (anteriorly) with a simultaneous advancement of the Inoue balloon system into the LV. The distal balloon is then gently inflated, the system retracted until there is resistance of contact with the mitral valve, and the balloon is inflated fully.

Immediate procedural success is most often defined as a final valve area $\geq 1.5\,cm^2$ without moderate or severe mitral regurgitation [22]. Other proposed indices of success include valve area : body surface area $\geq 1\,cm^2/m^2$, complete opening of at least one commissure, and no significant ($\geq$ grade 1 in the Sellers 0 to 4 classification) increase in mitral regurgitation relative to baseline [27].

Tips and tricks

Aside from case selection, an important element to the success of PTMV by the Inoue technique is appropriate balloon selection. Current manufacturer guidelines on balloon sizing are based on patient height, transthoracic echocardiographic findings of the mitral valve, and fluoroscopic presence of valvular calcification. The balloon reference size (RS) is best calculated according to a simple formula previously described [28]: patient height (in cm) is rounded to the nearest 10 cm and divided by 10, and 10 is added to yield the RS (in mm); e.g. if height = 148 cm, then RS = 150/10 + 10 = 25 mm. For pliable valves, a balloon catheter corresponding to the RS is used [29]. In contrast, in valves susceptible to iatrogenic severe mitral regurgitation (such as those severely calcified or with subvalvular lesions, with high Wilkins and Cormier scores), a balloon catheter one size smaller than an RS match is selected [29]. In the example of a 25 mm RS, a PTMC-26 Inoue catheter would be used for a pliable valve, whereas a PTMC-24 Inoue catheter is recommended for a "high-risk" valve. Inoue catheters are available in 2 mm size increments from PTMC-20 to PTMC-30.

Controlled stepwise inflation is important to avoid the severe complication of mitral regurgitation. This involves an understanding of pressure–volume relationships and the concept of the "high pressure" zone. The intra-balloon pressure transits from the "low pressure" to the "high pressure" zone as the balloon is inflated to within 2 mm of its nominal size, e.g. the 24–26 mm zone in a 26 mm balloon catheter (PTMC-26) [30]. The choice of initial inflation pressure is important and is influenced by the presence of pre-existing mitral regurgitation and whether the valve treated is "high risk", as has been discussed. In pliable valves the initial inflation size is (RS – 2) mm, and for "high risk" valves it is (RS – 4) mm. A stepwise dilation technique is recommended, with increments of 1 mm in the low pressure zone and 0.5 mm in the high pressure zone. The degree of mitral regurgitation (MR) should be assessed after each stepwise inflation and, if present, there should be 0.5 mm increments and no further inflations if the MR grade is ≥2+. While in the ventricle, the distal tip of the balloon is inflated and advanced back and forth, to ensure that it is free in the ventricle and not trapped in the chordae. This protects against accidental dilation within the subvalvular apparatus, which can cause severe MR.

Crossing the mitral valve can sometimes be challenging. In such cases a 0.025 or 0.018 inch wire can be used to advance through the balloon to the LV. In very large left atria, or when the transeptal puncture is too anterior, a reverse loop technique can be used to cross the mitral valve.

The imaging modality employed peri-procedurally is an important issue of contention. Some favor a local anesthesia, fluoroscopy-guided approach, with observation of transcatheter hemodynamics and use of TTE if necessary. However, this does not allow assessment of commissural splitting and characterization of any damage to the subvalvular apparatus, which can be clearly visualized by intra-procedural TEE. Although the latter strategy mandates general anesthesia in most cases, this is rarely an issue of concern with a good cardiac anesthesiologist and may help avoidance of complications, particularly in older patients treated in Western countries who often have less favorable valve anatomy.

Complications

Due to a refined case selection process and careful attention to procedural steps, PTMV has a high rate of success and a low complication rate. Important complications can occur and include cardiac tamponade, atrial septal defect, systemic embolism, severe MR (Fig. 19.7), emergent surgery, and death [31]. These complications have declined significantly with increasing global operator experience and a highly evolved technique and have declined to negligible rates overall [31]. The low procedural mortality is close to zero and usually occurs in the context of iatrogenic severe MR or tamponade. The routine use of echocardiography during the procedure and use of the stepwise dilation approach has minimized the complications of tamponade and iatrogenic mitral regurgitation.

Review of the literature

The natural history of treated and untreated disease has been well characterized. In developing countries, where rheumatic heart disease is prevalent, mitral stenosis tends to progress rapidly whereas in developed countries, where degeneration is more important in the pathophysiology, progression is more gradual [2]. Although there has been no randomized trial of PTMV versus medical therapy, the prognosis of untreated severe mitral stenosis is poor and is worsened by increasing NYHA status [2]. That said, PTMV has a reduced initial morbidity with short-term and medium-term survival similar to that recorded after open valvotomy [2]. Three small randomized studies of percutaneous mitral valvuloplasty have demonstrated results at least as good as those of closed surgical valvotomy [32–34]. One of these studies additionally demonstrated better symptomatic results with PTMV. Another had an additional comparator group of open surgical valvotomy, and although similar rates of restenosis were seen at 7-year follow-up with PTMV and open valvotomy, PTMV achieved lower rates of restenosis than closed commissurotomy [32].

Case selection, including the aforementioned echocardiographic scores, and center volume are important factors in rates of success in PTMV [35]. Procedural success varies from around 95% or more in optimal patients from high volume centers, to 80–85% in lower volume centers, and to less than 50–60% in patients with suboptimal anatomy [27]. Even in patients with good echocardiography scores and procedural success, the frequency of events progressively increases at 5 years following intervention with 62% requiring reintervention at 12 years of follow-up, but with a good rate of survival (82%) at this time point [36].

The available literature is dominated by the use of the Inoue device. Some non-randomized comparisons of the double balloon and Inoue balloon showed a higher likelihood of immediate optimal result with less iatrogenic mitral regurgitation [37,38], while others have shown no difference in the short or long term, with longer fluoroscopy times with the double balloon approach [39–43]. A randomized study comparing approaches showed no difference in immediate and 7-year outcomes between the double balloon and Inoue balloon [44]. Similarly, a single cylindrical versus Inoue balloon comparison showed no difference in efficacy but shorter procedures with fewer complications with the Inoue balloon [45]. A polyethylene balloon via

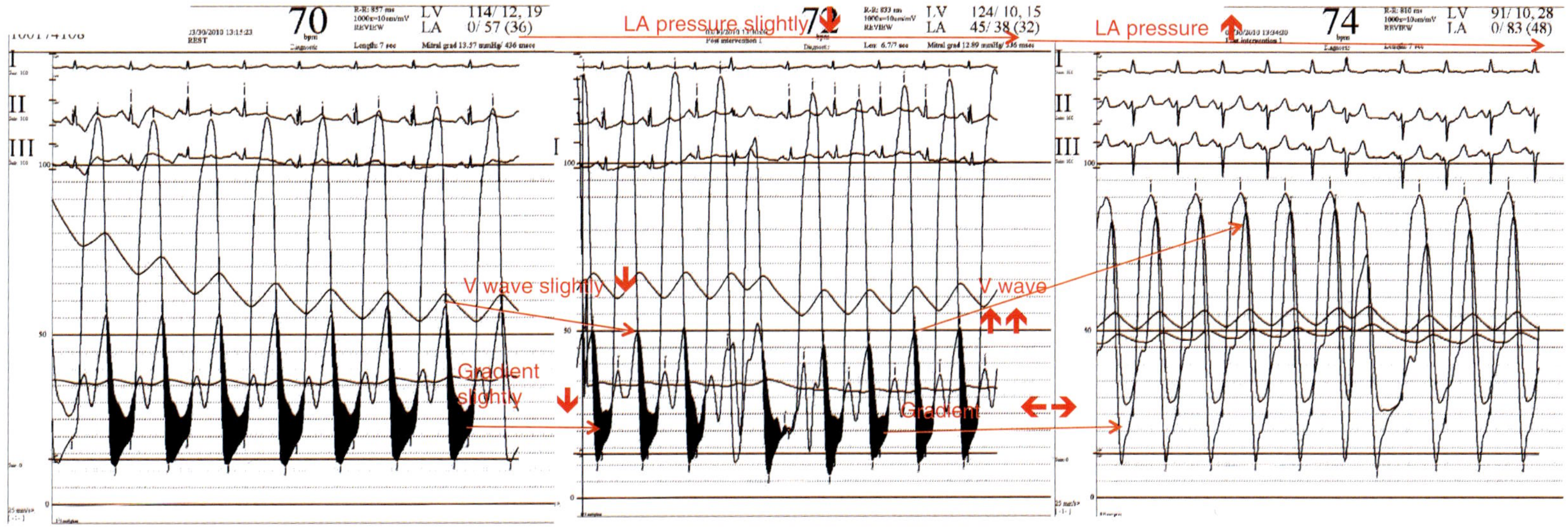

Fig. 19.7 Hemodynamics of PTMV complicated by severe mitral regurgitation. Pre PTMV tracing (left panel) shows a significant transmitral gradient (black shading). The V wave is likely elevated (57 mmHg) due to poor left atrial compliance associated with mitral stenosis. Initial dilation results in a reduction in this V wave to 38 mmHg, with a slight reduction in LA : LV gradient. Further mitral dilation (right panel) results in a huge increase in the V wave to 83 mmHg, indicative of severe mitral regurgitation. The transmitral gradient remained elevated due to the increased flow associated with severe MR. The patient was stabilized with an intra-aortic balloon pump and went for emergency surgery. Reproduced from Jilaihawi et al. [76] with permission from Elsevier.

the retrograde approach has also been used and compared to the Inoue technique, but had a lower mitral valve area achieved and a higher complication rate [46] with longer fluoroscopy times [47].

A non-randomized comparison of the Inoue balloon, metallic commissurotome, and multitrack double-balloon valvuloplasty showed no difference in immediate outcomes [48]: randomized comparisons of them have demonstrated similar results at immediate, short- and medium-term follow-up [49,50]. One study estimated the cost of a procedure with the metallic commissurotome to be a quarter of that of the Inoue technique [51].

Mitral regurgitation and available devices

The decline of rheumatic heart disease in developed countries has brought a decline in mitral stenosis but, in contrast, mitral regurgitation is a growing problem [52]. Moderate or severe mitral regurgitation is frequent and was thought to affect in excess of 2 million people in the USA in 2000; population aging and growth are expected to at least double this figure by 2030 [52]. Mitral regurgitation is due to failure of anterior and posterior leaflet coaptation leading to a regurgitation of left ventricular blood into the left atrium in systole. It is described according to causes and mechanisms. These are separately classified, with a particular cause producing regurgitation by a number of mechanisms [53]. Causes are etiologic descriptors of the pathophysiology and broadly classified as ischemic (due to consequences of ischemic heart disease) and non-ischemic. Non-ischemic causes include degenerative (myxomatous disease, leaflet degeneration, annular calcification), endocarditic, rheumatic, and less common miscellaneous causes (congenital, cardiomyopathy, inflammatory, drug-induced, trauma).

Mechanisms are anatomic descriptors and are classified as functional (mitral valve is structurally normal, regurgitation is caused by extrinsic valve deformation, such as annular dilation associated with LV remodeling) or organic (there is an abnormality intrinsic to the leaflets such as flail, prolapse, or restriction). The same organic/functional dichotomy for mechanisms of mitral regurgitation is often expressed as primary/secondary [54]. Another widely used mechanistic subclassification in the surgical literature is that of leaflet motion devised by Carpentier, who also first proposed lesion localization by A1–3 and P1–3 [55]. This subclassification is type I (normal leaflet motion), type II (excessive leaflet motion), and type III (restrictive leaflet motion) [55]. However, this classification has less relevance in the assessment of candidates for percutaneous mitral valve repair.

The severity of mitral regurgitation is often difficult to quantify. A combination of qualitative and quantitative criteria have been proposed by the American Society of Echocardiography guidelines (Table 19.2) [56]. Based on these criteria, MR can be graded as grade 1 to grade 4. Grade 3 and grade 4 are considered to be clinically significant.

Depending on cause and mechanism, medical therapy with diuretics, angiotensin-converting enzyme (ACE) inhibition, and beta-blockade for mitral regurgitation can provide some symptom relief, but no change has been consistently demonstrated on survival [53]. Cardiac resynchronization therapy has been used successfully to reduce MR whose underlying mechanism is functional and associated with significant dyssynchronous left ventricular dysfunction. For the most part, surgery is the mainstay of therapy for significant MR and, if feasible, surgical repair rather than replacement is the preferred treatment because of lower infection, better ventricular remodeling, and increased survival [57]. In the present era, there are several percutaneous repair techniques available, most of which are in the early phases and based on surgical principles; these can be broadly divided into annuloplasty approaches and leaflet repair [58]. Several technologies are emerging but only a few have undergone safety evaluations in man, and even fewer have been studied for efficacy (Table 19.3). In addition to repair technologies, companies are also working on percutaneous mitral valve replacement technologies which may have an important place for patients unsuitable for repair. These are early in their development and far from clinical studies at present. Interestingly, the Edwards Sapien transcatheter aortic valve (Edwards Lifesciences, Irvine, CA) has been effectively used by a transapical valve-in-valve approach for stenotic and regurgitant degenerated mitral bioprostheses [59,60].

Table 19.2 Severity grading of mitral regurgitation using qualitative and quantitative criteria proposed by the American Society of Echocardiography.

	Mild	*Moderate*		*Severe*
Specific signs of severity	Small central jet <4 cm² or <20% of LA area* Vena contracta width <0.3 cm No or minimal flow convergence	Signs of MR > mild present but no criteria for severe MR		Vena contracta width ≥0.7 cm with large central MR jet (area >40% of LA) or with a wall-impinging jet of any size, swirling in LA* Large flow convergence Systolic reversal in pulmonary veins Prominent flail MV leaflet or ruptured papillary muscle
Supportive signs	Systolic dominant flow in pulmonary veins A-wave-dominant mitral inflow pattern Soft density, parabolic CW Doppler MR signal Normal LV size	Intermediate signs/ findings		Dense, triangular CW Doppler MR jet E-wave-dominant mitral inflow (E >1.2 m/s) Enlarged LV and LA size (particularly when normal LV function is present)
Quantitative signs				
R vol (ml/beat)	<30	30–44	45–59	≥60
RF (%)	<30	30–39	40–49	≥50
EROA (cm²)	<0.2	0.2–0.29	0.3–0.39	≥0.4

Modified from Zoghbi et al. [56] with permission from Elsevier.
*At a Nyquist limit of 50–60 cm/s.
CW, continuous wave; EROA, effective regurgitant orifice area; LA, left atrium; LV, left ventricle; MR, mitral regurgitation; MV, mitral valve; R vol, regurgitant volume; RF, regurgitant fraction.

While percutaneous repair will be our primary focus for the remainder of this chapter, several devices have emerged for percutaneous annuloplasty that will be briefly discussed. Percutaneous annuloplasty devices may be divided into those that employ direct or indirect approaches. Indirect approaches exploit the anatomic proximity of the coronary sinus to the mitral valve. The coronary sinus partially encircles the posterior mitral leaflet, covering approximately two-thirds of its circumference (see Fig. 19.2). It is easily accessed via the right atrium by either the femoral or jugular venous approach and thus, with its simplicity, appeared an extremely attractive treatment modality initially. Devices used in this manner thus far in man include the Cardiac Dimensions Carillon device (Kirkland, WA), the Edwards Monarc device, and the Viacor PTMA device (Viacor Inc., Wilmington, MA).

All of the coronary sinus (indirect annuloplasty) devices have been subject to important limitations. The first of these is device fracture, with the unexpectedly high torsional forces in the coronary sinus. Secondly, an important problem encountered with these devices lies in the anatomic course of the coronary sinus; the coronary sinus crosses the path of the circumflex or an obtuse marginal branch in up to three-quarters of patients [9–11]. Heterogenous results have been achieved with these devices. In a study of the Viacor device only 9/27 patients actually had a device successfully implanted and only five of these had a reduction in MR [61]. The company has stopped further development of this device.

The Edwards Monarc device was evaluated in the EVOLUTION study in which the device was successfully implanted in 82% of patients [62]. The majority of patients had only 2+ MR and hence a reduction in MR was seen in only 41%, although a reduction in MR was seen in 86% of patients with MR ≥3+. Of those with coronary angiographic follow-up, 30% had some degree of coronary compression, which was significant (>50%) in 8%. Important lessons in case selection were

Table 19.3 Table of technologies: (I–IV) percutaneous mitral valve repair devices and (V) percutaneous mitral valve replacement devices.

Site of action	*Mechanism of action*	*Device*	*Status*	*Major limitations*
(I) Leaflets	(A) Edge-to-edge (leaflet plication)	MitraClip (Abbott Vascular, Santa Clara, CA)	Randomized trial data presented	Results when performed alone may not be durable. Possibility of iatrogenic MS
		MitraFlex (TransCardiac Therapeutics, LLC, Atlanta, GA)	Pre-clinical development	As for MitraClip
	(B) Space occupier (leaflet coaptation)	Percu-Pro Cardiosolutions Inc, West Bridgewater, MA	Phase 1 trial	Device thrombus formation. Residual MR or iatrogenic MS
	(C) Leaflet ablation	Thermocool (Biosense Webster, Inc., Diamond Bar, CA)	Animal models	Scarring not precise with residual MR. Leaflet/cardiac structure perforation
(II) Annulus	(A) Indirect annuloplasty			
	Coronary sinus approach (CS reshaping)	Monarc (Edwards Lifesciences, Irvine, CA)	FIM results. Feasibility study ongoing	CS at a distance from MA. Possibility of coronary artery compression
		Carillon (Cardiac Dimensions, Kirkland, WA)	FIM results. Feasibility study complete	As above
		Viacor (Viacor Inc., Wilmington, MA)	FIM results. Feasibility study ongoing	As above
	Asymmetric approach	St. Jude device St Jude Medical Inc., St Paul, MN	Animal models	CS at a distance from MA. Unequal tension on LA or MA. Device fracture or erosion, and thrombus formation
		NIH Cerclage technology (No manufacturer stated)	Animal models	CS at a distance from MA. Unequal tension on LA or MA
	(B) Direct annuloplasty			
	Percutaneous mechanical cinching	Mitralign (Mitralign, Inc., Tewksbury, MA)	FIM results	Only posterior MA cinching
		Accucinch GDS Guided Delivery Systems, Inc., Santa Clara, CA	FIM results	As above

(*Continued*)

Table 19.3 (*Cont'd*).

Site of action	*Mechanism of action*	*Device*	*Status*	*Major limitations*
	Percutaneous energy-mediated cinching	QuantumCor Quantumcor, Inc - San Clemente, CA	Animal models	Scarring not precise. Possible residual MR or atrogenic MS. Risk of cardiac structure perforation
		ReCor (ReCor Medical, Inc., Ronkonkoma, NY)	FIM results	As above; reduction in annular dimensions not accompanied by MR reduction
	Hybrid	Mitral solutions Mitral solutions, Fort Lauderdale, FL	Pre-clinical development	Not true "percutaneous" technique
		MiCardia MiCardia Corporation, Irvine, CA	Pre-clinical development	As above
(III) Chordal	(A) Transapical artificial chord	NeoChord NeoChord, Inc., Eden Prairie, MN MitraFlex TransCardiac Therapeutics, Atlanta, GA	Pre-clinical development	Residual leaflet prolapse or restriction with residual MR. Thrombus formation
	(B) Transapical–transeptal artificial chord	Babic (No manufacturer stated)	Pre-clinical development	As above
(IV) LV	LV (and MA) remodeling	Mardil-BACE Mardil Medical, Inc., Plymouth, MN	Temporary human implant	Requires minithoracotomy. Long-term effects unknown
(V) pMVR	Right minithoracotomy	Endovalve Endovalve, Inc., Princeton, NJ Herrmann prosthesis	Animal models	Anchoring challenges. LV outflow obstruction. Paravalvular leaks
	Transapical	Lutter prosthesis	Animal models	As above
	Transeptal	CardiaQ prosthesis	Pre-clinical development	As above

Adapted from Chiam et al. [83].

CS, coronary sinus; FIM, first-in-man; GDS, guided delivery system; LV, left ventricle/ventricular; MA, mitral annulus; MR, mitral regurgitation; MS, mitral stenosis; pMVR, percutaneous mitral valve replacement; NIH, National Institutes of Health.

implemented in the EVOLUTION II study but this was stopped by the sponsor due to slow enrollment [58]. The AMADEUS study evaluated the Cardiac Dimensions Carillon device, which was successfully implanted in 30 of the 48 patients enrolled [63]. Using quantitative measures, there was a 23% average reduction in MR, which was accompanied by significant improvements in NYHA status, 6-minute walk, and quality of life indices. Similar results for the Carillon were obtained with longer

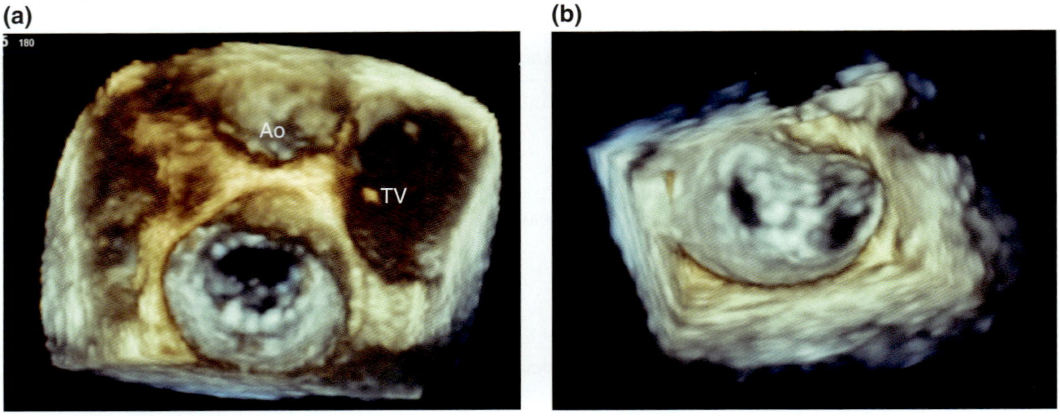

Fig. 19.8 Double orifice mitral valve repair. Demonstration by 3D TEE in the en face projection, with conversion of a single orifice (a) to a double orifice (b). Ao, aorta; TV, tricuspid valve.

follow-up in the TITAN study [64]. Studies ongoing for this device in grade 3–4+ functional MR include the INTEGRAL study in South America and the TITAN II study in Europe. The principal practical difference between the Monarc and Carillon devices is that although the Carillon achieves its maximal effect immediately, the Monarc requires several weeks for its spring to shorten fully.

The percutaneous direct annuloplasty approach avoids the potential problems of coronary compression but is technically more challenging. Two such devices are the Mitralign and the Guided Delivery Systems device (Boston, MA) [58]. They employ retrograde arterial access to the posterior mitral leaflet. In contrast to other percutaneous mitral devices, they are still early in their development with only preliminary first-In-man experiences. It should be noted that all percutaneous annuloplasty devices so far have treated patients with functional MR, for which surgical data are equally heterogeneous, often depending on whether the underlying cause is ischemic or non-ischemic [65,66].

Percutaneous leaflet repair has so far dominated the field of transcatheter therapies for mitral regurgitation, with the first data compared to surgery in a randomized trial [67]. These data will be discussed in some detail later in this chapter. Surgical leaflet repair has mainly used annuloplasty combined with leaflet resection for mitral regurgitation. It is likely that future percutaneous approaches for MR will combine both transcatheter annuloplasty and leaflet repair approaches. Although no transcatheter leaflet resection techniques are presently available, robotic mitral valve repair includes posterior leaflet resection on a frequent basis and is continuing to evolve rapidly as a minimally invasive approach [68]. In contrast to resection, a much less frequently used surgical approach is the double orifice, edge-to-edge repair, pioneered by Italian surgeon Ottavio Alfieri almost 20 years ago [69]. Despite only being performed in a small number of patients, durable clinical follow-up has been demonstrated up to 12 years post procedure, a compelling proof of concept for this technique [70].

Edge-to-edge, or more appropriately named double orifice (Fig. 19.8), percutaneous mitral valve repair has been employed in man using two devices. The Edwards Mobius device (Edwards Lifesciences, Irvine, CA) used a stitch delivered by the anterograde transeptal approach [71,72]. Because of "mixed results, procedural complexity, and a perceived limited patient population, the further investigation and device development has been suspended at present" [71].

Fortunately, this has not been the experience with the second device to employ a leaflet-to-leaflet repair approach for mitral regurgitation. The MitraClip device (Fig. 19.9) is a CE marked device that had been evaluated in a pivotal, randomized controlled trial. Although initially conceived for organic (primary) MR with malcoaptation, it has also been used effectively for functional (secondary) MR and, at least in Europe, is rapidly finding its place in the cardiologist's – and the surgeon's – armamentarium for treating mitral regurgitation.

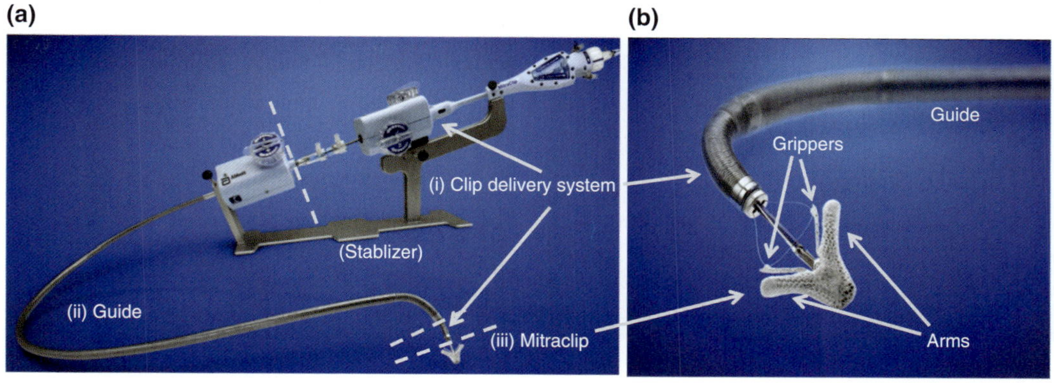

Fig. 19.9 The MitraClip system (Abbott Vascular, Santa Clara, CA). (a) The Evalve MitraClip system consisting of two principal components: (i) a clip delivery system (CDS) used to position and deploy the clip, and (ii) a steerable guide catheter. (iii) The MitraClip device is attached to the CDS. A stabilizer keeps the system precisely in position. (b) The MitraClip device. Reproduced from Jilaihawi et al. [82] with permission from Springer.

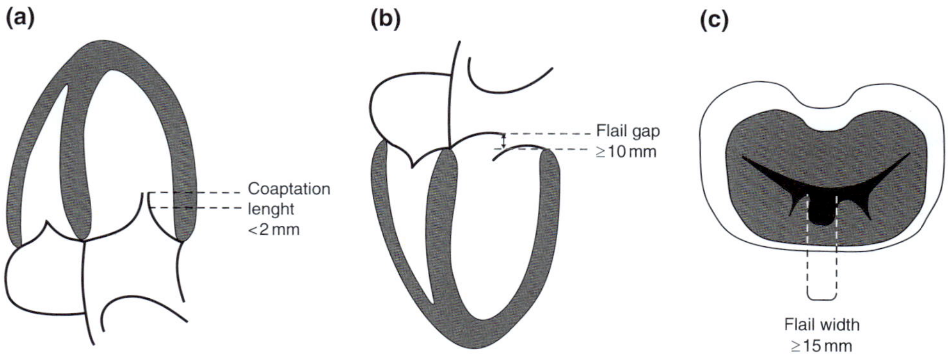

Fig. 19.10 Anatomic exclusion criteria for the MitraClip device: (a) insufficient coaptation length, (b) excessive flail gap, and (c) excessive flail width. Reproduced from Jilaihawi et al. [82] with permission from Springer.

In the remainder of this chapter we will discuss patient evaluation, procedural information, tips and tricks, complications, case examples, and the literature pertaining to this device.

MitraClip procedure

Patient evaluation

There are a number of important inclusion and exclusion criteria that must be fulfilled prior to MitraClip placement (Fig. 19.10). To optimize our results, it is our practice for the echocardiologists to review the two-dimensional and 3D TEE mitral valve morphology with the invasive cardiologists, collectively, off-line before the procedure. In order to facilitate a cohesive communication regarding anatomic suitability for the MitraClip procedure between echocardiologists, cardiac surgeons, and interventional cardiologists, imaging of the mitral valve is done in the surgical view.

This is facilitated by the 3D en face view, by live 3D zoom mode or full volume imaging, providing a rapid and clear anatomico-pathologic visualization of the mitral valve, permitting a definitive assessment of suitability for the procedure. This is coupled with 3D color to confirm the origin of the regurgitant jet and clearly define multiple and/or eccentric trajectories. In our experience 3D TEE clarifies the site of mitral valve prolapse in cases that can be ambiguous by two-dimensional TEE. Essentially, there must be significant (moderate to severe or greater) MR due to leaflet malcoaptation. It must originate from the central two-thirds of the

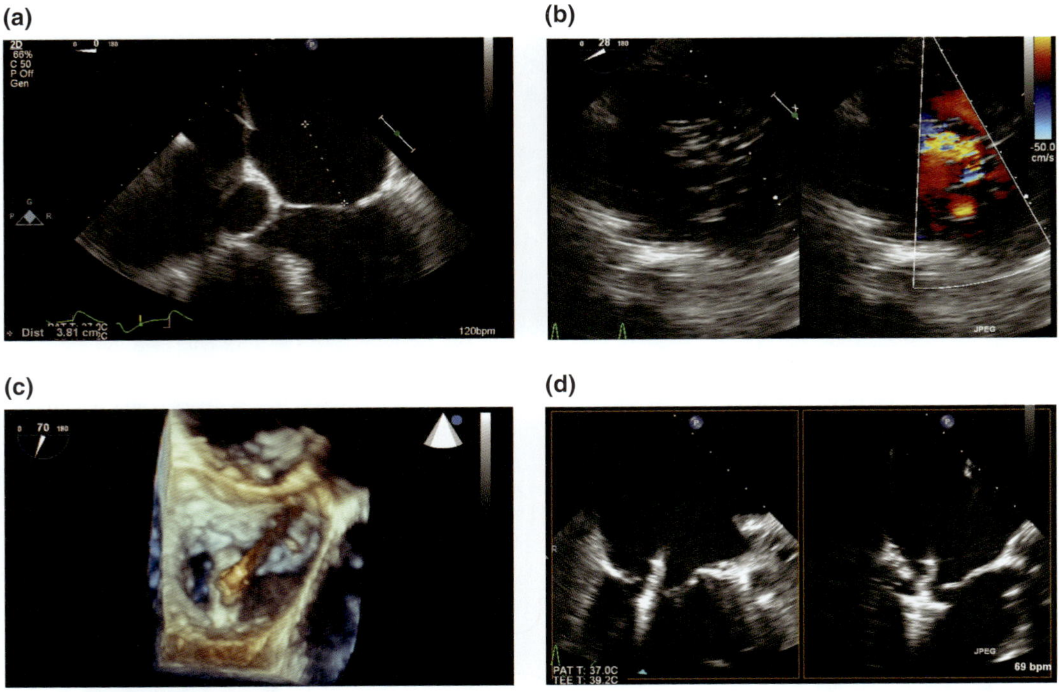

Fig. 19.11 Critical steps mandating TEE, preferably 3D TEE, in the MitraClip procedure. (a) Four-chamber view: optimal transeptal puncture height from the mitral valve annulus. (b) Transgastric view: demonstrates centrality of the regurgitant jet, and can also show clip orientation. (c) 3D en face view: clip orientation is clearly demonstrated. (d) X plane view: appropriate clip alignment and then grasping are demonstrated.

mitral valve (predominantly A2–P2 scallops). 3D scanning can clearly identify the location of malcoaptation and the underlying etiology, which may be degenerative (prolapse/flail) or have functional pathology (depressed LV function, restriction), but should not be rheumatic.

Important prerequisites for MitraClip use that can be assessed by two-dimensional or 3D techniques are significant MR, a sufficient leaflet tissue for mechanical coaptation (a coaptation length of at least 2 mm, flail gap <10 mm, and flail width <15 mm), and a mitral valve area over 4 cm^2, as there is an inevitable but small reduction in valve area on the transformation to a double orifice. Important exlusions are rheumatic disease and calcific leaflets.

In our experience, the most frequent cause of exclusion from the EVEREST (Endovascular Valve Edge-to-edge REpair STudy) I and II trials was insufficient MR, but commissural MR with, for instance, a lateral or medial prolapse detected on the screening 3D TEE, is not uncommon. A predominantly A2–P2 prolapse with some adjacent lateral or medial involvement can be effectively treated with a double clip technique and this can be inequivocally identified at baseline assessment with 3D TEE. Use of a double clip approach is not infrequent in our practice (see case examples, below) and expands the patient base of those suitable for the MitraClip.

Procedure and tips and tricks

The MitraClip procedure is a cath lab procedure using fluoroscopy and echocardiographic guidance. Online TEE, especially 3D TEE, is the most important imaging tool to guide the procedure (Fig. 19.11). Fluoroscopic "snap-shots" are used to complement the predominantly echo-guided procedure, and are of particular value in the orientation of a second clip, which is becoming increasingly common (Fig. 19.12). The integration of 3D TEE into our usual practice has dramatically shortened procedure time and increased efficiency. The multiplane capabilities of 3D TEE (X-plane) allows

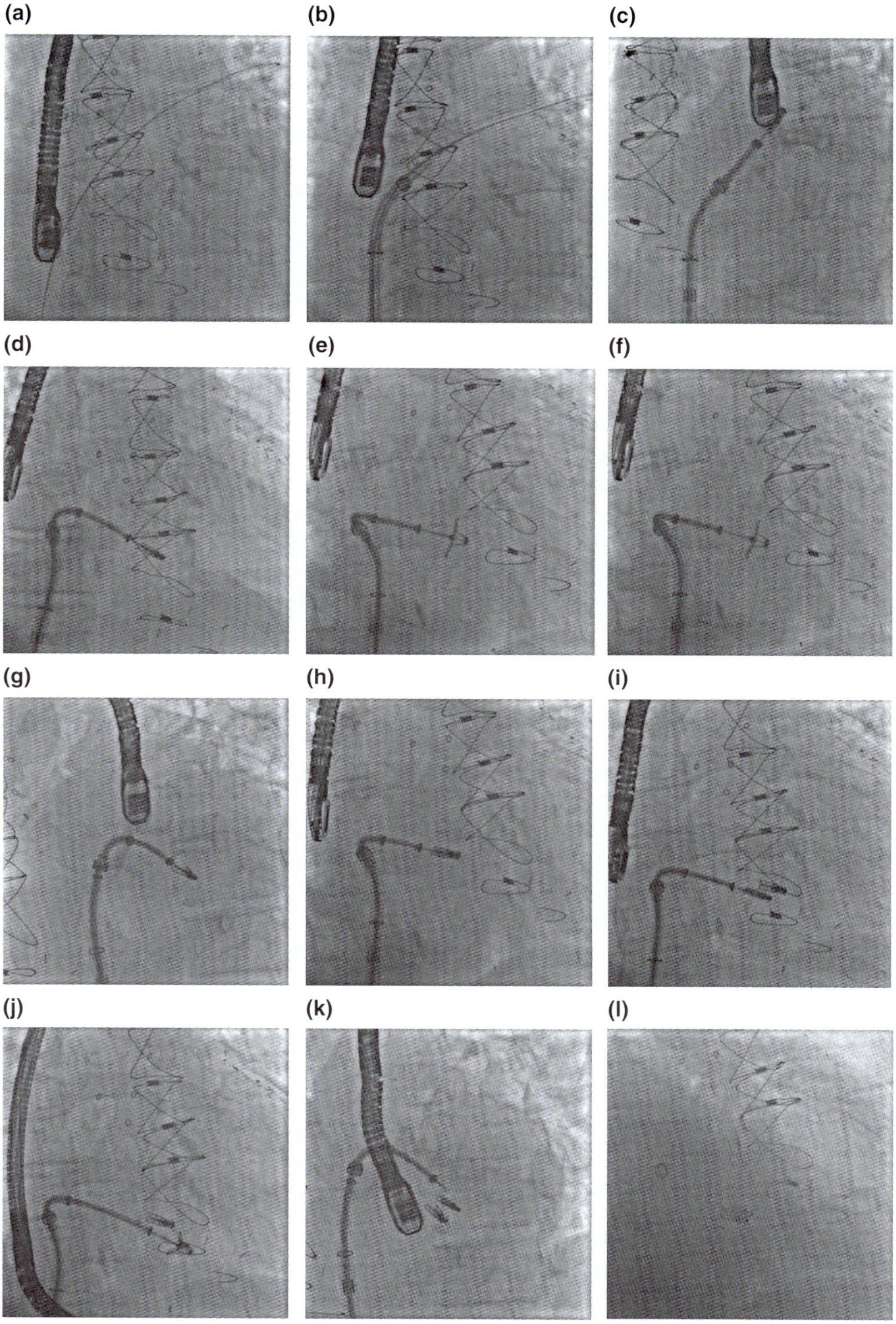

Fig. 19.12 Fluoroscopy in the MitraClip procedure. Although secondary to TEE, fluoroscopy is of confirmatory value throughout, and is especially useful for the orientation of a second clip. See text for further details. (a) Super-stiff wire placement in the left upper pulmonary vein, following transeptal puncture. (b) Advancement of the steerable guide over the wire. (c) Advancement of the clip delivery system (CDS) through the guide. (d) Downward deflection of the CDS. (e) Opening of the clip so that orientation may be seen on TEE. (f) Raising of the grippers. (g) Following grasp with the grippers, the clip is partially closed, and leaflet insertion is assessed by TEE. (h) The clip is fully closed and reduction in MR is visualized by TEE. (i) The first clip is deployed and the second advanced alongside, in a closed configuration. (j) The second clip is opened in the left ventricle. (k) The second clip is deployed. (l) The CDS is removed, leaving two clips.

two orthogonal planes to be shown at one time, which allows precise manipulation of catheters during the procedure.

The transeptal puncture is a crucial early step in the procedure. A good transeptal puncture will facilitate a straightforward procedure whereas a suboptimal puncture will prolong the procedure unnecessarily. Optimal imaging is fundamental to this. The bicaval and short axis views are used in combination with the four-chamber view (at the mid-esophageal level), which determines the "height" (which also incorporates an anterior–posterior dimension given the axis of the heart) from the mitral valve plane. The transeptal puncture is most optimally 3.5–4 cm above the line of coaptation of the leaflets. Accurate localization of the transeptal puncture can be achieved with multiplane TEE. In cases of degenerative mitral valve disease, where the line of coaptation is at or above the plane of the mitral annulus, the transeptal puncture needs to be posterior (and superior). In contrast, in cases of functional mitral valve disease where the line of coaptation is below the plane of the mitral annulus, the transeptal puncture should be more anterior (and inferior).

Following sucessful transeptal puncture, intravenous heparin is administered and activated clotting time (ACT) is monitored throughout the procedure, maintaining a level at around 250 s. A 0.035 inch Super-stiff exchange length guide wire is advanced through the transeptal catheter to the left upper pulmonary vein. The transeptal catheter is then removed and exchanged for the guide catheter. The MitraClip attached to the clip delivery system is then advanced through the guide catheter, into the left atrium. With the help of multiplane TEE, the MitraClip is then oriented appropriately over the mitral valve. The clip is opened and the arms are positioned perpendicularly to the leaflets using the en face 3D TEE projection. Once properly oriented, the clip is advanced to the LV, the clip delivery system is pulled back, and the leaflets are grasped by dropping the grippers. After confirmation of adequate grasping of the leaflets, the arms are closed, and the reduction in MR is assessed. Good grasping is assisted by holding the ventilator briefly and slow purposeful maneuvers. Optimal grasping can be confirmed both with live 3D and full volume echocardiography.

If there is no significant change in MR, the clip is repositioned. On the other hand, if the reduction is adequate, the clip is deployed. In cases of some residual MR on one side, a second clip can be deployed alongside the first. In addition to assessment of MR, mitral valve gradients are checked periodically throughout the procedure to ensure that there is no iatrogenic mitral stenosis.

Groin hemostasis is achieved by manual compression after the ACT has decreased appropriately. Preclosure with Perclose/Proglide devices (Abbott Vascular, Santa Clara, CA) or the "figure-of-8" suture technique can also be employed. After repair, it is recommended to give aspirin for 6 months and some operators also administer clopidogrel for 1 month. Infective endocarditis prophylaxis is recommended.

During the procedures it is ideal to treat all cases with a cardiac anesthesiologist monitoring and experienced echocardiographic imaging. In many high volume centers, the cardiac anesthesiologist is trained to facilitate both monitoring and echocardiographic guidance. It is important to note that the accurate assessment of MR pre and post procedure must be in the presence of normotension, and the anesthesiologist must therefore manipulate the blood pressure accordingly.

Evaluation of procedural success

The evaluation of MitraClip procedural success involves the following:

1 Clearly assessing leaflet insertion and device stability.

2 Reduction of mitral regurgitation.

3 Ensuring no significant gradient following clip deployment.

The EVEREST II study applied a primary composite endpoint for efficacy as freedom from death, from surgery for mitral valve dysfunction, and from grade 3+ or 4+ mitral regurgitation at 12 months [73]. Recommendations for evaluation of native valvular regurgitation have been clearly established and validated [56]. However, the presence of a double orifice presents new challenges. It is known that one cannot rely on jet penetration or jet area in this setting. Indeed, an in vitro model for the double orifice has recently demonstrated that color Doppler jet area overestimates regurgitant volume when multiple jets are present [74].

Moreover, quantitative tools for MR assessment, such as vena contracta, regurgitant orifice area by pisa formula, and regurgitant volume or fraction by the volumetric method have not been validated in the setting of a double orifice. Pulmonary vein flow reversal, an indicator of significant mitral regurgitation, is assessed at baseline and post MitraClip deployment. However, this is also influenced by left atrium (LA) and LV compliance and possibly also the presence of atrial fibrillation. Thus, in the absence of a substantiated framework for the assessment of residual MR in a double orifice, an integrative approach is employed incorporating a combination of a visual assessment of color flow Doppler, vena contracta, and pulmonary vein flow and their changes pre and post clip deployment. These parameters are scrutinized further with the pharmacologic increase in blood pressure with pressors following clip deployment.

With the creation of the double orifice, there is an inevitable immediate slight increase in mitral valve gradient [75,76]. However, there has been no documented case of significant mitral stenosis after the use of a MitraClip, even at 2 years follow-up [75]. Importantly, the gradient is not influenced by whether one or two clips are used [75].

Complications

The MitraClip is a remarkably safe procedure, with the majority of patients discharged the following day. Complications that can occur include tamponade (arising either from transeptal puncture or manipulation within the LA), iatrogenic atrial septal defect (especially if right atrial pressure is high, generating a right-to-left shunt; Fig. 19.13), LA thrombus and stroke, and clip detachment and embolization. Although 3D TEE is ideal, even two-dimensional TEE can identify thrombus and assess the interatrial septum post MitraClip, assessing the size of the shunt and evaluation disruption on either side of the septum.

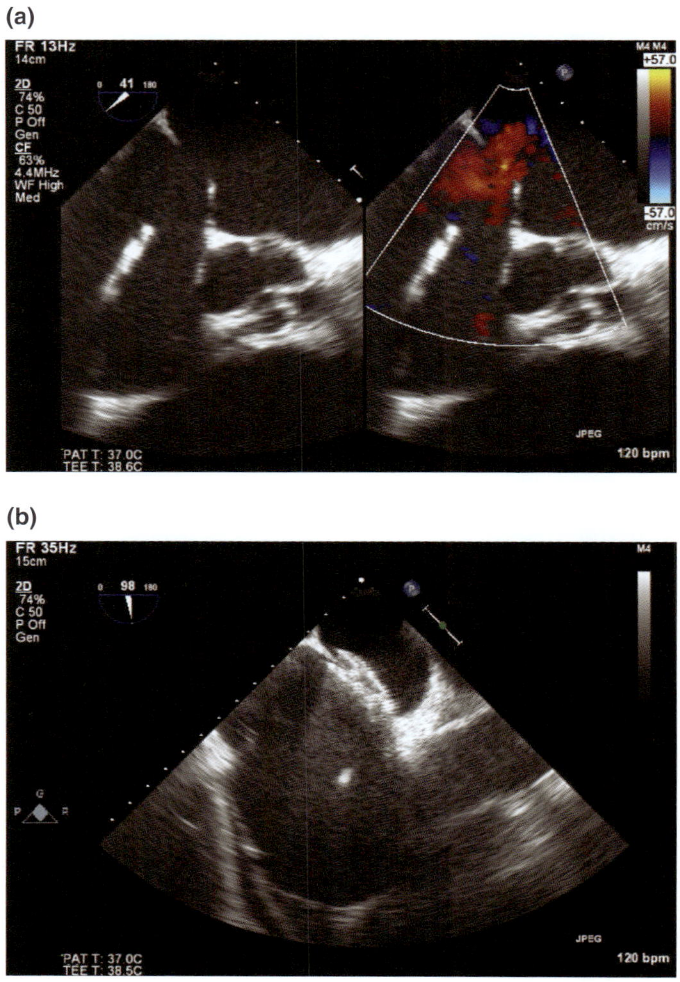

Fig. 19.13 Large iatrogenic atrial septum defect (ASD) following the MitraClip procedure. On removal of the guide, a large ASD was noted with a bidirectional shunt seen. (a) Notably, the patient had severe tricuspid regurgitation with bowing of the inter-atrial septum to the left atrium. (b) The defect was closed with an Amplatzer ASD occluder device.

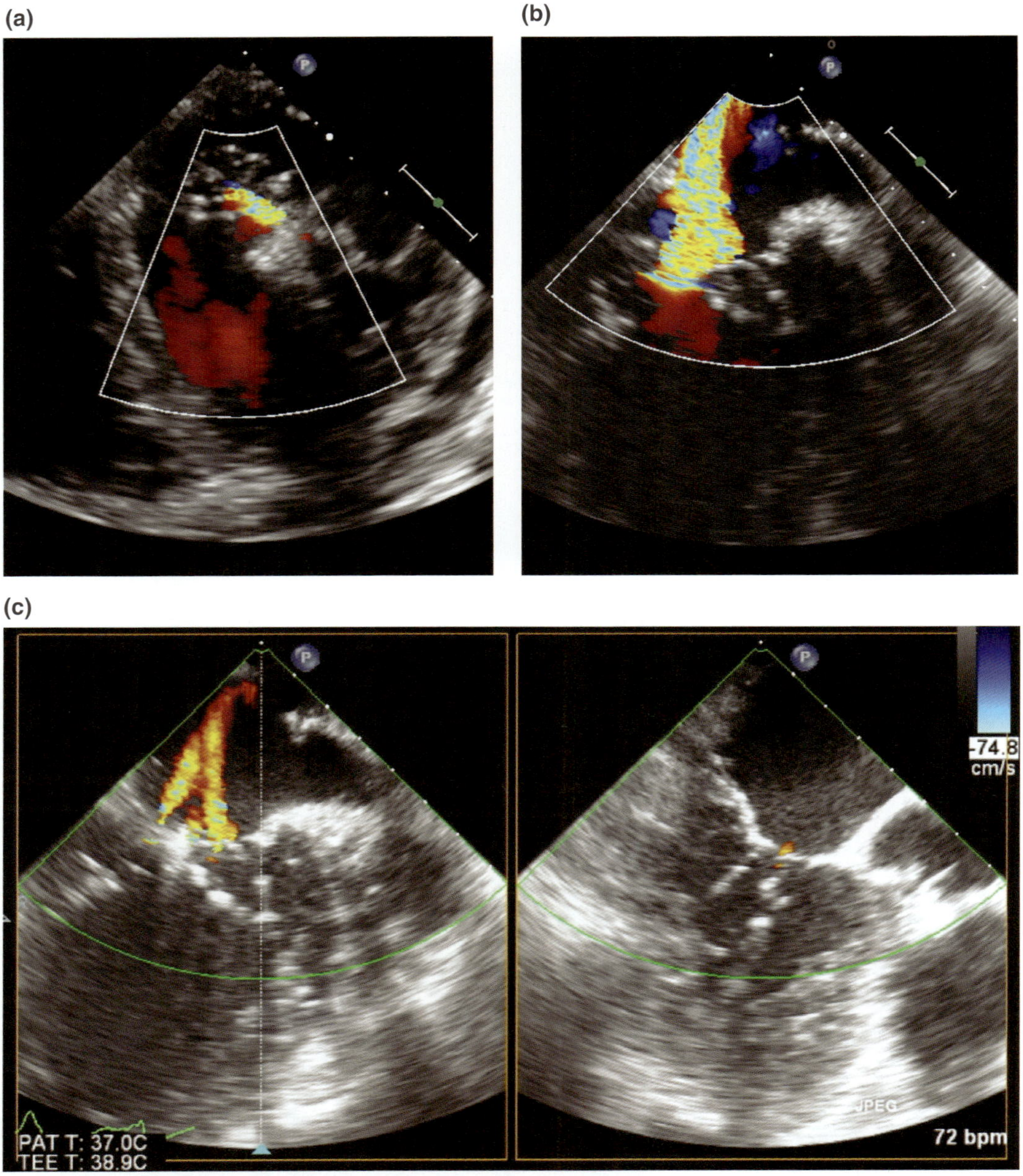

Fig. 19.14 Functional mitral regurgitation, showing a 55-year-old woman with end-stage renal disease, with non-ischemic cardiomyopathy with an ejection fraction of 25%. A central jet of MR is appreciated on the transgastric view of peri-procedural TEE (a), and appreciated as 4+ on the bicommissural view (b). One clip was deployed centrally between A2 and P2, with residual 1–2+ MR. A second clip was deployed lateral to the first. (c) X-plane post deployment of both clips revealed grade 1+ MR.

MitraClip case examples

See Figs 19.14–19.16 for some case examples of use of the MitraClip. Strikingly, the MitraClip can be applied to a wide variety of pathologies, both functional and organic mitral regurgitation.

Review of the literature

The MitraClip device remains investigational in the United States and has attained CE mark approval in 2008. The sum of clinical data currently available for this device includes that

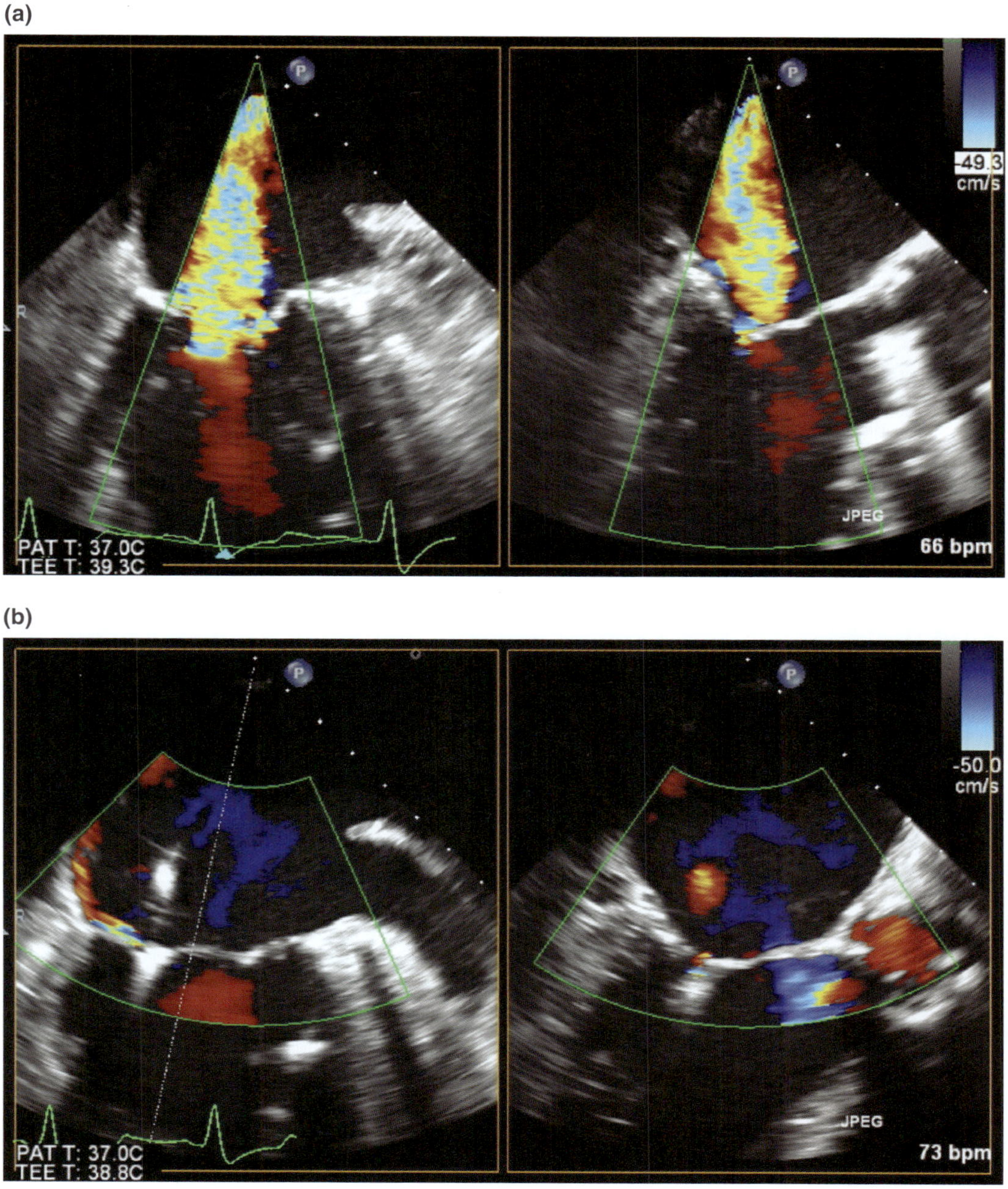

Fig. 19.15 Posterior leaflet restriction with severe MR, showing a 75-year-old man with multiple prior surgeries, including re-do coronary artery bypass graft and mechanical atrial valve replacement. There is a restricted posterior leaflet. The first clip is deployed central, the second just medial to the first. There was a reduction in MR from 4+ at baseline (a) to 1+ post procedure (b), as assessed on peri-procedural TEE.

from the EVEREST I and II clinical trials performed in North America and from the clinical studies following commercial approval in Europe and some countries in Asia (Table 19.4).

The initial EVEREST cohort included 107 anatomically suitable symptomatic patients with grade 3+/4+ MR from the initial pilot study and roll-in patients from the subsequent EVEREST II randomized study. Data evaluating the safety and

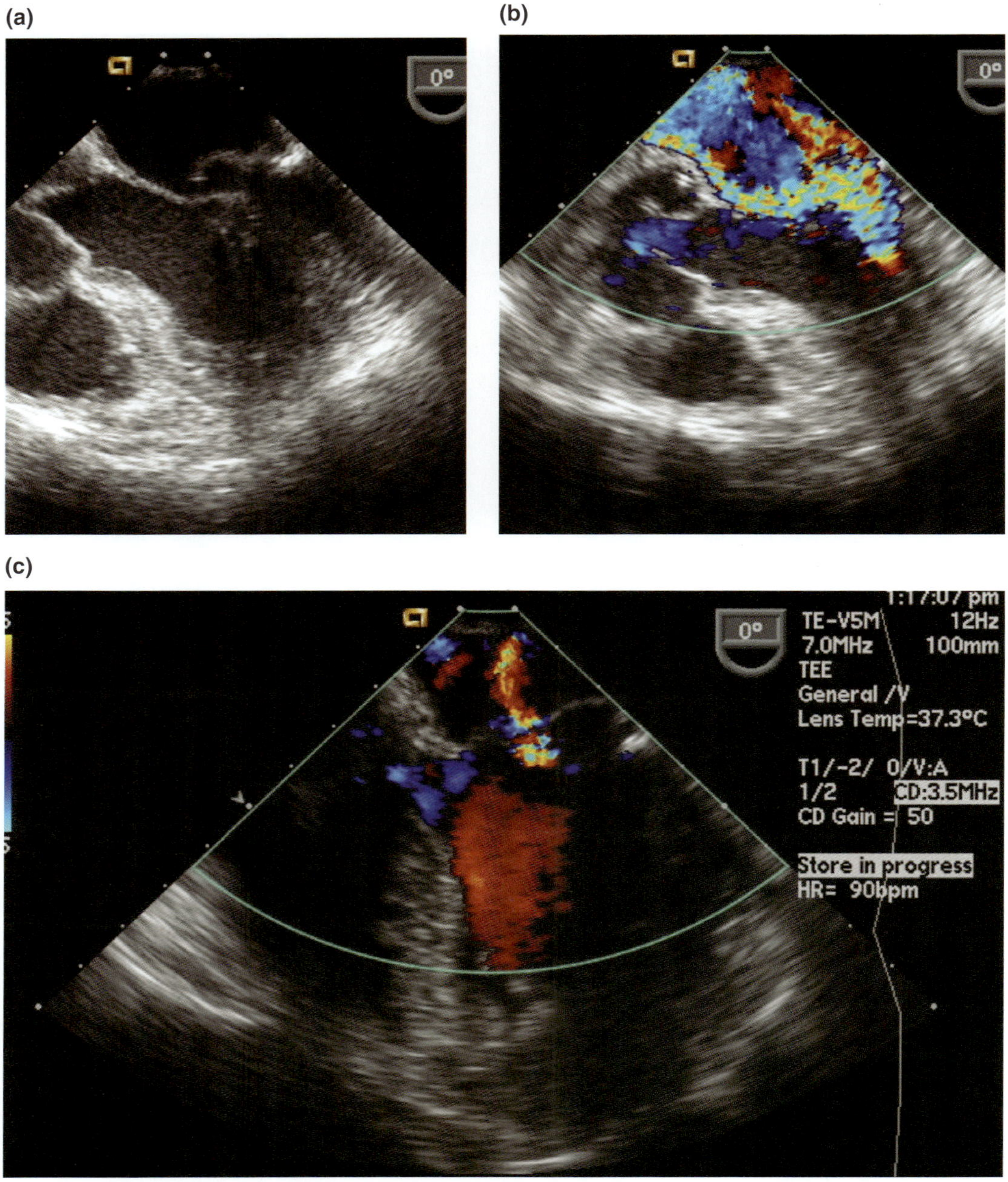

Fig. 19.16 Flail posterior leaflet, showing a 67-year-old man with chronic severe MR due to a flail posterior P2 leaflet (a, b). (c) After a double clip approach, the MR was reduced to grade 1–2+.

midterm durability of this study were reported by Feldman et al. in 2009 [77]. The primary success rate was 74%, with freedom from death and surgery rates of 90.1% and 76.3% at a median follow-up of 3.2 years. These encouraging results and low complication rate in this early experience confirmed the safety of this procedure.

The pivotal randomized controlled clinical trial, EVEREST II [73], compared the percutaneous MitraClip therapy with mitral valve surgery in 279 patients in a randomized fashion. Eligible patients were prospectively randomized to the MitraClip therapy or mitral valve surgery in a 2 to 1 ratio. Percutaneous repair was associated

Table 19.4 Data available to date for MitraClip use.

Study	*Population*	*n*
EVEREST I (feasibility)*	Non-randomized	55
EVEREST II*	Pre-randomization	60
EVEREST II	High-risk registry	78
EVEREST II (pivotal)	Randomized patients (2 : 1 MitraClip to surgery)	279 184 MitraClip
REALISM (continued access)	High risk and non-high risk	549
European Experience	Commercial	2113
Total MitraClip patients		3039

Data complete to March 28, 2011. Reproduced from Jilaihawi et al. [82] with permission from Springer.

with superior safety and similar improvements in clinical outcomes compared with conventional surgery, despite being less effective at reducing mitral regurgitation. This landmark study was unique in that it was the first prospective randomized trial comparing a percutaneous mitral repair technique with conventional surgery. The EVEREST II trial also incorporated a non-randomized high-risk arm evaluating patients at elevated surgical risk. In this arm, the MitraClip procedure was attempted in 78 patients. The observed mortality in this group was 7.7% at 30 days and this compared favorably to a mean predicted mortality by Society of Thoracic Surgeons (STS) score of 18.2%.

Despite the rapid growth of the MitraClip experience in Europe (Table 19.4), the data available from this thus far consist of a limited number of reports from a few non-randomized registries [78–80]. Amongst the patients treated, a significant proportion were those at high surgical risk, with congestive cardiac failure and depressed ejection fractions [78–80]. The data confirmed favorable outcomes in patients treated with an extremely low frequency of adverse events. Improvement in measures of MR, left ventricular dimensions, 6-minute walk distances, and *N*-terminal pro-brain natriuretic peptide plasma levels has been reported [80]. This provides further support for safety and efficacy in high-risk patients.

Conclusions

Transcatheter therapies for mitral valve disease have evolved to cater for changing epidemiologic patterns of disease. PTMV is a hugely successful evidence-based approach for the increasingly rare condition of rheumatic mitral stenosis. With the rise of age-related cardiac disease and parallel growth of mitral regurgitant disease, there is a need for a definitive transcatheter approach for this condition. Considerable headway has been made already to address this, particularly with the MitraClip, but this is a field that continues to evolve rapidly.

References

1 O'Gara P, Sugeng L, Lang R, et al. The role of imaging in chronic degenerative mitral regurgitation. JACC Cardiovasc Imaging 2008;1:221–37.

2 Chandrashekhar Y, Westaby S, Narula J. Mitral stenosis. Lancet 2009;374:1271–83.

3 Messika-Zeitoun D, Brochet E, Holmin C, et al. Three-dimensional evaluation of the mitral valve area and commissural opening before and after percutaneous mitral commissurotomy in patients with mitral stenosis. Eur Heart J 2007;28:72–9.

4 Salcedo EE, Quaife RA, Seres T, et al. A framework for systematic characterization of the mitral valve by real-time three-dimensional transesophageal echocardiography. J Am Soc Echocardiogr 2009;22:1087–99.

5 Eng MH, Salcedo EE, Quaife RA, et al. Implementation of real time three-dimensional transesophageal echocardiography in percutaneous mitral balloon valvuloplasty and structural heart disease interventions. Echocardiography 2009;26:958–66.

6 Flachskampf FA, Ropers D. Computed tomography to analyze mitral valve: an answer in search of a question. JACC Cardiovasc Imaging 2009;2:566–8.

7 Messika-Zeitoun D, Serfaty JM, Laissy JP, et al. Assessment of the mitral valve area in patients with mitral stenosis by multislice computed tomography. J Am Coll Cardiol 2006;48:411–13.

8 Delgado V, Tops LF, Schuijf JD, et al. Assessment of mitral valve anatomy and geometry with multislice computed tomography. JACC Cardiovasc Imaging 2009;2:556–65.

9 Tops LF, Van de Veire NR, Schuijf JD, et al. Noninvasive evaluation of coronary sinus anatomy and its relation to the mitral valve annulus: implications for percutaneous mitral annuloplasty. Circulation 2007;115:1426–32.

10 Maselli D, Guarracino F, Chiaramonti F, et al. Percutaneous mitral annuloplasty: an anatomic study of human coronary sinus and its relation with mitral valve annulus and coronary arteries. Circulation 2006;114:377–80.

11 Choure AJ, Garcia MJ, Hesse B, et al. In vivo analysis of the anatomical relationship of coronary sinus to mitral annulus and left circumflex coronary artery using cardiac multidetector computed tomography: implications for percutaneous coronary sinus mitral annuloplasty. J Am Coll Cardiol 2006;48:1938–45.
12 Foster GP, Dunn AK, Abraham S, et al. Accurate measurement of mitral annular dimensions by echocardiography: importance of correctly aligned imaging planes and anatomic landmarks. J Am Soc Echocardiogr 2009;22:458–63.
13 Chiribiri A, Kelle S, Kohler U, et al. Magnetic resonance cardiac vein imaging: relation to mitral valve annulus and left circumflex coronary artery. JACC Cardiovasc Imaging 2008;1:729–38.
14 Fujita N, Chazouilleres AF, Hartiala JJ, et al. Quantification of mitral regurgitation by velocity-encoded cine nuclear magnetic resonance imaging. J Am Coll Cardiol 1994;23:951–8.
15 Buchner S, Debl K, Poschenrieder F, et al. Cardiovascular magnetic resonance for direct assessment of anatomic regurgitant orifice in mitral regurgitation. Circ Cardiovasc Imaging 2008;1:148–55.
16 Chuang ML, Hibberd MG, Salton CJ, et al. Importance of imaging method over imaging modality in noninvasive determination of left ventricular volumes and ejection fraction: assessment by two- and three-dimensional echocardiography and magnetic resonance imaging. J Am Coll Cardiol 2000;35:477–84.
17 Han Y, Peters DC, Salton CJ, et al. Cardiovascular magnetic resonance characterization of mitral valve prolapse. JACC Cardiovasc Imaging 2008;1: 294–303.
18 Inoue K, Owaki T, Nakamura T, et al. Clinical application of transvenous mitral commissurotomy by a new balloon catheter. J Thorac Cardiovasc Surg 1984;87:394–402.
19 Bonow RO, Carabello BA, Kanu C, et al. ACC/AHA 2006 guidelines for the management of patients with valvular heart disease: a report of the American College of Cardiology/American Heart Association Task Force on Practice Guidelines (writing committee to revise the 1998 Guidelines for the Management of Patients With Valvular Heart Disease): developed in collaboration with the Society of Cardiovascular Anesthesiologists: endorsed by the Society for Cardiovascular Angiography and Interventions and the Society of Thoracic Surgeons. Circulation 2006;114:e84–231.
20 Wilkins GT, Weyman AE, Abascal VM, et al. Percutaneous balloon dilatation of the mitral valve: an analysis of echocardiographic variables related to outcome and the mechanism of dilatation. Br Heart J 1988;60:299–308.
21 Iung B, Cormier B, Ducimetiere P, et al. Immediate results of percutaneous mitral commissurotomy. A predictive model on a series of 1514 patients. Circulation 1996;94:2124–30.
22 Nobuyoshi M, Arita T, Shirai S, et al. Percutaneous balloon mitral valvuloplasty: a review. Circulation 2009;119:e211–19.
23 Lock JE, Khalilullah M, Shrivastava S, et al. Percutaneous catheter commissurotomy in rheumatic mitral stenosis. N Engl J Med 1985;313:1515–18.
24 Al Zaibag M, Ribeiro PA, Al Kasab S, et al. Percutaneous double-balloon mitral valvotomy for rheumatic mitral-valve stenosis. Lancet 1986;1:757–61.
25 Cribier A, Eltchaninoff H, Koning R, et al. Percutaneous mechanical mitral commissurotomy with a newly designed metallic valvulotome: immediate results of the initial experience in 153 patients. Circulation 1999; 99:793–9.
26 Eltchaninoff H, Tron C, Cribier A. Effectiveness of percutaneous mechanical mitral commissurotomy using the metallic commissurotome in patients with restenosis after balloon or previous surgical commissurotomy. Am J Cardiol 2003;91:425–8.
27 Vahanian A, Palacios IF. Percutaneous approaches to valvular disease. Circulation 2004;109:1572–9.
28 Lau KW, Hung JS. A simple balloon-sizing method in Inoue-balloon percutaneous transvenous mitral commissurotomy. Catheter Cardiovasc Diagn 1994;33:120–9; discussion 30–1.
29 Lau KW, Hung JS. Balloon-sizing method in Inoue mitral commissurotomy. Catheter Cardiovasc Diagn 1995; 35:183.
30 Inoue-balloon Percutaneous Transvenous Mitral Valvuloplasty. 2006. Available at www.ptmv.org.
31 Hung JS, Lau KW, Lo PH, et al. Complications of Inoue balloon mitral commissurotomy: impact of operator experience and evolving technique. Am Heart J 1999;138:114–21.
32 Ben Farhat M, Ayari M, Maatouk F, et al. Percutaneous balloon versus surgical closed and open mitral commissurotomy: seven-year follow-up results of a randomized trial. Circulation 1998;97:245–50.
33 Turi ZG, Reyes VP, Raju BS, et al. Percutaneous balloon versus surgical closed commissurotomy for mitral stenosis. A prospective, randomized trial. Circulation 1991;83:1179–85.
34 Patel JJ, Shama D, Mitha AS, et al. Balloon valvuloplasty versus closed commissurotomy for pliable mitral stenosis: a prospective hemodynamic study. J Am Coll Cardiol 1991;18:1318–22.
35 National Heart, Lung, and Blood Institute Balloon Valvuloplasty Registry Participants. Multicenter experience with balloon mitral commissurotomy. NHLBI Balloon Valvuloplasty Registry Report on immediate and 30-day follow-up results. Circulation 1992;85: 448–61.
36 Palacios IF, Sanchez PL, Harrell LC, et al. Which patients benefit from percutaneous mitral balloon valvuloplasty?

Prevalvuloplasty and postvalvuloplasty variables that predict long-term outcome. Circulation 2002; 105:1465–71.
37 Leon MN, Harrell LC, Simosa HF, et al. Comparison of immediate and long-term results of mitral balloon valvotomy with the double-balloon versus Inoue techniques. Am J Cardiol 1999;83:1356–63.
38 Ruiz CE, Zhang HP, Macaya C, et al. Comparison of Inoue single-balloon versus double-balloon technique for percutaneous mitral valvotomy. Am Heart J 1992;123:942–7.
39 Sharma S, Loya YS, Desai DM, et al. Percutaneous mitral valvotomy using Inoue and double balloon technique: comparison of clinical and hemodynamic short term results in 350 cases. Catheter Cardiovasc Diagn 1993; 29:18–23.
40 Gerardin B, Losay J, Leriche H, et al. [Percutaneous mitral valvulotomy: comparison of 2 techniques in 100 matched-pair patients]. Arch Mal Coeur Vaiss 1992;85:1799–803.
41 Abdullah M, Halim M, Rajendran V, et al. Comparison between single (Inoue) and double balloon mitral valvuloplasty: immediate and short-term results. Am Heart J 1992;123:1581–8.
42 Zhang HP, Gamra H, Allen JW, et al. Comparison of late outcome between Inoue balloon and double-balloon techniques for percutaneous mitral valvotomy in a matched study. Am Heart J 1995;130:340–4.
43 Trevino AJ, Ibarra M, Garcia A, et al. Immediate and long-term results of balloon mitral commissurotomy for rheumatic mitral stenosis: comparison between Inoue and double-balloon techniques. Am Heart J 1996;131:530–6.
44 Kang DH, Park SW, Song JK, et al. Long-term clinical and echocardiographic outcome of percutaneous mitral valvuloplasty: randomized comparison of Inoue and double-balloon techniques. J Am Coll Cardiol 2000;35:169–75.
45 Shaw TR, Turnbull CM, Currie P, et al. A comparison of cylindrical and Inoue balloon techniques for mitral valvotomy in patients in the United Kingdom. Br Heart J 1994;72:486–91.
46 Bahl VK, Chandra S, Jhamb DK, et al. Balloon mitral valvotomy: comparison between antegrade Inoue and retrograde non-transseptal techniques. Eur Heart J 1997;18:1765–70.
47 Iakovou I, Pavlides G, Voudris V, et al. Outcome of percutaneous mitral balloon valvuloplasty: comparison of the inoue and retrograde non-transseptal techniques. A single-center experience. J Invasive Cardiol 2002; 14:522–6.
48 Sharieff S, Aamir K, Sharieff W, et al. Comparison of Inoue balloon, metallic commissurotome and multi-track double-balloon valvuloplasty in the treatment of rheumatic mitral stenosis. J Invasive Cardiol 2008; 20:521–5.
49 Bhat A, Harikrishnan S, Tharakan JM, et al. Comparison of percutaneous transmitral commissurotomy with Inoue balloon technique and metallic commissurotomy: immediate and short-term follow-up results of a randomized study. Am Heart J 2002; 144:1074–80.
50 Guerios EE, Bueno RR, Nercolini DC, et al. Randomized comparison between Inoue balloon and metallic commissurotome in the treatment of rheumatic mitral stenosis: immediate results and 6-month and 3-year follow-up. Catheter Cardiovasc Interv 2005;64:301–11.
51 Zaki AM, Kasem HH, Bakhoum S, et al. Comparison of early results of percutaneous metallic mitral commissurotome with Inoue balloon technique in patients with high mitral echocardiographic scores. Catheter Cardiovasc Interv 2002;57:312–17.
52 Nkomo VT, Gardin JM, Skelton TN, et al. Burden of valvular heart diseases: a population-based study. Lancet 2006;368:1005–11.
53 Enriquez-Sarano M, Akins CW, Vahanian A. Mitral regurgitation. Lancet 2009;373:1382–94.
54 Carabello BA. The current therapy for mitral regurgitation. J Am Coll Cardiol 2008;52:319–26.
55 Carpentier A. Cardiac valve surgery – the "French correction". J Thorac Cardiovasc Surg 1983;86: 323–37.
56 Zoghbi WA, Enriquez-Sarano M, Foster E, et al. Recommendations for evaluation of the severity of native valvular regurgitation with two-dimensional and Doppler echocardiography. J Am Soc Echocardiogr 2003;16:777–802.
57 Fedak PW, McCarthy PM, Bonow RO. Evolving concepts and technologies in mitral valve repair. Circulation 2008;117:963–74.
58 Feldman T, Cilingiroglu M. Percutaneous leaflet repair and annuloplasty for mitral regurgitation. J Am Coll Cardiol 2011;57:529–37.
59 Cheung A, Webb JG, Wong DR, et al. Transapical transcatheter mitral valve-in-valve implantation in a human. Ann Thorac Surg 2009;87:e18–20.
60 Webb JG, Wood DA, Ye J, et al. Transcatheter valve-in-valve implantation for failed bioprosthetic heart valves. Circulation 2010;121:1848–57.
61 Sack S, Kahlert P, Bilodeau L, et al. Percutaneous transvenous mitral annuloplasty: initial human experience with a novel coronary sinus implant device. Circ Cardiovasc Interv 2009;2:277–84.
62 Harnek J, Webb JG, Kuck K-H, et al. Transcatheter implantation of the MONARC coronary sinus device for mitral regurgitation: 1-year results from the EVOLUTION Phase I Study (clinical evaluation of the Edwards Lifesciences Percutaneous Mitral Annuloplasty System for the treatment of mitral regurgitation). J Am Coll Cardiol Interv 2011;4:115–22.
63 Schofer J, Siminiak T, Haude M, et al. Percutaneous mitral annuloplasty for functional mitral regurgitation:

results of the CARILLON Mitral Annuloplasty Device European Union Study. Circulation 2009;120:326–33.

64 Hoppe UC. Abstracts of the European Society of Cardiology Congress, 28 August – 1 September 2010, Stockholm, Sweden. Eur Heart J 2010;31(Suppl 1):160–1.

65 Bach DS, Bolling SF. Improvement following correction of secondary mitral regurgitation in end-stage cardiomyopathy with mitral annuloplasty. Am J Cardiol 1996;78:966–9.

66 Mihaljevic T, Lam BK, Rajeswaran J, et al. Impact of mitral valve annuloplasty combined with revascularization in patients with functional ischemic mitral regurgitation. J Am Coll Cardiol 2007;49:2191–201.

67 Feldman T, Foster E, Glower DG, et al. Percutaneous repair or surgery for mitral regurgitation. N Engl J Med 2011;364:1395–406.

68 Cheng W, Fontana GP, De Robertis MA, et al. Is robotic mitral valve repair a reproducible approach? J Thorac Cardiovasc Surg 2010;139:628–33.

69 Alfieri O, Maisano F, De Bonis M, et al. The double-orifice technique in mitral valve repair: a simple solution for complex problems. J Thorac Cardiovasc Surg 2001;122: 674–81.

70 Maisano F, Vigano G, Blasio A, et al. Surgical isolated edge-to-edge mitral valve repair without annuloplasty: clinical proof of the principle for an endovascular approach. EuroIntervention 2006;2:181–6.

71 Mack MJ. Percutaneous treatment of mitral regurgitation: So near, yet so far! J Thorac Cardiovasc Surg 2008;135:237–9.

72 Webb JG, Maisano F, Vahanian A, et al. Percutaneous suture edge-to-edge repair of the mitral valve. EuroIntervention 2009;5:86–9.

73 Feldman T, Foster E, Glower DG, et al. Percutaneous repair or surgery for mitral regurgitation. N Engl J Med 2011;364:1395–406.

74 Lin BA, Forouhar AS, Pahlevan NM, et al. Color Doppler jet area overestimates regurgitant volume when multiple jets are present. J Am Soc Echocardiogr 2010;23:993–1000.

75 Herrmann HC, Kar S, Siegel R, et al. Effect of percutaneous mitral repair with the MitraClip device on mitral valve area and gradient. EuroIntervention 2009; 4:437–42.

76 Jilaihawi H, Makkar R, Hussaini A, et al. Contemporary application of cardiovascular hemodynamics: transcatheter mitral valve interventions. Cardiol Clin 2011;29:201–9.

77 Feldman T, Kar S, Rinaldi M, et al. Percutaneous mitral repair with the MitraClip system: safety and midterm durability in the initial EVEREST (Endovascular Valve Edge-to-Edge REpair Study) cohort. J Am Coll Cardiol 2009;54:686–94.

78 Tamburino C, Ussia GP, Maisano F, et al. Percutaneous mitral valve repair with the MitraClip system: acute results from a real world setting. Eur Heart J 2010;31:1382–9.

79 Franzen O, Baldus S, Rudolph V, et al. Acute outcomes of MitraClip therapy for mitral regurgitation in high-surgical-risk patients: emphasis on adverse valve morphology and severe left ventricular dysfunction. Eur Heart J 2010;31:1373–81.

80 Franzen O, van der Heyden J, Baldus S, et al. MitraClip(R) therapy in patients with end-stage systolic heart failure. Eur J Heart Fail 2011;13:569–76.

81 Castillo JG, Solis J, Gonzalez-Pinto A, et al. [Surgical echocardiography of the mitral valve]. Rev Esp Cardiol 2011;64:1169–81.

82 Jilaihawi H, Hussaini A, Kar S. MitraClip: a novel percutaneous approach to mitral valve repair. J Zhejiang Univ Sci B 2011;12:633–7.

83 Chiam PT, Ruiz CE. Percutaneous transcatheter mitral valve repair: a classification of the technology. JACC Cardiovasc Interv 2011;4:1–13.

20

CHAPTER 20

Real-time magnetic resonance imaging guidance in cardiac surgery

Ming Li, Dumitru Mazilu & Keith A. Horvath
Cardiothoracic Surgery Research Program, National Heart, Lung and Blood Institute, National Institutes of Health, Bethesda, MD, USA

Introduction

Minimally invasive cardiac surgery usually requires emptying of the heart to allow visualization of the surgical field [1]. To facilitate this visualization and permit surgical correction of intracardiac structures, cardiopulmonary bypass is employed but carries risk and can lead to adverse effects [2–4]. Real-time magnetic resonance imaging (rtMRI) techniques have been previously described for intravascular guidance [5,6] and may be immediately applicable to provide vision in a beating heart with circulating blood to guide the surgeon in a minimally invasive cardiac surgery environment.

MRI provides better image quality and a complete view of the entire thorax, more so than other competing imaging methods such as fluoroscopy/angiography, in which many anatomic structures are not visible, and echocardiography, in which the field of view is small. Vascular as well as soft tissue visualization can easily be performed simultaneously with MRI. As a result of the clarity of MRI, image interpretation is easy for anyone familiar with the surgical anatomy. New generations of open, wide, and short bore magnetic resonance scanners and the real-time sequences provide intraoperative guidance for minimally invasive cardiac surgery. Moreover, MRI-guided surgery allows direct functional assessments to be made before, during, and immediately after an intervention that are not obtainable by conventional imaging alone.

However, operative rtMRI guidance has stringent requirements for surgical instruments and devices. Typically, devices that are used during interventions, such as catheters and wires, are not designed to be magnetic resonance visible or compatible as they often contain ferromagnetic materials or long electrical conductors. In this chapter, we illustrate the interactive rtMRI, MRI compatibility of the instruments and devices, and device tracking techniques. We also present a promising example of MRI-guided cardiac surgery, specifically, transapical aortic valve replacement under rtMRI.

Interactive real-time magnetic resonance imaging

With recent technologic advances, including changeable magnetic field gradients, multichannel receiver coils, and advanced computing systems, rtMRI is applicable in the clinical scanner. Scanners can provide real-time images of acceptable quality in excess of 10 frames per second. One of the strengths of rtMRI is the ability to interactively adjust image

Endovascular and Hybrid Therapies for Structural Heart and Aortic Disease, First Edition.
Edited by Jacques Kpodonu and Raoul Bonan.

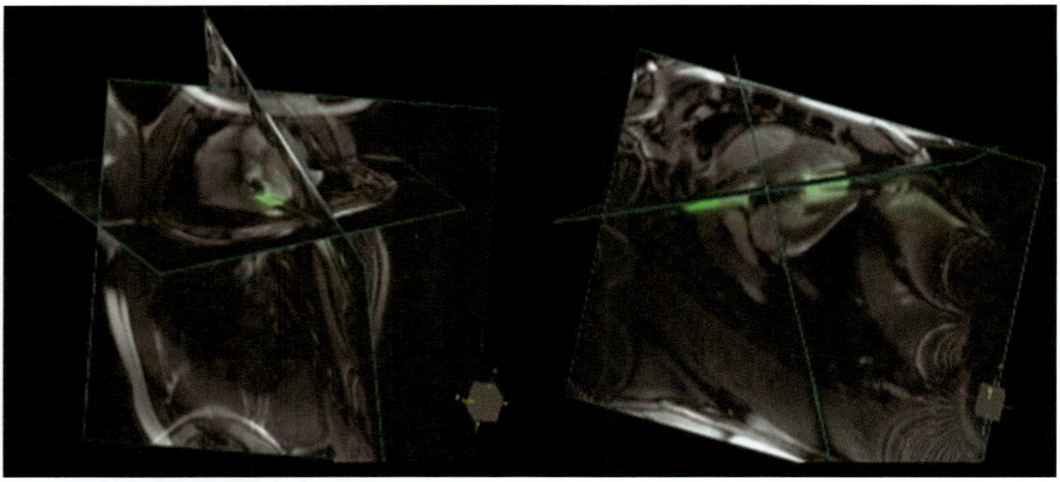

Fig. 20.1 Real-time MRI provides superior visualization for implanting the aortic valve prosthesis. Snapshots show multiple image planes displayed at their relative 3D position. The 3D rendering provides 3D anatomic information.

acquisition, reconstruction, and display parameters during the scan. These interactive features accommodate image contrast, image plane orientations, acquisition speed, spatial resolution, temporal resolution, 3D rendering, and device tracking [7–10]. The ability to change these imaging and display parameters during a scan may be used as the physician advances from one stage to another during a procedure.

Some magnetic resonance (MR) scanner manufacturers provide an interactive interface for adjusting imaging planes and some parameters during a real-time scan. At the National Heart, Lung and Blood Institute (NHLBI) an rtMRI interactive system was developed and used in interventional procedures [11–14]. This system consists of an interactive user interface, an operating room large screen display, specialized pulse sequences, and customized image reconstruction software. A computer with multiple high-performance central processing units and graphics card is connected by gigabit Ethernet to a commercial reconstruction computer of a clinical 1.5-T scanner (Sonata, Avanto or Espree Siemens Medical Systems). With this system, multiple oblique planes can be imaged and displayed simultaneously at their respective 3D locations (Fig. 20.1). High-quality images are obtained at approximately five frames per second, depending on imaging parameters, with low latency. The 3D rendering can be rotated on the in-room display to match the orientation of the patient. Image slices can be repositioned, disabled, or enabled as needed. The MRI tissue contrast can be interactively channeled by toggling saturation pulses off/on to highlight injected T1-shortening contrast agent. Devices incorporating small receiver coils can be displayed with color highlight for visual tracking.

Magnetic resonance compatibility of the instruments and devices

Three basic features for high-quality MRI are high and homogenous magnetic fields, fast-switching magnetic field gradients, and radiofrequency (RF) pulses. These extreme environmental conditions require adequate materials for the instruments and devices that can be safely manipulated inside the scanner without interfering with the imaging quality. The strong magnetic fields make ferromagnetic materials dangerous projectiles. The homogeneity of the main magnetic field is strongly affected by ferromagnetic materials inside the MRI scanner, resulting in substantial distortion of images. The generation of eddy currents inside conductive materials due to fast-switching gradient magnetic fields may alter the local homogeneity of the main magnetic field and severely affect the quality and linearity of MR images, causing image artifacts. Moreover, eddy currents and RF pulses may cause unwanted heating of conductive materials. Devices containing closed metallic loops should be avoided in the MRI environment.

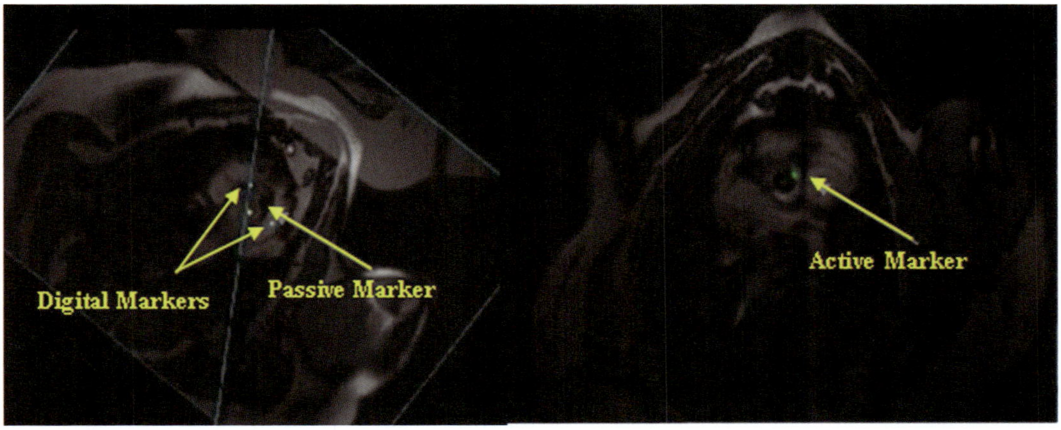

Fig. 20.2 Device tracking. The passive marker shows a black signal in MRI. The active marker shows a bright signal and highlighted in green. These markers are used to indicate the orientation of the prosthesis in an MRI-guided aortic valve implantation procedure. The coronary ostia locations are digitally marked.

Materials suitable for MR-compatible devices are non-magnetic and non-conductive. Plastics, ceramics, and composite materials are frequently used. Some metals are also used in the MRI environment. Based on their reaction in a magnetic field, metals can be characterized into three categories: ferromagnetic, paramagnetic, and diamagnetic materials. Ferromagnetic materials, such as iron, magnetic stainless steel, cobalt, and nickel, exhibit a strong attraction to magnetic fields. These materials are not MRI safe and should be totally avoided in the MRI environment. Paramagnetic metals have a small and positive susceptibility to magnetic fields; hence they require some compromise when they are to be used inside MR scanners and close to imaging areas. Diamagnetic metals have a very weak and negative susceptibility to magnetic fields. Copper, silver, and gold are diamagnetic. They are MRI safe, and will not affect the homogeneity of static magnetic field when they are placed close to a MR scanner. They have very limited or negligible image artifacts even if they are located close to imaging areas. The MR compatibility of certain types of materials and devices has been reported in references [15–17]. In order to be suitable for medical devices, these materials should also be biocompatible and sterilizable.

Device tracking

A crucial requirement for an MR-guided procedure is reliable tracking of the inserted instruments and devices to navigate inside a beating heart. The devices can be made visible by incorporating markers, such as "active" coils, or "passive" elements causing signal voids (e.g. steel) or signal enhancement (e.g. gadolinium).

Passive markers made of paramagnetic materials can be located in the imaging volume using the contrast obtained from the distortion or signal void [18,19]. The paramagnetic material typically appears as a dark feature in MR images. The nitinol guide wire appears as a dark curve in MR images. Small austenitic stainless steel fragments welded on the side of the stent can show the orientation of the expended stent (Fig. 20.2a) [20]. If the imaging field of view is particularly cluttered, such as in vascular areas around the heart, this type of passive marker can be difficult to locate. Another type of passive marker is a contrast agent. Catheters filled with gladolinium-diethylenetriaminepentacetate Gd-DTPA) are evident by bright signal from the lumen [21]. The principal advantage of passive markers is the fact that there is no concern about generating unwanted heating.

Active markers are small MR receiver coils. The signal from the coil is bright in the image and can be color highlighted (Fig. 20.2b). The receiver coils can be manufactured into different shapes for different purposes. Flexible, long, and narrow receiver coils incorporated on a guide wire or invasive device will allow the entire length of the device to be receptive to MR signal [22]. Small focal coils can be used for tracking individual points [23,24]. Kocaturk and colleagues developed a loopless antenna configuration that imparts interventional MR catheters with satisfactory mechanical and imaging characteristics. This compact loopless antenna design can be generalized to visualize the whole shaft of any general purpose polymer catheter to perform safe interventional procedures [25]. Active markers are advantageous since they provide positive image contrast, and if the device exits the imaging plane it may be easily located using projection imaging methods. One limitation of active markers is the potential heating of the coils and the long connecting signal cables.

MRI-guided transapical aortic valve replacement

We investigated the surgical procedure in which rtMRI is used to guide the placement of a prosthetic aortic valve in the beating heart via direct apical access. Our group first used a commercially available platinum-iridium stent (Cheatham Platinum, NuMed, Hopkinton, NY) for supporting conventional aortic prosthesis. A two-stage balloon-tipped catheter (NuMed) made of plastic is used for expanding the balloon-expandable stented prosthesis [20]. In this section, we illustrate the specially designed self-expanding stent and delivery device, and detail the surgical procedure of using these devices in aortic valve replacement under rtMRI guidance on an animal study.

Stents and devices

We designed and developed a new self-expanding stent (Fig. 20.3) to accommodate conventional aortic bioprostheses, such as the Toronto SPV (St. Jude Medical, Minneapolis, MN) or Freestyle (Medtronic, Minneapolis, MN), whose clinical durability and success rates are already proven. The stent will expand without external force and can be crimped before it is allowed to expand. The stent is a cylinder made of a biocompatible nickel-titanium alloy (nitinol), which assumes a "pre-programmed" final configuration upon release from the delivery device and exposed to body temperature. The stent has nine rods – three of which are used to align with the commissures of the prosthetic valve. A repeating chevron pattern along the length of the cylinder and flared ends ensures perfusion through the stent where needed and better fixation to the aorta and annulus. It is created with different diameters to accommodate 21–25 mm stentless prosthetic valves that match the patients' aortic size. At the distal end of the stent, there are three small round extensions. Any one of these extensions is used to accommodate a small austenitic stainless steel fragment ($0.09 \times 0.254 \times 0.6$ mm), which serves as a passive marker indicating the orientation of the stented prosthesis in MRI. At the proximal end of the stent, there is another set of three small round extensions. These extensions, or so called grasping members, are used to retrieve and reposition the stent as well as to prevent unexpected motion of the stent during deployment. The stent can be retrieved if it has been partially released, but cannot be retrieved once it has been completely released.

A delivery device (Fig. 20.4) was developed for holding and delivering the self-expanding stented prosthesis. The length of the delivery device is 60 cm and it consists of a straight plastic rod, outside of which is a sheath protecting the stented prosthesis before it is deployed. The diameter of the delivery device is 9.5 mm and fits into a 10 mm trocar. The inner rod has a central channel for a guide wire and stent-retrieving device. The translation and rotation of the delivery device directly relate to the translation and rotation of the loaded stented prosthesis. A small rubber gasket is used to prevent blood leakage from the central channel. The plastic rod can move back and forth inside the sheath. An active guide wire is embedded in a groove on the sheath. There is a handle on the inner rod and the sheath, respectively, for the surgeon to hold and manipulate the delivery device. In a procedure with the self-expanding stent, the loaded delivery device will first go into the ascending aorta and the edge of the inner rod is placed at the aorta annulus level. The retraction of the sheath will let the crimped stent expand and affix to the desired position.

Stent retrieving is carried out by holding a grasping member with a specially designed retrieving device presented. The retrieving device is a loop

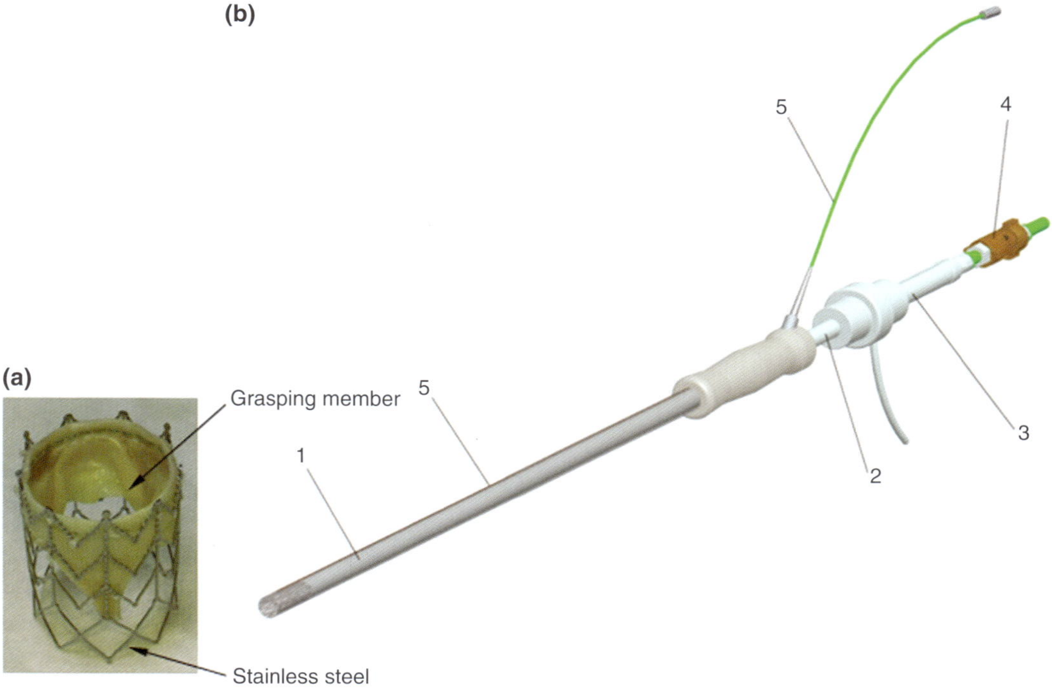

Fig. 20.3 (a) A Medtronic Freestyle valve sewn inside the nitinol self-expanding stent. A small piece of stainless steel welded on the small round extension of the distal end of the stent serves as a passive marker indicating the orientation of the prosthesis. The grasping member of the proximal end is used for retrieval and repositioning of the stent. (b) A CAD drawing of the delivery device with loop coil and antenna. The sheath with handle (1) protects and retains the prosthesis compressed until deployment. linner rod with handle (2) pushes the prosthesis for deployment. The inner channel of the inner rod provides access for the loop snare wire (4). The end spacer with dimension protection (3), protects the end valve and ensures the exact dimension for the loop snare wire. The loop coil antenna (5) is fixed into the groove cut on the exterior tube of the valve delivery system. The delivery device is made of nylon and delrin.

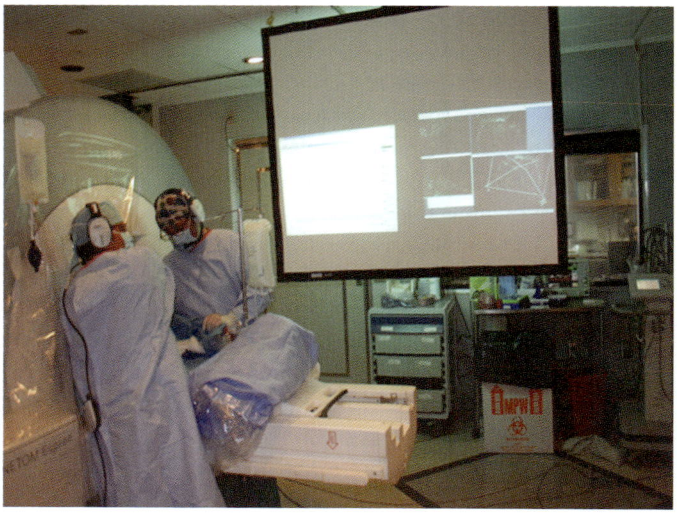

Fig. 20.4 Using real-time MRI as projected onto the screen, the surgeon advances the delivery device into the left ventricle. He can then precisely position the prosthetic valve for deployment.

snare wire. A thin nitinol wire is folded and forms the loop, which then lassoes a grasping member of the stent. The folded wire is housed inside and protected by a 2 mm diameter flexible nititol tube. This device can pass through the central channel of the delivery device. Before the procedure, the stented prosthesis is held and locked by the retrieving device and loaded inside the delivery device. By pulling the retrieving device, the surgeon can retrieve the stent back into the delivery device before the stent is fully deployed. Once the prosthesis is deployed, the surgeon can release the stent by unlocking the loop.

Procedure

A 1.5 T Magnetom Espree (Siemens) with a shorter and wider bore has been used for imaging. This magnet design gives a clearance of up to 30 cm above the chest of the supine patient, and the short design allows easy surgical access. The imaging gradients and amplifiers of the new system yield the same quality and nearly the same scanning performance as that of the standard cardiac MR scanners, and high-quality images can be obtained in real time with low latency.

Preoperative preparation

After the subject was intubated and anesthetized, the physician placed the trocar into the apex of the heart. Specifically using standard titanium surgical instruments via a 6 cm subxiphoid incision, the pericardium was opened and the apex of the heart was exposed. Two concentric pursestrings were placed around the apex, through which a 10 mm trocar was inserted into the left ventricle. Typical time to complete this part of the procedure was 15–20 minutes. Standard MR sequences were performed to obtain the orientation of the heart, evaluate ventricular and valve function, and locate the native valve annulus and the origin of the coronary arteries. Pre-scanning also allows setting up scan planes to be used for real-time imaging during valve implantation and follow-up myocardial perfusion and aortic flow imaging. Three imaging planes were prescribed for real-time imaging during implantation. Two of these planes were positioned to provide long axis views of the left ventricle, showing the right coronary artery and left main coronary artery origins, respectively. The other plane provided an axial view of the aortic valve. The coronary ostia and aortic annulus location were digitally marked. These digital marks remained visible at all times in the 3D rendering and were used for anatomic reference.

Based on the preoperative image, an appropriate size prosthesis was selected and mounted on a self-expanding stent of matching size. The stented valve was then compressed and placed inside the outer sheath at the distal end of the delivery device. The prosthesis was aligned with the active guide wire that is embedded in the sheath of the delivery device.

Valve implantation

The surgeon viewed the real-time imaging on a projection screen while manipulating the deployment device within the animal in the magnet. The prosthetic valve and delivery system were advanced through the trocar. During implantation, the axial slice was shifted as needed to visualize the device and to guide proper orientation of rhw commissures with the help of the passive marker. The long axis views were interactively modified to show the path of the delivery device, while keeping the coronary origins in view. Both the active wire and the passive marker were used to identify the location and orientation of the prosthesis. The surgeon was in direct contact with the scanner operator by means of headphones and a microphone (Magnacoustics, Atlantic Beach, NY) to request changes in the imaging planes as needed (Fig. 20.5; Video 20.1).

The loaded delivery device was first advanced into the ascending aorta. The retraction of the sheath allows the crimped prosthesis to expand and affix to the desired position. Upon release of the stent by retraction of the outer sheath, the chevron-like nitinol cylinder together with bioprosthetic valve expanded to its pre-programmed diameter. Retracting and repositioning of the prosthesis is possible before the stent is fully advanced outside of the sheath. After deployment, the delivery device was removed from the trocar. During the procedure, the animals were monitored with an electrocardiogram, oxygen saturation, end-tidal carbon dioxide, systemic and left ventricular blood pressure, and arterial blood gas analysis.

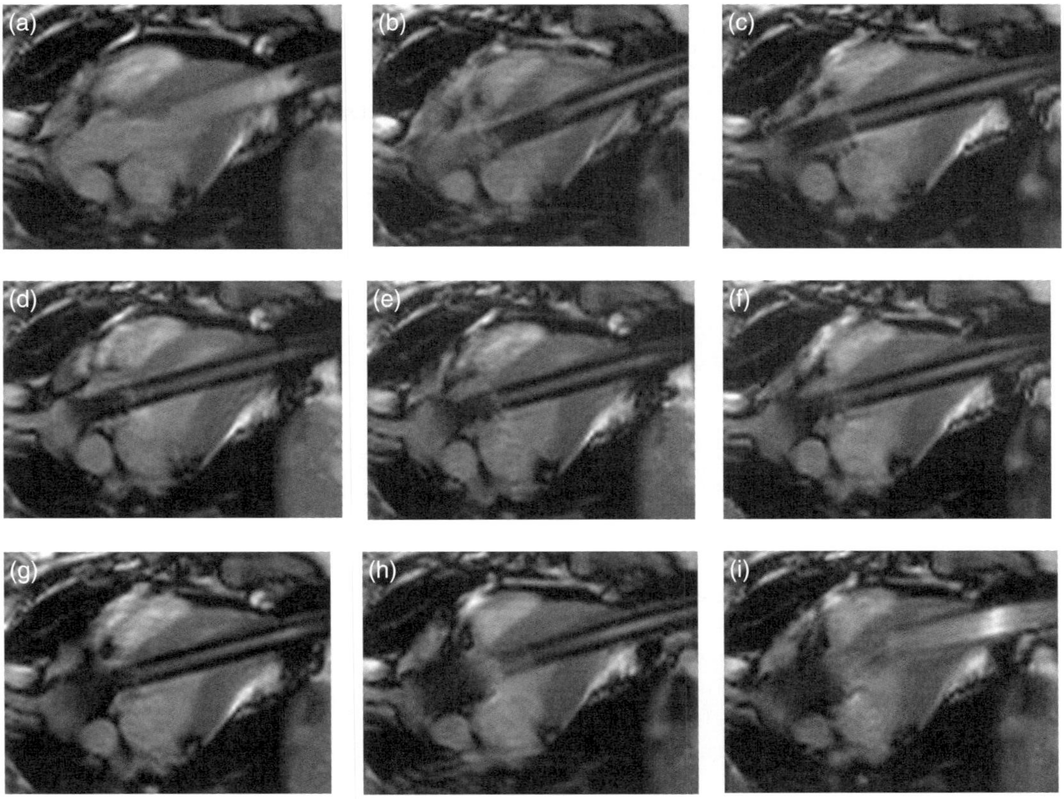

Fig.20.5 Selected frames from real-time MRI displayed within the scan room, showing the deployment of the self-expanding stented prosthetic valve. (a) The stented prosthesis is inserted inside the trocar. (b) The stented prosthesis is advanced to the end of the trocar. (c) The prosthesis is inserted across the native valve and aligned with the coronary ostia and aortic annulus. (d–g) Sequence of prosthesis expansion; during this period, the prosthesis can be retrieved. (h) The prosthesis is fully deployed. (i) The delivery device is removed from the trocar.

The average time from introduction of the self-expanding prosthesis into the trocar to the stent being fully expanded (deployment time) was 60 ± 14 seconds (mean ± SD). The time was significantly shorter with the self-expandable stent than with the balloon-expandable prosthesis, which had a time of 74 ± 18 seconds (mean ± SD) [26]. The procedures using balloon-expandable prostheses take a slightly longer time because of the time used for staging the balloon inflation and the difficulty in orienting the valve, knowing that once the balloon was completely inflated there was no margin to allow for adjustment.

Post-placement validation

After placement of the valve, the trocar was removed and the apex closed with pursestring sutures. Post-placement images were acquired to confirm the positions of the prostheses and valvular and heart function. In addition to anatomic confirmation of adequate placement of the prosthetic valve in relation to the aortic annulus and the coronary arteries, functional assessment of the valve and left ventricle was also obtained with MRI. Gated cine-MRI was used to assess mitral valve function and myocardial function. Phase contrast cine-MRI was used to identify flow through the new valve as well as intravalvular or paravalvular regurgitation (Fig. 20.6). An MR first-pass perfusion scan was performed during intravenous injection of Gd-DTPA contrast agent to confirm that myocardial blood flow was intact to all segments of the myocardium (Fig. 20.7) [27].

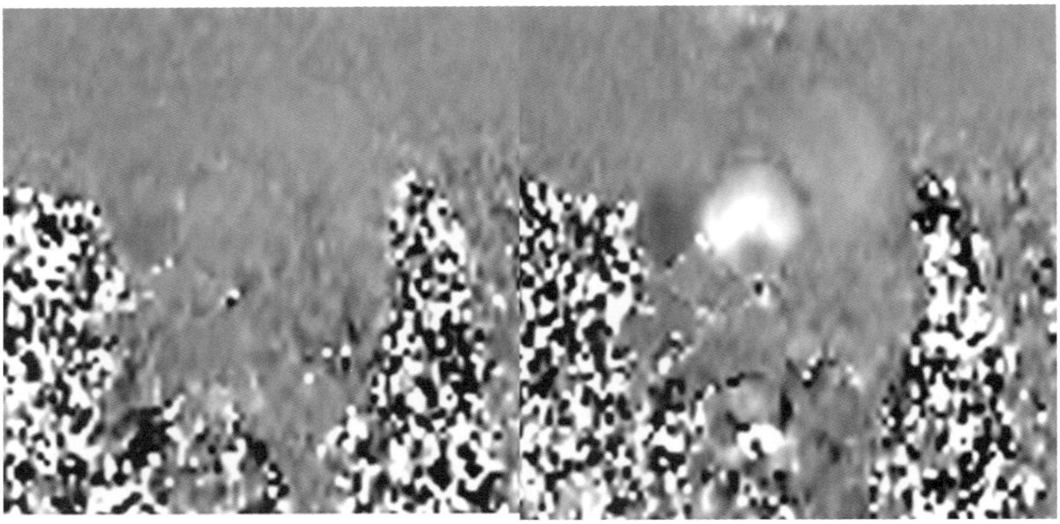

Fig. 20.6 Short axis frames from a cine phase contrast scan depicting the blood flow through the aorta and atria after trocar removal and chest closure. These scans are used to confirm adequate valve opening and blood flow through the prosthetic valve and to identify intravalvular or paravalvular regurgitation. Left: diastole; right: systole.

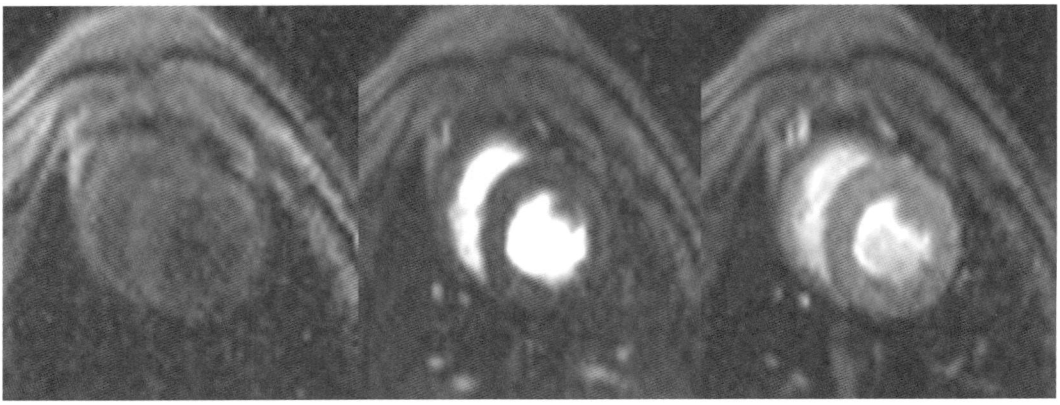

Fig. 20.7 A first-pass perfusion scan was performed during intravenous injection of Gd-DTPA contrast agent to confirm that myocardial blood flow was intact to all segments of the myocardium. Left to right represent a different time after venous injection of Gd-DTPA.

Conclusions

The distinct advantage of MRI for guiding cardiac surgery is that the surgeon can see "through" the blood, and thus all of the morphological landmarks for positioning the device are visible. Calcification does not interfere with MRI. The short and wide magnet makes it possible to have high-performance rtMRI to provide superb guidance while the prosthetic valve is being manipulated and placed. In addition to the anatomic detail, MRI provides the ability to analyze myocardial function and perfusion. MRI-guided surgery allows direct functional assessments to be made before, during, and immediately after valve implantation that are not obtainable by conventional imaging alone.

The combination of real-time non-invasive, non-contrast imaging that can provide both anatomic details and functional assessments will enable the use of minimally invasive approaches that may provide patients with a less morbid and more durable solution to structural heart disease.

Expansion of rtMRI guidance to facilitate other types of cardiac surgical procedures, including mitral, pulmonary, and tricuspid valve replacements or repairs, should be considered to minimize trauma and enhance patient benefit.

References

1 Buffolo E, Gerola L. Minimally invasive bypass grafting: a historical perspective. In: Goldstein DJ, Oz MC (eds) Minimally Invasive Cardiac Surgery, 2nd edn. Totowa, NJ: Humana Press, 2004, pp. 45–51.
2 Kirklin JK, Westaby S, Blackstone EH, et al. Complement and the damaging effects of cardiopulmonary bypass. J Thorac Cardiovasc Surg 1983;86(6):845–57.
3 Kestin AS, Valeri CR, Khuri SF, et al. The platelet function defect of cardiopulmonary bypass. Blood 1993;82(1):107–17
4 Kozik DJ, Tweddell JS. Characterizing the inflammatory response to cardiopulmonary bypass in children. Ann Thorac Surg 2006;81(6):S2347–54.
5 Henk CB, Higgins CB, Saeed M. Endovascular interventional MRI. J Magn Reson Imaging 2005;22:451–60.
6 Lederman RJ. Cardiovascular interventional magnetic resonance imaging. Circulation 2005;112:3009–17.
7 Derbyshire JA, Wright GA, Henkelman RM, et al. Dynamic scan-plane tracking using MR position monitoring. J Magn Reson Imaging 1998;8:924–32.
8 Bock M, Volz S, Zuhlsdorff S, et al. MR-guided intravascular procedures: real-time parameter control and automated slice positioning with active tracking coils. J Magn Reson Imaging 2004;19:580–9.
9 Elgort DR, Wong EY, Hillenbrand CM, et al. Real-time catheter tracking and adaptive imaging. J Magn Reson Imaging 2003;18:621–6.
10 Kuehne T. Cardiac interventions guided by magnetic resonance imaging. Heart Metab 2007;34:19–23.
11 Guttman MA, Kellman P, Dick AJ, et al. Real-time accelerated interactive MRI with adaptive TSENSE and UNFOLD. Magn Reson Med 2003;50:315–21.
12 Guttman MA, Lederman RJ, Sorger JM, et al. Real-time volume rendered MRI for interventional guidance. J Cardiovasc Magn Reson 2002;4:431–42.
13 Lederman RJ. Cardiovascular interventional magnetic resonance imaging. Circulation 2005;112:3009–17.
14 Guttman MA, Raval AN, Lederman RJ, et al. Real-time catheter-directed MRA with effective background suppression and persistent rendering. J Magn Reson Imaging 2008;28(2):538–42.
15 Chinzei K, Kikinis R, Jolesz F. MR Compatibility of mechatronic devices: design criteria. Proc MICCAI '99 Lecture Notes Computer Sci 1999;1679:1020–31.
16 Schenck JF. MR safety at high magnetic fields. Magn Reson Imaging Clin North Am 1998;6:715–30.
17 Schenck JF. Safety of strong, static magnetic fields. J Magn Reson Imaging 2000;12:2–19.
18 Bakker CJ, Bos C, Weinmann HJ. Passive tracking of catheters and guidewires by contrast-enhanced MR fluoroscopy. Magn Reson Med 2001;45:17–23.
19 Buecker A, Spuentrup E, Schmitz-Rode T, et al. Use of a nonmetallic guide wire for magnetic resonance-guided coronary artery catheterization. Invest Radiol 2004; 39:656–60.
20 Horvath KA, Mazilu D, Guttman M, et al. Midterm results of transapical aortic valve replacement via real-time magnetic resonance imaging guidance. J Thorac Cardiovasc Surg 2010;139(2):424–30.
21 Omary RA, Unal O, Koscielski DS, et al. Real-time MR imaging-guided passive catheter tracking with use of gadolinium-filled catheters. J Vasc Interv Radiol 2000;11:1079–85.
22 Ocali O, Atalar E. Intravascular magnetic resonance imaging using a loopless catheter antenna. Magn Reson Med 1997;37(1):112–18.
23 Kuehne T, Fahrig R, Butts K. Pair of resonant fiducial markers for localization of endovascular catheters at all catheter orientations. J Magn Reson Imaging 2003;17(5):620–4.
24 Quick HH, Zenge MO, Kuehl H, et al. Interventional magnetic resonance angiography with no strings attached: wireless active catheter visualization. Magn Reson Med 2005;53(2):446–55.
25 Kocaturk O, Saikus CE, Guttman MA, et al. Whole shaft visibility and mechanical performance for active MR catheters using copper-nitinol braided polymer tubes. J Cardiovasc Magn Reson 2009;11:29.
26 Horvath KA, Mazilu D, Kocaturk O, et al. Transapical aortic valve replacement under real-time magnetic resonance imaging guidance: experimental results with balloon-expandable and self-expanding stents. Eur J Cardiothorac Surg 2011;39(6):822–8.
27 Kellman P, Derbyshire JA, Agyeman KO, et al. Extended coverage first-pass perfusion imaging using slice-interleaved TSENSE. Magn Reson Med 2004;51:200–4.

Videoclip

This chapter contains the following videoclip:

Video 20.1 Transapical aortic valve replacement under MRI guidance.

It can be accessed at www.wiley.com/go/Valverepair.

21

CHAPTER 21

Patent ductus arteriosus

Dabit Arzamendi[1] *& Mark Reisman*[2]

[1] Interventional Cardiology and Structural Heart Intervention, Department of Cardiology, Hospital de la Santa Creu i Sant Pau, Barcelona, Spain

[2] Swedish Heart and Vascular Institute, Swedish Medical Center, Seattle, WA, USA

Introduction

The patent ductus arteriosus (PDA) is an essential fetal structure that connects the roof of the pulmonary artery to the proximal descending aorta and only becomes abnormal if it remains open in term infants older than 3 months [1]. Isolated PDA is found in around one in 2000 full-term infants, with girls affected about twice as often as boys [2,3]. The size and shape of the PDA vary greatly and impact on clinical severity (ranging from asymptomatic patients to Eisenmenger's syndrome) and on the type of occluding device when catheter intervention is considered.

Patent ductus arteriosus anatomy

The ductus arteriosus is a vessel communication connecting the proximal left pulmonary artery to the descending aorta that in fetal life, when the lungs are not functional, diverts the right ventricular cardiac output away from the high-resistance pulmonary vascular bed to the systemic circulation. This function ceases to exist after delivery, a functional closure occurs within 48 hours postpartum, and complete anatomic closure with fibrosis occurs during the next 2–3 weeks. However in one in 2000 full-term infants the ductus arteriosus remains patent and in the majority of cases there is no identifiable cause. Persistence of the duct is associated with chromosomal aberrations (trisomy 21 and 18, Rubinstein–Taybi, CHARGE), asphyxia at birth, birth at high altitude, and congenital rubella [1,4].

The duct's pulmonary orifice is located just leftward from the pulmonary artery bifurcation and the aortic orifice (the ampulla) is on the medial side of the aorta, at the level or just distal to the origin of the left subclavian artery (Fig. 21.1). In most of the cases the ampulla is wider and progressively narrows to the pulmonary artery end. The narrowing at the pulmonary orifice is due to the fact that the duct begins to close spontaneously from the pulmonary end [5], leaving a diverticulum on the aortic side (Kommerell's diverticulum). The ductus arterious is connected to the left pulmonary artery even in the presence of a right aortic arch. Rarely, however, it connects to the right pulmonary artery. Bilateral PDA has very rarely been observed. The width diameter of the PDA is measured at its narrowest point and it is not greater than 4 mm in 78% of patients.

The arterial duct can present in a variety of sizes and configurations. Krichenko et al. classified the duct following its configuration in the lateral angiogram [6]:

- The type A or conical duct has a well-defined aortic ampulla and constriction near the pulmonary artery end. This is the most frequent one.
- Type B is a large duct with a window-like structure, which is very short in length.
- Type C is a tubular duct without any constriction.
- Type D is a complex duct with multiple constrictions.

Endovascular and Hybrid Therapies for Structural Heart and Aortic Disease, First Edition.
Edited by Jacques Kpodonu and Raoul Bonan.

- The type E or elongated duct has constriction remote from the edge of the trachea as viewed on lateral angiography

This classification system allows the interventionalist to assess the size and configuration of the duct and select the most suitable occlusion device. There are other anatomic factors to take into consideration before the closure: in pediatric patients the duct is more elastic, while in adulthood it may develop atherosclerotic lesions and become more calcified and fragile. Moreover large ducts, although rare, are more frequently observed in adults and they may be dilated in an aneurysm-like manner.

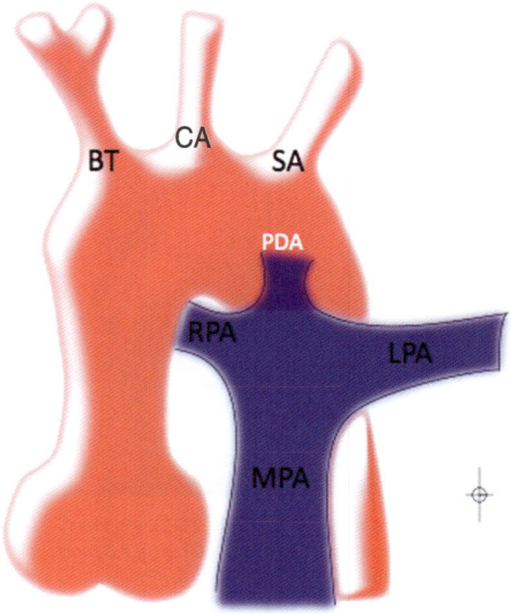

Fig. 21.1 Location of a patent ductus arteriosus (PDA). BT, brachiocephalic trunk; CA, carotid artery; LPA, left pulmonary artery; MPA, main pulmonary artery; RPA, right pulmonary artery; SA, subclavian artery.

Patent ductus arteriosus detection

Isolated PDA is generally fully diagnosed by echocardiography and is considered a class III indication for a computed tomography (CT) scan or magnetic resonance imaging (MRI) [7]. However both CT and MRI can provide more precise anatomic and morphological details of the PDA.

Transthoracic echocardiography

Transthoracic echocardiography (TTE) is the method of choice to confirm PDA and to characterize the hemodynamic significance of the PDA [8].

Confirm the ductal patency

The duct is directly observed in the parasternal short axis view and suprasternal projection and is shown as continuous flow from the aorta to the pulmonary artery bifurcation or to the left pulmonary artery (Fig. 21.2). In the suprasternal view, a pulsed Doppler signal shows diastolic reverse flow in the descending aorta under the site of duct

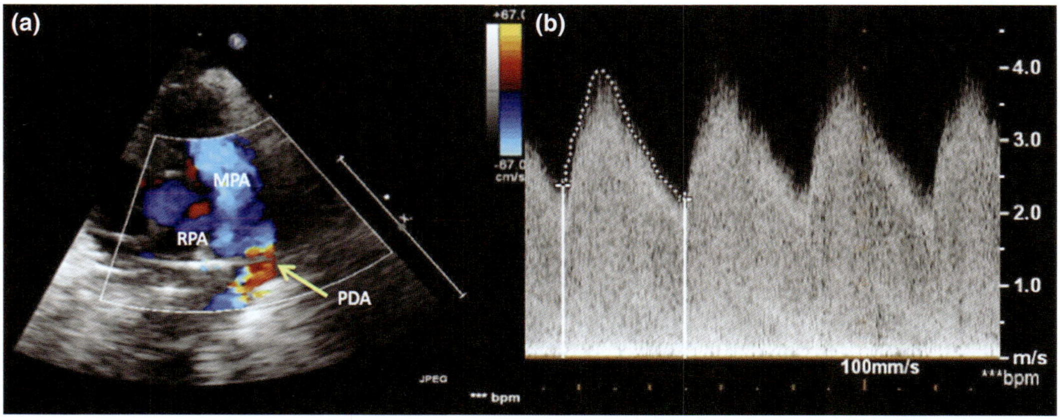

Fig. 21.2 (a) Patent arterial duct, seen by two-dimensional echocardiography, suprasternal view. The patent ductus arteriosus (PDA) is observed as a turbulent flow with color Doppler from the aorta to the pulmonary artery bifurcation. MPA, main pulmonary artery; RPA, right pulmonary artery. (b) Continuous Doppler examination from the suprasternal view, showing a continuous systolic flow of higher velocities, with the flow directed from the aorta to the pulmonary artery.

origin, and diastolic forward flow in the aortic arch above the duct origin. Right in the duct, continuous (systolic–diastolic) flow will be detected (Fig. 21.2).

Characterize the hemodynamic significance

1 *Ductal size*. The ductal size is normally the main determinant of echocardiographic significance. A PDA is commonly considered hemodynamically significant when transductal diameter is >1.5 mm [9,10]. For percutaneous closure, the minimal diameter and the diameter of the ampulla have to be measured.

2 *Characterization of the flow pattern and direction*. The direction and volume of the transductal shunt is dependent on transductal (pulmonary versus systemic) resistance. The PDA can be designated as closing/restrictive or unrestrictive and pulsatile according to pulse-wave Doppler flow patterns. Patients with unrestrictive ductus will have a large left-to-right shunt with a pulsatile flow pattern and the highest velocity at end systole (peak systolic velocity is usually less than 1.5 m/s and the ratio of peak systolic : diastolic velocity can be as high as 4 : 1) [11,12]. In patients with restrictive PDA, the flow velocity increases as blood accelerates across a narrower vessel leading to a reduction in the peak systolic : diastolic ratio.

3 *Pulmonary artery flow*. The presence of a large PDA leads to diastolic flow in the main branches of the pulmonary artery with a turbulent systolic flow pattern. There are no direct measures of the increased amount of pulmonary blood flow; however, left heart size and flow are useful surrogate determinants of the magnitude of the flow and its impact.

Therefore, TTE is a helpful tool to diagnose the presence of PDA, to determine the hemodynamic severity (ductus size, restrictive/unrestrictive, left ventricle size) and to measure the required diameters for the futher percutaneous closure. Transesophageal echocardiography and contrast echocardiography may be helpful in some cases, but TEE is the gold standard for PDA diagnosis.

Magnetic resonance imaging and computerized tomography scans

Computed tomography and MRI can provide more precise anatomic and morphological details of the patent ductus arteriosus. Using multiplanar CT

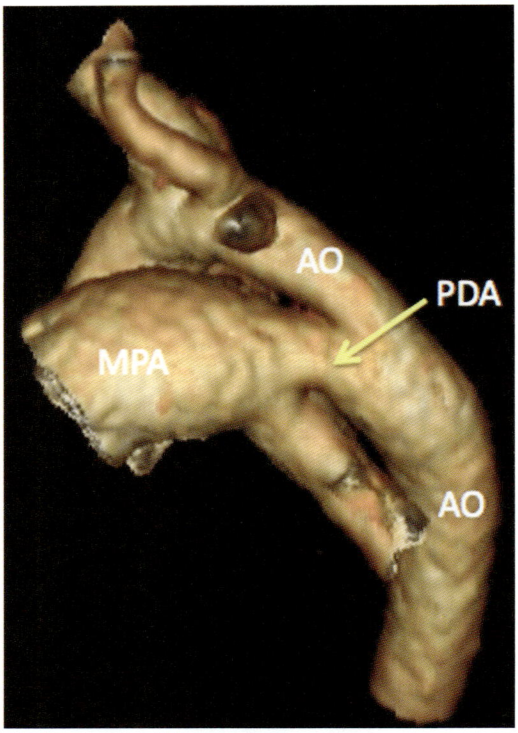

Fig. 21.3 Patent ductus arteriousus (PDA), seen by CT scan, sagittal view, showing a large PDA (arrow). AO, aorta; MPA, main pulmonary artery.

reformations, the location, caliber, length, and morphology of the PDA can be assessed in isolated defects as well in complex malformations. In adult patients, the presence and degree of calcifications of the wall of the PDA can be shown (Fig. 21.3)

MRI is useful particularly in the case of aneurysm formation or in association with a potential coexisting great artery anomaly. Cine-MRI and MRI-phase velocity cine acquisitions can respectively visualize the flow jet into the main pulmonary artery and assess the amount of shunt (QP/QS) (Figs 21.4 and 21.5)

Patient evaluation

Patient clinical and TEE evaluation is necessary to ascertain the severity of the PDA and to determine when the PDA needs to be closed. PDA in adulthood can be divided, by their size and clinical severity, into:

- Clinically silent duct ("silent PDA"). This is detectable only by echocardiography, with no heart murmurs audible.

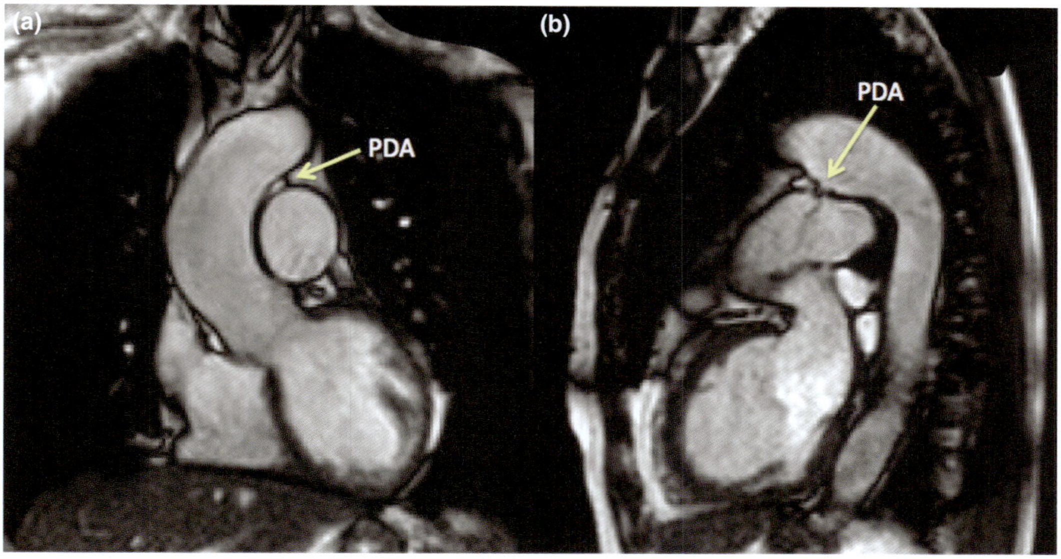

Fig. 21.4 Patent ductus arteriosus (PDA), seen by MRI. (a) Coronal view showing a small PDA (arrow). (b) Sagittal view.

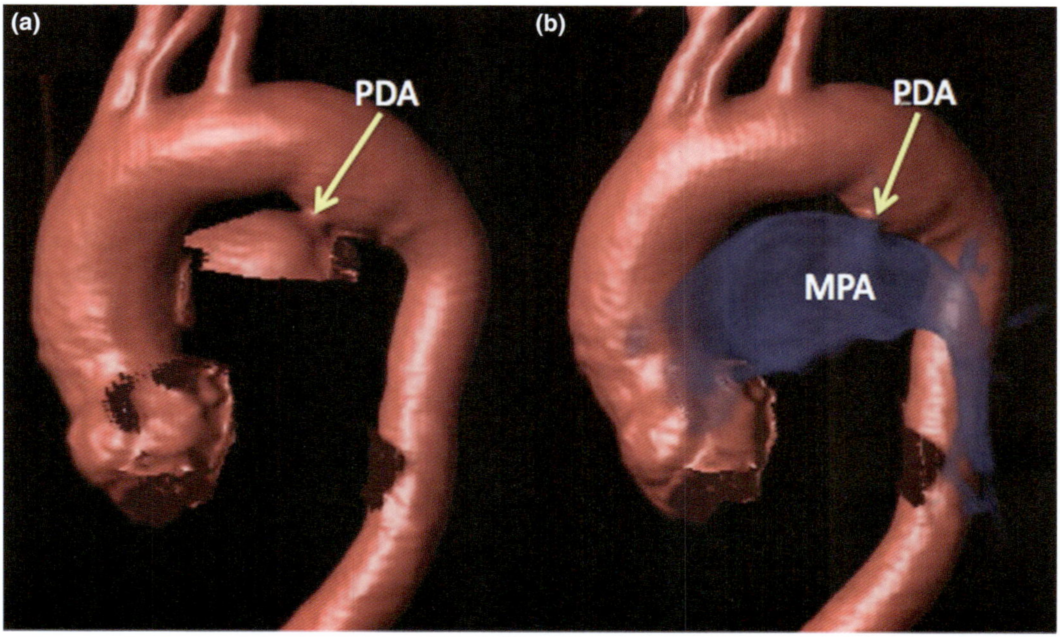

Fig. 21.5 Patent ductus arteriosus (PDA), seen by MRI 3D reconstruction. (a) Saggital view of the PDA (arrow). (b) The main pulmonary artery (MPA) is included.

- Small PDA. There is an audible long ejection or a continuous murmur, radiating to the back. It causes negligible hemodynamic change, the left ventricular size is normal, and there is no pulmonary hypertension. A small PDA is asymptomatic in adulthood.
- Moderate PDA. There is an audible continuous murmur and wide pulse arterial pressure (as in aortic regurgitation). It causes enlargement of the left atrium and left ventricle and some degree of pulmonary hypertension (usually reversible). Adults with moderate ducts are asymptomatic

in about 25% of cases, while the remaining ones experience dispnea, palpitations, or atypical chest pain [13].

- Large PDA. This does not usually occur in adults unless associated with Eisenmenger's syndrome. PDA with a significant left-to-right shunt can result in left heart failure; however, such cases are rare as most ducts are closed during childhood.
- Eisenmenger's syndrome. A continuous murmur is absent; there is severe, irreversible pulmonary hypertension, differentiated hypoxemia and cyanosis (lower body saturations lower than right arm saturations), and toe clubbing. Patients may show relatively few symptoms, and are free of pronounced exertional dyspnea as the respiratory centers are not exposed to hypoxia. During exercise, patients may complain of lower limb fatigability or pain, with the latter associated with hypertrophic osteoarthropathy. In the end stage, the patient may show signs of right heart decompensation.

The PDA should be closed, with the exception of the presence of silent tiny duct and the presence of severe, irreversible pulmonary vascular disease. There are a number of indications for PDA closure [7].

- Closure is indicated in both symptomatic and asymptomatic patients with significant left-to-right shunting (subsequent enlargement of the left ventricle) through a moderate to large PDA in the absence of fairly significant pulmonary hypertension.
- The occurrence of an episode of endarteritis, irrespective of the size of the PDA, indicates the need for closure.
- There has not been unanimity in terms of the indication for intervention in patients with a small PDA without volume load of the left ventricle. There is no hemodynamic reason to close the PDA and the risk for endocarditis is low. A strategy for closure is usually advocated in children and young adults because of the low risk of device closure.
- If pulmonary hypertension is present (pulmonary arterial pressure more than two-thirds of systemic arterial pressure or pulmonary arteriolar resistance exceeding two-thirds of systemic arteriolar resistance), there must be a net left-to-right shunt of 1.5 : 1 or more, or evidence of pulmonary artery reactivity with reversibility studies or, in highly selected cases, lung biopsy evidence that pulmonary arterial changes are potentially reversible.

The following associated lesions should be looked for, especially in pediatric patients:

- Coarctation of the aorta and a ventricular septal defect are the most common.
- Vascular ring (usually in the setting of a left-sided PDA with right aortic arch) may occur.
- PDA is universally present at birth in patients with congenital heart disease associated with limited or interrupted pulmonary or systemic blood flow (such as in patients with pulmonary atresia or the hypoplastic left heart syndrome). The circulation under these circumstances is PDA dependent, and patency of the PDA is critical to survival until surgery is performed.

Closure devices and procedural information

Catheter-based PDA closure has become the method of choice. Several systems for duct closure have been developed and are presented in the Table 21.1. The choice of the device will depend on the size of the PDA: routinely, small ducts (<2–3 mm) are closed with coils while larger ones (>3 mm) are closed with the Amplatzer ductal occluder, since the risk of coil embolism is high for these cases [14].

For PDA closure, femoral arterial and venous access is obtained preferably in almost all cases. Typically, a 4 Fr sheath is placed into the artery, and a 6 Fr sheath into the vein. Heparin (75 IU/kg) and antibiotic prophylaxis (cefazolin 25 mg/kg) are given at the appropriate times. A standard catheterization is then performed and in patients with PDA and pulmonary hypertension, hemodynamic testing is appropriate prior to closure to check reversibility of pulmonary resistance after oxygen/vasodilator administration and, in some centers, the duct is occluded transiently with a balloon and pulmonary/systemic pressure measure (if pulmonary pressure decreases after balloon inflation, but systemic pressure stands stable, the PDA closure is feasible). The initial angiogram is taken in straight posteroanterior (PA) and lateral projections; an alternative view is 30–40° right anterior oblique (RAO). The narrowest portion of

Table 21.1 Advantages and disadvantages of different devices.

	Device description	*Size (mm)*	*Advantages*	*Disadvantages*	*Photograph*
Gianturco, Jackson and Flippercoils	The coils are usually covered with Dacron strands to increase thrombogenicity	3–20 mm in diameter, and may be introduced through 4 or 5 Fr non-tapered angiographic catheters with an inner lumen of 0.035 inches	• Easy to deliver • Low cost	• Pulmonary embolism • Difficult in large PDAs	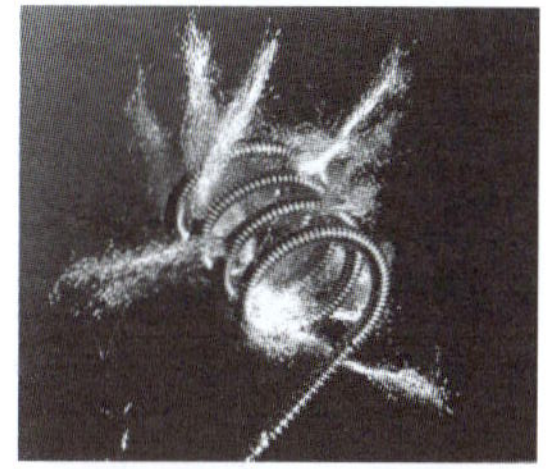
Amplatzer duct occluder (AGA Medical)	Nitinol wire mesh shaped into a cylindrical plug with a flared collar to secure the duct occluder in the PDA	5, 6, 8, 10, 12, 14, and 16 mm	• Most used • Easy to retrieve	• Late corrosion • Allergy to nickel • 6–8 Fr delivery system	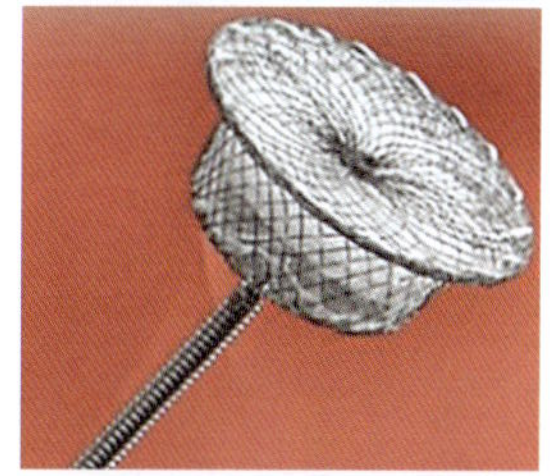
Amplatzer duct occluder II (AGA Medical)	Multilayered, flexible, nitinol wire mesh shaped into a cylindrical waist with retention disks on either end to secure it in the PDA. The device configuration is a central waist with two retention disks	3–6 mm diameter and 4–6 mm in length	• 4 Fr delivery system • Possible to deliver it from the aorta or the pulmonary artery	• Late corrosion • Allergy to nickel	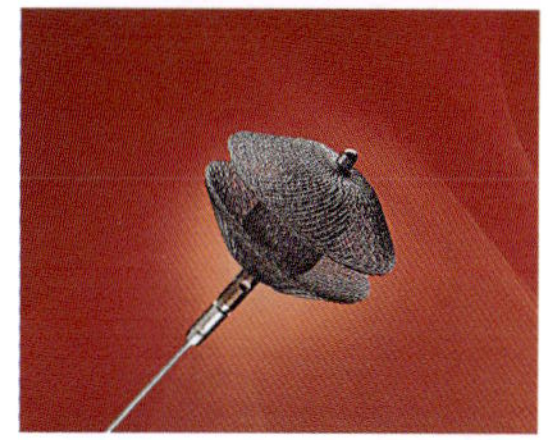
Nit-Occlud (pfm AG)	Nitinol coil especially designed for PDA closure. Graduated stiffness from aortal to proximal windings for optimal adaptation to ductus anatomy	9–22 mm in diameter and 5–12 mm in length	• Available for large PDAs • 4–5 Fr delivery system	• Limited experience	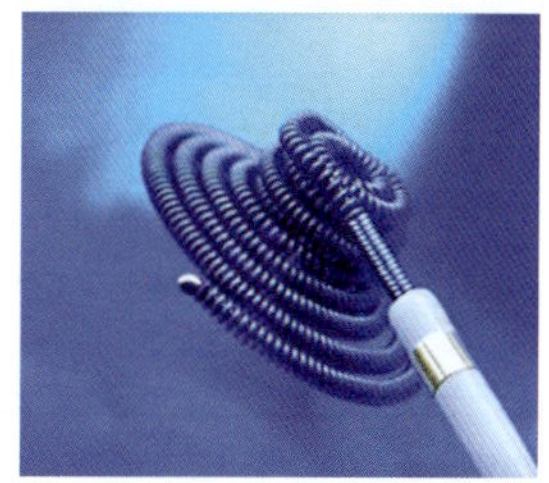

PDA is measured, as well as the size and length of the ampulla, and the morphology of the duct is evaluated. It is crucial to measure the PDA minimum diameter during systole, as this measurement can be 30% larger than the diastolic dimension. Then the closure device is chosen.

Coil occlusion

For PDA occlusion with a coil, the retrograde approach is used routinely. The PDA is then crossed with a 0.035 inch wire through an end-hole catheter (JR2, multipurpose, or cobra catheter) and the catheter is advanced over the wire into the main pulmonary artery (the position should be confirmed by pressure transduction).

A coil for occlusion is chosen based on consideration of the duct's morphology, length, and size. Every coil has three measurements: (i) the coil wire size; (ii) the diameter of the coil as it loops; and (iii) the length of the coil. The coil is usually chosen to have a diameter of at least twofold the diameter of the duct and a length that will produce approximately four loops ($\pi \times$ diameter $\times$ 4). Usually a 0.038 inch coil is chosen because it is stronger and more stable than the 0.035 inch one. A straight wire of the same caliber as the coil is then inserted through the plastic-covered end of the cartridge. The coil is advanced and a single loop is extruded, then the catheter and wire are pulled back together until the loop is at the desired location at the pulmonary artery side. The wire is now kept stable as the catheter is withdrawn, uncovering the aortic end of the coil; finally the coil is delivered.

After 10 minutes, an angiogram is performed in the descending aorta. If there is no flow through the PDA or just a small amount of smoke oozing through the coil, the procedure is complete. If there is a jet of residual flow through the coil, a second coil is implanted and intravenous protamine may be administered.

The definition of a successful transcatheter PDA occlusion is permanent complete PDA closure without creating obstruction (from the coil) to the aorta or pulmonary artery. Immediate complete occlusion is obtained in 59% of patients, and this increases to 95–100% at1-year follow-up [14,15]. Failure to implant the coil is uncommon; when it does occur, it has been related to a large PDA minimal diameter (>4 mm) and short PDA length [16,17].

Closure with an Amplatzer duct occluder

The Amplatzer duct occluder (ADO; AGA Medical Corp., Golden Valley, MN) is a self-expanding occlusion device made from nitinol wires configured into a mesh framework; there is polyester fabric inside the device to help induce thrombosis. It has been approved for patients older than 6 months and weighing more than 6 kg, and is generally used only in a PDA with a minimum diameter of at least 2–2.5 mm, with a sufficiently large aortic ductal ampulla to prevent the device from protruding out into the lumen of the descending aorta.

Venous access is necessary for device delivery, although the new ADO II device is symmetric on both sides and it could be delivered retrograde from the pulmonary artery into the aorta. Routinely the device is delivered through the vein and the arterial access is used for the angiographic control. The ADO size is selected such that the smallest device diameter should be at least 2 mm larger than the smallest PDA diameter. The long sheath is introduced over a J-tipped guide wire positioned in the descending abdominal aorta. The retention skirt is first deployed in the proximal descending aorta and then the sheath and device are pulled simultaneously until the retention disk contacts the ampulla; an angiogram may be performed to assess device position. The remaining portion of the device can be deployed by unsheathing the device under tension. Any pulmonary artery or aortic obstruction should be evaluated if suspected. When position is confirmed the device is released. If the device position is suboptimal, the device is pulled back into the sheath, the sheath is redeployed into the aorta, and the implant procedure is repeated. The device can easily be repositioned numerous times or removed and replaced with another size device. A post implant angiogram is performed to confirm device position and make sure there is no residual jet leak; a small amount of smoke oozing through the device is often seen and should resolve spontaneously (Fig. 21.6).

Immediate complete occlusion is obtained in 44–56% of patients. The number of complete closures rises to 66–76% within 24 hours, to 94.6–100% at 6 months, with 100% of completely closed ducts after 1 year [18–20].

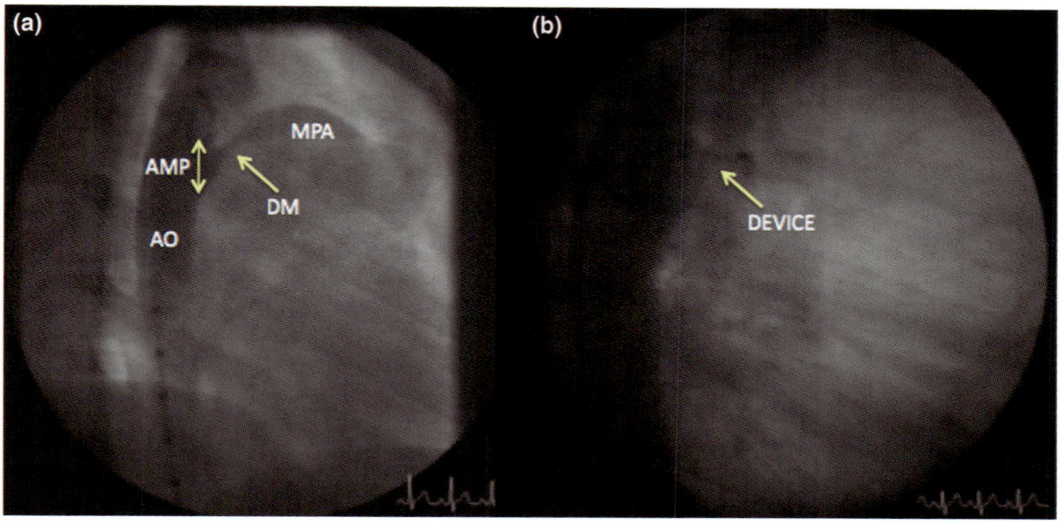

Fig. 21.6 Patent ductus arteriosus (PDA), seen by angiogram, lateral view. (a) Type A PDA, where the ampulla (AMP) is well defined and the diameter decreases at the pulmonary end. AO, aorta; DM, minimal diameter of the duct; MPA, main pulmonary artery. (b) Closure with an ADO II device.

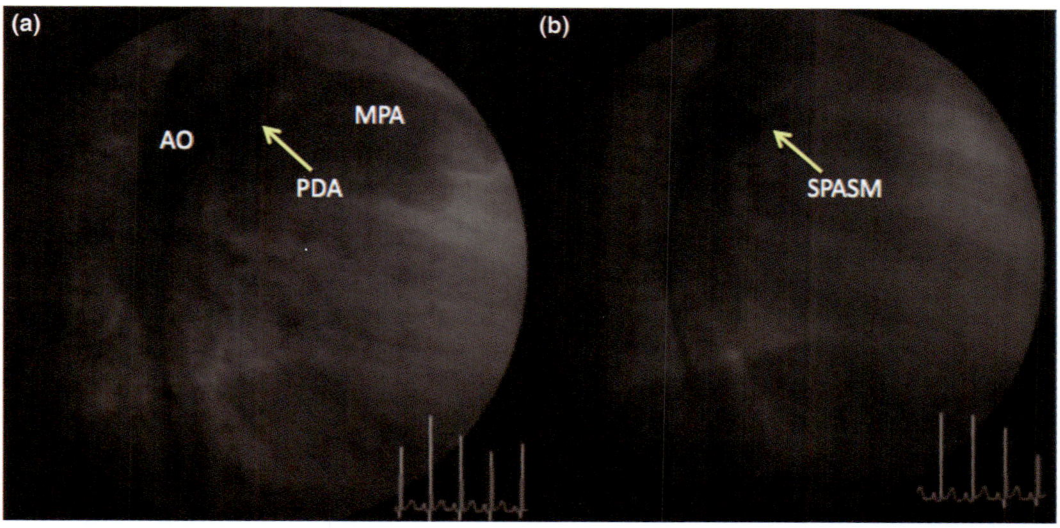

Fig. 21.7 Patent ductus arteriosus (PDA), seen by angiogram, lateral view. (a) Large type C PDA. AO, aorta; MPA, main pulmonary artery. (b) After manipulation with the catheter a severe spasm of the PDA is observed.

Challenging anatomy

The ADO is a less suitable device for more tubular type PDAs, especially if the largest diameter is seen in the central portion of the PDA. In these circumstances, the Amplatzer vascular plug II may be more suitable. However, caution has to be applied for this indication, because the lack of Dacron in these devices may prevent complete occlusion in moderate-sized high–low PDAs [21].

Complications

With the devices available today, closure of the standard PDA in a child should have virtually zero mortality and extremely minimal morbidity. Coil embolization has been one of the most frequent complications prior to introduction of the ADO, but this complication can be virtually eliminated if coils are exclusively used in very small PDAs.

The incidence of reported major complications varies from 0% to 2.3%, with the overall rate of adverse events being 4.8% [8,22]. Rare complications that have been described include partial occlusion of the left pulmonary artery, aortic obstruction, as well as devvice embolization [8,23,24]. Vascular complications and/or blood loss requiring transfusion have been reported in 0.3% of cases and hemolysis secondary to a residual shunt has been observed in about 0.5% of patients [22,25]. In some cases during manipulation ductus spasm can be observed and it is necessary to administer vasodilators to measure correctly the diameter of the PDA (Fig. 21.7).

The risk of infectious endarteritis is low in the absence of Eisenmenger's syndrome. According to the guidelines of the American Heart Association, endocarditis prophylaxis is no longer recommended in patients with PDA and absence of a history of infectious endocarditis and cyanosis [26]. In patients with a residual shunt after closure and Eisenmenger's syndrome, the risk of infectious endocarditis/endarteritis is present and requires antibiotic prevention.

References

1 Benson LN, Cowan KN. The arterial duct: its persistence and its patency. In: Anderson RHBE, Macartney FJ, Rigby ML, Shinebourne EA, Tynan M (eds) Paediatric Cardiology. London: Churchill Livingstone, 2002, pp. 1405–59.

2 Mullins CE, Pagotto L. Patent ductus arteriosus. In: Garson AJBJ, Bricker JT, Fisher DJ, Neish SR (eds) The Science and Practice of Pediatric Cardiology. Baltimore: Williams & Wilkins, 1998, pp. 1181–97.

3 Perloff JK. The Clinical Recognition of Congenital Heart Disease. Philadelphia: Saunders/Elsevier, 1994.

4 Nora JJ. Multifactorial inheritance hypothesis for the etiology of congenital heart diseases. The genetic-environmental interaction. Circulation 1968;38:604–17.

5 Smallhorn JF, Gow R, Olley PM, et al. Combined noninvasive assessment of the patent ductus arteriosus in the preterm infant before and after indomethacin treatment. Am J Cardiol 1984;54:1300–4.

6 Krichenko A, Benson LN, Burrows P, et al. Angiographic classification of the isolated, persistently patent ductus arteriosus and implications for percutaneous catheter occlusion. Am J Cardiol 1989;63:877–80.

7 Warnes CA, Williams RG, Bashore TM, et al. ACC/AHA 2008 guidelines for the management of adults with congenital heart disease: a report of the American College of Cardiology/American Heart Association Task Force on Practice Guidelines (writing committee to develop guidelines on the management of adults with congenital heart disease). Developed in collaboration with the American Society of Echocardiography, Heart Rhythm Society, International Society for Adult Congenital Heart Disease, Society for Cardiovascular Angiography and Interventions, and Society of Thoracic Surgeons. J Am Coll Cardiol 2008;52: e1–121.

8 Masura J, Tittel P, Gavora P, et al. Long-term outcome of transcatheter patent ductus arteriosus closure using Amplatzer duct occluders. Am Heart J 2006;151:755 e7–755 e10.

9 Evans N. Current controversies in the diagnosis and treatment of patent ductus arteriosus in preterm infants. Adv Neonatal Care 2003;3:168–77.

10 Evans N, Iyer P. Longitudinal changes in the diameter of the ductus arteriosus in ventilated preterm infants: correlation with respiratory outcomes. Arch Dis Child Fetal Neonatal Ed 1995;72:F156–61.

11 Su BH, Peng CT, Tsai CH. Echocardiographic flow pattern of patent ductus arteriosus: a guide to indomethacin treatment in premature infants. Arch Dis Child Fetal Neonatal Ed 1999;81:F197–200.

12 McNamara PJ, Sehgal A. Towards rational management of the patent ductus arteriosus: the need for disease staging. Arch Dis Child Fetal Neonatal Ed 2007;92:F424–7.

13 Harrison DA, Benson LN, Lazzam C, et al. Percutaneous catheter closure of the persistently patent ductus arteriosus in the adult. Am J Cardiol 1996;77:1094–7.

14 Wang JK, Liau CS, Huang JJ, et al. Transcatheter closure of patent ductus arteriosus using Gianturco coils in adolescents and adults. Catheter Cardiovasc Interv 2002;55:513–18.

15 Zellers TM, Wylie KD, Moake L. Transcatheter coil occlusion of the small patent ductus arteriosus (<4 mm): improved results with a "multiple coil-no residual shunt" strategy. Catheter Cardiovasc Interv 2000;49:307–13.

16 Shim D, Beekman RH, 3rd. Transcatheter management of patent ductus arteriosus. Pediatr Cardiol 1998;19: 67–71; discussion 72–3.

17 Moore JW, George L, Kirkpatrick SE, et al. Percutaneous closure of the small patent ductus arteriosus using occluding spring coils. J Am Coll Cardiol 1994;23: 759–65.

18 Faella HJ, Hijazi ZM. Closure of the patent ductus arteriosus with the amplatzer PDA device: immediate results of the international clinical trial. Catheter Cardiovasc Interv 2000;51:50–4.

19 Podnar T, Gavora P, Masura J. Percutaneous closure of patent ductus arteriosus: complementary use of

detachable Cook patent ductus arteriosus coils and Amplatzer duct occluders. Eur J Pediatr 2000;159:293–6.
20 Thanopoulos BD, Hakim FA, Hiari A, et al. Patent ductus arteriosus equipment and technique. Amplatzer duct occluder: intermediate-term follow-up and technical considerations. J Interv Cardiol 2001;14:247–54.
21 Javois AJ, Husayni TS, Thoele D, et al. Inadvertent stenting of patent ductus arteriosus with Amplatzer Vascular Plug. Catheter Cardiovasc Interv 2006;67: 485–9.
22 Pass RH, Hijazi Z, Hsu DT, et al. Multicenter USA Amplatzer patent ductus arteriosus occlusion device trial: initial and one-year results. J Am Coll Cardiol 2004;44:513–19.
23 Shahabuddin S, Atiq M, Hamid M, et al. Surgical removal of an embolised patent ductus arteriosus amplatzer occluding device in a 4-year-old girl. Interact Cardiovasc Thorac Surg 2007;6:572–3.
24 McMullan DM, Moulick A, Jonas RA. Late embolization of Amplatzer patent ductus arteriosus occlusion device with thoracic aorta embedment. Ann Thorac Surg 2007; 83:1177–9.
25 Joseph G, Mandalay A, Zacharias TU, et al. Severe intravascular hemolysis after transcatheter closure of a large patent ductus arteriosus using the Amplatzer duct occluder: successful resolution by intradevice coil deployment. Catheter Cardiovasc Interv 2002;55:245–9.
26 Wilson W, Taubert KA, Gewitz M, et al. Prevention of infective endocarditis: guidelines from the American Heart Association: a guideline from the American Heart Association Rheumatic Fever, Endocarditis, and Kawasaki Disease Committee, Council on Cardiovascular Disease in the Young, and the Council on Clinical Cardiology, Council on Cardiovascular Surgery and Anesthesia, and the Quality of Care and Outcomes Research Interdisciplinary Working Group. Circulation 2007;116:1736–54.

22

CHAPTER 22
Patent foramen ovale

Dabit Arzamendi[1] *& Mark Reisman*[2]

[1] Interventional Cardiology and Structural Heart Intervention, Department of Cardiology, Hospital de la Santa Creu i Sant Pau, Barcelona, Spain

[2] Swedish Heart and Vascular Institute, Swedish Medical Center, Seattle, WA, USA

Introduction

A patent foramen ovale (PFO) is a vestige of the fetal circulation and results from the lack of fusion of the septum primum and septum secundum. PFO is a found in up to 25% of unselected adults [1], and most are discovered incidentally and have no clinical consequences. However, association of PFO with various clinical conditions such as embolic stroke [2], platypnea-orthodeoxia syndrome [3], decompression sickness in divers [4] and migraine [5] have been reported. Percutaneous closure of a PFO has been shown to be an effective and safe procedure [6].

Patent foramen ovale anatomy

In the fetal circulation the atrial septum is composed by the fusion of two septa, the septum primum and secundum, that allow a communication between the right and left atria through an oval-shaped tunnel called the foramen ovale. The foramen ovale plays an important role in fetal circulation, whereby oxygenated blood from the umbilical veins and inferior vena cava is preferentially directed through the Eustachian valve and foramen to the left atrium and systemic circulation. At birth, the right heart pressure and pulmonary vascular resistance drop as the pulmonary arterioles open in reaction to oxygen filling the alveolus. Left atrial pressure rises as the amount of blood returning from the lung increases. Either or both mechanisms may cause the foramen to close. This fusion is complete by age 2 years in about 75% of individuals, but remains patent in 25% [1,7,8]. The reasons PFOs fail to close are unknown, but they likely relate to multifactorial inheritance [9,10].

Heterogeneity of size and morphology are pertinent to interventional device closure selection. The mechanism for closure of the oval foramen can be likened to that of a door closing against a doorframe. When the valve (septum primum) is large enough to overlap the muscular rim or limbus (septum secundum) that is located on the right atrial side of the septum and is completely adherent to the infolded superior and inferior margins of the muscular rim (septum secundum), the septum is totally intact. In some cases the patency of the oval foramen is due to an adequate valve that is not completely adherent to the muscular rim (competent valve). In other cases the valve is large enough to occlude the foramen, but owing to factors like changes in atrial pressures/volume causing stretched atrial walls and/or aneurysmal flap valve, the PFO becomes apparent. In these cases the retraction of the valve in aneurysmal deformation can allow the valve to herniate into the right or left atrium (incompetent valve) [11]. The length of the PFO tunnel ranges from 3 to 24 mm, with a mean length of 9 mm [12–14]. Greater PFO size increases the risk of paradoxal embolism (Fig. 22.1).

Endovascular and Hybrid Therapies for Structural Heart and Aortic Disease, First Edition.
Edited by Jacques Kpodonu and Raoul Bonan.

A PFO is associated with several anatomic anomalies. A common association is atrial septal aneurysm (ASA), where part or all of the atrial septum shows aneurysmal dilation protruding into either atria [15,16]. ASA is defined as phasic septal excursion of at least 15 mm during the cardiorespiratory cycle [17]. The prevalence of ASA is 1% in autopsy-based studies [18] and 2.2–4% in transesophageal echocardiographic studies [19,20]. The prevalence of ASA is greater among patients with embolic events [21–24] and 60% of patients with ASA have an associated PFO [20,22]. Additionally, the PFOs seen in the presence of ASA tend to be larger compared with those seen without associated ASA (Fig. 22.2) [25,26]. Thus, the association of ASA with embolic events is likely based on the high prevalence of large PFOs.

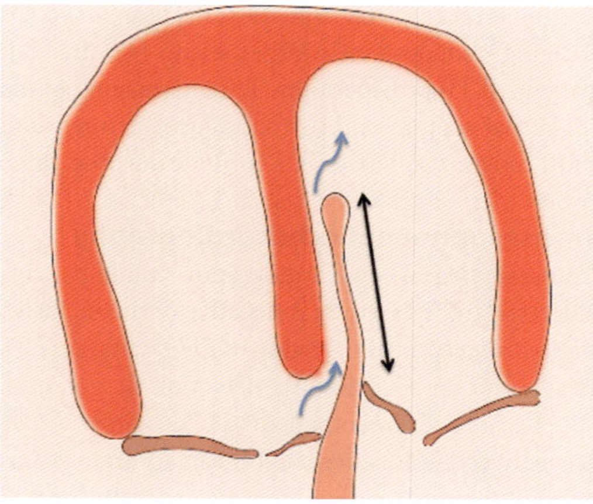

Fig. 22.1 Design of a patent foramen ovale. The black arrow delimits the tunnel length of the foramen. The blue arrows represent the flow passing through the PFO from the right atrium to the left atrium.

The Chiari network is a remnant of the right valve of the sinus venosus, and its role is poorly understood [27]. It originates from a region of the Eustachian and Thebesian valves with attachment to the upper wall of the right atrium or atrial septum. The prevalence of the Chiari network is 2–3% [28] and is associated with the presence of a PFO [29].The Eustachian valve is a membrane-like structure in the right atrium, a remnant of the right valve of the sinus venosus that directs blood flow from the inferior vena cava to the fossa ovalis area in the fetus [30]. Among adults, a Eustachian valve can cause a significant right-to-left shunt in the presence of an interatrial communication by altering the blood flow pattern [31,32]. A prominent Eustachian valve is also more commonly found among patients with presumed paradoxical embolism than in control patients [33]. Therefore, the presence of atrial anatomic variants that can promote flow from the inferior vena cava toward the PFO may increase the chance of paradoxical embolization beyond that associated with PFO size.

Patent foramen ovale detection

Transthoracic echocardiography (TTE), transesophageal echocardiography (TEE), and transcranial Doppler (TCD) ultrasound are commonly

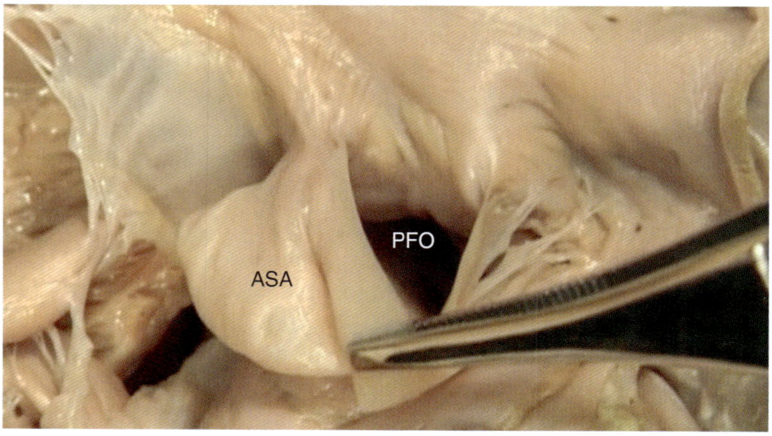

Fig. 22.2 Pathology exam of a left atrium. A large septal aneurysm (ASA) is observed associated to a large patent foramen ovale (PFO).

used to detect and assess PFOs. Intracardiac echocardiography (ICE) can be a useful tool during PFO closure in the cath lab.

Transcranial Doppler

Transcranial Doppler is a non-invasive test for diagnosing the presence of a PFO. This technique has high sensitivity in detecting PFO [34]. An ultrasound probe is placed over the middle cerebral artery with concomitant venous administration of an echo-contrast medium not passing through the pulmonary capillary bed and registers micro bubbles passing into the cerebral circulation. The principal limitations of TCD are that it only indicates the existence of right-to-left shunting, does not distinguish between intracardiac or extracardiac shunting, and provides no anatomic information about PFO. Thus, the echocardiogram remains the gold standard to detect a PFO, as it shows both the presence and the location of the shunt.

Transthoracic echocardiography

Since Doppler color-flow only detects 5–10% of interatrial shunts, a contrast study is needed for PFO detection. Intravenous injection of saline mixed with air greatly enhances the diagnosis of right-to-left shunts by permitting visualization of microbubbles in the chambers of the left side of the heart that would otherwise be filtered by the lung capillaries. To increase diagnostic sensitivity the injection should be performed both at rest and with maneuvers that increase right atrial pressure (i.e. Valsalva, coughing) [35,36]. PFO is judged to be present with the visualization of microbubbles in the left atrium within three cardiac cycles from the right atrial opacification [37]. When microbubbles are observed after the third beat this may correspond to intrapulmonary shunting.

Quantification of the number of bubbles appearing in the left atrium is not feasible because the number of bubbles depends on many factors (differences in the amount of bubbles injected, speed with which they are injected, variations in blood flow pattern in cardiac chambers, contrast material injected into the lower extremities has a higher chance of crossing a PFO) [38–41]. It was shown that in any PFO, right-to-left shunting varies considerably, and that the magnitude of contrast shunting does not necessarily correlate with the true anatomic size of the PFO [14]. However, some echocardiography laboratories classify severity as complete left chamber opacification, almost complete opacification, or slight opacification [42].

The principal limitation of TTE is its relatively poor sensitivity compared to TEE (20% versus 42%) [8], plus with TEE it is possible to delineate the structure of the interatrial septum and the PFO.

For guiding percutaneous closure of a PFO, TTE has the advantage of offering multiple planes to evaluate the device and atrial septum. However, it has limited ability to interrogate the lower rim of atrial septal tissue above the inferior vena cava after device placement, because the device interferes with imaging in virtually all planes. In addition, the septum is relatively far from the transducer and color imaging is suboptimal in large patients [43]. In adult patients, TTE provides more limited imaging of the interatrial septum and surrounding structures, and most centers use TEE or ICE to guide the procedure.

Transesophageal echocardiography

Transesophageal echocardiography should be considered if the TTE study is negative or inconclusive but a strong clinical suspicion of PFO remains. TEE is superior to TTE for the detection of potential sources of cardioembolism (57% versus 27%, respectively) [44], since it allows an accurate evaluation of the cardiac structures: presence of thrombi in the left atrial appendage; spontaneous echo contrast in the left atrium; left ventricular thrombi in the presence of impaired kinetics; atherosclerotic plaques in the aorta. With TEE it is also possible to do a more complete evaluation of the PFO anatomy than is actually pertinent for the percutaneous closure: detailed assessment of the interatrial septum (see Fig. 22.2); tunnel length, measuring the maximum opening diameter of the communicating channel at the entrance into the left atrium [33] (long tunnels represent a problem for devices with a fixed distance between the right and left atrial components [11]) (Fig. 22.3); the presence of ASA and/or Chiari network, etc.

During the intervention, TEE is useful in determining the size of the device to be implanted and provides direct visual guidance in device deployment and avoids interference with other structures (Figs 22.4 and 22.5). However, TEE is poorly tolerated by patients in the supine position and

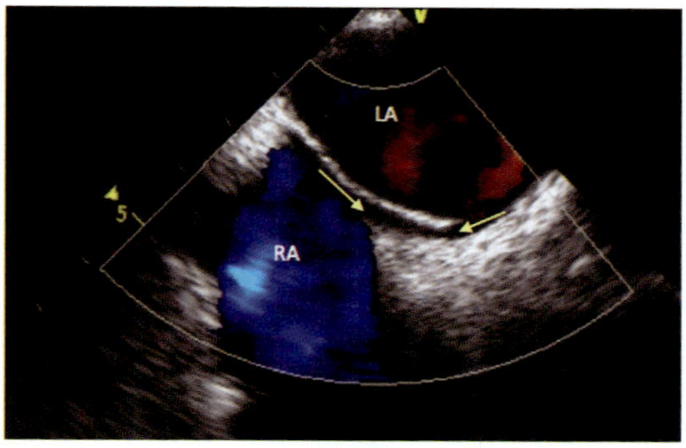

Fig. 22.3 Transesophageal echo, longitudinal view, showing measurement of the length of patent foramen ovale; the tunnel is delimited by the arrows. LA, left atrium; RA, right atrium.

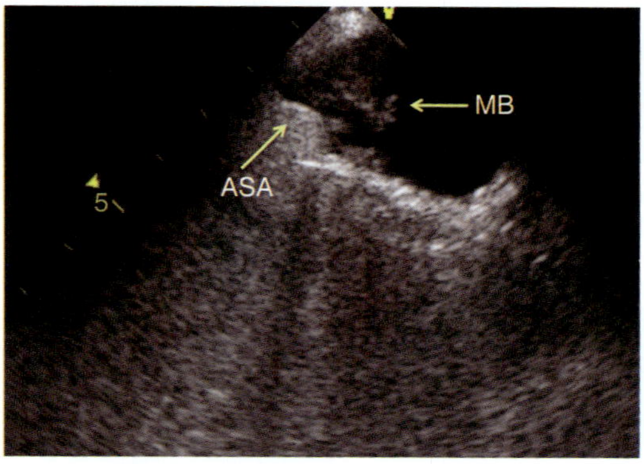

Fig. 22.4 Positive contrast echocardiography showing microbubbles (MB) crossing the interatrial septum with an aneurysm (ASA) via a patent foramen ovale from the right atrium to the left atrium.

requires conscious sedation (with attendant aspiration risk in supine patients) or general anesthesia, which lengthens the procedure; it is also associated with 0.2% of serious complications (including bronchospasm, hypoxia, arrhythmias, upper gastrointestinal trauma, and bleeding) [45]. Moreover this approach requires a dedicated echocardiographer to perform the TEE while the operator performs the closure procedure, as well as anesthesia support personnel if general anesthesia is used.

Intracardiac echocardiography

Intracardiac echocardiography has become the imaging standard for atrial septal closure procedures in many centers [46–52]. ICE provides imaging of the interatrial septum and surrounding structures that is comparable with TEE but does not require additional sedation or general anesthesia to perform (Fig. 22.6). ICE enables characterization of the PFO, tunnel, septum, and shunting and is useful in percutaneous closure device deployment (Fig. 22.7). Compared with guidance using TEE, ICE has been shown to improve patient comfort, shorten both procedure and fluoroscopy times, and offer comparable cost with TEE-guided interventions [48–50]. Moreover, it can be an alternative to TEE in selected patients with absolute contraindication to TEE (esophagectomy). Currently available ICE systems provide a single-use 8–10 Fr phased-array intracardiac ultrasound-equipped catheter and require additional 8–11 Fr venous access. Most of the complications are related to the vascular access (hematoma, bleeding), but other complications such as cardiac perforation, arrhythmia, or thromboembolism have been also described [43].

Patient evaluation

Since indications for PFO closure remain controversial, previous evaluation of the patient and determination of the indication for PFO closure are essential. PFOs have been related to different pathologies.

Cryptogenic stroke

Approximately 40% of ischemic strokes are considered cryptogenic (i.e. no apparent cause) [46]. The first publication to mention the possible relationship of a cerebrovascular event with the presence of PFO was reported by Julius Cohnheim, a German pathologist, in 1877 who reported the case of a young woman who died of a stroke and he hypothesized that the clot passed through the PFO [53]. However, the association between PFO and cryptogenic stroke remains controversial, since paradoxical embolism is rarely a proven diagnosis but rather one of suspicion [2,21,54–62]. Possible mechanisms for this association include:

- Formation of thrombus in the foramen ovale canal as a consequence of stasis and minimal pressure differences between the atria (these data are anecdotal and based on surgical observations) [63,64].
- Paradoxical embolism, with the passage of thrombus from the peripheral venous system to

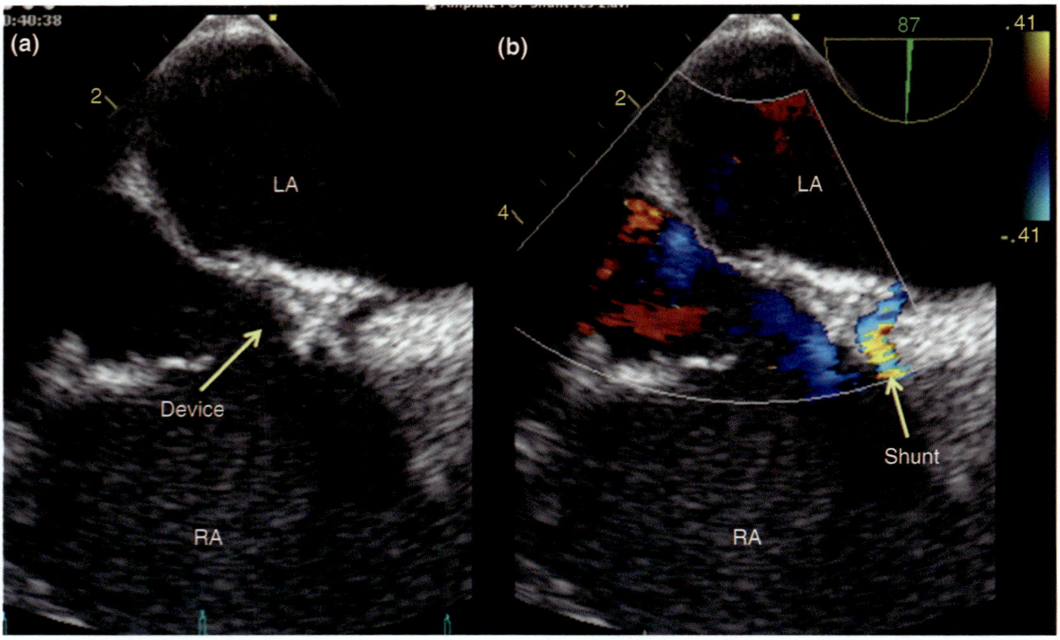

Fig. 22.5 Transesophageal echo after device implantation. (a) Color Doppler showing a residual shunt in the aortic rim. (b) A BioStar device has been implanted in the PFO. LA, left atrium; RA, right atrium.

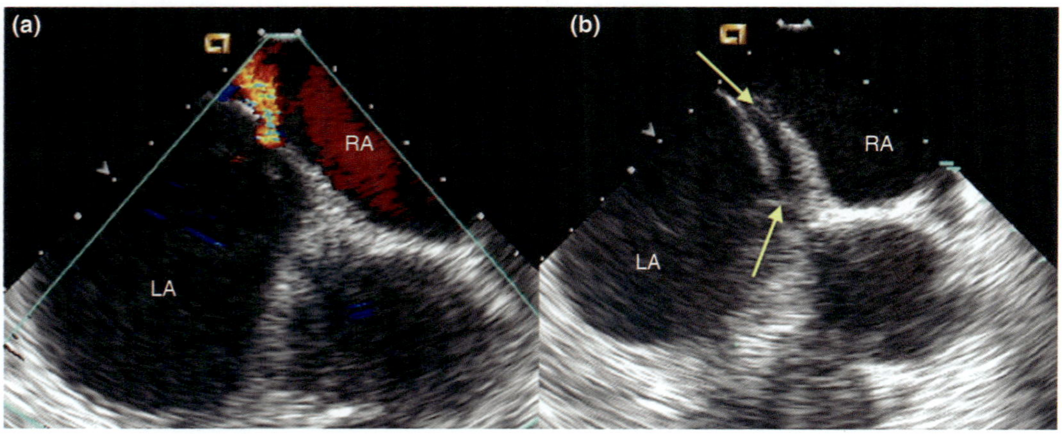

Fig. 22.6 Intracardiac echocardiography. (a) The anatomy of the foramen is well assessed; the arrows delimit the length of the tunnel. (b) A spontaneous shunt through the foramen can be observed with colour Doppler from the right atrium (RA) to the left atrium (LA).

left cardiac cavities through the PFO. Thus, paradoxical embolism requires:

- A favorable pressure gradient for right-to-left shunting. Such a gradient normally occurs only transiently, in early systole [65]. Moreover, conditions that promote right-to-left shunting, such as pulmonary hypertension or Valsalva-inducing activities, are rarely documented in patients with stroke who have a patent foramen ovale [66].
- Source of thrombus. The source of the thrombus rarely is revealed in the evaluation of patients with cryptogenic stroke and PFO [66]. The reportedly low rate of detection of deep vein thrombosis may reflect delays in imaging (after the initiation of

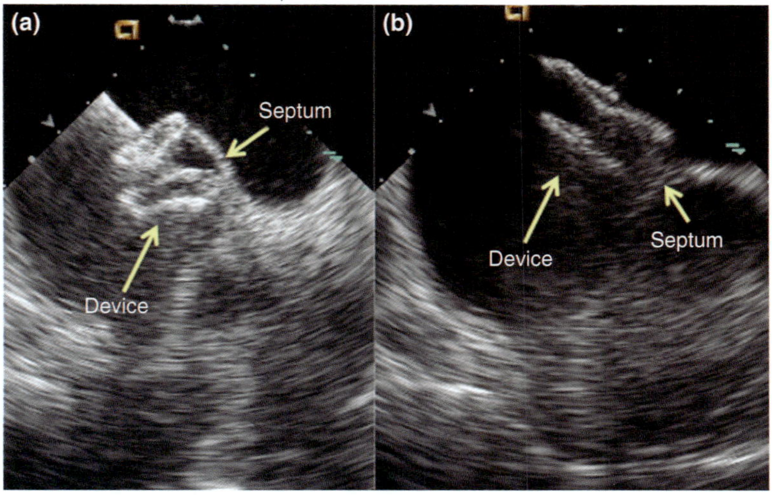

Fig. 22.7 Intracardiac echocardiography during device deployment. (a) The device is well deployed in the septum. (b) The device is approached to the septum from the left atrium.

anticoagulation) [67], due to complete thrombus migration, inability to detect residual thrombus, or undetected thrombosis in a calf or pelvic vein [68,69]. Indeed, small embolic fragments (1 mm in diameter) are sufficient to cause a clinical stroke [70].

Adding to the mechanistic uncertainty, population-wide figures suggest that the yearly risk of cryptogenic stroke in healthy persons with PFO may be as low as 0.1% [71]. This observation suggests that additional factors might be necessary to increase the associated risk of stroke, some related to the patient itself and some others related to the PFO features.

1 *Patient-associated risk factors*:
- Age <55 years. The prevalence of PFO is five-fold increased among patients 55 years old or younger with cryptogenic stroke compared to stroke-free controls [2,72]. In older patients, other cardiovascular factors might be involved in the etiology of the stroke and PFO will be involved in a lower percentage of events.
- Concurrent risk factors for venous thromboembolism, such as trauma, recent surgery, use of oral contraceptives, and hypercoagulable states [73]. The presence of hypercoagulable states is not a *conditio sine qua non* for the diagnosis of cryptogenic stroke associated with PFO, but increases the chance of having a thrombotic event that could promote cryptogenic stroke. The two most common genetic risk factors for venous thrombosis, factor V Leiden and prothrombin G20210A gene mutation, have been associated with a fourfold increased risk of cerebral ischemia in PFO patients [74,75]. These data indicate that coexistence of a PFO and inherited hypercoagulable states may identify subjects at higher risk for paradoxical embolism.

2 *Features of the patent foramen ovale*:
- Large anatomic defect (>5 mm) between the primum and secundum septa [42,76,77].
- Increased right-to-left shunting or shunting at rest [61,62,78].
- Increased septal mobility and the presence of an atrial septal aneurysm [54,58,61].

Therefore prior to PFO closure, patients have to be extensively studied to assess that PFO is the main cause behind the cryptogenic stroke.

1 *Neurologic study*. It is necessary to determinate the cause of stroke and rule out hemorrhage with computerized tomography (CT) or magnetic resonance imaging (MRI). Carotid ultrasound also has to be performed to rule out a possible atheroembolic origin of the stroke.

2 *Cardiologic study*. TEE should be considered in order to get information about other possible sources of the emboli (appendage, left ventricle, aorta) and we can get a detailed assessment of the PFO for the future closure.

3 *Vascular study*. A Doppler ultrasound should be performed to exclude deep vein thrombosis in the lower limbs and, alternatively, pelvic vein visualization by MRI/cardiac CT or venography should be done.
4 *Hematologic study*. To exclude thrombophilic states coagulation testing – including prothrombin and activated partial thromboplastin times, antiphospholipid antibodies, fibrinogen, protein C, protein S, activated protein C resistance, and antithrombin – is undertaken. Genetic analyses for inherited prothrombotic conditions including the G1691A mutation in the factor V (FV) gene, the G20210A mutation in the prothrombin (PT) gene, and the C677T mutation in the methylene tetrahydrofolate reductase (MTHFR) gene should also be performed.

The American Academy of Neurology considers evidence to be insufficient for them to take a position on the efficacy of percutaneous or surgical closure, and American Heart Association/American Stroke Association guidelines consider data are insufficient to recommend PFO closure in patients with a first episode. However, they do recommend considering closure in patients who, although receiving medical treatment, present a second episode (class IIb, evidence C) [79]. In the absence of results from randomized studies, in patients with cryptogenic infarction and PFO, percutaneous closure could be considered the treatment of choice for those receiving medical treatment who experience recurrent stroke, who are contraindicated for medical treatment and who have PFOs with high anatomic risk (ASA or hypermobile septum, long tunnel, right-to-left spontaneous shunting).

Platypnea-orthodeoxia syndrome

The platypnea-orthodeoxia syndrome (POS) comprises both dyspnea (platypnea) and arterial desaturation in the upright position with improvement in the supine position (orthodeoxia). Right-to-left cardiac or pulmonary shunting can cause the syndrome, in intracardiac shunting through a PFO; postural hypoxemia seems to be a consequence of redirecting flow in the inferior vena cava towards the interatrial septum due to the distortion of anatomic relations. Blood may flow from right to left at the atrial level even when right heart pressure is normal [44], as typically occurs with persistent Eustachian valves. This syndrome usually occurs in the elderly and has been associated with aortic root dilation, aorta elongation, kyphoscoliosis, spine compression fracture, pericardial effusion, right-sided pneumonectomy, and diaphragmatic paralysis [80].

Diagnosis of PFO with POS should be by tilt-test, measuring arterial saturation in different positions, and contrast echocardiography, which should show intracardiac shunting [81].

The definitive treatment for this syndrome is PFO closure [3,81]. Currently, percutaneous closure could be considered the treatment of choice, with an initial success rate of nearly 100%, significant increase in oxygen saturation, and low incidence of complications [82–84].

Migraine

Migraine headache is a benign recurring syndrome of headache, nausea, vomiting, and/or other symptoms of neurologic dysfunction and has been associated with PFO. There are different hypotheses to explain this pathology: some suggest that circulating serotonin and prostaglandins, normally removed in the lungs, may trigger migraine by reaching the brain through the PFO [85]; others have postulated that is caused by the passage of small venous emboli through the PFO, thus stroke and migraine would represent a continuum of vascular complications caused by focal and transient hypoperfusion [86].

In fact, migraine is a risk factor for cryptogenic stroke [87], especially in young patients without cardiovascular factors. Moreover, migraine with aura also develops as a complication of injury to large vessels (acute vertebral or carotid artery dissections) suggesting that ischemic events might cause migraine [88].

PFO has been found to be more prevalent among patients suffering from migraine with aura, ranging from 41% to 72% [89]. Several non-randomized studies showed a significant relationship between PFO closure and improvement of migraine [90], with migraine resolution or significant improvement in 70–76% of cases [91,92]. However, in the only published randomized double-blinded study, the MIST trial [93], no significant differences were observed either in the primary endpoint of migraine headache cessation (4.1% in both groups, $P = 0.51$), or in the secondary endpoint of 50% reduction in days with headache. But several issues have been raised regarding the quality of shunt diagnosis and closure performance in this study: no PFO was found in the 6.8% of catheterized patients, PFO was defined as the appearance of bubbles in the left atrium five beats later than their appearance in the right atrium, and moderate to large residual shunt was observed in 5.8% of the cases. For the above-mentioned reasons, the MIST trial should be considered inconclusive.

Therefore, the relationship between headache and right-to-left shunt remains poorly characterized and current available data are insufficient to recommend PFO closure in these patients. Larger studies of PFO and headache are underway, as are randomized trials of PFO closure and migraine headache relief.

Decompression sickness

Decompression sickness describes a condition arising from the precipitation of dissolved gasses into bubbles inside the body on depressurization during ascent after a scuba dive. Type 1 decompression sickness is composed of localized joint pain, musculoskeletal pain, and/or skin rash. Type 2 decompression sickness consists of neurologic symptoms (limb tingling, paresthesias, severe headache with mental confusion, paraplegia, loss of consciousness, audiovestibular symptoms, dyspnea with chest pain). The PFO at rest is significantly associated with type 2 decompression sickness.

PFO has been found to increase by five times the risk of major decompression illness and the risk increases with increasing PFO size [4]. It is more frequent in those with right-to-left shunting at rest, ASA and larger PFO.

The current European clinical fitness for diving practice does not include PFO screening before diving, as the absolute risk is very low and most patients recover completely after recompression treatment. Divers with symptoms of decompression illness or ischemic brain lesions should be advised to abstain from diving. Divers with a PFO associated with high-risk anatomy (ASA, wide patency diameter) must be advised of the risk in continuing to scuba dive, and PFO closure has been proposed for this indication [94].

Devices and procedural information

Many devices have been used for PFO closure, but most of them were not designed specifically for this use, and consequently we are still lacking the ideal device. We summarize the different devices available at the moment and their principal characteristics. The ideal device should take into account many factors.

- The delivery system should have a small sheath diameter in order to reduce the risk of vein thrombosis, especially in those patients who present with thrombophlebitis and those with thrombophilic disorders. At the moment most of the devices require an 8–9 Fr sheath for device deployment.
- It should be possible to deliver the device with one easy maneuver and it should be easy to retrieve. Ideally it should be possible to deliver the device completely to evaluate the final position of the device and the residual shunt, with the possibility of retrieving it if the position and/or the size of the device are not right.
- The delivery system should be adaptable to the morphology of the PFO. It should be possible to completely close the PFO irrespective of the presence of ASA or long tunnels.
- The system should be minimally thrombogenic and bioabsorbable. The surface of the device should minimize platelet adhesion and, especially, the formation of platelet aggregates. Ideally the material should be eliminated progressively, with minimal inflammatory reaction and should leave no residual or a minimal amount of material.

For PFO closure there are some common steps regardless of the device chosen. The PFO is crossed under fluoroscopy with a multipurpose 5 Fr catheter or is advanced gently a 0.035 inch J wire. Once the catheter is placed in the left superior pulmonary vein an extra-stiff 260 cm length wire is advanced though it. Then the catheter is exchanged for a long 8–11 Fr introducer. The PFO occluder device is released through the sheath following the specific recommendations for each device. All procedures are done by monitoring fluoroscopy, preferably in a left anterior oblique (LAO) craniocaudal projection 40-35 projection. When TEE is used, patients need deep sedation or general anesthesia. Monitoring with ICE avoids the need for intubation and reduces the procedural time.

At the end of the procedure and before releasing the device, it is necessary to check the position of the device, the presence of residual shunts, and to do different maneuvers to assure the stability of the device. All patients should receive 70 IU of heparin during the procedure. Aspirin ± clopidogrelare given before the procedure and for the next 6 months. We also recommend endocarditis prophylaxis for the next 6 months. At the end of the procedure the long sheath has to be removed followed by manual compression. Depending on operator experience, a vascular closure device can be used.

Before discharging the patient we recommend a reassessment of the patient with echocardiography and electrocardiography. For those in whom the PFO has not been perfectly occluded, a TEE should be done after 3 months.

Challenging anatomy

In most of cases PFO closure is a straightforward procedure, but in some situations we can find challenging anatomy:

1 *Long tunnels.* Long tunnels represent a problem for devices with a fixed distance between the right and the left atrial components, as there is the potential for both disks to be partially deployed within the tunnel. In these cases there are different possible solutions:

- Use new devices with an adjustable tunnel size (Premere).
- In some cases transeptal puncture can be really useful. Once the transeptal puncture is done the delivery sheath is advanced through the new transeptal hole and the device is implanted in this position, avoiding the PFO tunnel.
- Detunnelization. With this technique the aim is to turn the PFO into an atrial septal defect (ASD). A 25 mm sizing balloon is advanced through the PFO and is inflated to 20 mm, completely obliterating the morphology of the tunnel and turning it into a true ASD. Then the PFO or ASD device is implanted.

2 *Atrial septum aneurysm.* For large aneurysms, where there is a marked excess of tissue, both the transeptal and detunnelization techniques can be used.

Complications

The rate of major complications has been estimated at 1.5%, including death, hemorrhage requiring blood transfusion, cardiac tamponade, need for surgery, and massive fatal pulmonary emboli. Minor complications include bleeding not requiring transfusion, peri-procedural atrial arrhythmias, transient atrioventricular node block, device arm fractures, device embolization with successful catheter retrieval, asymptomatic device thrombosis, need for recatheterization, symptomatic air embolism, transient ST-segment elevation, arteriovenous fistula formation, and femoral hematoma. These have been reported in 7.9% of cases [6].

The rate of complications varies depending on the devices, but in general major complications have been infrequent and the overall safety and results of the devices have compared favorably with standard open surgical repair [95].

References

1 Hagen PT, Scholz DG, Edwards WD. Incidence and size of patent foramen ovale during the first 10 decades of life: an autopsy study of 965 normal hearts. Mayo Clin Proc 1984;59:17–20.

2 Lechat P, Mas JL, Lascault G, et al. Prevalence of patent foramen ovale in patients with stroke. N Engl J Med 1988;318:1148–52.

3 Medina A, de Lezo JS, Caballero E, et al. Platypnea-orthodeoxia due to aortic elongation. Circulation 2001;104:741.

4 Torti SR, Billinger M, Schwerzmann M, et al. Risk of decompression illness among 230 divers in relation to the presence and size of patent foramen ovale. Eur Heart J 2004;25:1014–20.

5 Anzola GP, Magoni M, Guindani M, et al. Potential source of cerebral embolism in migraine with aura: a transcranial Doppler study. Neurology 1999;52:1622–5.

6 Khairy P, O'Donnell CP, Landzberg MJ. Transcatheter closure versus medical therapy of patent foramen ovale and presumed paradoxical thromboemboli: a systematic review. Ann Intern Med 2003;139:753–60.

7 Meissner I, Whisnant JP, Khandheria BK, et al. Prevalence of potential risk factors for stroke assessed by transesophageal echocardiography and carotid ultrasonography: the SPARC study. Stroke prevention: assessment of risk in a community. Mayo Clin Proc 1999;74:862–9.

8 Homma S, Sacco RL. Patent foramen ovale and stroke. Circulation 2005;112:1063–72.
9 Hara H, Virmani R, Ladich E, et al. Patent foramen ovale: current pathology, pathophysiology, and clinical status. J Am Coll Cardiol 2005;46:1768–76.
10 Clark EB. Pathogenetic mechanisms of congenital cardiovascular malformations revisited. Semin Perinatol 1996;20:465–72.
11 Ho SY, McCarthy KP, Rigby ML. Morphological features pertinent to interventional closure of patent oval foramen. J Interv Cardiol 2003;16:33–8.
12 Marshall AC, Lock JE. Structural and compliant anatomy of the patent foramen ovale in patients undergoing transcatheter closure. Am Heart J 2000;140:303–7.
13 Sievert H, Horvath K, Zadan E, et al. Patent foramen ovale closure in patients with transient ischemia attack/stroke. J Interv Cardiol 2001;14:261–6.
14 Pinto FJ. When and how to diagnose patent foramen ovale. Heart 2005;91:438–40.
15 Marazanof M, Roudaut R, Cohen A, et al. Atrial septal aneurysm. Morphological characteristics in a large population: pathological associations. A French multicenter study on 259 patients investigated by transoesophageal echocardiography. Int J Cardiol 1995;52:59–65.
16 Olivares-Reyes A, Chan S, Lazar EJ, et al. Atrial septal aneurysm: a new classification in two hundred five adults. J Am Soc Echocardiogr 1997;10:644–56.
17 Hanley PC, Tajik AJ, Hynes JK, et al. Diagnosis and classification of atrial septal aneurysm by two-dimensional echocardiography: report of 80 consecutive cases. J Am Coll Cardiol 1985;6:1370–82.
18 Silver MD, Dorsey JS. Aneurysms of the septum primum in adults. Arch Pathol Lab Med 1978;102:62–5.
19 Agmon Y, Khandheria BK, Meissner I, et al. Frequency of atrial septal aneurysms in patients with cerebral ischemic events. Circulation 1999;99:1942–4.
20 Pearson AC, Nagelhout D, Castello R, et al. Atrial septal aneurysm and stroke: a transesophageal echocardiographic study. J Am Coll Cardiol 1991;18:1223–9.
21 Di Tullio M, Sacco RL, Gopal A, et al. Patent foramen ovale as a risk factor for cryptogenic stroke. Ann Intern Med 1992;117:461–5.
22 Zabalgoitia-Reyes M, Herrera C, Gandhi DK, et al. A possible mechanism for neurologic ischemic events in patients with atrial septal aneurysm. Am J Cardiol 1990;66:761–4.
23 Mirode A, Tribouilloy C, Boey S, et al. [Aneurysm of the interatrial septum. Contribution of transesophageal echography. Relation with systemic embolic complications]. Ann Cardiol Angeiol (Paris) 1993;42:7–12.
24 Albers GW, Comess KA, DeRook FA, et al. Transesophageal echocardiographic findings in stroke subtypes. Stroke 1994;25: 23–8.
25 Homma S, Sacco RL, Di Tullio MR, et al. Atrial anatomy in non-cardioembolic stroke patients: effect of medical therapy. J Am Coll Cardiol 2003;42:1066–72.
26 Fox ER, Picard MH, Chow CM, et al. Interatrial septal mobility predicts larger shunts across patent foramen ovales: an analysis with transmitral Doppler scanning. Am Heart J 2003;145:730–6.
27 Werner JA, Cheitlin MD, Gross BW, et al. Echocardiographic appearance of the Chiari network: differentiation from right-heart pathology. Circulation 1981;63:1104–9.
28 Chiari H. About network development in the right side of the heart. Beitr Pathol Anat 1897;22:1–10.
29 Schneider B, Hofmann T, Justen MH, et al. Chiari's network: normal anatomic variant or risk factor for arterial embolic events? J Am Coll Cardiol 1995;26:203–10.
30 Hickie JB. The valve of the inferior vena cava. Br Heart J 1956;18:320–6.
31 Morishita Y, Yamashita M, Yamada K, et al. Cyanosis in atrial septal defect due to persistent eustachian valve. Ann Thorac Surg 1985;40:614–16.
32 Raffa H, al-Ibrahim K, Kayali MT, et al. Central cyanosis due to prominence of the eustachian and thebesian valves. Ann Thorac Surg 1992;54:159–60.
33 Schuchlenz HW, Saurer G, Weihs W, et al. Persisting eustachian valve in adults: relation to patent foramen ovale and cerebrovascular events. J Am Soc Echocardiogr 2004;17:231–3.
34 Jauss M, Zanette E. Detection of right-to-left shunt with ultrasound contrast agent and transcranial Doppler sonography. Cerebrovasc Dis 2000;10:490–6.
35 Ha JW, Shin MS, Kang S, et al. Enhanced detection of right-to-left shunt through patent foramen ovale by transthoracic contrast echocardiography using harmonic imaging. Am J Cardiol 2001;87:669–71, A11.
36 Kronik G, Slany J, Moesslacher H. Contrast M-mode echocardiography in diagnosis of atrial septal defect in acyanotic patients. Circulation 1979;59:372–8.
37 Homma S, Di Tullio MR, Sacco RL, et al. Characteristics of patent foramen ovale associated with cryptogenic stroke. A biplane transesophageal echocardiographic study. Stroke 1994;25:582–6.
38 Hamann GF, Schatzer-Klotz D, Frohlig G, et al. Femoral injection of echo contrast medium may increase the sensitivity of testing for a patent foramen ovale. Neurology 1998;50:1423–8.
39 Droste DW, Lakemeier S, Wichter T, et al. Optimizing the technique of contrast transcranial Doppler ultrasound in the detection of right-to-left shunts. Stroke 2002; 33:2211–16.
40 Droste DW, Kriete JU, Stypmann J, et al. Contrast transcranial Doppler ultrasound in the detection of right-to-left shunts: comparison of different procedures and different contrast agents. Stroke 1999;30:1827–32.
41 Devuyst G, Piechowski-Jozwiak B, Karapanayiotides T, et al. Controlled contrast transcranial Doppler and arterial blood gas analysis to quantify shunt through patent foramen ovale. Stroke 2004;35:859–63.

42 Schuchlenz HW, Weihs W, Horner S, et al. The association between the diameter of a patent foramen ovale and the risk of embolic cerebrovascular events. Am J Med 2000;109:456–62.
43 Silvestry FE, Kerber RE, Brook MM, et al. Echocardiography-guided interventions. J Am Soc Echocardiogr 2009;22:213–31; quiz 316–17.
44 Rahmatullah AF, Rahko PS, Stein JH. Transesophageal echocardiography for the evaluation and management of patients with cerebral ischemia. Clin Cardiol 1999;22:391–6.
45 Daniel WG, Erbel R, Kasper W, et al. Safety of transesophageal echocardiography. A multicenter survey of 10,419 examinations. Circulation 1991;83:817–21.
46 Sacco RL, Ellenberg JH, Mohr JP, et al. Infarcts of undetermined cause: the NINCDS Stroke Data Bank. Ann Neurol 1989;25:382–90.
47 Bartel T, Konorza T, Arjumand J, et al. Intracardiac echocardiography is superior to conventional monitoring for guiding device closure of interatrial communications. Circulation 2003;107:795–7.
48 Boccalandro F, Baptista E, Muench A, et al. Comparison of intracardiac echocardiography versus transesophageal echocardiography guidance for percutaneous transcatheter closure of atrial septal defect. Am J Cardiol 2004;93:437–40.
49 Rhodes JF, Jr., Qureshi AM, Preminger TJ, et al. Intracardiac echocardiography during transcatheter interventions for congenital heart disease. Am J Cardiol 2003;92:1482–4.
50 Mullen MJ, Dias BF, Walker F, et al. Intracardiac echocardiography guided device closure of atrial septal defects. J Am Coll Cardiol 2003;41:285–92.
51 Butera G, Chessa M, Bossone E, et al. Transcatheter closure of atrial septal defect under combined transesophageal and intracardiac echocardiography. Echocardiography 2003;20:389–90.
52 Hijazi Z, Wang Z, Cao Q, et al. Transcatheter closure of atrial septal defects and patent foramen ovale under intracardiac echocardiographic guidance: feasibility and comparison with transesophageal echocardiography. Catheter Cardiovasc Interv 2001;52:194–9.
53 Cohnheim J. Thrombose und embolie. Vorlesungen über allgemeine Pathologie 1887;1:165–230.
54 Steiner MM, Di Tullio MR, Rundek T, et al. Patent foramen ovale size and embolic brain imaging findings among patients with ischemic stroke. Stroke 1998;29:944–8.
55 Handke M, Harloff A, Olschewski M, et al. Patent foramen ovale and cryptogenic stroke in older patients. N Engl J Med 2007;357:2262–8.
56 Hausmann D, Mugge A, Becht I, et al. Diagnosis of patent foramen ovale by transesophageal echocardiography and association with cerebral and peripheral embolic events. Am J Cardiol 1992;70:668–72.
57 Jones EF, Calafiore P, Donnan GA, et al. Evidence that patent foramen ovale is not a risk factor for cerebral ischemia in the elderly. Am J Cardiol 1994;74:596–9.
58 Mas JL, Arquizan C, Lamy C, et al. Recurrent cerebrovascular events associated with patent foramen ovale, atrial septal aneurysm, or both. N Engl J Med 2001; 345:1740–6.
59 Homma S, Sacco RL, Di Tullio MR, et al. Effect of medical treatment in stroke patients with patent foramen ovale: patent foramen ovale in Cryptogenic Stroke Study. Circulation 2002;105:2625–31.
60 Meissner I, Khandheria BK, Heit JA, et al. Patent foramen ovale: innocent or guilty? Evidence from a prospective population-based study. J Am Coll Cardiol 2006; 47:440–5.
61 Di Tullio MR, Sacco RL, Sciacca RR, et al. Patent foramen ovale and the risk of ischemic stroke in a multiethnic population. J Am Coll Cardiol 2007;49:797–802.
62 De Castro S, Cartoni D, Fiorelli M, et al. Morphological and functional characteristics of patent foramen ovale and their embolic implications. Stroke 2000;31:2407–13.
63 Falk V, Walther T, Krankenberg H, et al. Trapped thrombus in a patent foramen ovale. Thorac Cardiovasc Surg 1997;45:90–2.
64 Caes FL, Van Belleghem YV, Missault LH, et al. Surgical treatment of impending paradoxical embolism through patent foramen ovale. Ann Thorac Surg 1995;59:1559–61.
65 Eggebrecht H, Naber CK, Plato C, et al. Analysis of fossa ovalis membrane velocities by transesophageal Doppler tissue echocardiography: a novel approach to functional assessment of patent foramen ovale. J Am Soc Echocardiogr 2004;17:1161–6.
66 Falk RH. PFO or UFO? The role of a patent foramen ovale in cryptogenic stroke. Am Heart J 1991;121:1264–6.
67 Stollberger C, Slany J, Schuster I, et al. The prevalence of deep venous thrombosis in patients with suspected paradoxical embolism. Ann Intern Med 1993;119:461–5.
68 Kiernan TJ, Yan BP, Cubeddu RJ, et al. May-Thurner syndrome in patients with cryptogenic stroke and patent foramen ovale: an important clinical association. Stroke 2009;40:1502–4.
69 Cramer SC, Rordorf G, Maki JH, et al. Increased pelvic vein thrombi in cryptogenic stroke: results of the Paradoxical Emboli from Large Veins in Ischemic Stroke (PELVIS) study. Stroke 2004;35:46–50.
70 Mohr JP. Cryptogenic stroke. N Engl J Med 1988;318:1197–8.
71 Lock JE. Patent foramen ovale is indicted, but the case hasn't gone to trial. Circulation 2000;101:838.
72 Overell JR, Bone I, Lees KR. Interatrial septal abnormalities and stroke: a meta-analysis of case-control studies. Neurology 2000;55:1172–9.
73 Chaturvedi S. Coagulation abnormalities in adults with cryptogenic stroke and patent foramen ovale. J Neurol Sci 1998;160:158–60.
74 Pezzini A, Del Zotto E, Magoni M, et al. Inherited thrombophilic disorders in young adults with ischemic stroke and patent foramen ovale. Stroke 2003;34:28–33.

75 Karttunen V, Hiltunen L, Rasi V, et al. Factor V Leiden and prothrombin gene mutation may predispose to paradoxical embolism in subjects with patent foramen ovale. Blood Coagul Fibrinolysis 2003;14:261–8.
76 Devuyst G, Despland PA, Bogousslavsky J, et al. Complementarity of contrast transcranial Doppler and contrast transesophageal echocardiography for the detection of patent foramen ovale in stroke patients. Eur Neurol 1997;38:21–5.
77 Mesa D, Franco M, Suarez de Lezo J, et al. [Prevalence of patent foramen ovale in young patients with cerebral ischemic accident of unknown origin]. Rev Esp Cardiol 2003;56:662–8.
78 Serena J, Segura T, Perez-Ayuso MJ, et al. The need to quantify right-to-left shunt in acute ischemic stroke: a case-control study. Stroke 1998;29:1322–8.
79 Sacco RL, Adams R, Albers G, et al. Guidelines for prevention of stroke in patients with ischemic stroke or transient ischemic attack: a statement for healthcare professionals from the American Heart Association/American Stroke Association Council on Stroke: co-sponsored by the Council on Cardiovascular Radiology and Intervention: the American Academy of Neurology affirms the value of this guideline. Circulation 2006;113:e409–49.
80 Godart F, Rey C, Prat A, et al. Atrial right-to-left shunting causing severe hypoxaemia despite normal right-sided pressures. Report of 11 consecutive cases corrected by percutaneous closure. Eur Heart J 2000;21:483–9.
81 Cheng TO. Transcatheter closure of patent foramen ovale: a definitive treatment for platypnea-orthodeoxia. Catheter Cardiovasc Interv 2000;51:120.
82 Delgado G, Inglessis I, Martin-Herrero F, et al. Management of platypnea-orthodeoxia syndrome by transcatheter closure of atrial communication: hemodynamic characteristics, clinical and echocardiographic outcome. J Invasive Cardiol 2004;16:578–82.
83 Guerin P, Lambert V, Godart F, et al. Transcatheter closure of patent foramen ovale in patients with platypnea-orthodeoxia: results of a multicentric French registry. Cardiovasc Intervent Radiol 2005;28:164–8.
84 Ortega Trujillo JR, Suarez de Lezo Herreros de Tejada J, Garcia Quintana A, et al. [Transcatheter closure of patent foramen ovale in patients with platypnea-orthodeoxia]. Rev Esp Cardiol 2006;59:78–81.
85 Kruit MC, van Buchem MA, Hofman PA, et al. Migraine as a risk factor for subclinical brain lesions. JAMA 2004;291:427–34.
86 Dalkara T, Nozari A, Moskowitz MA. Migraine aura pathophysiology: the role of blood vessels and microembolisation. Lancet Neurol 2010;9:309–317.
87 Etminan M, Takkouche B, Isorna FC, et al. Risk of ischaemic stroke in people with migraine: systematic review and meta-analysis of observational studies. Br Med J 2005;330:63.
88 Tzourio C, Benslamia L, Guillon B, et al. Migraine and the risk of cervical artery dissection: a case-control study. Neurology 2002;59:435–7.
89 Schwedt TJ, Demaerschalk BM, Dodick DW. Patent foramen ovale and migraine: a quantitative systematic review. Cephalalgia 2008;28:531–40.
90 Morandi E, Anzola GP, Angeli S, et al. Transcatheter closure of patent foramen ovale: a new migraine treatment? J Interv Cardiol 2003;16:39–42.
91 Reisman M, Christofferson RD, Jesurum J, et al. Migraine headache relief after transcatheter closure of patent foramen ovale. J Am Coll Cardiol 2005;45:493–5.
92 Azarbal B, Tobis J, Suh W, et al. Association of interatrial shunts and migraine headaches: impact of transcatheter closure. J Am Coll Cardiol 2005;45:489–92.
93 Dowson A, Mullen MJ, Peatfield R, et al. Migraine Intervention With STARFlex Technology (MIST) trial: a prospective, multicenter, double-blind, sham-controlled trial to evaluate the effectiveness of patent foramen ovale closure with STARFlex septal repair implant to resolve refractory migraine headache. Circulation 2008;117:1397–404.
94 Cartoni D, De Castro S, Valente G, et al. Identification of professional scuba divers with patent foramen ovale at risk for decompression illness. Am J Cardiol 2004;94:270–3.
95 Du ZD, Hijazi ZM, Kleinman CS, et al. Comparison between transcatheter and surgical closure of secundum atrial septal defect in children and adults: results of a multicenter nonrandomized trial. J Am Coll Cardiol 2002;39:1836–44.

23

CHAPTER 23

Articulated Robotic MedProbe snake robot for single port surgery

Marco A. Zenati[1], Mohsen Mahvash[2] & Howie Choset[3]

[1] Harvard Medical School, Boston, MA, USA

[2] Division of Cardiothoracic Surgery, BHS, Medical Robotics and Computer Assisted Surgery (MRCAS) Laboratory, Harvard Medical School, Boston, MA, USA

[3] Robotics Institute, Carnegie Mellon University, Pittsburgh, PA, USA

Introduction

The Articulated Robotic MedProbe (ARM) system (Fig. 23.1) is the result of collaboration initiated in 1996 between the University of Pittsburgh Medical Center (UPMC) and Carnegie Mellon University's Robotics Institute (CMU). Dr. Zenati, who initiated this collaboration, is a cardiothoracic surgeon and a pioneer of minimally invasive cardiac surgery; he was the first surgeon in the United States to perform robotic coronary bypass surgery on the beating heart using the ZEUS robotic system from Computer Motion at UPMC in 2000 [1]. Because of this early involvement with robotic surgery, a partnership was formed with CMU (Professor Takeo Kanade) to develop the next generation of robotic surgical systems. The first result of this collaboration with Dr. Cam Riviere was the HeartLander crawling robot in 2001 [2], an inchworm-like robot that uses suction to adhere to the surface of the beating heart. Locomotion is image guided and can be semiautonomous [3]. The HeartLander is used for epicardial left ventricular injection of regenerative material and for pacing lead placement [4].

Realizing the limitations of commercially available surgical robots due to the rigid nature of the operating arms, a collaboration was initiated by Dr. Zenati in 2003 with the group of Professor Howie Choset at CMU. Choset's group has significant experience with snake robots for a variety of non-medical tasks, including search-and-rescue, jet engine inspection, and industrial and defence applications. Dr. Alon Wolf also joined the team and a novel medical snake robot was conceived and prototypes fabricated. A 5-year NIH/NHLBI R01 grant entitled "Articulated Robot for Epicardial Interventions" enabled the development of subxiphoid single port epicardial interventions on the beating heart.

ARM snake robot

The ARM robotic system is a snake robot platform that features highly articulated multilink catheters allowing minimally invasive procedures in target organs located deep within the body and otherwise difficult or previously impossible to reach through a single port [5,6]. The ARM contains multiple open device channels to accept a variety of flexible surgical and interventional tools as well as on-board visualization. The platform enables physicians to operate through non-linear circuitous paths, self-supported and through a single access point into the body. The ARM's flexibility and motion is gained from its numerous mechanical linkages (>30) with two concentric mechanisms.

Endovascular and Hybrid Therapies for Structural Heart and Aortic Disease, First Edition.
Edited by Jacques Kpodonu and Raoul Bonan.

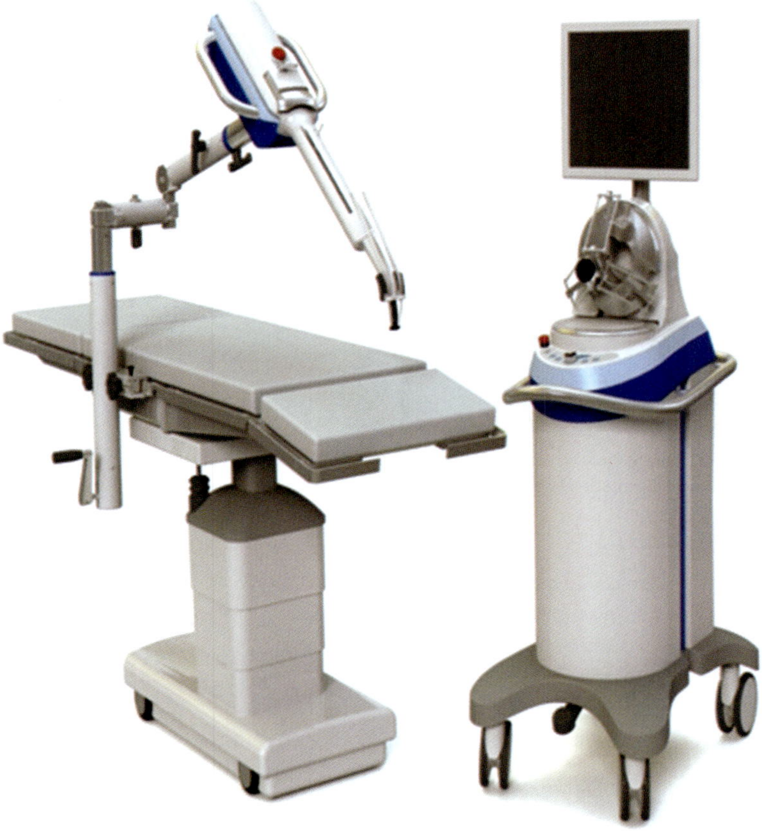

Fig. 23.1 The ARM snake robot. Courtesy of Cardiorobotics, Inc., Rynham, MA.

Each mechanism can be placed into a rigid or flexible state. By employing a patented "follow-the-leader" movement strategy with these two alternate states (rigid or flexible), the ARM can be directed into any shape through the relative orientation of its linkages. The multijointed ARM is disposable to ensure sterility, whereas the physician console and feeder unit are reusable. In addition to the core system there are a number of accessories: (i) a support stand, which attaches to the operating table and enables easy positioning of the ARM into the clinical site of interest; (ii) a camera system, incorporated into the distal tip, employs a near high-definition CMOS camera and LED lamps for high-quality visualization of the surgical site; and (iii) hand-held surgical tools, dedicated for use with the ARM, allowing rotation and articulation, in addition to triangulation towards the surgical site. The surgeon retains tactile feedback from the tools, enabling more efficient and safe retraction, dissection, and excision of tissue for the desired clinical application. A key distinguishing feature of the ARM, which differs from a "next generation flexible endoscope" is that it contains multiple degrees of freedom distributed across its length and it is self-supporting. When compared to the 7 degrees of freedom of movement possible using the human arm, the robotic ARM's greater than 30 degrees of freedom enhance the physician's ability to access, visualize, and perform interventions in hard to reach anatomic targets.

The ARM accepts an operator-defined input to generate a unique shape in 3D space (Fig. 23.2). The ARM can track along this curvilinear 3D path and return to points along the path or take a new shape as defined by the operator. One shape can be "remembered" at a time. This core property allows the ARM to work outside the constraints of a natural lumen, such as the oropharynx, or on the surface of an organ, such as the heart. The ARM's

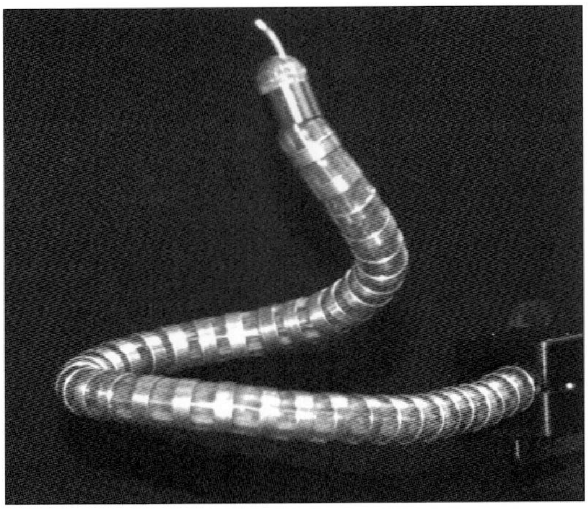

Fig. 23.2 The ARM snake robot is able to assume complex 3D shapes. The radiofrequency ablation catheter is shown protruding from the tip.

exact shape and location can remain static allowing it to hover in place without any tremor while delicate procedures are being performed at its distal end, and then automatically retract along the exact same path from where it came to protect the delicate anatomic structures and surrounding tissues from compression or friction damage [7,8]. Additionally, the ARM not only supports its own weight but can support additional loads and be used to exert force on tissues itself such as for dissection or retraction or via tools delivered through its channels. Conversely, the ARM can become limp, allowing it to take the shape of the surrounding structures. In this state the ARM will lie in a hand as a soft braided rope, which is an important safety feature [9, 10].

Cardiorobotics, Inc.

Cardiorobotics is a Delaware "C" Corporation originally formed in 2005 (as Innovention Technologies LLC) by the inventors of the ARM technology and is currently based in Rynham, MA. They are Howie Choset PhD, Associate Professor of Robotics at CMU, Marco Zenati MD, Professor of Surgery at Harvard Medical School in Boston, and Alon Wolf PhD, Associate Professor at Technion Institute in Israel. Dr. Zenati was on the medical faculty at UPMC at the time he and Drs Choset and Wolf developed the first generation medical "snake robotics" platform in-licensed by the Company. Cardiorobotics has exclusive worldwide licences for its ARM technologies from CMU as well as additional development of its own intellectual property portfolio. The company's development history includes the completed development and production of its clinical prototype, and in 2009 receiving the Institutional Review Board (IRB) approval from the NA Homolka Hospital in the Czech Republic and approval from the Czech Republic Ministry of Health to begin human trials. In February 2010, the first patient was successfully enrolled in the clinical trial and discharged without any adverse event 1 day later. In June 2010, another two patients were successfully enrolled and discharged without any adverse events. The company has also completed the design of its market entry prototypes and has validated the product specifications against surgeons' requirements.

First human use of the ARM snake robot

The first human use (FHU) trial of the clinical prototype of the ARM robotic system was initiated in February 2010 and successfully completed in June 2010 with a total of three patients having been enrolled [11]. The FHU procedures were all performed at the Na Homolce Hospital in Prague by Dr. Neuzil (a leading cardiac electrophysiologist) and Dr. Czerny (a cardiac surgeon). Na Homolce Hospital is a major center of excellence in cardiovascular medicine in Europe. The physicians were able to perform all elements of the clinical protocol without incident and the cases were completed in less than 5 hours from initial access to skin closure per approved protocol. All patients were discharged home 1–2 days later without any adverse events reported. During these procedures, a J&J CARTO mapping and ablation catheter was used successfully through the ARM's instrument channel. Up to 200 recordings from the patient's beating heart surface using the CARTO mapping electrodes demonstrated that the ARM could be safely manipulated within the pericardial space from a small single subxiphoid port and over the heart's ventricular surfaces in a human with no induced hemodynamic changes in the heart. The clinical prototype of the ARM was also able to integrate well with high-tech imaging modalities frequently used by interventionalists, such as intracardiac echocardiography (ICE), fluoroscopy, electroanatomic mapping (CARTO), and direct endoscopic visualization.

Future of the ARM snake robot: the next generation catheter

Traditionally, a catheter has been defined as a small device capable of entering the arterial or venous circulation and performing diagnostic or therapeutic interventions. However, a variety of catheters are also used outside the blood stream (in the urinary tract, gastrointestinal tract, etc.). Catheter-based therapy is expanding at a rapid pace and complex interventions are now carried out routinely, including transcatheter aortic valve implantation (TAVI) and thoracic endovascular aortic repair (TEVAR) for aneurysm repair. A first generation robotic catheter system (Sensei, Hansen Medical, Mountain View, CA) is being tested to facilitate complex intravascular interventions. The ARM snake robot's current outside diameter (12 mm) is adequate for subxiphoid epicardial interventions but smaller sizes are being developed which will enable complex intravascular procedures [12].

References

1 Zenati MA. Robotic heart surgery. Cardiol Rev 2001;9:287–94.

2 Patronik NA, Zenati MA, Riviere CN. Crawling on the heart: a mobile robotic device for minimally invasive cardiac interventions. Lect Notes Computer Sci 2004;3217:9–16.

3 Ota T, Patronik NA, Schwartzman D, et al. Minimally invasive epicardial injections using a novel semi-autonomous robotic device. Circulation 2008;118(Suppl I):S115–20.

4 Chapman MP, Lopez Gonzales JL, Goyette B, et al. Application of the HeartLander crawling robot for injection of a thermally sensitive anti-remodeling agent formyocardial infarction therapy. Conf Proc IEEE Eng Med Biol Soc 2010;1:5428–31.

5 Ota T, Degani A, Zubiate B, et al. Epicardial atrial ablation using a novel articulated robotic medical probe via a percutaneous subxiphoid approach. Innovations 2006;1(6):335–40.

6 Ota T, Degani A, Schwartzman D, et al. A highly articulated robotic surgical system for minimally invasive surgery. Ann Thorac Surg 2009;87:1253–6.

7 Zenati MA, Yokota T, Schwartzman D, et al. Model-guided epicardial interventions using a novel "snake" robot (CARDIO-ARM) through a subxiphoid port access. In: Proceedings of the 14th International IASTED Conference on Robotics and Applications, 2009, pp. 242–6.

8 Chapman MP, Zenati MA. A highly articulated robotic system (CardioARM) is safer than a rigid system for intrapericardial intervention in a porcine model. Paper presented at Proceedings of the IEEE International Conference on Robotics and Automation (ICRA), Workshop on "Snakes, Worms and Catheters: Continuum and Serpentine Robots for Minimally Invasive Surgery", Anchorage, Alaska, May 3, 2010.

9 Choset H, Zenati MA, Ota T, et al. Enabling medical robotics for the next generation of minimally invasive procedures: minimally invasive cardiac surgery with single port access. In: Rosen J, Hannaford B, Satava RM (eds) Surgical Robotics: systems, applications and visions. New York: Springer, 2010, p. 257.

10 Tully S, Kantor S, Zenati MA, et al. Image guidance and semi autonomous navigation for robot assisted epicardial interventions. Paper presented at Proceedings or the International Society for Minimally Invasive Cardiac Surgery, Annual Meeting, Washington, DC, June 2011.

11 Neuzil P, Reddy V, Zenati MA, et al. Single-port subxiphoid access epicardial ablation using "snake" robotic system. Paper presented at Proceedings of the International Society for Minimally Invasive Cardiac Surgery (ISMICS), 2010 Annual Meeting, Berlin, Germany, June 2010.

12 Choset H, Zenati MA. Enabling medical robotics for the next generation of minimally invasive procedures. Paper presented a t Proceedings of the IEEE/ICRA, Anchorage, Alaska, May 2010.

Index

Endovascular and Hybrid Therapies for Structural Heart and Aortic Disease, First Edition.
Edited by Jacques Kpodonu and Raoul Bonan.